Pharmacokinetic-Pharmacodynamic Modeling and Simulation

Pharmacokinetic-Pharmacodynamic Modeling and Simulation

Peter L. Bonate, PhD, FCP

Genzyme Corporation
San Antonio, TX USA

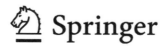 Springer

Peter Bonate
Genzyme Oncology
San Antonio, TX 78229
USA
peter.bonate@genzyme.com

Library of Congress Control Number: 2005928491

ISBN-10: 0-387-27197-X   e-ISBN: 0-387-27199-6
ISBN-13: 978-0387-27197-2

Printed on acid-free paper.

Printed in the United States of America.

9 8 7 6 5 4 3

springer.com

TABLE OF CONTENTS

PREFACE

This book is written for the pharmacokineticist who performs pharmacokinetic-pharmacodynamic modeling and is occasionally asked to model data that may have nothing to do with pharmacokinetics, but may be important in other areas of drug development. The emphasis of this book is on modeling in drug development since that is my own area of expertise and because ultimately all pharmacokinetic-pharmacodynamic modeling is applied to the therapeutic use of drugs in clinical practice. Throughout this book, pharmacokinetic and pharmacodynamic models will be used without derivation and little in the way of explanation. It is expected the reader has basic knowledge of pharmacokinetics and simple pharmacodynamic models. If not, the reader is referred to Gibaldi and Perrier (1982), Wagner (1993), or Shargel and Yu (1999) for background material. The reader is also expected to have had a 1-year introductory course in statistics that covers basics of probability, regression, and analysis of variance. A 1-semester course in matrix algebra is desired but not needed.

The material in this text begins with a broad overview of modeling, which I call 'The Art of Modeling'. This chapter is meant to introduce some of the broad topics associated with modeling, such as model selection criterion, model validation, the importance of good communication, and ethics. The next chapter is linear regression, which is the foundation for most parametric modeling. From there nonlinear regression is covered, followed by variance models, weighting, and transformations. Lastly, case studies in linear and nonlinear models are presented to illustrate the theory that was

presented in the previous chapters. In the material presented to this point, a key assumption is that each subject contributes a single observation to the data set. Next, the book moves to mixed effects models, which allow for multiple observations to be measured on the same individual. The next chapter is linear mixed effects models, which is meant as a brief introduction to the topic. Next is the theory of nonlinear mixed effects models, which form the foundation for population pharmacokinetic-pharmacodynamic modeling. This is followed by a chapter on practical issues in nonlinear mixed effects modeling, such as how weight, genetic, or racial information is incorporated into a model. The last chapter in this section presents some case studies on population pharmacokinetic-pharmacodynamic modeling. A key concept in this book is the inter-relatedness between the material. For example, nonlinear mixed effects models are simply extensions of linear mixed effects models, which are themselves extensions of linear models, etc. Thus, in order to understand the more complex chapters, it is necessary to understand the foundation material, e.g., what is a variance model and how are they used, how can a linear covariate model be built into a nonlinear mixed effects model, etc.

I wrote this book to be as reader-friendly as possible. Those parts of the book that are non-technical are written in an almost conversational tone with anecdotes and interesting quotes interspersed throughout. I love quotations and each chapter begins with one I thought especially poignant about the forthcoming material in the chapter. When mathematics are needed, I tried to make those sections self-contained. Variables are defined in each chapter so the reader does not have to search for "now what is G again?"

John of Salisbury (1115–1180), a twelfth century English philosopher and historian, once wrote:

> *We are like dwarves sitting on the shoulders of giants. We see more, and things more distant than they did, not because our sight is superior or because we are taller than they, but because they raise us up, and by their great stature add to ours.*

I would like to thank the many giants that helped me understand things I was unclear about during the writing of this text and the reviewers that took the time to read the chapters and offer their opinions on how each could be improved. Without your help I would have been lost in many places. I would like to ask that if you do spot any mistakes or typographical errors to please contact me at peter.bonate@gmail.com.

I would also like to thank my wife, Diana, for her encouragement and my children, Robyn and Ryan, for reminding me that there is indeed more to life than writing "Daddy's Big Book of Science", which is what they called this while I was writing it.

Peter L. Bonate
Genzyme Corporation
San Antonio, Texas
June 2005

REVIEWERS

In a book such as this, it is impossible for one person to be an expert on everything. I could not have done this endeavor without the help of others. I would like to thank the following individuals who took the time to review the chapters.

Leon Aarons, PhD
Senior Lecture
School of Pharmacy and Pharmaceutical
  Sciences
University of Manchester
Manchester, UK

Jeff Barrett, PhD, FCP
Clinical Pharmacology & Therapeutics
Children's Hospital of Philadelphia
Philadelphia, PA USA

Seth Berry, PharmD
Associate Scientist
Quintiles Transnational Corp.
Kansas City, MO USA

Marie Davidian, PhD
Professor
Department of Statistics
North Carolina State University
Raleigh, NC USA

Johan Gabrielsson, PhD
Senior Principle Scientist
AstraZeneca
Sodertalje, Sweden

Danny R. Howard, PhD
Global Head, Pharmacokinetics
Novartis Pharmaceutical Corp.
East Hanover, NJ USA

Howard Lee, PhD, MD
Assistant Professor
Assoc. Director for the Clinical Investigation
Core Center for Clinical Pharmacology
Department of Medicine
University of Pittsburgh
Pittsburgh, PA USA

Bernd Meibohm, PhD, FCP
Associate Professor of Pharmaceutical Sciences
College of Pharmacy
University of Tennessee
Memphis, TN USA

Diane Mould, PhD
Projections Research, Inc.
Phoenixville, PA USA

David Ruppert, PhD
Professor of Engineering
School of Operations Research and Industrial
    Engineering
Cornell University
Ithaca, NY USA

Dan Weiner, PhD
Sr. Vice President
Business Development

Pharsight Corporation
Research Triangle Park, NC USA

Paolo Vicini, PhD
Associate Professor
Bioengineering
University of Washington
Seattle, WA USA

Jianjun Alan Xiao, PhD
Research Fellow
Merck & Co.
West Point, PA USA

Chapter 1

The Art of Modeling

Drawn by my eager wish, desirous of seeing the great confusion of the various strange forms created by ingenious nature, I wandered for some time among the shadowed cliffs, and came to the entrance of a great cavern. I remained before it for a while, stupefied, and ignorant of the existence of such a thing, with my back bent and my left hand resting on my knee, and shading my eyes with my right, with lids lowered and closed, and often bending this way and that to see whether I could discern anything within; but that was denied me by the great darkness inside. And after I stayed a while, suddenly there arose in me two things, fear and desire—fear because of the menacing dark cave, and desire to see whether there were any miraculous things within.

—Leonardo da Vinci (1452–1519), Renaissance scientist and philosopher

INTRODUCTION

The focus of this book is primarily on the development of pharmacokinetic and pharmacokinetic-pharmacodynamic models. Models that are reported in the literature are not picked out of thin air. Useful models take time and effort and what is rarely shown is the process that went into developing that model. The purpose of this chapter is to discuss model development, to explain the process, and to introduce concepts that will be used throughout this book. Those criteria used to select a model extend to whether the model is a linear model or a nonlinear mixed effects model and that is why this material is provided first. If the reader can understand what makes a good or validated model, then the particular type of model is irrelevant.

WHAT IS A MODEL AND WHY ARE THEY MADE?

A system is a collection of objects that interact to create a unified whole, such as a cell culture system, a rat, or a human. The type of models that are of interest in this book are mathematical models that represent the system of interest and "*can be used to explore the structure and behavior of the system*" (Wastney et al., 1997). A more simplistic definition might be that a mathematical model defines how you think your data were generated. Most famous mathematical models can be found in chemistry and physics, such as:

- Boyle's law, $PV = $ constant, which states that for a given mass at fixed temperature the pressure (P) times the volume (V) of a gas is a constant;
- Newton's second law of motion, $F = ma$, which states that the force (F) acting on an object is equal to its mass (m) times its acceleration (a); and
- $E = mc^2$, perhaps the most famous equation of the last century, which most people believe has to do with Einstein's theory of relativity, but in actuality has nothing to do with it. This equation is founded on the basis that matter and energy are really different forms of the same thing and states that that the amount of energy (E) that could be produced is equal to the mass (m) of an atom times the speed of light (c) squared.

1

Mathematical models in biology tend to be more complex, but are all based on the same foundations used to develop models in the more physically oriented sciences.

In defining a mathematical model it is helpful to distinguish between the various components of the model. Models are built using experimentally derived data. This so-called data generating process is dependent on system inputs, system dynamics, and the device used to measure the output from a system (Fig. 1.1). But in addition to these systematic processes are the sources of error that confound our measurements. These errors may be measurement errors but also include process noise that is part of the system. One goal of mathematical modeling is to differentiate the "information" or systematic component in the system from the noise or random components in the system, i.e.,

DATA = SYSTEMATIC COMPONENT + ERROR.

Hence, models usually consist of a structural model or systematic component plus a statistical model that describes the error component of the model. Early in the modeling process the focus may lie with the systematic component and then move to a more holistic approach involving the error components. For example, the 1-compartment model after bolus administration is

$$C = \frac{D}{V} \exp\left(-\frac{CL}{V}t\right) + \varepsilon. \qquad (1.1)$$

The first term on the right hand side of Eq. (1.1) is the structural model having two inputs (also called independent variables), D (dose) and t (time), and one output (also called the dependent variable), C (concentration). The variables V (volume of distribution) and CL (clearance) are referred to as model parameters which must be estimated from the observed concentration data. The second term in Eq. (1.1) is the error component (also called the variance model). ε represents the deviation between model predicted concentrations and observed concentrations.

Modeling is done for a number of reasons depending on the point of view. Scientifically, modeling "provides a systematic way of organizing data and observations of a system at the cell, tissue, organ, or whole animal (human) levels" and "affords the opportunity to better understand and predict physiological phenomena" (Epstein, 1994). Financially, companies utilize modeling as a way to better leverage business decisions and this has been shown to result in substantial cost savings over traditional experiments (Van Buskirk, 2000). And on a personal level, modelers model because it's fun and challenging.

Beyond characterizing data, once a model is developed, it can be used to answer "what if" questions—a process known as simulation. Hence, modeling and simulation (M&S) are often used in the same breath by modelers. But there are many important differences between modeling and simulation. A model looks back in time. Given a set of outputs (data), the model attempts to find a set of parameters that explain the data generating process. Simulation looks forward in time. Given a model and a set of parameters, what happens if the inputs are varied. In simulation, the model is fixed and the inputs are varied. In modeling, the inputs and outputs are fixed, but what happens in between is varied. More about the differences between M&S will become evident using examples throughout the book.

The implementation of mathematics into biology, physiology, pharmacology, and medicine is not new, but its use has grown in the last three decades as computer speeds have increased and scientists have begun to see the power of modeling to answer scientific questions. A conference was held in 1989 at the National Institutes of Health called "Modeling in Biomedical Research: An Assessment of Current and Potential Approaches." One conclusion from that conference was that "*biomedical research will be most effectively advanced by the continued application of a combination of models—mathematical, computer, physical, cell, tissue culture and animal—in a complementary and interactive manner.*"

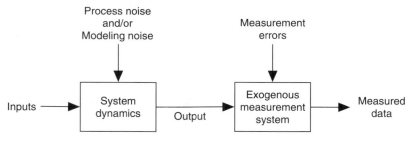

Figure 1.1 Diagram of the system under study. Redrawn with from DiStefano and Landaw (1984). Reprinted with permission from The American Physiological Society, Copyright 1984.

Today, the interplay between these different types of models has never been greater. As scientists become more "mathletic" and as the drive to decrease the use of living animals in medical research increases, mathematical models will play an increasingly important part of medical research.

The use of modeling in drug development, for which many of the examples in this book have been culled, is also becoming increasingly important. Aarons et al. (2001) and Balant and Gex-Fabry (2000) present comprehensive reviews on the applications and use of M&S in drug development. The cost to develop a new drug in 2003 was estimated at 802 million dollars (DiMasi, Hansen, and Grabowski, 2003). Clearly, drug companies must find ways to reduce costs and expedite getting a drug to market. Two recent papers written by financial advisors suggest that M&S will play a "vital role" in drug development by enabling scientists to predict how drugs will act in whole systems, organs, and at the sub-cellular level, to predict clinical trial outcomes before they are actually conducted, and to adapt clinical trials on the fly as patient data is accumulated without compromising its statistical validity, thereby lowering costs and potentially speeding development (IBM Business Consulting Services, 2003; PricewaterhouseCoopers, 1999).

These reports also criticize the pharmaceutical industry for slowly adopting M&S as a research and development tool. Perhaps drug companies have failed to routinely implement M&S as part of the development process because modelers have failed to show that the methodology can indeed lower the cost of drug development, expedite development time, or result in faster and more efficient approval times by regulatory agencies. Thankfully, regulatory agencies have issued recent guidances advocating a more integral role for M&S in the development process through the establishment of exposure-response relationships thereby forcing drug companies to increase the role of M&S in the development of drugs (United States Department of Health and Human Services et al., 2003). Currently, however, M&S groups within industry tend to be fringe or splinter groups, usually within the clinical pharmacology or clinical pharmacokinetics department, that operate sporadically on drug development projects or in cases where they are called in to "save" failed clinical trials. But, if the financial advisors are correct, then the role of M&S in drug development will only increase over time, to the benefit of those who love to model and to the company as well.

One theme that will be stressed throughout this book is the concept that there is and can never be a true model for a biological system. Biological systems are inherently nonlinear of potentially infinite dimension with feedback loops, possibly circadian variation, and are exceedingly complex with sometimes very tight control. It is folly to think that given the limited number of subjects and number of observations collected per subject in clinical or preclinical studies that the true model could be uncovered and its parameters estimated with any degree of precision. No modeler could ever develop a model with the degree of precision that explains such a system in the presence of the many uncontrolled variables that influence the data generating process. However, it may be possible that a reasonable approximation or simplification to the true data generating model could be developed.

Because the true model can never be identified, there can never be a "right" model. Box (1976) stated, in one of the most famous adages in pharmacokinetics, that *"all models are wrong, some are useful."* This quote is made time and again, yet it is not uncommon to hear pharmacokineticists talk about the "right model" or even worse "the wrong model." All models are wrong—there is no right model. Granted some models are better than others, but models are really in the eye of the beholder. A modeler may choose one model over another, especially when the model is complex, because along the model development process there are many forks in the road. One modeler may choose one path, whereas another may choose another path. At the end of the process, each modeler may have a model that is different from the other modeler, each with equal credibility. So which model is the right model? Well, neither is.

There is a famous film director from Japan named Kurosawa who directed a movie called Rashomon (1950). The story itself is violent, involving rape and murder, but is told in flashbacks from the point of view of each of the participants. With each narrator the characters are essentially the same, as are most of the details, but each person's story is different. In the end, Kurosawa never reveals what truly happened. The point is that reality is relative. Each modeler views a model from a different point of view, each of which may be a valid interpretation of the data, none of which may be correct. In Rashomon, all the presenters could be telling the truth or none of them could be telling the truth. This is called the Rashomon effect—there may be a multitude of models that describe a set of data giving the same degree of predictability and error (Breiman, 2002). The tendency in our profession to use the phrase "the right model" needs to be changed. Should the term "better model" be used? "Is there a better model?" "Model A is better than Model B." Consider the case where a model is developed. New data is collected and the original model is revised to explain the new data. Does the development of the second model mean that the first model was wrong? Certainly not, it means the second model is better.

It is unfortunate that as a profession we choose to sabotage ourselves with a poor choice of words to professionals outside our field. We need to move beyond using the phrase "the right model" since those outside our profession may not understand the nuances between "the right model," "the best model," "a better model," or "the wrong model." In doing so, we will avoid confusion and add credibility to our results.

MODELING AS PROBLEM SOLVING

Modeling is an exercise in problem solving and there are steps that can be taken to maximize the probability of solving the problem. The following outlines the steps for effective problem solving:

1. One of Steven Covey's "7 *Habits for Highly Effective People*" (1989) is to "*begin with the end in mind.*" This is a good modeling advice. Recognize and define the problem. Define your destination before you go off on a modeling adventure. What use do you want your model to serve? If you are part of a team, such as a project team in a pharmaceutical company, get team members to agree to the problem and how you have defined it before you go off to solve it.

2. Analyze the problem. What data are available to solve the problem? Given the data available can the problem be solved? Has proper attention to study design and data collection been done to achieve the objective? Question whether a model is even necessary. Perhaps a noncompartmental analysis of the data will suffice instead. If the goal is to model multiple-dose data from single dose data, then something simple like the superposition principle may be useful.

3. Identify alternative solutions. Review past solutions for current problems. Perhaps something that you are trying to do has already been done and reported in the literature for a different drug. Sometimes it is possible to break a complex problem into a series of simpler problems. Sometimes you will need to be creative though and possibly need to brainstorm with others.

4. Evaluate the possible solutions. Define criteria for choosing a solution. Is time more important than cost? What is the most cost- and time-effective alternative to answer the question? Understand who will use the results and what will be the best way to communicate those results. Perhaps modeling is not the optimal solution.

5. Decide on a solution, keeping in mind that rarely will any single solution be perfect. Identify limitations of all proposed solutions.

6. Visualize the steps needed to get there. We have all heard stories of how great athletes visualize a race or a game beforehand to provide a competitive edge over their opponents. They visualize the steps leading to winning the event, such as starting from a runner's block, and then visualize the actual winning of the event, such as crossing the finish line. Modeling is no different. For example, suppose the goal is to identify those patient characteristics, like age, that might be predictive of exposure for a new drug. It will be useful to plan the steps needed to achieve the goal, such as collecting all the relevant data, developing a pharmacokinetic model, and then using linear regression to examine the relationship between area under the curve (a measure of exposure) and patient characteristics. Having a strategy before you start will always lead you to the finish line faster than starting without a strategy.

7. Implement the strategy by building a solution incrementally. Don't try to solve the problem all at once. If no solution can be found, try reformulating the problem. Examine the assumptions and look for hidden constraints. Perhaps some of the assumptions are unnecessary or are overly complex.

8. Remember that there are other alternatives, ones that you did not examine, so try to avoid totally focusing on the one solution you implemented. Take time to reflect at the completion of a project. What hurdles occurred during the process? What would you do differently next time if the same hurdle occurs? What would you do differently in general?

Despite the best plans, roadblocks are often encountered in developing complex models. For example, a modeler may envision what the model should look like but once the model is actually fit to the data, the parameter estimates may be poorly estimated or the goodness of fit of the model is poor, in which case, another model is often needed. It is not uncommon though for the modeler to be uncertain about what that next model should be. Hence, the modeler encounters a mental roadblock.

Getting past the roadblock is what separates a good modeler from a great modeler, an inexperienced modeler from an experienced modeler. Often the solution can be drawn from past experience from models or methods seen in the literature. Sometimes, though, creativity and insight are required, another aspect that makes modeling an art. Hewlett-Packard published a short series of on-line articles on how inventors invent. Thirteen of their best inventors were interviewed and asked how they overcome roadblocks and get creative. Most replied the same thing: switch gears and do something else. Many replied that their creative obstacles were overcome, even inspired some said, while doing something mundane, like sleeping, showering, or simply walking down the hallway. Others thought that bouncing ideas off colleagues were useful.

Modeling can be very rewarding to the modeler, as is solving any complex problem. But it is easy to "spin your wheels" and lose focus or get caught in obstacles that seem insurmountable. Just remember, to remain focused on the end result, but stay flexible and open to new ideas that may develop during the process. As McCullough and Nelder (1989) put it—don't fall in love with your models. It is easy to get "locked into" a model and build a model out of pure nonsense.

TYPE OF MODELS

Models represent the system under study. But no system is measured without error. Humans have yet to create a device that measures something with absolute certainty (recall Fig. 1.1). Rescigno and Beck (1987) call the system to be studied the primary system, and what is used to study the primary system by the investigator the secondary system. Under these definitions, a model can be considered a type of secondary system used to test properties of the primary system. To form a model, a set of inputs and outputs must be available. Inputs perturb the system in some manner. For example, if the system under study were a human, then administering a dose of drug into the subject would represent the input. The blood samples used for pharmacokinetic analysis and any pharmacodynamic endpoints that are measured would then represent the set of outputs. Both the inputs and outputs cannot be measured perfectly and are subject to error, both systematic and random in nature. It is typically assumed that the input errors are negligible. When the input errors are not this gives rise to a special class of models called error-in-variables models, which will be discussed in the chapter on Linear Models and Regression.

Models can be classified into many different categories. Using the nomenclature of DiStefano and Landaw (1984), pharmacokinetic models can generally be broken down into two types: models of data and models of systems. Models of data, usually referred to as empirical models, require few assumptions about the data generating mechanism. Examples include allometric scaling and sum of exponentials used to characterize a concentration-time profile. Empirical models are useful when little is known about the underlying physical process from which the data are generated yet one still must make some conclusions regarding the data. While empirical models may be useful at prediction they should not be extrapolated.

Model of systems, or mechanistic models, are based on physical and physiological principles and should have as many features of the system incorporated into the model as the data allow (Thakur, 1991). Factors such as transport to tissues dependent on blood flow, kinetics of receptor binding, and intracellular diffusion processes may all play a role. These models usually take the form of differential equations or partial differential equations based on mass-balance, product-precursor, or mass-action principles. Examples of mechanistic models include physiological-based pharmacokinetic models where the transport into and out of tissues is modeled as a function of blood flow and permeability between the blood and tissue. While one places greater trust in mechanistic models because they are based on theory, an analyst should always ask the question "What if the theory is wrong?" for then a mechanistic model may not be representing the system. Some models may also be hybrid models, mechanistic in places where the physiology and pharmacology of the system are understood and empirical in places that are still black boxes.

Models of systems can also be categorized into various types based on the attributes of the system, including:

- Time-variant vs. time-invariant,
- Deterministic vs. stochastic,
- Static vs. dynamic,
- Lumped vs. distributed,
- Linear vs. nonlinear, and
- Continuous vs. discrete.

Each of these categories can then be combined into more descriptive categories, e.g., a nonlinear, time-variant system or a static, time-invariant discrete system.

Time-variant means that the parameters of the system change over time, such as an autoinduction process that increases a drug's hepatic clearance with repeated administration. Time-invariant or stationary parameters do not change over time. It is typically assumed that a drug's pharmacokinetics are stationary over time so that the principle of superposition[1] applies. With a static model, the output depends only on the input and does

---

[1] Superposition was developed in physics to explain the behavior of waves that pass simultaneously through the same region in space. In pharmacokinetics, superposition states that concentration-time profiles passing through the same relative region in time are additive. For example, if two doses are taken 24 hours apart and the concentration 6 hours and 30 hours after the first dose was 100 and 10 ng/mL, respectively, then the concentration 6 hours after the second dose (which is 30 hours after the first dose) would be equal to 110 ng/mL (100 ng/mL + 10 ng/mL). Thron (1974) presents a comprehensive review of linearity and the meaning of superposition.

not vary over time. In the analysis of kinetic systems, static models are restricted to steady-state conditions and one example is the physiological modeling of circulatory systems. In contrast, the output of a dynamic system changes over time. In a lumped system, the various organs are "lumped" into single groups. The classic example is a compartmental system. In a 1-compartment model the entire body is treated as a single compartment. In a 2-compartment model the richly perfused organs are treated as the central compartment with the slowly perfused, poorly distributed organs, like fat and skin, treated as the peripheral compartment. In a distributed system, the spatial aspects of a system are built into the model. Rarely are these seen in the pharmacokinetics field since their solution typically requires partial differential equations, which few pharmacokineticists are familiar with and few software packages are equipped to solve.

All biological systems are complex, nonlinear systems. Model or function nonlinearity is defined when the derivative of a model with respect to a model parameter depends on any parameter in the model, such as when clearance follows Michaelis–Menten kinetics, or when the derivative does not exist, such as a change-point model. Estimation of parameters in a nonlinear system is more difficult than a linear system and often involves numerical optimization techniques. System nonlinearity can arise when the rate of change in a component of the system depends on the state of another component in the system, such as might arise when a component of the system shows feedback. Even though nonlinearity applies to all physiological and pharmacokinetic systems, often a useful assumption is one of linearity. For example, the dose of a drug given may result in drug concentrations much less than the Michaelis constant for metabolism, in which case the system can be approximated by a linear one. Most drugs are assumed to have linear pharmacokinetics, although some drugs, like many anti-cancer agents, demonstrate nonlinear behavior. Sometimes a nonlinear equation can be transformed to a linear one, such as the Lineweaver–Burke transformation of the Hill equation in enzyme kinetics, although this is not recommended because the transformation often distorts the distribution of the random error component of the model (Garfinkel and Fegley, 1984).

Models are also classified into whether they are deterministic or stochastic. Stochastic (Greek for "guess") systems involve chance or probability, whereas a deterministic system does not. In a deterministic model no randomness is assumed to be present, an assumption that is clearly not realistic. Stochastic models assume random variability and take into account that variability. There is no such thing as a deterministic model—all

measurements have some error associated with them and, as such, are stochastic models by definition. However, deterministic models are useful to understand the properties of a system in the absence of natural variation. Simulations may be done using the systematic component of a model to understand the behavior of the system under different conditions.

Two types of models are usually seen in pharmacokinetics: a pharmacokinetic model, which relates dose and dosing frequency to drug concentrations, and a pharmacodynamic model, which relates drug concentrations to an effect, such as change in stomach pH, a physiologic marker, such a glucose concentration, or an outcome, such as absence or presence of an adverse event. The pharmacokinetic model predicts the concentration-time profile of the drug in the sampled biological fluid, usually plasma or serum after the administered dose. The pharmacodynamic model predicts the observed effect given the concentration provided by the pharmacokinetic model. Derendorf and Meibohm (1999) review pharmacokinetic/pharmacodynamic relationships and provide some useful classifications for these models. The pharmacokinetic and pharmacodynamic model may be either mechanistic or empirical or both.

PROPERTIES OF A USEFUL MODEL

Models are either useful or less useful. So what makes one model more useful than another? Rescigno, Beck, and Thakur (1987) state that models should be judged by three points of view: retrodiction, prediction, and understanding. Retrodiction is simply the ability to recall what happened in an experiment—does the model conform to the original data from the primary system, i.e., is the model consistent with experimental knowledge. The model must also be predictive. What will happen in future experiments? Lastly, does the model increase our understanding of the primary system under study or does the model increase our understanding of the grand primary system. For example, suppose the model is one of renal transport kinetics. Does the model increase our understanding of the physiology of the kidney? If the model does not help us decide how to answer questions about the primary system or how it fits into the world, the model may be of little value.

These properties reported by Rescigno, Beck, and Thakur (1987) should, however, be treated as a minimal set of properties for a useful model. Table 1.1 presents some other properties of a useful model. Foremost is that the model is actually used and even more importantly, is used to make a decision. Modeling for the sake of modeling, while useful for educational purposes and

Table 1.1 Properties of a useful model.

- Ability characterize the observed data and to include the most important features of the data.
- Makes accurate and precise predictions.
- Increases understanding of the system.
- The model is actually used.
- The model is completed on time.
- Logically consistent, plausible.
- Validated by empirical observations.
- Robust to small changes in the data.
- Appropriate level of precision and detail.
- As simple as possible.
- Judged on what it is intended to do.
- Has flexibility.
- Is effective as a communication tool.
- Serves many different purposes.
- May allow for extrapolation outside the data range.

possible publication, is of no practical value if the model is not used by anyone. Second, the model should be logically consistent, which means that the model has mathematical and biological plausibility. For example, are the parameters related to clearance consistent with organ blood flow? Is the pharmacodynamic model consistent with the known biology of the system? Are the parameter estimates unique, consistent, and precisely estimated? If the parameters are not precisely defined, certain aspects of the model may be overparameterized or the data set itself may be insufficient to obtain precise parameter estimates, in which case more data must be collected.

Third, is the model validated? Model validation is a contentious topic and will be discussed in more detail throughout the book and later in the chapter. Some would argue that a model is only useful if it has been validated, while others may argue that there are situations where an exploratory model is very useful. Generally, the degree of validation is dependent on the field of interest (engineering may require more validation than biomedical sciences) and application of the model. Related to validation is flexibility, which is another property of a useful model. Can more data be added to the model without having to change its structure? If so, the model is more useful than one that changes every time more data is added.

The next two properties, appropriate level of detail and as simple as possible, are two sides of the same coin because model detail increases at the expense of simplicity. Modeler's refer to this aspect of model development as Occam's razor. Formulated by William of Occam in the late Middle ages in response to increasingly complex theories being developed without an increase in predictability, Occam's razor is considered today to be one of the fundamental philosophies of modeling—the so-called principle of parsimony (Domingos, 1999). As ori-

ginally stated, "*Entities should not be multiplied beyond necessity*," the theory has mutated into many other familiar forms, such as Einstein's quote "*Everything should be made as simple as possible, but not simpler.*" In basic terms, Occam's razor states that the simplest model should be chosen. By choosing the simpler model, those concepts or variables not needed to explain the data are eliminated, thereby reducing the chance for redundancies, inconsistencies, or ambiguities in the model. But what exactly is the simplest model is not entirely clear. One common interpretation is if two models fit a data set equally well, choose the model with the smaller number of estimable parameters. But modeling is not always that easy. Sometimes a more complex model will be chosen because it is more consistent with theory.

Models should be judged on what they were intended to do. For example, if a model was developed in young adults and has good accuracy and prediction under different dosing regimens, should the model be deemed inadequate when it is applied to geriatric patients and does not predict with any degree of accuracy? Similarly, if a model characterizes one aspect of the data well but fails to characterize another aspect of the data, is the model still a good model? These philosophical questions should probably be answered on a case by case basis and different individuals may answer them differently. In the latter example, it may be that the system is quite complex and the modeler is really interested only in making predictions about that part of the system. In this case, the model can still be of value. In the former example, the model is still a good model, just one that it is not very generalized.

For a model to be useful, it must be developed on-time. A great solution that is arrived at too late is of no value to anyone. It is better to have a model that can provide rough answers in a useable time frame than an elegant model that is done too late. Also, models that are completed late look unfavorably upon the modeler and next time may not be assigned a project or worse, the use of a model in the future to solve a problem may not be considered as an option by the project team. This latter consequence reflects badly on modelers all over, not just on the modeler who was late, because then project teams see modeling as taking too many man-hours and being unreliable.

A useful model is one that serves as an effective communication tool. Often pharmacokineticists are asked by project teams in the pharmaceutical industry to interpret safety or efficacy data in relation to drug concentrations. Is there a relationship between the two? A quantitative approach to the problem would be to develop a model relating drug concentrations to effect (exposure-response). The model can then be presented to the team as evidence that indeed there is a predictable, controllable relationship between dose or concentration and outcome. Unfortunately many managers and people on project teams are neither math literate nor pharmacokinetic literate so the pharmacokineticist is caught between Scylla and Charybdis. A complex model, which may be needed for complex data, may be just as difficult to communicate as presenting the data itself. Still, a complex model presented effectively by a model communicator (pun intended) can be very compelling and aid in decision-making. More will be discussed on model communication later in the chapter.

Lastly, a useful model should serve many different purposes. The model may be used to characterize data for a report or publication, may be used to better understand the system under study, may be used to make predictions for future studies, or all of the above. The more purposes a model can serve the more useful it will become.

As an example, consider the data plotted in Fig. 1.2. The observed data were simulated using the model

$$C = 8 \exp(-0.3t) + 2 \exp(-0.01t) + \varepsilon \qquad (1.2)$$

where ε is normally distributed random error with mean zero and variance 4. As already stated, there may be a multitude of models that describe a set of data each with equal predictability and error (Rashomon effect). Four models were fit to the data

$$C = \beta_1 + \beta_2 \frac{1}{t} + \beta_3 \frac{1}{t^2} \qquad (1.3)$$

$$C = \beta_1 + \beta_2 \frac{1}{t} + \beta_3 \frac{1}{t^2} + \beta_4 \frac{1}{t^3} \qquad (1.4)$$

$$C = \beta_1 + \beta_2 \frac{1}{t} + \beta_3 \frac{1}{t^2} + \beta_4 \frac{1}{t^3} + \beta_5 \frac{1}{t^4} \qquad (1.5)$$

$$C = A \exp(-\alpha t) + B \exp(-\beta t). \qquad (1.6)$$

Equations (1.3)–(1.5) are inverse polynomials up to fourth degree and have estimable parameters β. Equation (1.6) is the model used to generate the data and has estimable parameters $\{A, \alpha, B, \beta\}$.

Which model is more useful? Table 1.2 shows the residual sum of squares (which will be discussed in greater detail later) for each model. For now, the smaller the residual sum of squares, the "better" the model. In theory, one would expect that the form of the equation

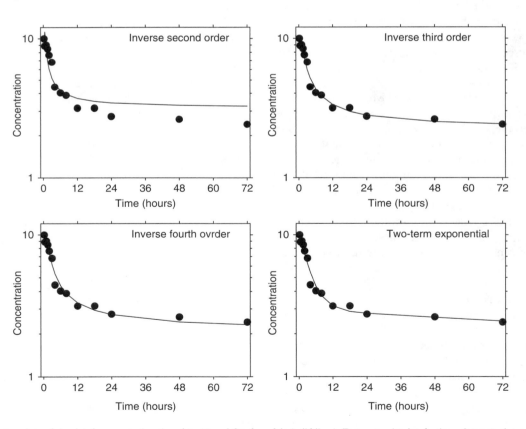

Figure 1.2 Scatter plots of simulated concentration-time data (●) and fitted models (solid lines). Data were simulated using a 2-term polyexponential model and were fit with inverse order polynomials up to degree four and to a 2-term exponential equation. The residual sum of squares for each model is shown in Table 2.

Table 1.2 Summary statistics for models fit to the data shown in Fig. 1.2.

Model	Number of estimable parameters	Residual sum of squares
Second order inverse polynomial	3	15.7
Third order inverse polynomial	4	1.80
Fourth order inverse polynomial	5	1.61
Two-term exponential model	4	2.47

used to generate the data would result in the best model. In other words, one would expect Eq. (1.6) to be the superior model to the other models since it is of the same form as data generating model. However, both Eqs. (1.4) and (1.5) resulted in smaller residual sum of squares than Eq. (1.6) which means these inverse polynomial models better predicted the observed concentrations than the exponential model. Occam's razor would lead us to choose Equation (1.4) over Eq. (1.5) since the former has fewer estimable parameters. This example illustrates why there is no such thing as a right model. Equation (1.4) is clearly the wrong model, but it in fact has better predictive properties than the equation used to generate the data. If interest were solely in being able to make predictions about the data at some point in time, say at 36 hours post-dose when no samples were collected, an inverse polynomial may be more useful as it will be more accurate than an exponential model.

So why aren't inverse polynomials used more frequently if they can have better predictive properties than exponential equations? The polyexponential equation is consistent with the theory for an n-compartmental system, which is one of the properties of a useful model. In this particular case, a two-term exponential equation is consistent with a 2-compartment model following bolus intravenous administration. The model parameters from the two-term exponential equation also directly translate to pharmacokinetic parameters, such as volume of distribution. There is no similar theory for inverse polynomials—they are strictly empirical equations. The parameters of an inverse polynomial have no physiological meaning. A useful model may also allow for extrapolations outside the range of data measured. For example, given a two-term exponential model [Eq. (1.6)] the limits for such a model are A+B when time equals zero and zero when time goes to infinity. This is what one would expect. Following bolus administration, concentrations are at their maximal and finite in value at time equal zero. As time goes towards infinity, all the drug in the body is eventually removed and concentrations approach zero. But for an inverse polynomial, at time equal zero, the dependent variable is undefined because inverse time (i.e., 1/0) does not exist. Taking the limit as time approaches zero, the dependent variable blows up towards infinity, which clearly is not possible as drug concentrations in the body must be finite since a finite amount of drug is given. At the other end of the time scale, when time approaches infinity, the dependent variable approaches the intercept term (β_1) because all the inverse time terms approach zero. So, the inverse polynomial model predicts concentrations to remain in the body infinitely equal in concentration to the model intercept. These concepts are illustrated in Fig 1.3. This example illustrates the hazards of extrapolating an empirical model outside the data range. So, despite better predictive properties, pharmacokineticists rely on models with pharmacokinetic interpretations that are consistent with theory.

In summary, a useful model, like the concept of a good model, is in the eye of the beholder. The model may fail at predicting certain aspects of the data, but if the modeler is not concerned with that portion of the data that is unexplainable, the model may still have value. Another modeler may argue, however, that the model is not useful since it fails to explain all aspects of the data. In another case, a modeler may also be quite satisfied at developing a model given the data on hand, but a project team may find the model to be useless if it cannot be used to help guide clinical development. Modelers must ever strive to make their models useful.

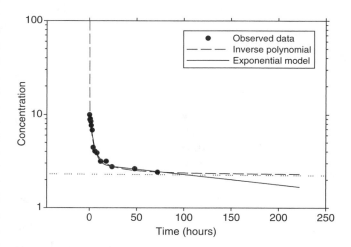

Figure 1.3 Extrapolation of the cubic inverse polynomial model and exponential model as time goes to zero and infinity. Observed data are denoted by ●. The solid line denotes the two-term exponential model, while the dashed line indicates the inverse polynomial of degree three. The dotted line denotes the intercept of the inverse polynomial model. In terms of residual sum of squares, the inverse polynomial model is the superior model but does not allow for extrapolation beyond the observed data range nor does the inverse polynomial model terms have any physiological meaning.

THE MODEL DEVELOPMENT PROCESS

Mesterton-Gibbons (1989) describes the modeling process as being as simple as ABC. Clearly that's not true, but it does make for a nice, catchy mnemonic. 'A' is for assume. Often there is inadequate information at the outset to solve a problem, except for the most simplest cases, so assumptions are needed right from the beginning. These assumptions may be in the form of parameter values, or model structure, or distributional assumptions, like the distribution of the model residuals. A model that has poor predictability may not be a poor model at all. Indeed, the problem may simply be that the assumptions are wrong. Next, 'B' is for borrow. Few models are developed in a vacuum. Most models are based on other models. Hence, knowledge is borrowed from the literature, from previous experience, or from colleagues and then a starting model is built to evaluate. 'C' is then to criticize the model and the assumptions the model was predicated upon. Modeling is iterative. If the model does not meet our needs then we go back to 'A,' modify our assumptions, and then start over again, hopefully learning from what we have just done.

While clever, most books on modeling don't use this simple mnemonic and instead present a more formal process initially proposed by Box and Hill (1967). They stated that the process of model-building can be thought to involve three stages:

1. Identification of the model,
2. Fitting the model, and
3. Diagnostically check the adequacy of the fit.

Although these stages have been repeatedly reported throughout the statistical literature, they are really only the middle part of the process. Chatfield (1988) expanded the number of stages to five, which include the original three by Box and Hill:

1. Look at the data,
2. Formulate a sensible model,
3. Fit the model to the data,
4. Diagnostically check the adequacy of the fit, and
5. Present the results and conclusions.

Models are not static—they change over time as more data and experience with the drug are accumulated. Basic assumptions made about a model may later be shown to be inaccurate. Hence, a more comprehensive model development process is:

1. Analyze the problem,
2. Identify relevant variables to collect,
3. Perform the experiment and collect data,
4. Look at, clean the data, and format for modeling,
5. Formulate a model,
6. Fit the model to the data,
7. Diagnostically check the adequacy of the fit,
8. Validate the model,
9. Update the model as appropriate (go back to Step 5),
10. Interpret the results, and
11. Communicate the results.

Figure 1.4 illustrates this process graphically.

The first step of the process should be to identify the problem, which has already been extensively discussed. The next step is to identify the relevant variables to collect. Data are usually not cheap to collect. There is ordinarily a fine line between money available to perform an experiment and the cost of collecting data. We want to collect as much data as possible, but if a variable is not needed then perhaps it should not be collected. Once the variables to be collected are identified, the accuracy and bias of the measurement methods should be examined because collected data are of no value if it is biased or inaccurate. Sometimes, however, the modeler is not involved in choosing which variables to collect and is brought in to analyze data after an experiment is already completed. It may be that the data needed to solve the problem was not collected or that only some of the data were collected, in which case some creative thinking may be needed to obtain a solution.

The next step is to perform the experiment and collect the data. Whether the data is a small scale animal study or a large scale clinical trial, the basics of data collection are the same. The validity of the results of any study are dependent on the quality of data collected. Therefore, data collection, whether stored electronically or on paper, must be designed to ensure high quality. Two keys to good quality are randomization and blinding, although in practice sometimes neither of these can be done. Document everything from a regulatory point of view; if it isn't documented, it never happened.

Rarely, however, will the data be in a format suitable for analysis. The more complex the data, the more pre-processing will be needed to put the data in a format suitable for analysis. The next step then is to look at the data and clean as needed. Check the quality of the data. Have the data been entered to suitable precision, for instance, two places behind the decimal? Perform descriptive statistics and look at histograms to examine for discordant results. It is not uncommon in large clinical multi-national clinical trials for clinical chemistry data to be of different units between the United States

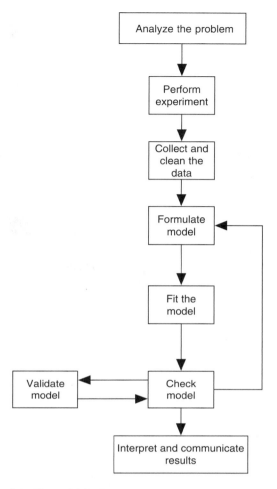

Figure 1.4 The model development process.

interpreted and presented, either in written or oral format. This process of model development is an empirical one, dependent on the data set used to build the model. Sometimes this is referred to as exploratory data analysis, data mining, or data dredging. Rare is the model in drug development built on theory, and then tested using experimental data—the so-called confirmatory model.

For particularly complex models, such as multi-compartment, multiple input-output experiments, one trick to modeling such data is to break the model down into subsystems. So for instance, suppose concentration-time data for parent drug and metabolite are available and it is known the metabolite is formed by irreversible metabolism of parent drug. One way to model the data is to first define and fit a model for parent drug, ignoring the metabolite. Then once that model is identified, analyze the metabolite data using a forcing function based on the parent concentration-time profile as the input to the metabolite model. Once both models are identified, combine them together and then re-fit the joint model. A similar approach can be made for pharmacokinetic-pharmacodynamic models where the pharmacodynamic model is a simple function of the concentration data. First, find the pharmacokinetic model and fix the model parameters. Then find the pharmacodynamic model keeping the pharmacokinetic model fixed. Once both models are fitted, combine the models and fit the joint model simultaneously.

Within the empirical model development framework, model development iterates until a suitable model is chosen. But model development may also occur globally across researchers. An excellent example of between-scientist model development is with the models used to characterize the pharmacokinetics of paclitaxel (Taxol®), an agent that is used in the treatment of various cancers. Paclitaxel is a poorly soluble drug given by infusion and formulated in a mixture of alcohol and a polyoxyethylated castor oil called Cremophor EL (50/50, v/v). Early studies reported that paclitaxel pharmacokinetics could be characterized by a 2-compartment model with first-order elimination (Brown et al., 1991; Longnecker et al., 1987; Wierkin et al., 1987). Large between-subject variability was observed in the parameter estimates, e.g., clearance ranged from 53 to 1260 mL/min/m^2 (Longnecker et al., 1987). Model predicted concentrations were judged to be reasonably close to observed concentrations and later studies, using noncompartmental analysis, produced similar pharmacokinetic estimates (Grem et al., 1987; Wiernik et al., 1987). But these early studies used long infusion times, 6 to 26 hours in length.

When paclitaxel was given as short infusion, hypersensitivity reactions typically occurred. Hence, paclitaxel was typically given by prolonged infusion. It was specu-

and Europe. Merging of data must then be transformed to a common unit before analysis can proceed. Data may have been wrongly entered into the computer. It is not uncommon to clean a data set and do an initial model fitting to the data only to find that something was missed and more data cleaning is needed. Whatever cleaning is done to the data should be documented in whatever final report is written on the analysis. Also, what quality control checks were made on the data should be documented. If data need to be transformed prior to analysis, such as a log-transformation on a dependent variable, then this too should be clearly documented in the report.

Once the data is cleaned and placed in a suitable format for analysis, herein begins the typical stages of model development reported by most books. Model development tends to be iterative in that a base model is chosen and evaluated. If the model is rejected, a new model is generated and evaluated. Once a suitable model is chosen, the model is validated to examine its generalizability. When a final model is found, the results are lated that decreasing the length of infusion and premedicating with a corticosteroid and anti-histamine would decrease the occurrence of hypersensitivity reactions, and be more convenient for the patient. In a clinical study testing this hypothesis, the shorter infusion with premedication did indeed result in a lower incidence of hypersensitivity reactions and was also shown to be less neutropenic (Eisenhauer et al., 1994). Unfortunately, paclitaxel concentrations were not determined in this study. In a similar repeated study that did measure paclitaxel plasma concentrations, when paclitaxel was given as either a 3 or 24 hour infusion, systemic clearance estimates after the 24 hour infusion were greater than after the 3 hour infusion (Huizing et al., 1993). A 3-compartment model was now more consistent with the data, which the authors attributed to having a more sensitive analytical assay thereby detecting the presence of another phase in the concentration-time profile. The authors also speculated that saturable pharmacokinetics was occurring but did not attempt to include this phenomenon in their model.

Dose-dependent clearance and distribution was then later observed in a Phase 1 study in children with solid tumors (Sonnichsen et al., 1994). In a study in adults with ovarian cancer, Gianni et al. (1995) used a 3-compartment model with saturable intercompartmental clearance into Compartment 2 and saturable, Michaelis–Menten elimination kinetics from the central compartment to describe the kinetics after 3 hour and 24 hour infusion. Now at this point one would typically assume that the mechanism for nonlinear elimination from the central compartment is either saturable protein binding or saturable metabolism. But the story is not that simple. Sparreboom et al. (1996a) speculated that since Cremophor EL is known to form micelles in aqueous solution, even many hours after dilution below the critical micellular concentration, and can modulate P-glycoprotein efflux, that the nonlinearity in pharmacokinetics was not due to paclitaxel, but due to the vehicle, Cremophor EL. This hypothesis was later confirmed in a study in mice (Sparreboom et al., 1996b).

An *in vitro* study was then conducted with human red blood cells (RBCs) which showed that the blood to plasma ratio in the absence of Cremophor EL was 1.07, but after the addition of Cremophor EL giving concentrations similar to those seen at the end of a 3 hour infusion of $175 \, mg/m^2$ paclitaxel, the blood to plasma ratio decreased to 0.69 (Sparreboom et al., 1999). Hence, Cremophor EL decreased the unbound fraction of paclitaxel available for distribution into tissues in a concentration-dependent manner, which explains the saturable tissue distribution phenomenon in multi-compartmental models. The presence of many compartments within the blood that paclitaxel may distribute into (unbound, plasma protein bound, RBCs, and Cremophor EL-derived micelles) also explains the nonlinear elimination kinetics from the central compartment. Current models now measure paclitaxel in each of these blood compartments and use a 3-compartment model with saturable elimination and saturable tissue distribution due to saturable transport, which is quite different than the first model developed for paclitaxel (Henningsson et al., 2001; van Zuylen et al., 2001). But the story is not over. Karlsson et al. (1997) have argued that, using plasma paclitaxel concentrations as the dependent variable, the current model for saturable tissue distribution due to saturable transport cannot be kinetically distinguished from a model with linear transport processes but with saturable, noninstantaneous tissue binding. So the modeling process continues. This example illustrates how since 1987 the pharmacokinetic models for paclitaxel have changed from simple linear pharmacokinetic models to complex nonlinear ones. Is there a universal model for paclitaxel pharmacokinetics? Yes. Will it ever be found? Maybe. Meanwhile, science and modeling progress.

GOODNESS OF FIT CRITERIA

Once a model is developed, the next step is to either assess how "good" the model is or to compare the model to alternative models in order to determine which model is "better." The words "good" and "better" are used because they are meant to represent semi-quantitative terms that intuitively one has a feeling for, but cannot really be defined. Goodness of fit criteria are either graphical in nature or are presented as some metric, like the coefficient of determination (R^2, which will be discussed later). Metric-like criteria have an advantage in that they are quantifiable. For example, a model with an R^2 of 0.9 can be judged superior to a model with an R^2 of 0.3, all other things being equal. However, few things beat a good graphical analysis to demonstrate the validity of a model and with today's software packages one would be remiss if these graphics were not examined on a routine basis.

Residuals and Residual Analysis

If Y is the observed data vector and $\hat{Y}$ is the model predicted data vector, ordinary residuals are the difference between observed and model predicted values

$$e_i = Y_i - \hat{Y}_i \qquad (1.7)$$

where i = 1, 2, ..., n. Positive residuals indicate that the model underpredicts the observation, whereas negative residuals indicate that model overpredicts the observation. Residuals are usually assumed to be independent, normally distributed with mean zero and variance σ^2 if the model is appropriate. The examination of residuals as part of the model evaluation process is referred to as residual analysis, which is useful because it can aid in isolating outliers or erroneous data points, i.e., observations that are discordant from the others, can aid in determining if the model assumptions are wrong or whether a different structural model should be used, and can aid in detecting observations that exert undue influence on the reported model parameters. Other types of residuals exist, such as Studentized or weighted residuals (which will be discussed later in the chapter).

An unbiased model should have residuals whose mean value is near zero. For a linear model the residuals always sum to zero, but for a nonlinear model this is not always the case. Conceptually one metric of goodness of fit is the squared difference between observed and predicted values, which has many different names, including the squared residuals, the sum of squares error (SSE), the residual sum of squares, or error sum of squares

$$SSE = \sum_{i=1}^{n}\left(Y_i - \hat{Y}_i\right)^2 = \sum_{i=1}^{n} e_i^2. \qquad (1.8)$$

The problem with SSE is that SSE decreases as the number of model parameters increases. Alternatively one could calculate the variance of the residuals called the mean square error (MSE)

$$MSE = \frac{SSE}{n - p} \qquad (1.9)$$

where p is the total number of estimable parameters in the model and the denominator is collectively referred to as the *degrees of freedom*[2]. MSE is an unbiased estimate of the error variance term σ^2 if the model is appropriate.

The residuals themselves also contain important information on the quality of the model and a large

part of model evaluation consists of residual analysis. Most residual analyses involve graphical examination of systematic trends or departures from the expected values. The following plots are often created and examined after model creation:

1. Scatter plot of predicted value (ordinate) versus residual (abscissa). No systematic trend in the residuals should be observed with the data appearing as a shotgun blast. Systematic trends are indicative of model misspecification. See Fig. 1.5 for an example.

2. Plot of absolute or squared residuals versus predicted value. Again, no systematic trend in the residuals should be observed and the plot should appear as a shotgun blast. Heteroscedasticity or misspecification of the variance model is evident if a positive trend in squared or absolute residuals with increasing predicted

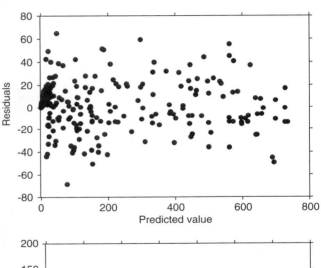

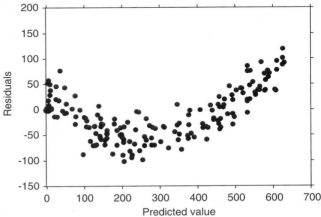

Figure 1.5 Sample residual plot. Paired (x, Y) data were simulated using the model $Y = 13 + 1.25x + 0.265x^2$. To each Y value was added random error from a normal distribution with mean zero and standard deviation 25. The top plot is a plot ordinary residuals versus predicted values when the fitted model was a second-order polynomial, the same model as the data-generating model. The bottom plot is the same plot when the fitted model was linear model (no quadratic term). Residual plots should appear as a shotgun blast (like the top plot) with no systematic trend (like the bottom plot).

---

[2] Defining degrees of freedom in a simple manner is difficult. First consider that there are n "pieces of information" contained within a data set having n observations. From these n pieces of information, either a parameter or variability can be estimated with each item being estimated decreasing the information in the data set by one degree of freedom. The degrees of freedom then is the number of pieces of information less all the estimated items. For example, given a data set in which the mean was estimated, the degrees of freedom then is n − 1. With a model having p-estimable parameters, the degrees of freedom is n − p.

values is observed. More will be discussed on this plot in the chapter on Variance Models, Weighting, and Transformations.

3. The residuals should also be uncorrelated so that if the residuals, e_1, e_2, e_3, etc., are lagged and plotted, i.e., e_1 vs. e_2, e_2 vs. e_3, etc., there should be no trend in the plot. When the residuals are correlated, such a process is termed 'autocorrelation' and unfortunately, this plot is rarely examined in pharmacokinetic/pharmacodynamic models.

4. A histogram of residuals. The histogram should show approximate normality with the center of mass located near zero (Fig. 1.6). Histograms, while easy to generate, do not easily detect subtle deviations from normality. More on histogram analysis is presented elsewhere in this chapter.

5. Normal probability plots or, half-normal plots are recommended instead of histograms for detecting deviations from normality. For a normally distributed random variable X with mean 0 and variance σ^2, a

good approximation to the expected value of the ith observation is

$$E(X_i) = \sqrt{MSE}\left[\Phi^{-1}\left(\frac{i - 0.375}{n + 0.25}\right)\right] \qquad (1.10)$$

where $\Phi^{-1}(f)$ denotes the fth percentile of the standard normal distribution. A standard normal plot plots the expected value of the residual against the value of the residual itself (ordered from smallest to largest). One criticism of the normal plot is what has been called 'supernormality' (Atkinson, 1985) in that residuals from non-normal distributions will tend to appear more normal than they truly are. Thus an adequate normal plot in and of itself is not confirmatory for a normal distribution. A modification of the normal plot, used to combat supernormality, is the half-normal plot where

$$\sqrt{MSE}\left[\Phi^{-1}\left(\frac{n + i + 0.5}{2n + 9/8}\right)\right] \qquad (1.11)$$

is plotted against the absolute value of the ith residual, again sorted from smallest to largest. Half-normal plots tend to show more sensitivity to kurtosis at the expense of not showing skewness but are more sensitive at detecting outliers and influential observations than normal plots.

6. Another type of plot, called a QQ (quantile-quantile) plot, plots the residuals ordered from smallest to largest against

$$\Phi^{-1}\left(\frac{i - 0.5}{n}\right). \qquad (1.12)$$

Normal, half-normal, and QQ plots that are linear are consistent with normality, whereas non-normal distributions tend to have systematic deviations from linearity. It should be noted that some software packages omit the $\sqrt{MSE}$ term in Eq. (1.10) since this omission has no impact on the nature of the plot, simply a change in intercept. Atkinson (1981) suggests plotting a "envelope" around the plot using simulation to aid in the interpretation of the plot but no software packages do this and so the reader is referred there for more details.

Figure 1.7 presents an example of the normal, half-normal, and QQ plot for simulated data from a normal, chi-squared distribution with four degrees of freedom, and Student's T-distribution with four degrees of freedom. It must be stressed that these plots are not always conclusive and that with small sample sizes normality can easily be mistaken for non-normality.

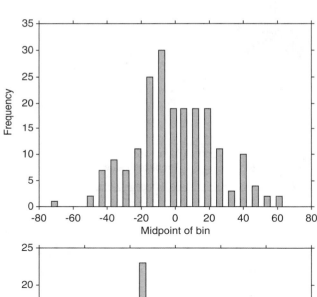

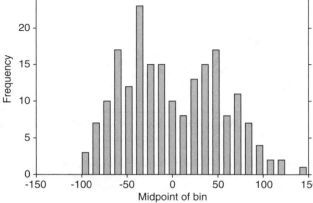

Figure 1.6 Histogram of residuals from data in Fig. 1.5. Top plot is quadratic model. Bottom plot is plot of linear model.

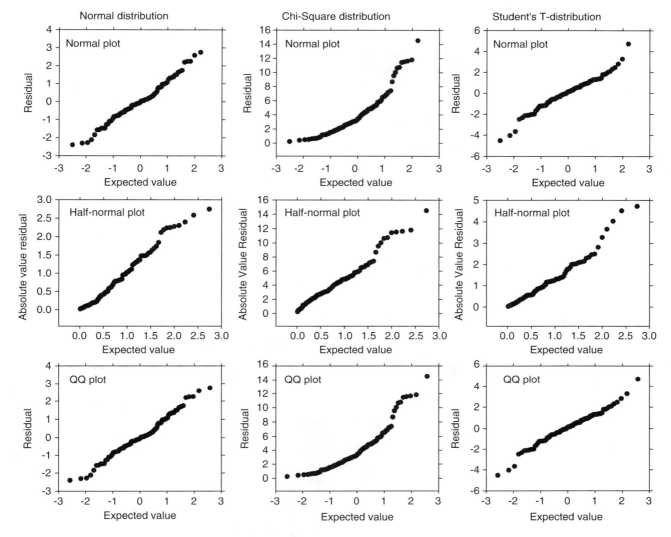

Figure 1.7 Normal, half-normal, and QQ plots for 100 simulated observations from a normal distribution (left), chi-squared distribution with four degrees of freedom (middle), and student's T-distribution with four degrees of freedom (right). If the data are consistent with a normal distribution, the resulting plots should all show approximate linearity with no curvatures. The normal plot and QQ plot are usually indistinguishable. The half-normal plot is usually more sensitive at detecting departures from normality than the normal or QQ plot.

7. A plot of residuals against explanatory variables not included in the model is useful to detect whether the explanatory variable should be included in the model. The plot should show no systematic trend if the explanatory variable is not predictive, but if the plot shows a systematic trend then this is evidence that perhaps the variable should be included in the model.

8. If one of the independent variables is time, a scatter plot of residuals versus time is useful. The plot should show random variation centered around zero. Systematic trends in the plot indicate the model does not predict the time trend accurately. More formally a runs test or Durbin–Watson test can be performed to test for lack of randomness.

9. If multiple observations are available on each sampling unit, such as a subject in a clinical trial, a plot of residuals versus subject number may be informative at detecting systematic deviations between subjects. Each subject's residuals should be centered around zero with approximately the same variance. Subjects that show systematic deviance from the model will tend to have all residuals above or below the zero line. This plot becomes more useful as the number of observations per subject increases because with a small number of

observations per subject, the sensitivity of the plot at detecting deviance from the model decreases.

Many of the plots just suggested are not limited to ordinary residuals. Weighted residuals, partial residuals, studentized residuals, and others can all be used to aid in model diagnostics. Beyond residual plots, other plots are also informative and can help in detecting model inadequacies. One notable plot is a scatter plot of observed versus predicted values usually with the line of unity overlaid on the plot (Fig. 1.8). The model should show random variation around the line of unity. Systematic deviations from the line indicate model misspecification whereas if the variance of the predicted values increases as the observed values increase then the variance model may be inappropriate.

While informal, an informative graph can be helpful in detecting gross violations of the model assumptions. A graph is also an effective means to communicate

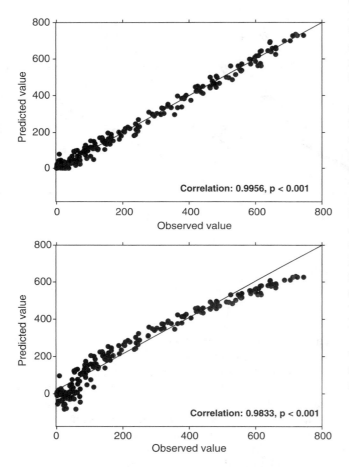

Figure 1.8 Plot of observed versus predicted values for the data in Fig. 1.5. The top plot shows reasonable goodness of fit while the bottom plot shows a systematic trend suggesting the model is not a reasonable approximation to the data. Solid line is line of unity. Note that both plots have very high correlation coefficients, despite one having a systematic trend from the line of unity.

how well a model performs. Subtle differences between two competing models, however, usually cannot be differentiated by the basis of graphics unless the two models are highly dissimilar. It should also be noted that data transformations (which will be discussed in later chapters) may also affect these plots considerably. For further details on residual analysis the reader is referred to Atkinson (1985) or Cook and Weisberg (1982).

Goodness of Fit Metrics

Along with graphical assessment one may present metrics, actual numbers, that attempt to quantify the goodness of fit of the model. Two such metrics were presented in the previous section, SSE and MSE, and in this section other metrics will be presented. Formal hypothesis tests may be done on these metrics, such as comparing the metric from one model against another. However, many test statistics based on these metrics tend to be sensitive to the assumption of the underlying distribution, e.g., normally distributed, such that the results from these tests should be treated with skepticism (Cook and Weisberg, 1982).

Common modifications to SSE and MSE lead to a class of metrics called discrimination functions. These functions, like the Akaike Information Criteria (AIC), are then used to choose between competing models. One problem with functions like the AIC and MSE is that the actual value of the function is impossible to interpret without some frame of reference. For instance, how can one interpret a MSE or an AIC of 45? Is that a good or bad? Further, some discrimination functions are designed to be maximized whereas others are designed to be minimized. In this book, the model with the smallest discrimination function is superior to all other models having the same number of estimable parameters, unless otherwise noted. This class of functions will be discussed in greater detail in the section on Model Selection Criteria.

Three goodness of fit metrics bear particular attention: the coefficient of determination, the correlation coefficient, and the concordance coefficient. The coefficient of determination (R^2) is simply

$$R^2 = 1 - \frac{SSE}{SST} = 1 - \frac{\sum_{i=1}^{n}\left(Y_i - \hat{Y}_i\right)^2}{\sum_{i=1}^{n}\left(Y_i - \overline{Y}\right)^2}. \quad (1.13)$$

where $\overline{Y}$ is the mean of the observed Y values. The reason R^2 is so often used is its ease of interpretation— it explains the proportion of variation "explained" by the model and ranges from 0 to 1 with 1 being a perfect fit to the data. Still what constitutes a good R^2 is debatable and depends on what is being measured. The R^2 for an analytical assay should be very high, probably greater than 0.98, while an R^2 greater than 0.4 may be acceptable some cases, like correlating apparent oral clearance to creatinine clearance.

R^2 is not perfect and has many flaws. Many cautionary notes have been written on the misuse of R^2 (Healy, 1984; Kvalseth, 1985). For example, with linear models having no-intercept or with nonlinear models, it may be possible for SSE to be larger than SST leading R^2 to be negative. R^2 is also influenced by the range of the observations with the wider the range of the independent variable, the larger R^2 tends to be (Helland, 1987). Further, when additional terms are added to a model, R^2 will always increase because SSE will always decrease. Since R^2 can be artificially increased due to additional model parameters, an adjusted R^2 is often used that adjusts R^2 for the additional degrees of freedom

$$R_{adj}^2 = 1 - \left(\frac{n-1}{n-p}\right)\frac{SSE}{SST}. \qquad (1.14)$$

Thus, the adjusted R^2 may decrease when additional terms are added to the model and they do not contribute to the goodness of fit.

Related to the coefficient of determination is the correlation coefficient, ρ, which is almost exclusively used in the association between two variables, X and Y. In relation to goodness of fit, X is the observed dependent variable, e.g., plasma drug concentrations, and Y is the model predicted dependent variable, e.g., predicted plasma drug concentrations, such as the plot shown in Figure 8. In the case of two variables ρ has maximum likelihood estimator

$$\hat{\rho} = r = \frac{\sum\limits_{i=1}^{n}(Y_i - \overline{Y})(X_i - \overline{X})}{\sqrt{\sum\limits_{i=1}^{n}(X_i - \overline{X})^2 \sum\limits_{i=1}^{n}(Y_i - \overline{Y})^2}}. \qquad (1.15)$$

r is a biased estimator for ρ, but becomes less biased as n goes to infinity. Since the covariance between two random variables is bounded by the product of the individual standard deviations, ρ is bounded by ± 1. r is also called Pearson's correlation coefficient for his pioneering work in this area, although the symbol 'r' was first noted by Sir Frances Galton for his work on regression towards the mean (which he called reversion) (Pearson, 1920; Zar, 1984).

Pearson's product-moment correlation coefficient, often simply referred to as the correlation coefficient, r, has two interesting properties. First,

$$\sqrt{R^2} = \pm r. \qquad (1.16)$$

Similarly, the maximum likelihood estimate for ρ^2 is R^2, which is why the coefficient of determination is usually mentioned in the same breath as the correlation coefficient. Second, r is scale invariant. If X and/or Y is multiplied by 10 or 1000, r does not change.

The correlation coefficient, r, is probably the most misused statistic in science. Much has been written criticizing the reporting of correlation coefficients. Foremost is the argument that X and Y must be *bivariate normal* for correlation results to be valid (Analytical Methods Committee and Royal Society of Chemistry, 1988), which is not exactly correct. The interpretation of the correlation coefficient depends on whether X and Y is random or fixed. If X and Y are random, then indeed they should be bivariate normal and r is an estimate of ρ, the population correlation coefficient. However, if x is fixed and Y is a function of x, then r is interpreted as the square root of the coefficient of determination. In both instances, the correlation coefficients are identical. However, the interpretation is subtly different.

Second, reporting of correlation coefficients without a graphical depiction of the data can be exceedingly misleading. Figure 1.9 shows four plots with misleading correlation coefficients [these examples were suggested by Harmatz and Greenblatt (1992)]. In all four cases, the correlation coefficients were highly significant, but clearly there is something going on in the underlying structure of the data. The bottom left plot also shows how a single data point can produce a highly significant correlation coefficient.

Third, correlation coefficients have been criticized for their use in assessing goodness of fit (Harmatz and Greenblatt, 1992). Correlation coefficients are a measure of association, not a measure of goodness of fit. A model may have a high correlation but still have poor predictive qualities. One particular area where correlation coefficients have been abused is in the assessment of linearity of an analytical method for measuring drug concentrations in biological fluids. The correlation coefficient does not indicate linearity or lack thereof. Figure 1.10 shows an example of a scatter plot where nonlinearity is occurring at high concentrations, but still leads to an exceedingly significant correlation coefficient. Another area where correlations are inappropriately used is in the assessment of dose proportionality in clinical studies of new chemical entities.

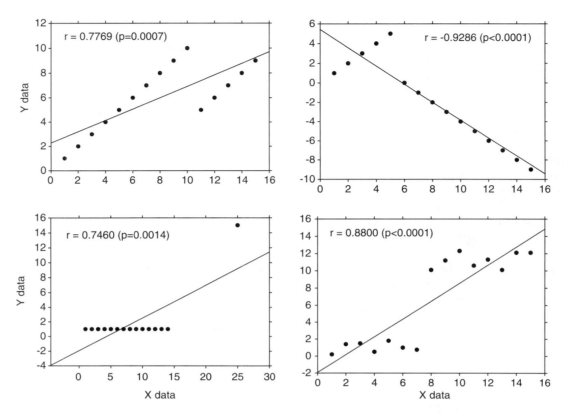

Figure 1.9 Example plots of misleading correlation coefficients suggested by Harmatz and Greenblatt (1992). Note that, in contrast to R^2, the correlation coefficient is independent of the scale of the X- and Y-axes.

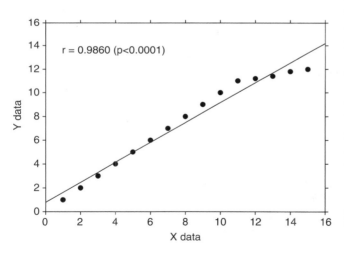

Figure 1.10 Example of a misleading correlation coefficient used in assessing linearity. The correlation coefficient for the simple linear model is quite high ($r = 0.9860$) but notice that the model systematically overpredicts higher concentrations, while underpredicts concentrations in the middle of the data range. This model shows systematic bias in its prediction despite having an excellent correlation.

Fourth, the correlation coefficient is reported not for their magnitude, but for their significance, e.g., $p < 0.01$. Tests of this nature are simply testing whether the correlation coefficient equals zero or not. Since the significance of a correlation coefficient is dependent on the sample size, large sample sizes easily can lead to significant correlations. For example, a correlation coefficient of 0.20, which under a linear model indicates that 4% of the variance is explained by the predictor variables, becomes significant at $p \leq 0.05$ when the sample size is more than 100. A more relevant hypothesis test is the one-sided null hypothesis that the correlation is greater than some value deemed by the analyst to have value, such as $\rho > 0.95$.

One other point needs mentioning in regard to correlation, and that is **correlation does not imply causality**. These last words are highlighted to stress their importance. Table 1.3 presents the nine tenets for causality as presented by Hill (1965). Correlation by its nature implies that X and Y can be reversed without loss of generality. Causality implies cause and effect. Just because a significant correlation has been detected between X and Y, it is entirely possible that the relationship is not

Table 1.3 Basic tenets of causality as proposed by Hill (1965).

Tenet	Meaning
• Strength of association	A high correlation between the causal variable and outcome is needed.
• Consistency	The results should be repeatable and consistent across studies.
• Specificity	The outcome is specific for the causal variable.
• Temporality	Changes in the causal variable should lead to changes in the outcome variable.
• Biological gradient	The more intense the causal variable the more intense the outcome variable.
• Biologic plausibility	There should be biological basis for the cause and effect.
• Biologic coherence	Implies a cause-and-effect interpretation.
• Experimental evidence	Experimental evidence supports the theory and is consistent with causality.
• Analogy	Similar to other cause-and-effect outcomes.

Note: Hill originally applied these criteria to the causality between risk factors and disease in epidemiology. These criteria have been modified to reflect causality between a causal variable and outcome variable in general.

due to an unknown, unobservable variable Z. For example, if X acts on Z and Z acts on Y, but Z is unobservable, an artifactual relationship between X and Y may exist. Still, it is easy to lose sight of the fact that just because a variable is correlated with another does not mean that a causal relationship exists.

Sheiner and Beal (1981) have pointed out the errors involved in using the correlation coefficient to assess the goodness of fit (GOF) in pharmacokinetic models. Pearson's correlation coefficient overestimates the predictability of the model because it represents the "best" linear line between two variables. A more appropriate estimator would be a measure of the deviation from the line of unity because if a model perfectly predicts the observed data then all the predicted values should be equal to all the observed values and a scatter plot of observed vs. predicted values should form a straight line whose origin is at the point (0,0) and whose slope is equal to a 45° line. Any deviation from this line represents both random and systemic error.

At the time the Sheiner and Beal (1981) paper was published, there were no good measures to assess the deviation from a 45° line. Lin (1989) developed the concordance coefficient to assess the reproducibility of two assay methods and was designed to correct some of the problems associated with the correlation coefficient, thereby measuring what Sheiner and Beal (1981) proposed almost 10 years earlier. The concordance coefficient (ρ_c) between X and Y measures the degree of agreement between X and Y by assessing the degree to which data pairs fall on the 45° line through the origin and can be estimated by

$$\hat{\rho}_c = \frac{2S_{xy}}{S_x^2 + S_y^2 + (\overline{X} - \overline{Y})^2}.$$ (1.17)

where

$$S_x^2 = \frac{\sum_{i=1}^{n} (X_i - \overline{X})^2}{n},$$ (1.18)

$$S_Y^2 = \frac{\sum_{i=1}^{n} (Y_i - \overline{Y})^2}{n}, \text{ and}$$ (1.19)

$$S_{xy} = \frac{\sum_{i=1}^{n} (X_i - \overline{X})(Y_i - \overline{Y})}{n}.$$ (1.20)

The concordance coefficient has the following properties:

1. $-1 \le |\rho| \le \rho_c \le |\rho| \le 1$,
2. $\rho_c = 0$ if and only if $\rho = 0$,
3. $\rho_c = \rho$ if and only if $\mu_x = \mu_y$ and $\sigma_x = \sigma_y$,
4. $\rho_c = \pm 1$ if and only if readings are in perfect agreement or perfect reversal, and
5. $|\rho_c|$ can be < 1 even if $|\rho| = 1$.

The reader is referred to Lin (1981) for details on calculating the variance of the concordance coefficient, which is not easily done. One disadvantage to the concordance coefficient is that, like the correlation coefficient and coefficient of determination, there are no guidelines as to what constitutes good agreement between observed and predicted values. This is left to the analyst to decide. Similarly the concordance coefficient can be just as misleading as a correlation coefficient and all the caveats regarding use of the correlation coefficient apply to the concordance coefficient as well. Vonesh, Chinchilli, and Pu (1996) present the use of concordance coefficient in population models.

In summary, the measures presented in this section represent metrics that assess the goodness of fit in a model but say nothing about prediction. The coefficient of determination, correlation coefficient, and concordance coefficient cannot not recommended as a means to guide the choice between two competing models. This is not to state that these metric should not be used—they should. But any goodness of fit metric must also be presented with corresponding graphical analysis of the goodness of fit.

MODEL SELECTION

General Comments

In modeling, observed data is frequently taken and a model developed, which is then used to draw inferences about the data used to develop the model—a circular process to be sure. In order for valid inference to be drawn, however, a proper model must be used. But what is the proper model? In pharmacokinetic modeling, one often has a set of candidate models to choose from, such as a 1-, 2-, or 3-compartment model after bolus administration. Which model is most appropriate? With today's software it's is an easy matter to obtain parameter estimates for most any model. Choosing an appropriate model is often far more difficult than estimating the parameters of a model. It is the choice of model, the formulation of the model, where science and intuition meet and therein lies the art of modeling.

The choice of model should be based on biological, physiological, and pharmacokinetic plausibility. For example, compartmental models may be used because of their basis in theory and plausibility. It is easy to conceptualize that a drug that distributes more slowly into poorly perfused tissues than rapidly perfused tissues will show multi-phasic concentration-time profiles. Alternatively, the E_{max} equation, one of the most commonly used equations in pharmacodynamic modeling, can be developed based on mass balance principles and receptor binding kinetics.

Unfortunately, not enough time is spent teaching students to think critically about the models they are using. Most mathematics and statistics classes focus on the mechanics of a calculation or the derivation of a statistical test. When a model is used to illustrate the calculation or derivation, little to no time is spent on why that particular model is used. We should not delude ourselves, however, into believing that once we have understood how a model was developed and that this model is the "true" model. It may be in physics or chemistry that elementary equations may be true, such as Boyle's law, but in biology, the mathematics of the system are so complex and probably nonlinear in nature with multiple feedback loops, that the true model may

never be known. At best, it can hoped that a model is found that provides a good "approximation" to the data. Besides even if the appropriate structure of a biological model could be identified, the number of parameters to estimate would be untenable for any optimization algorithm. Hence, approximating models are used, which are generally much simpler than the data generating process.

Choosing Compartmental Models

Pharmacokinetic models are typically modeled by examining the number of phases in the concentration-time profile after single dose administration with the number of compartments equaling the number of phases. If after bolus administration or after extravascular administration and absorption is essentially completed, the concentration-time profile when plotted on a log-scale shows only one phase, a 1-compartment open model is chosen. If two phases are shown, a 2-compartment open model is chosen.

Wagner (1975) has discussed at length the difficulties associated with formulating pharmacokinetic models. For instance, with a triexponential concentration-time profile after single dose intravenous administration, which is consistent with a 3-compartment open model, there are 13 such models to choose from. There are only three such models for the more common two compartment open model. If sampling is only done from the central compartment, however, one cannot unambiguously determine which of the 2-compartment open models apply. This is known as model indistinguishability, which was referred to more generally as the Rashomon effect.

Suppose one does a study wherein a single dose of the drug is given both orally and intravenously on two separate occasions and finds that the oral concentration-time data were best fit using a four-term polyexponential equation, whereas after intravenous administration the concentration-time profile was best fit with a two-term polyexponential equation. In this case there are 27 possible compartmental models to choose from. Whereas most books on pharmacokinetics present the 1- and 2-compartment model, the situation is clearly not that simple (see Wagner's (1993) text for examples).

So how then does a pharmacokineticist choose an appropriate compartmental model? Wagner suggests collecting the following data to aid in choosing a class of model:

1. Serial drug concentrations of parent drug after single dose bolus intravenous administration of different doses with sampling commencing early after dosing to capture rapidly equilibrating compartments, and sam-

pling long enough to capture the terminal elimination phase with at least four data points or long enough to estimate the maximal velocity and Michaelis constant if the elimination kinetics of the drug are nonlinear.

2. Serial drug concentrations following single dose extravascular administration of different doses given as a solution (not as a formulated tablet, capsule, etc.) at amounts low enough so as to not precipitate in the gastrointestinal tract.

3. Measurement of major metabolites (see Baille et al. (2002) for a discussion on what constitutes a major metabolite) at the same time and in the same matrix as parent drug when experiments (1) and (2) are conducted.

4. Measurement of parent drug and major metabolites in urine collected over the same intervals as experiments (1) and (2).

Still, even with following Wagner's guidelines it may be that many different models fit the data equally well. The situations becomes more complex when variables other than time are included in the model, such as in a population pharmacokinetic analysis. Often then it is of interest to compare a number of different models because the analyst is unclear which model is the more appropriate model when different models fit almost equally to the same data. For example, the E_{max} model is routinely used to analyze hyperbolic data, but it is not the only model that can be used. A Weibull model can be used with equal success and justification. One method that can be used to discriminate between rival models is to run another experiment, changing the conditions and seeing how the model predictions perform, although this may be unpractical due to time or fiscal constraints. Another alternative is to base model selection on some a priori criterion.

Bias versus Variance Tradeoff

As the number of parameters in a model increases, the "closeness" of the predicted values to the observed values increases, but at the expense of estimating the model parameters. In other words, the residual sum of squares decreases as more parameters are added into a model, but the ability to precisely estimate those model parameters also decreases. When too many parameters are included in a model the model is said to be "overfitted" or "overparameterized," whereas when too few parameters are included, the model is said to be "underfitted." Overfitting produces parameter estimates that have larger variances than the simpler model, both in the parameter estimates and in predicted values. Underfitting results in biased parameter estimates and biased prediction estimates. As model complexity increases,

generalizability increases to a point and then begins to decrease. In others words, the ability of the model to predict not just the observed data but other data generated using the same data generating process increases to a maximum and then decreases as the model becomes more and more dependent on the data upon which the model was predicated. These concepts are illustrated in Fig. 1.11.

An appropriate model is one that compromises between a model with biased estimates and a model with large variances—the so-called bias-variance trade-off (Myers, 1986). In general, a model that is slightly overfit is preferred to a model that is underfit because biased parameter estimates are a greater evil than large variance estimates. When bias and variance are optimized, the resulting model will tend to have good generalizability. Unfortunately, many model selection criteria, like the Bayesian Information Criteria (BIC), tend to choose the simpler model over the more complex model such that these models tend to choose underfit models more often.

To further illustrate the bias-variance trade-off, consider the concentration-time (C, t) data in Fig. 1.12. The data were simulated using a two-exponent model

$$C = 200 \exp(-0.25t) + 50 \exp(-0.03t) \qquad (1.21)$$

with log-normal random error having a coefficient of variation of 27% added. Exponential models of order 1, 2, and 3 were then fit to the data

$$C = A \exp(-\alpha t) \qquad (1.22)$$
$$C = A \exp(-\alpha t) + B \exp(-\beta t) \qquad (1.23)$$
$$C = A \exp(-\alpha t) + B \exp(-\beta t) + C \exp(\gamma t) \qquad (1.24)$$

using nonlinear regression with weights equal to inverse concentration. The model fits are shown in Fig. 1.12. Table 1.4 presents the goodness of fit statistics, parameter estimates, and variance estimates for each model. With each model the degrees of freedom decreases because more and more "information" in the data is used to estimate the model parameters. Recall that the error sum of squares (SSE) estimates the closeness of the observed and predicted values with smaller generally being better for models with the same number of estimable parameters. Clearly the 1-exponent model was not a good fit to the data, although the parameter estimates were precisely estimated, thus illustrating that precise parameter estimation alone is not a good indicator of goodness of fit.

The two-exponent model significantly decreased the SSE and also resulted in precise parameter estimates. The goodness of fit of the three-exponent model looked

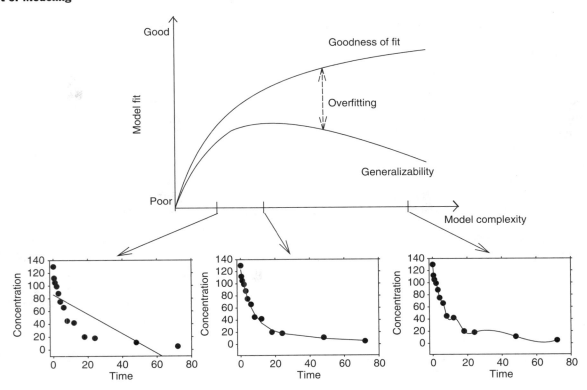

Figure 1.11   Relationship between goodness of fit and generalizability as a function of model complexity. The Y-axis represents any measure of goodness of fit, where a larger value represents a better fit. The three graphs at the bottom indicate how goodness of fit improves as model complexity increases. In the left graph, the complexity of the model does not match the observed data. In the middle graph, there is a good balance between complexity and goodness of fit. In the right graph, the model is more complex than the data; the model is a good fit to the data but overfits the data. Figure reprinted and modified with permission from Pitt and Myung (2002) with permission from Elsevier Science, Copyright, 2002.

virtually the same as the two-exponent model but had a smaller SSE, which one might think is a better thing. But look at the cost invoked by estimating these two add-

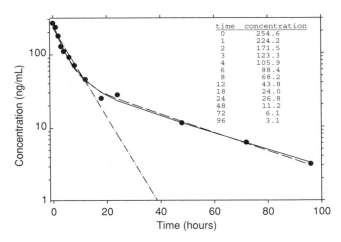

Figure 1.12   Scatter plot of data used to illustrate bias versus variance trade-off. The dashed-dotted line is the fit to a one-exponent model. The dashed line is the fit to a two-exponent model and the solid line is the line of fit to a three-exponent model. Data were fit using nonlinear linear regression with weights equal to inverse concentration.

itional parameters. The estimate of the residual variance (MSE) has increased compared to the two-exponent model and the standard error of the parameter estimates has vastly increased. The standard error of the parameter estimates was so wide with the 3-compartment model that only one parameter (γ) was precisely estimated. This example illustrates the concept that an underfit model produces a more biased model but an overfit model produces larger variances.

Model Discrimination Criteria

There are three schools of thought on selection of models: frequentist, information-theoretic, and Bayesian. The Bayesian paradigm for model selection has not yet penetrated the pharmacokinetics arena and as such will not be discussed here. The reader is referred to Hoeting et al., (1999) for a useful review paper. Frequentists rely on using probability to select a model and model development under this approach looks like the branches of a tree. A base model is developed and then one or more alternative models are developed. The alternative models are then compared to the base model and if one of the alternative models is statistically a

Table 1.4 Summary of parameter estimates and goodness of fit statistics after fitting exponential equations to the data in Fig. 1.12.

	One-exponent	Two-exponent	Three-exponent
SSE	52.85	6.55	6.04
DF	11	9	7
MSE	4.80	0.73	0.86
Parameter	Estimate (SE)	Estimate (SE)	Estimate (SE)
A	223.5 (20.7)	212.7 (12.2)	85.9 (327.2)
α	0.14 (0.0194)	0.268 (0.0295)	0.468 (0.904)
B		46.3 (8.6)	138.4 (314)
β		0.0286 (0.00482)	0.191 (0.242)
C			39.2 (21.5)
γ			0.0261 (0.0091)

Data for the one-exponent model were fit to the equation $Y = A \times \exp(-\alpha t)$. Data for the two-exponent model were fit to the equation $Y = A \times \exp(-\alpha t) + B \times \exp(-\beta t)$. Data for the three-exponent model were fit to the equation $Y = A \times \exp(-\alpha t) + B \times \exp(-\beta t) + C \times \exp(-\gamma t)$. All data were fit using nonlinear regression with inverse concentration as the weights. Legend: SE, standard error of the parameter estimate; SSE, sum of squares error; DF, degrees of freedom; MSE, mean square error.

better fit than the base model then the alternative model becomes the new base model. This process is repeated until a final model is developed. A classic example of this approach is forward stepwise linear regression.

Frequentist model selection is based on two models being nested. A nested model is where one model can be written as a simplification of another model. For example,

$$Y = Ae^{-\alpha t} \qquad (1.25)$$

is nested within

$$Y = Ae^{-\alpha t} + Be^{-\beta t} \qquad (1.26)$$

when $B = 0$. The model in Eq. (1.26) is referred to as the full model, whereas the model in Eq. (1.25) is referred to as the reduced model. By definition, the full model has more model parameters than the reduced model. But,

$$Y = \frac{E_{max}x}{EC_{50} + x} \qquad (1.27)$$

and

$$Y = A(1 - e^{-kx}) \qquad (1.28)$$

are non-nested models since neither model is a simplification of the other.

The F-test and likelihood ratio test (LRT) are the frequentist methods of choice for testing nested models.

Given two nested models, the full model having f-parameters with residual sum of squares SSE_f and the reduced model having r-parameters with residual sum of squares SSE_r, such that $f > r$, then the F-test

$$F = \frac{\left(\dfrac{SSE_r - SSE_f}{f - r}\right)}{\left(\dfrac{SSE_f}{n - f}\right)} \qquad (1.29)$$

is distributed as an F-distribution with f-r and n-f degrees of freedom. The null hypothesis is that the reduced model is the superior model, while the alternative hypothesis is that the full model is the superior model. The full model is chosen as the superior model if the p-value[3] associated with F is less than or equal to some critical value (denoted α), usually 0.05 or 0.01. α is also called the Type I error rate, which is the probability of declaring a null hypothesis false given that it is in fact true. From a frequentist's perspective, α ensures that at most $\alpha \times 100\%$ of the all true null hypotheses will be rejected by standard null hypothesis testing procedures in the long run. For nonlinear models, the F-test is only approximate and dependent on the degree of intrinsic nonlinearity in the model, which fortunately is usually small in most of the models dealt with in pharmacokinetics and can therefore be ignored (Bates and Watts, 1988).

Related to the F-test is the likelihood ratio test, which derives from the Neyman–Pearson test. Likelihoods and log-likelihoods are discussed in the appendix of the book. Given two nested models estimated using maximum likelihood, the full model having f-parameters with likelihood L_f and the reduced model having r-parameters with likelihood L_r, such that $f > r$, then the general likelihood ratio test is

$$\lambda = \frac{L_r}{L_f}. \qquad (1.30)$$

If the maximum likelihood estimates of the full and reduced models are normally distributed then for large n, $-2Ln(\lambda)$ is distributed as a chi-squared random variable with f-r degrees of freedom. An approximate size α test then is to declare the full model the superior model if

---

[3] The p-value is sometimes mistaken as the probability that the null hypothesis is true or as evidence against the null hypothesis, both of which are incorrect. Formally, a p-value is defined as probability of observing data at least as contradictory to the null hypothesis H_0 as the observed data given the assumption that H_0 is true. The reader is referred to Hubbard and Bayarri (and commentary) (2003) for a very interesting discussion on p-values and critical levels from Fisher's and Neyman–Pearson's point of view.

$-2\text{Ln}(\lambda)$ is greater than or equal to the chi-squared value associated f-r degrees of freedom and critical value α (Bain and Engelhardt, 1987). If LL_f and LL_r are the log-likelihoods for the full and reduced models, respectively, then an alternative form of the likelihood ratio test is given by

$$\text{LRT} = 2(LL_f - LL_r) \qquad (1.31)$$

which is approximately distributed as a chi-squared random variable with f-r degrees of freedom. An approximate size α test then is to declare the full model the superior model if the LRT is greater than or equal to the chi-squared value associated f-r degrees of freedom and critical value α (Buse, 1982). For example, for 1 degree of freedom difference between the full and reduced models, a critical value of 3.84 is required for 0.05 level significance or 6.63 for 0.01 level significance.

But the frequentist approach to model selection is not without its faults. Foremost is that there is no easy way of comparing non-nested models with different numbers of parameters. If two non-nested models have the same number of parameters, choose the model with the smallest residual sum of squares. For non-nested models with unequal numbers of parameters, Royston and Thompson (1995) present a method should one be needed, but the test statistic is not easily computed using standard pharmacokinetic software. Second, the choice of α is arbitrary. There is nothing magical about 0.05 or 0.01, although their use is ubiquitous in the statistical literature, with 0.05 being the most common criteria. Third, α does not remain fixed when repeated hypothesis tests are performed, like when many different models are compared. The overall Type I error rate (often referred to as the familywise error rate, ζ) for k independent hypothesis tests tested at significance level α is given by

$$\zeta = 1 - (1 - \alpha)^k. \qquad (1.32)$$

The familywise Type I error rate increases with repeated hypothesis testing, a phenomenon referred to as multiplicity, leading the analyst to falsely choose a model with more parameters. For example, the Type I error rate increases to 0.0975 with two model comparisons, and there is a 1 in 4 chance of choosing an overparameterized model with six model comparisons.

As an aside, the error rate in Eq. (1.32) assumes that the hypothesis tests are independent. Although this assumption has never been proven in the regression literature, model development using stepwise methods undoubtedly produces multiple hypothesis tests which are correlated, probably in relation to the degree of correlation between predictor variables used in a model. In the case where two statistical tests are correl-

ated the Type I error rate using Eq. (1.32) is overestimated. If Test 1 has Type I error rate α_1 and Test 2 has Type I error rate α_2, then the familywise Type I error rate is bounded by the inequality $\alpha_1 \leq \zeta \leq 1 - (1 - \alpha_1)(1 - \alpha_2)$. See Moye (2003) for further details on multiple testing.

One conservative approach to controlling Type I error rate is to use Bonferroni-corrected α-levels. Under this paradigm, reject the null hypothesis if the observed p-value is less than α/k, where k is the kth hypothesis tested. Clearly, however, for many hypothesis tests, it would be nearly impossible to find a statistically significant model. Therefore, most modelers fix α at some small value, usually 0.01 or 0.001, in the hopes of reducing the Type I error rate.

As Burnham and Anderson (2002), in their seminal book on model selection, state: "*How does one interpret dozens of P-values, from tests with differing power, to arrive at a good model?*" Good question. Because of the problems associated with the frequentist approach, some modelers prefer to take an information-theoretic approach to model selection. Under this approach, data can be partitioned into information and noise and it is the model's job to separate the two. Kullback–Leibler (Kullback, 1987) proposed that given the true model, denoted f(x), where x is the set of all independent variables that predict some variable Y, and given an approximating model to f(x) called $g_i(x|\theta)$, where i denotes that the approximating model is one of many possible approximating models and θ is set of parameters in the model g, then, if f and g are continuous functions, the Kullback–Leibler Information measure equals

$$I(f,g) = \int f(x)\text{Ln}\left(\frac{f(x)}{g(x|\theta)}\right)dx \qquad (1.33)$$

which broadly quantifies the information lost when g is used to approximate f. I(f,g) is the "distance" or discrepancy from g to f and is sometimes called relative entropy. I(f, g) must always be a positive number greater than or equal to zero. In other words, information will always be lost unless g equals f. Kullback–Leibler's result has formed the basis of information theory which has application in economics, computer science, physics, communications, and statistics.

Unfortunately, Kullback–Leibler cannot be applied directly to data because g must be known with certainty, something that can never be done except in simulations. Akaike[4] (1973) proposed the use of Kullback–Leibler

---

[4] Akaike is often mispronounced by pharmacokineticists as "Ah-chi-key" but the correct pronunciation is "Ah-kay-e-kay."

distance as the basis for model selection. Akaike showed when x and Y are drawn from the same joint distribution the critical issue to estimate Kullback–Leibler distance was to estimate the double expectation

$$E_Y E_x \left\{ Ln \left[g(x|\hat{\theta}) \right] \right\} \tag{1.34}$$

where $\hat{\theta}$ is the maximum likelihood estimate of θ and both expectations are taken with respect to the true model f. Akaike, who then came up with this next thought while taking a seat on a commuter train, proposed that the double expectation could be estimated from the empirical log-likelihood at its maximum point, denoted LL($\hat{\theta}$|data). For notational purposes, however, LL($\hat{\theta}$|data) will be denoted as LL. Mathematically, however, this results in overestimation of the double expectation. Under certain conditions, however, the degree of bias equals p, the number of estimable model parameters. Hence, an asymptotic approximately unbiased estimator for Eq. (1.34) would be

$$LL - p. \tag{1.35}$$

Akaike then defined *an* Information Criterion (AIC) by multiplying Eq. (1.35) by −2 to take "*historical reasons into account*" giving

$$AIC = -2LL + 2p. \tag{1.36}$$

Hence, Akaike, who considered the AIC "…*a natural extension of the maximum likelihood principle*," created an empirical function that linked Kullback–Leibler distance to maximum likelihood, thereby allowing information theory to be used as a practical tool in data analysis and model selection.

Akaike based his derivation on a large sample size. Hurvich and Tsai (1989) have proposed a second-order bias adjustment for small, more realistic sample sizes. Their criterion, the corrected AIC called AICc, consists of the AIC plus an additional nonstochastic penalty term

$$AICc = AIC + \frac{2p(p+1)}{n-p-1}. \tag{1.37}$$

The additional term prevents the size of the model from exceeding the sample size. AICc appears to have better sensitivity at detecting the true model structure for small sample sizes. Using Monte Carlo simulation of linear regression models with three parameters having a sample size of ten, the AICc correctly identified the number of model parameters 96% of the time compared to 36% with the AIC. When the sample size was increased to 20, the model structure was correctly identified 88% of the

time with AICc and 64% with AIC. It is recommended that AICc be used whenever n/p < 40. Unfortunately, the AICc has not been implemented in any pharmacokinetic software package so the analyst will have to manually calculate its value.

Akaike's criterion and its derivations has been called by some [see Verbeke and Molenberghs (2000) for example] as a minimization function plus a penalty term for the number of parameters being estimated. As more model parameters are added to a model, −2LL tends to decrease but 2 p increases. Hence, AIC may decrease to a point as more parameters are added to a model but eventually the penalty term dominates the equation and AIC begins to increase. Conceptually this fits into the concept of bias-variance trade-off or the trade-off between overfitting and underfitting.

To apply the AIC (or AICc), one fits a set of models, computes the AIC for each model, and then chooses the model with the smallest AIC. Hence, the model with the smallest AIC is the model that has the lowest degree of information lost between the true model and the approximating model. But it is important to remember that AIC only selects the best model from a set of models. AIC does not select the true model nor can it find a better model from other untested models.

AIC and AICc are used in practice by computing the AIC for each model in a set of models, identifying the model with the smallest AIC[5], and computing the AIC differences

$$\Delta AIC_i = AIC_i - AIC_{min}. \tag{1.38}$$

AIC differences represent the loss of information relative to the "best" model in the set. Given a set of R models, one of them must be best in a Kullback–Leibler sense. To better interpret the AIC differences, Akaike weights can be formed

$$w_i = \frac{\exp\left(-\frac{1}{2}\Delta AIC_i\right)}{\sum_{i=1}^{R} \exp\left(-\frac{1}{2}\Delta AIC_i\right)} \tag{1.39}$$

where the sum of the weights will equal 1. In a Bayesian sense, an Akaike weight can be interpreted as the posterior model probability. A model with a large Akaike weight is evidence that that model is best in a Kullback–Leibler sense. The ratio of Akaike weights between two competing models is sometimes called an evidence ratio. For example, two models have weights 0.25 and 0.15 with a corresponding evidence ratio of 1.67, which is not exceedingly large. Hence, the weight

---

[5] AIC and AICc will be used interchangeably hereafter.

of evidence for the model with the larger Akaike weight is not convincing. But two models having weights 0.25 and 0.01 have an evidence ratio of 25, which provides more convincing evidence that the former model is a better model.

In the case of least squares (which will be discussed in greater detail in the next chapter), assuming normally distributed random errors, where the residuals are normally distributed with mean zero and have variance σ^2, the log likelihood is given by

$$LL = -\frac{n}{2}Ln(2\pi) - \frac{n}{2}Ln\left[\frac{\sum\limits_{i=1}^{n}\left[Y_i - \hat{Y}_i\right]^2}{n}\right] - \frac{n}{2}. \quad (1.40)$$

Hence, the AIC is

$$AIC = -2\left[-\frac{n}{2}Ln(2\pi) - \frac{n}{2}Ln\left[\frac{\sum\limits_{i=1}^{n}[Y_i - \hat{Y}_i]^2}{n}\right] - \frac{n}{2}\right] + 2p$$

$$= [nLn[\hat{\sigma}^2] + nLn(2\pi) + n] + 2p \quad (1.41)$$

where $\hat{\sigma}^2$ denotes that the residual variance is estimated from the maximum likelihood estimate given the data and model. Since the term $(n \times Ln(2\pi) + n)$ are constants, a more simplified version is

$$AIC = nLn(\hat{\sigma}^2) + 2p. \quad (1.42)$$

Two errors are usually made in the estimation of AIC using Eq. (1.41). One is that $\hat{\sigma}^2$ in Eq. (1.42) is the maximum likelihood estimate of σ^2

$$\hat{\sigma}^2 = \frac{\sum\limits_{i=1}^{n}(Y_i - \hat{Y}_i)^2}{n} \quad (1.43)$$

and not the unbiased mean square error (MSE) estimate of σ^2 calculated using Eq. (1.9). Second, p includes all estimable parameters, including variance components. Hence, for a simple nonlinear model p should include all structural parameters plus one for estimating σ^2. Interestingly, in population pharmacokinetics, variance components are included in the AIC calculation, but for simple nonlinear regression problems the variance components are usually forgotten in the calculation. Luckily, in the case of simple nonlinear regression problems, when computing the difference in AIC values between two competing models, the forgotten variance components cancel out.

Akaike allowed for the existence of other AIC-like criteria that could be derived by making different assumptions regarding the distribution of the data. Schwarz (1978), in a Bayesian context, developed the Bayesian Information Criteria (BIC), which is also called the Schwarz Information Criteria (SIC) or Schwarz's criteria (SC), as

$$BIC = -2LL + pLn(n) \quad (1.44)$$

assuming equal probability for each model and that every possible parameter value under the model has equal probability (i.e., diffuse priors). BIC tends to be more conservative than AIC and more often chooses the simpler model. BIC is not an estimate of Kullback–Leibler information, but weights and evidence ratios similar to AIC can be computed using Eq. (1.39) after substituting BIC for AIC. The main advantage of the BIC is that if the set of models contains the true data generating model, the BIC will converge to probability 1 in choosing the true model as $n \to \infty$, a property known as consistency. In contrast, the AIC is not consistent in the sense that BIC is.

Yamaoka et al. (1978) proposed using an AIC-like criteria for choosing pharmacokinetic models. They defined AIC assuming normally distributed random errors with zero mean and variance σ^2 as

$$AIC = nLn(SSE) + 2p \quad (1.45)$$

for the ordinary least squares case or

$$AIC = nLn(SSE_w) + 2p \quad (1.46)$$

for the weighted least squares case. A BIC-like criteria can also be developed as

$$BIC = nLn(SSE) + pLn(n). \quad (1.47)$$

The AIC used by Yamaoka et al. is not the exact AIC reported by Akaike but is slightly different. However, its use is valid if all the models under consideration all have the same log-likelihood function. Yamaoka et al. (1978) demonstrated the use of the AIC by distinguishing between mono-exponential, bi-exponential, and tri-exponential equations. However, not all software packages use this definition. For example, WinNonlin (Pharsight Corp., Cary NC) uses Eq. (1.45) with p equal to only the number of structural model parameters and does not include the estimated residual variance. SAAM II (SAAM Institute, Seattle, WA) calculates the AIC as

$$AIC = \frac{[-LL + (p + q)]}{n} \quad (1.48)$$

where p is the number of structural model parameters estimated and q is the number of estimated variance components. In the dataset in Fig. 1.12, WinNonlin reports an AIC of 69.77, while SAAM II reports an AIC of 3.22 after fitting a two-exponential model to the data with weights equal to inverse concentration. Neither program computes a second-order AIC for small sample sizes.

Burnham and Anderson (2002) raise a number of issues regarding the AIC that bear repeating. First, the AIC cannot be used to compare different datasets. AIC can only be compared using the same data set, otherwise a modeler is comparing apples to oranges. Second, AIC values cannot be compared on the same dataset if one of the models was based on a transformation of the dependent variable. For example, it is unfair to compare the AIC based on Y to another model based on Ln(Y), even if they are the same dataset. Third, only the AIC value calculated using all parts of Eq. (1.36) can be used to compare models with different error structures. AIC values calculated using AIC-like statistics, such as Eq. (1.45), cannot be used with models having different error structures. For example, a modeler should not compare a model fit assuming normally distributed random errors to one assuming log-normal random errors using Eq. (1.45) since the models have different log-likelihood functions. Fourth, AIC can be used to compare non-nested models, which is an extreme advantage over the frequentist approach that has no such easily calculated test for comparisons. Fifth, AIC is not a "test," there are no p-values or statistical power or α-levels associated with a particular value of AIC. Sixth, AIC is invariant to 1:1 transformations of the dependent variable. Lastly, the value of an AIC tells nothing about how good the model is. The exact value of an AIC is meaningless—worth only derives when comparing an AIC to another AIC.

In the pharmacokinetic literature, the F-test and AIC are often presented as independent model selection criteria with the F-test being used with nested models and the AIC being used with non-nested models. Using these criteria in this manner is not entirely appropriate. The AIC and F-test are not independent nor is the AIC limited to non-nested models. To see how the AIC and F-test are related, consider two models with n-observations. The full model has f-degrees of freedom and residual sum of squares SSE_f. The reduced model has r-degrees of freedom and residual sum of squares SSE_r. The F-test comparing the reduced model to the full model is then

$$F = \frac{\left(\dfrac{SSE_r - SSE_f}{f - r}\right)}{\left(\dfrac{SSE_f}{n - f}\right)}. \tag{1.49}$$

Now consider the AIC for the two models,

$$AIC_f = nLn(SSE_f) + 2f \tag{1.50}$$

$$AIC_r = nLn(SSE_r) + 2r. \tag{1.51}$$

Let

$$\begin{aligned} \Delta AIC &= AIC_f - AIC_r \\ &= nLn(SSE_f) + 2f - nLn(SSE_r) - 2r \end{aligned}. \tag{1.52}$$

The full model is superior to the reduced model if

$$AIC_f < AIC_r \text{ or } \Delta AIC < 0. \tag{1.53}$$

Equation (1.52) can be simplified to

$$\Delta AIC = n\left[Ln\left(\frac{SSE_f}{SSE_r}\right)\right] + 2(f - r). \tag{1.54}$$

Substituting Eq. (1.49) into Eq. (1.54) and using a little algebra shows that

$$\Delta AIC = 2(f - r) - n\left[Ln\left(\frac{F(f - r)}{(n - f)} + 1\right)\right]. \tag{1.55}$$

What this equation shows is that the F-test and AIC are not independent and that given one of them the other can be determined. These equations also show that sometimes the two criteria can lead to different conclusions. Suppose a modeler fit an E_{max} model with two estimable parameters and a sigmoid E_{max} model with three estimable parameters to a data set with 14 observations, such as might be the case when fitting a pharmacodynamic model to individual data. In this case, an F-test greater than 3.84 is required to declare the sigmoid E_{max} model the superior model at the 0.05 level, which is equivalent to a ΔAIC of -2.19. An F-test value less than 3.84 is considered to be not statistically significant at the 0.05 level and the reduced model is chosen as the superior model. However, any ΔAIC less than 0, even values between 0 and -2.19, is still considered to be indicative that the full model is the superior model. Hence, the possibility exists for the two criteria to reach different conclusions.

To further illustrate that information-theoretic approaches and frequentist approaches may reach different conclusions, consider the case where the full model has log-likelihood LL_f and f-estimable parameters while the reduced model has log-likelihood LL_r and r-estimable parameters. The likelihood ratio test is then

$$LRT = -2(LL_r - LL_f) \tag{1.56}$$

with f−r degrees of freedom or equivalently

$$\text{LRT} = \text{AIC}_r - \text{AIC}_f + 2(f - r). \qquad (1.57)$$

Now consider the case where $\text{AIC}_r = \text{AIC}_f$, then the likelihood ratio test simplifies to

$$\text{LRT} = 2(f - r). \qquad (1.58)$$

A difference of 1 degree of freedom between the full and reduced model corresponds to a LRT of 2 with a corresponding p-value of 0.157, leading one to conclude that the reduced model is the superior model. This conclusion concurs with using the ΔAIC approach to model selection. But, Eq. (1.58) shows that the LRT increases, and its corresponding p-value decreases, as the degrees of freedom f−r increases. For example, with 8 degrees of freedom, the LRT is 16 with a corresponding p-value of 0.042 which, if one uses an α-level of 0.05, would lead to the conclusion that the full model is the superior model. In contrast, the ΔAIC approach would still favor the reduced model. Hence, the LRT leads to strong rejection of the simpler model in favor of the more complex model when there is a large degree of freedom difference between nested models. More extreme differences between the two approaches can be seen if one lets $\text{AIC}_r = \text{AIC}_f - x$, where x varies from 0 to 4. In this case the LRT becomes

$$\text{LRT} = 2(f - r) - x. \qquad (1.59)$$

Suppose now f−r is 20, that is the full model has 20 more estimable parameters than the reduced model and x = 4. The LRT is then 36 with 20 degrees of freedom, a p-value of 0.0154. Using an α-level of 0.05, this value of LRT would be strong evidence that the full model is the superior model. The AIC approach however clearly supports the reduced model. These examples indicate that in choosing an α-level for model selection, the degrees of freedom and sample size should be taken into account (Burnham and Anderson, 2002; Lindsey, 1999).

Ludden et al. (1994) have compared the ability of the AIC calculated using Eq. (1.45), BIC calculated using Eq. (1.47), and F-test to select the correct pharmacokinetic model using Monte Carlo simulation. They did not examine the use of AICc in model selection, which is unfortunate, since that would have been a more relevant criteria than AIC. They showed that the three tests do not always agree in their choice for the correct model, which is expected. The F-test tends to select the simplest model more often than does the AIC or BIC, even if the more complex model is the correct model. The AIC tends to select the complex model more often than the BIC when the complex model is correct. But the BIC tends to select the simpler model more often than the AIC when the simpler model is correct. Thus, the BIC tends to select the simpler model regardless of which model is correct, i.e., the BIC is conservative. Also, if the BIC selects the more complex model then so will the AIC. Similarly, if the F-test chooses the complex model then so will the BIC. The bottom line from their study is that when the more complex model is the correct model, then the AIC and BIC will be better at selecting it, but when the simpler model is correct, the F-test tends to select it more often than the AIC and BIC. Unfortunately, this is of little help to the analyst in having to choose a model. When two models are distinguishable and a reasonable sampling scheme is used, the authors-concluded F-test, AIC, and BIC all perform equally well and any criterion can be used. But for most situations, the authors conclude that, it would be prudent to use the AIC or BIC as model selection criterion.

A Note on Inference

Inference is the act of drawing conclusions from a model, be it making a prediction about a concentration at a particular time, such as the maximal concentration at the end of an infusion, or the average of some pharmacokinetic parameter, like clearance. These inferences are referred to as point estimates because they are estimates of the true value. Since these estimates are not known with certainty they have some error associated with them. For this reason confidence intervals, prediction intervals, or simply the error of the point estimate are included to show what the degree of precision was in the estimation. With models that are developed iteratively until some final optimal model is developed, the estimate of the error associated with inference is conditional on the final model. When inferences from a model are drawn, modelers typically act as though this were the true model. However, because the final model is uncertain (there may be other equally valid models, just this particular one was chosen) all point estimates error predicated on the final model will be underestimated (Chatfield, 1995). As such, the confidence interval or prediction interval around some estimate will be overly optimistic, as will the standard error of all parameters in a model.

Unfortunately there is nothing in statistical theory that allows determination of the correct error estimate taking into account model uncertainty. Bayesian model averaging has been advocated as one such solution, but this methodology is not without criticism and is not an adequate solution at this point in time. At this point the only advice that can be given is to be aware of model uncertainty and recognize it as a limitation of iterative model development.

Closing Notes

Model development should not proceed through blind devotion to model discrimination criteria. These criteria should be thought of as guidelines, rather than rules. Unfortunately, this advice does not sit well with some modelers because it allows for subjectivity and modeler bias to creep into model development. The author argues that blind devotion to model discrimination criteria fails to allow for expert opinion in model development. Table 1.5 presents some hints for successful model development. Models should be selected based on the totality of evidence: residual plots, goodness of fit plots, precise and plausible parameter estimates, reasonable and valid model assumptions, and proper judgment. Before modeling think about the problem and if you do not understand the problem or the biology of the system, ask an expert or read on your own about the subject matter.

It should also be recognized that collecting more data may not necessarily alleviate model selection biases. Newly collected data may not be fully exchangeable with the current data set (an observation that has profound implications for model validation) and so model development based on more data may not lead to the same model or the same conclusions. Lastly, a model based on data can never be proven. No amount of data can prove a model is correct, no matter how simple. A model can only be disproved.

IDENTIFIABILITY OF COMPARTMENTAL MODELS

With the plethora of modern modeling software it is a simple matter to write any differential equation and solve it to suitable numerical accuracy. Indeed, with some software (e.g., SAAM II, Madonna, Stella) it is not even necessary to write differential equations any longer, models can be simply generated using a graphical

Table 1.5 Hints for successful model development as presented by Cross and Moscardini (1985).

- Remember that no model represents the complete system. Base models on the totality of evidence.
- Models are usually built with some purpose in mind. Keep that purpose in mind during the development process and be careful if the model is used for something other than for what it was intended.
- Do not fall in love with your model.
- Don't distort the data to fit the model.
- Do not extrapolate beyond the region of validity of your model.
- Be flexible. Listen to the experts and be willing to change the model based on new information.
- Talk to the experts to understand the system.
- Do not retain discarded models, but always keep them in mind.
- Be willing to think outside the box.

user interface. But being able to write a model and then estimate the model parameters given a set of data is not always possible. Two types of identifiability issues arise. One is structural identifiability, first defined by Bellman and Astrom (1970), which refers to uniquely estimating a model's parameters given a model and ideal, error-free data. The other is numerical identifiability, which refers to accurate and precise estimation of a structurally identifiable model's parameters given real, observed data. It may be that in theory a model is structurally identifiable but the data is such that, in practice, the parameters of the model cannot be estimated. If a model is not structurally identifiable then a model will not be numerically identifiable. Similarly, a model that is numerically identifiable does not necessarily mean the model is structurally identifiable.

These concepts are best illustrated by example. Consider the case where a drug administered by bolus administration follows a 1-compartment model. Now suppose the nurse fails to record the dose administered. The model is given by the familiar equation

$$C = \frac{D}{V} \exp\left(-\frac{CL}{V}t\right) \tag{1.60}$$

where C is concentration, D dose, V volume of distribution, CL clearance, and t time. This model has three estimable parameters: D, CL, and V. To estimate volume of distribution one may take the log-transformed concentrations plotted against time

$$Ln(C) = Ln\left(\frac{D}{V}\right) - \frac{CL}{V}t \tag{1.61}$$

and extrapolate to time 0

$$Ln(C_0) = Ln\left(\frac{D}{V}\right). \tag{1.62}$$

If the dose was known then V can easily be solved. But neither dose nor volume of distribution is known in this case, so estimating volume of distribution uniquely cannot be done irregardless of how much data is collected. This latter point is extremely important. No matter how much data is collected in *a given experiment*, the parameters of an unidentifiable model can never be uniquely solved. The outcome is binary; the model is either identifiable or it is not. However, sometimes it is possible to change the experiment and collect different data, such as urine in addition to plasma, to make a model identifiable. This will be discussed shortly.

This example is kind of artificial in the sense that rarely is the administered dose not known. A more reasonable example would be Model A shown in Fig. 1.13. In this model, drug is sampled and dosed from the central compartment but elimination occurs both from the central and peripheral compartment. Such a model might be postulated for a drug that is eliminated from the central compartment and has irreversible transfer to a peripheral site where it is metabolized. In this case the model is

$$C = \frac{D}{V} \exp^{-(k_{10}+k_{12})t} \qquad (1.63)$$

where k_{10} is the rate constant of elimination from the central compartment and k_{12} is the rate constant of loss from the central compartment to the peripheral compartment. Log-transformation

$$Ln(C) = \theta_1 - \theta_2 t \qquad (1.64)$$

shows two model parameters β_1 and β_2 where

$$\theta_1 = Ln\left(\frac{D}{V}\right) \qquad (1.65)$$

$$\theta_2 = k_{10} + k_{12}. \qquad (1.66)$$

Knowing the dose administered V can be solved. But knowing θ_2 one cannot obtain a unique estimate of k_{10} and k_{12}, only their sum can be obtained. No matter how many data points are obtained during the elimination phase of this drug will allow k_{10} and k_{12} to be uniquely

identified. The lesson here is that whenever a model includes two eliminating peripheral compartments, while the input is in any other compartment, the model should have an observation from at least one of the eliminating compartments (Slob, Janssen, and van den Hof, 1997). In this example, data collected from either Compartment 2 or Compartment 3 would render the model identifiable. What should be striking about these two examples is that they are simple models, not very complex, and yet the model parameters are unidentifiable.

Another type of identifiability relates to a model that is identifiable but the parameters are not unique. The classic example of this is the 1-compartment model after extravascular administration assuming complete bioavailability

$$C = \frac{D}{V}\left[\frac{k_a}{k_a - k_{10}}\right]\left[e^{-k_{10}t} - e^{-k_a t}\right] \qquad (1.67)$$

where k_a and k_{10} are the absorption and elimination rate constants, respectively. This model can be written equivalently as

$$C = \theta_0\left[e^{-\theta_1 t} - e^{-\theta_2 t}\right] \qquad (1.68)$$

where

$$\theta_0 = \frac{D}{V}\left[\frac{k_a}{k_a - k_{10}}\right], \qquad (1.69)$$

$\theta_1 = k_{10}$, and $\theta_2 = k_a$. So then fitting Eq. 1.68 one obtains the solution for V as

$$V = \frac{D}{\theta_0}\left[\frac{\theta_2}{\theta_2 - \theta_1}\right]. \qquad (1.70)$$

But, Eq. 1.68 can also be written as

$$C = -\theta_0\left[e^{-\theta_2 t} - e^{-\theta_1 t}\right] \qquad (1.71)$$

with solution for V of

$$V = -\frac{D}{\theta_0}\left[\frac{\theta_2}{\theta_2 - \theta_1}\right]. \qquad (1.72)$$

Hence, the two solutions

$$[k_{10}, k_a, V] = \left[\theta_1, \theta_2, \frac{D}{\theta_0}\left(\frac{\theta_2}{\theta_2 - \theta_1}\right)\right] \qquad (1.73)$$

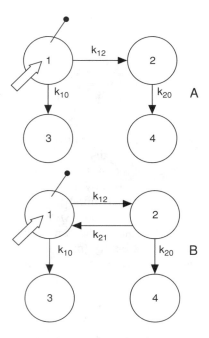

Figure 1.13   Examples of structurally unidentifiable models.

$$[k_{10}, k_a, V] = \left[\theta_2, \theta_1, -\frac{D}{\theta_0}\left(\frac{\theta_2}{\theta_1 - \theta_2}\right)\right] \quad (1.74)$$

provide identical concentration-time profiles for a drug.

For example, a drug with parameters [1, 0.05, 100] provides an identical concentration-time profile as [0.05, 1, 5]. Thus, even though k_a and k_{10} are uniquely identifiable they are indistinguishable in the absence of further information, such as knowledge of what V is. In most situations and without conscious effort, to distinguish between the two outcomes it is assumed that absorption is faster than elimination, $k_a \gg k_{10}$, and that Eq. 1.68 is the solution. In case where $k_{10} \gg k_a$ this is referred to as flip-flop kinetics and Eq. is the solution. Only in the case where both intravenous and extravascular data are obtained can k_a and k_{10} be uniquely determined (Chan and Gibaldi, 1985). All other cases are based on the assumption of which rate constant is larger, absorption or elimination.

As $k_a \to k_{10}$ the issue of numerical identifiability becomes important. Since the denominator of Eq. 1.68 contains the term $k_a - k_{10}$, as $k_a \to k_{10}$ then $k_a - k_{10} \to 0$ and $k_a/(k_a - k_{10}) \to \infty$. Dividing by zero will quickly occur. even with a double-precision processor on a computer, which is not definable, and even before zero is reached, significant digits will be lost in the calculation (Acton, 1996). The problem can be solved by reformulating the problem. Taking the limit as $k_a \to k_{10}$ Eq. can be approximated by

$$C = \frac{Dk't}{V}\left(e^{-k't}\right) \quad (1.75)$$

where k' is a hybrid estimate of k_a and k_{10} (Zhi, 1990).

Numerical identifiability also becomes a problem with a poorly or inadequately designed experiment. For example, a drug may exhibit multi-exponential kinetics but due to analytical assay limitations or a sampling schedule that stops sampling too early, one or more later phases may not be identifiable. Alternatively, if sampling is started too late, a rapid distribution phase may be missed after bolus administration. In these cases, the model is identifiable but the data are such that all the model components cannot be estimated. Attempting to fit the more complex model to data that do not support such a model may result in optimization problems that either do not truly optimize or result in parameter estimates that are unstable and highly variable.

Having understood the problem, a more formal definition of identifiability can be made. A compartmental model is structurally identifiable (or sometimes called globally identifiable) if every estimable parameter in the model is uniquely identifiable everywhere in the parameter space. A model is locally identifiable if a parameter is identifiable in a constrained region of the parameter space. A great deal of mathematics is needed to solve more complex problems to an exact solution of whether a model is identifiable or not and many papers have been written on the topic (Cobelli and DeStefano, 1980; Evans et al., 2001; Godfrey, Chapman, and Vajda, 1994). Even with symbolic mathematical software, such as MathCad (Mathsoft, Cambridge, MA) or Mathematica (Wolfram Research, Champaign, IL) the equations can be too difficult to solve. Still, most identifiability issues can be identified a priori using some simple rules and a simulation based approach to identifiability.

In order for a model to be identifiable, all compartments must be input and output reachable. An input reachable compartment has at least one path leading from some input. Output reachable refers to all compartments must somehow be connected to an observed compartment. Figure 1.14 presents an example of a model with input and output reachability problems and is therefore unidentifiability. Compartment 2 in Model A shown in Fig. 1.13 is output unreachable and therefore unidentifiable. Input and output reachability are necessary conditions for identifiability but are not sufficient. A model that is input and output reachable may still not be identifiable (see Model B in Fig. 1.13). If

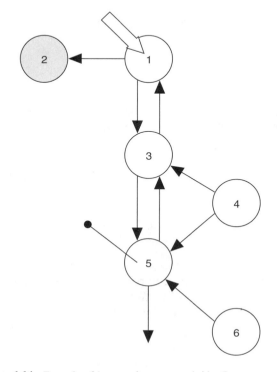

Figure 1.14 Example of input and output reachable. Compartment 6 is input unreachable. Compartment 2 is output unreachable. This model is unidentifiable.

either input or output reachability is not met, the model is unidentifiable. A more stringent criteria for identifiability is that the model is strongly connected, i.e., starting in any compartment material can pass to any other compartment by some path. A model that is strongly connected has input-output reachability.

A necessary and sufficient condition for identifiability is the concept that with p-estimable parameters at least p-solvable relations can be generated. Traditionally, for linear compartment models this involves using Laplace transforms. For example, going back to the 1-compartment model after first-order absorption with complete bioavailability, the model can be written in state-space notation as

$$\frac{dX_0}{dt} = -k_a X_0$$
$$\frac{dX_1}{dt} = k_a X_0 - k_{10} X_1 \qquad (1.76)$$
$$C = \frac{X_1}{V}$$

with initial conditions $X_0(0) = D$ and $X_1(0) = 0$ where X_0 represents the absorption compartment and X_1 is the central compartment. In Laplace notation

$$\begin{aligned} s\overline{X}_0 - D &= -k_a \overline{X}_0 \\ s\overline{X}_1 &= k_a \overline{X}_0 - k_{10} \overline{X}_1 \end{aligned} \qquad (1.77)$$

Solving for $\overline{X}_0$ and $\overline{X}_1$ and then substituting $\overline{X}_0$ into $\overline{X}_1$ gives

$$\overline{X}_1 = \frac{k_a D}{(s + k_a)(s + k_{10})}. \qquad (1.78)$$

Since a concentration is being measured, then the Laplace transform of the observation function needs to be scaled by 1/V.

Central to the use of Laplace transforms for identifiability analysis is the concept of the transfer function H(s) defined as

$$H(s) = \left\{ \frac{\mathcal{L}[y(t, p)]}{\mathcal{L}[u(t, p)]} \right\} \qquad (1.79)$$

where $\mathcal{L}[y(t, p)]$ denotes the Laplace transfer function for the measuring compartment observation and $\mathcal{L}[u(t, p)]$ is the input function in Laplace notation. Letting $\mathcal{L}[u(t, p)] = D$ and $\mathcal{L}[y(t, p)]$ equal Eq. (1.78), then

$$H(s) = \frac{\left[\dfrac{Dk_a}{V(s + k_a)(s + k_{10})} \right]}{D} = \frac{k_a}{V(s + k_a)(s + k_{10})} \qquad (1.80)$$

which is equivalent to

$$H(s) = \frac{B}{s^2 + A_2 s + A_1} \qquad (1.81)$$

where

$$B = \frac{k_a}{V}, \qquad (1.82)$$
$$A_2 = k_a + k_{10}, \text{ and} \qquad (1.83)$$
$$A_1 = k_a k_{el}. \qquad (1.84)$$

The coefficients of the powers of s in Eq. (1.81) are called the moment invariants and are functions of the parameters of the models. Models with equivalent moment invariants are indistinguishable kinetically (a true Rashomon effect), and will be detailed further momentarily. As can be seen there are three equations [Eqs. (1.82)–(1.84)] and three unknowns so all the parameters are uniquely identifiable but there are two solutions to k_a and k_{10}, so this model is locally identifiable.

Now consider what happens when bioavailability (F) is incomplete and unknown. Equation (1.67) is modified to

$$C = \frac{FD}{V} \left[\frac{k_a}{k_a - k_{10}} \right] \left[e^{-k_{10}t} - e^{-k_a t} \right] \qquad (1.85)$$

and the resulting transfer function is

$$H(s) = \frac{\left[\dfrac{FDk_a}{V(s + k_a)(s + k_{10})} \right]}{D} = \frac{Fk_a}{V(s + k_a)(s + k_{10})} \qquad (1.86)$$

which can be written as

$$H(s) = \frac{B}{s^2 + A_2 s + A_1} \qquad (1.87)$$

where now

$$B = \frac{k_a F}{V} \qquad (1.88)$$

and A_1 and A_2 are the same as before. Now there are three equations but four unknowns. Hence, this model is unidentifiable, unless either V or F is known.

As might be apparent, this method is tedious and quickly becomes cumbersome. Other methods, such as determining the rank of the Jacobian matrix (Jacquez, 1996) or Taylor series expansion for nonlinear compartment models (Chappell, Godfrey, and Vajda, 1990), are even more difficult and cumbersome to perform. There are a few software programs that have been written, such as IDENT (Jacquez and Perry, 1990), IDEXMIN (Merino et al., 1996), and Globi (Audoly et al., 1998) that determine whether a model is identifiable. These programs all have different algorithms and front-end interfaces but should all give the same result in the end.

An easier approach to test for identifiability, however, is to first test for input-output reachability and then use an empirical test. Failure on either test indicates the model is probably unidentifiable. First, write the model you wish to fit in some modeling software program. Then simulate lots of data without random error using the same input-output design as your experiment so that numerical identifiability is not an issue. It does not matter what the model parameters are, but make them physiologically plausible. Then fit the model to the simulated data using the parameters used to simulate the data as starting values. If the model is identifiable, convergence is achieved rapidly, within a few iterations. The residual sum of squares should be nearly zero and the precision of the parameter estimates should be very tight. If the model is unidentifiable two things may happen. One is that the model may not converge as it bounces around the parameter space looking for an optimum. The other is that convergence is achieved, but the parameters have large standard errors despite the model having a small residual sum of squares.

For example, concentration-time data using Model A in Fig. 1.13 was simulated after a unit dose with the following parameters: $V = 1$, $k_{10} = 0.15$, $k_{12} = 0.05$, and $k_{20} = 0.05$. Two hundred and fifty (250) data points were simulated on the time interval 0 to 24. The units of the parameters and time are irrelevant. The model was then fit in SAAM II, version 1.1, and WinNonlin Professional, Version 4.0. SAAM II never could achieve convergence and in the end the program indicated the covariance matrix was unreliable. No estimates of the final parameters could be obtained. WinNonlin achieved convergence after two iterations with the following results (estimate $\pm$ standard error of estimate): $V = 1.0 \pm 7E - 5$, $k_{12} = 0.04857 \pm 0.06324$, $k_{20} = 0.05 \pm 0$, and $k_{10} = 0.1514 \pm 0.06327$. The fit is almost perfect with a residual sum of squares of 9E-6. As expected, V was precisely estimated. The precision of k_{12} and k_{10} was quite poor with coefficients of variation greater than 40%. k_{20} did not even change from the starting value.

In a second fitting attempt, when k_{20} was changed to an initial condition of 0.5, the final parameter estimate was 0.5 ± 0. Jacquez (1990) refers to k_{20} as a nonsensical parameter (or unobservable parameter) since this parameter has no influence on the observations of the experiment. It is easy to see why this is so. Loss of drug from Compartment 1, the measuring compartment, is irreversible via k_{10} and k_{12}. Whatever happens once

the drug leaves Compartment 1 has no impact on what happens in Compartment 1. In general, whenever a parameter does not change from its starting value, one should change the starting value for the parameter in question to a number of different values. If after optimization the parameter does not ever change from its starting value, this is a good indication the parameter is nonsensical and the model is unidentifiable.

This example illustrates what may happen when an unidentifiable model is fit to data. The model may fail to converge or if it does, large standard errors of the parameter estimates may be observed despite an excellent goodness of fit. If the latter happens during model development then this is a good indication that the model is unidentifiable.

A subtle concept, not readily apparent from the transfer function [Eq. (1.79)], is that model identifiability also depends on the shape of the input function, $\mathcal{L}[u(t, p)]$ (Godfrey, Jones, and Brown, 1980). This property can be exploited, in the case of a single measurement system, to make a model identifiable by the addition of another input into the system. But care must be made in what is the shape of the second input. A second input having the same shape as the first input will not make an unidentifiable model identifiable. If, for example, a second bolus input into Compartment 2 of Model B in Fig. 1.13 were added at the same time as the bolus input into Compartment 1, the model will still remain unidentifiable. If, however, the input into Compartment 1 is a bolus and the input into Compartment 2 is an infusion the model will become globally identifiable. But, if the inputs are reversed and the input into Compartment 1 is an infusion and the input into Compartment 2 is a bolus, the model becomes globally identifiable only if there is an independent estimate of the volume of distribution of the central compartment. Hence, one way to make an unidentifiable model identifiable is to use another route of administration.

Another approach to make a model identifiable is to change the experimental design and collect additional data from another compartment. But this may not always resolve the problem. One common perception is that collecting urine is a useful aid in resolving identifiability problems. This is true only if the rate constants from all other losses from the central compartment are known. For example, if loss in Compartment 1 via k_{10} in Model A in Fig. 1.13 were entirely to urine, collecting urine from Compartment 3, in addition to the sample from Compartment 1, would not resolve the model's unidentifiability because k_{20} still remains nonsensical. In Model B in Fig. 1.13, suppose Compartments 3 and 4 represent urine, i.e., loss from Compartments 1 and 2 is entirely by renal elimination. Collecting urine from Compartments 3 and 4, in addition to Compartment 1, would resolve the model's unidentifiability, but measuring only from Compartment 3 or from Compartment 4 would still keep the model unidentifiable.

Similarly, measuring a metabolite may or may not be helpful. For example, suppose Compartment 2 in Model A in Fig. 1.13 represented a metabolite. Measuring metabolite concentrations from Compartment 2, in addition to the sample collected from Compartment 1, does not resolve either model's unidentifiability. The only way to resolve this model's unidentifiability is to collect samples from all compartments simultaneously. Metabolite data is helpful only if the rate constants for loss from other compartments is known (Godfrey, Jones, and Brown, 1980).

Identifiability is not a common problem in pharmacokinetics since the type of models that are usually dealt with are mammillary compartment models, in which all the peripheral compartments are directly connected to the central compartment and drug elimination occurs only from the central compartment (Model A in Fig. 1.15). Under this single input-single output scheme, all mammillary compartment models are identifiable. If, however, transfer to any peripheral compartment is unidirectional or irreversible, the model will become unidentifiable (Model B in Fig. 1.15). The model will become identifiable if a sample is collected from the compartment having irreversible gain from the central compartment, e.g., Compartment 2 in Model B. If the transfer between compartments is reversible, i.e., material can flow to the peripheral compartment from the central compartment and then back to the central compartment, and if only one peripheral compartment has irreversible loss from the compartment the model is identifiable (Model C in Fig. 1.15). But if two or more peripheral compartments have irreversible loss from them, the model will become unidentifiable (Model D in Fig. 1.15). Only by collecting measurements from all the outputs of the peripheral compartments will the model become identifiable (Model E in Fig. 1.15). If the loss to any peripheral compartment from the central compartment is irreversible and any peripheral compartment has irreversible loss, the model is unidentifiable (Model F and G in Fig. 1.15). If the peripheral compartment having irreversible loss is the same compartment that has irreversible gain from the central compartment, the model can be made identifiable by collecting measurements from the output of the peripheral compartment (Model H in Fig. 1.15). If, however, the peripheral compartment with irreversible loss is different than the peripheral compartment having irreversible gain from the central compartment (Model F in Fig. 1.15), then samples must be collected from both the peripheral compartment having irreversible gain and from the output of the

peripheral compartment having irreversible loss (Model I in Fig. 1.15). Collecting measurements from the peripheral compartments is insufficient to make the model identifiable. It should be noted that these results apply to extravascular administration, as well.

While not related to identifiability directly, the issue of model indistinguishability is often spoken of in the same breath. First recognized as a problem by Wagner (1975) and then formalized by Godfrey and colleagues (1989; 1994), model indistinguishability analysis refers to the generation of the complete class of models that can produce identical output profiles given the input structure of the experiment and proposed reference model. In other words, for a given compartmental model there may be other different compartmental model that can produce the identical output as the one that was observed. This phenomenon was referred to earlier as the Rashomon effect, but when dealing specifically with compartmental models the term "indistinguishability" will be used. Indistinguishability analysis is exceedingly difficult for models with more than two compartments and unfortunately there is no software program that will automate the analysis.

Indistinguishability is usually checked by three different methods: similarity transformation, examination of the Laplace transforms, and geometric evaluation. The latter two methods are the most common and those will be the methods used herein. As a simple example, consider Model B in Fig. 1.13. The Laplace transform of the observation compartment is

$$\mathcal{L}[y(t,p)] = \frac{\frac{1}{V}(s - k_{22})}{(s - k_{11})(s - k_{22}) - k_{12}k_{21}}$$
$$= \frac{\frac{1}{V}(s - k_{22})}{s^2 - (k_{22} + k_{11})s - k_{12}k_{21} + k_{12}k_{21}} \quad (1.89)$$

where $k_{22} = (k_{21} + k_{20})$ and $k_{11} = (k_{12} + k_{10})$. All the coefficients of the powers of s (including s^0) in the numerator and denominator of the Laplace transforms of all observations compartments, after canceling any common factors and ensuring that the highest power of s in the denominator is unity, are called the moment invariants (Godfrey and Chapman, 1989). The input-output behavior of a model is determined by the moment invariants so models that have similar moment invariants are kinetically indistinguishable. This model has three moment invariants: $-k_{22}$, $-k_{11} + k_{12}$, and $k_{11}k_{22} - k_{12}k_{21}$. The Laplace transform method for indistinguishability then examines all other models, identifiable or not, for whether they have the same set of moment invariants.

For two compartment models there are only a few possibilities, but for more compartments the method

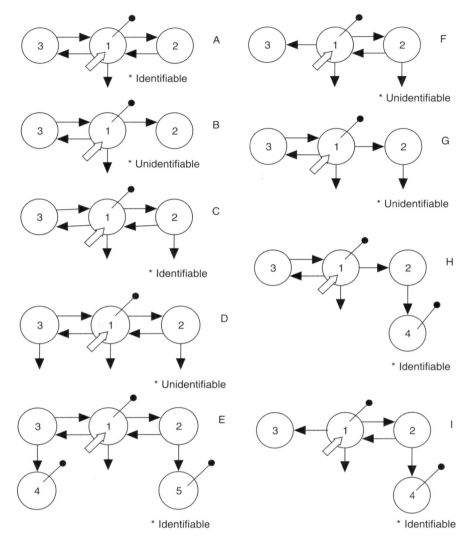

Figure 1.15 Identifiable and unidentifiable 3-compartment mammillary models.

becomes cumbersome. Returning to Model B in Fig. 1.13, there are two indistinguishable models which are shown in Fig. 1.16. To further illustrate that these models are in fact indistinguishable from the reference model, concentration-time data were simulated assuming a bolus input of 1 and a volume of distribution of 1. Since volume of distribution is uniquely identified in the reference model its value is irrelevant. The models shown in Fig. 1.16 were then fit to the simulated data. The model parameters used to simulate the data and the final parameter estimates after model fitting are shown in Table 1.6. Both of the indistinguishable models perfectly fit the data, but the parameter estimates are different than the data generating model. If one had to choose between models, expert knowledge would be important in making a decision.

For more than 2-compartments, Laplace transform and similarity transformation become unwieldy because the number of possible models rapidly becomes enormous. Zhang, Collins, and King (1991) present an example using isoniazid and its metabolite, whose pharmacokinetic profiles can be described using a 4-compartment model as shown in Fig. 1.17. With such a model having 4-compartments there are 11,440 candidate models to evaluate. To reduce the number of models to evaluate Godfrey and Chapman (1989) present some geometrical rules that must occur for a model to indistinguishable. Given an n-compartment system with all paths leading to and from a compartment being present, except those known a priori not to be present, the following rules must be met for a candidate model to be indistinguishable:

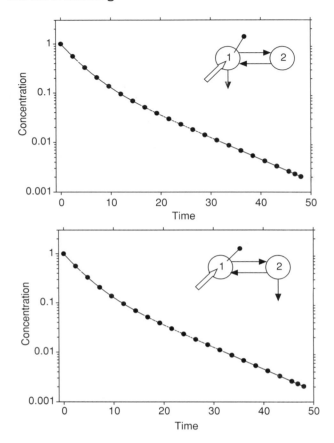

Figure 1.16 Two indistinguishable compartmental models fit (solid lines) to the concentration-time profiles simulated under Model B in Fig. 1.13 (the reference model). Data were simulated using the reference model with unit bolus and volume of distribution equal to 1. The models were then fit to the simulated data. The analysis could not distinguish between the models.

1. The length of the shorted path from a perturbed[6] compartment to an observed compartment must be preserved. In this example, the observed compartment and the perturbed compartment are the same for isoniazid, while Compartment 3 can be reached in by a path length of 1.

2. The number of compartments with a path to a given observed compartment is preserved. In this example, only Compartment 2 has a path to Compartment 1, while only Compartment 4 has a path to Compartment 3. Hence, Compartment 1 and Compartment 3 can only have 1 path returning to them.

3. The number of compartments that can be reached from any perturbed compartment is preserved. In this example, only Compartment 1 is perturbed and all compartments can be reached from Compartment 1. Hence, all compartments must remain reachable from Compartment 1.

---

[6] A perturbed compartment is one in which material is added to the compartment to push the system from steady-state, following which the system returns to steady-state (Jacquez, 1996).

Table 1.6 Model parameters used for simulation of data in Fig. 1.16 (Reference model) and final parameter estimates for the two indistinguishable models.

Model	k_{01}	k_{12}	k_{11}	k_{20}
Reference model	0.10	0.15	0.05	0.10
Model 1	0.20	0.05	0.15	—
Model 2	—	0.03	0.25	0.12

4. The number of traps must be preserved, a trap being a compartment that has no outflow from it (Compartment 2 in Fig. 1.14 is a trap). There are no traps in the reference model so there can be no traps in the indistinguishable models.

Following these geometrical rules the number of possible indistinguishable models is reduced to 40. Examination of the moment invariants for these models revealed 18 indistinguishable models (see Fig. 1.18) from the reference model, all of which were globally identifiable. These models might then be further reduced by knowing, for example, that conversion to the metabolite cannot occur from the parent drug's peripheral compartment to the metabolite's central compartment. Future experiments could then be designed to determine which model better characterizes the data. As can be seen, indistinguishability analysis is not easy, but should be considered for multi-compartment, multi-output models.

Most pharmacokineticists rarely concern themselves with identifiability or indistinguishability. Some may never even have heard of these terms. But with pharmacokinetic-pharmacodynamic models becoming more and more mechanistic, e.g., Jusko's now 6th-generation corticosteroid model (Ramakrishnan et al., 2002), issues in identifiability and model indistinguishability will become more commonplace. While this section is far from exhaustive in the recognition and remediation of these problems, hopefully the reader will have an appreciation of these concepts and have

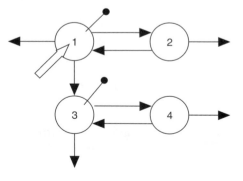

Figure 1.17 The pharmacokinetic model used to describe the concentration-time profile for isoniazid and its metabolite. Isoniazid is administered into Compartment 1 where it is irreversibly metabolized forming Compartment 3. Both parent and metabolite concentrations are measured (Compartment 1 and 3, respectively) and conform to a 2-compartment model.

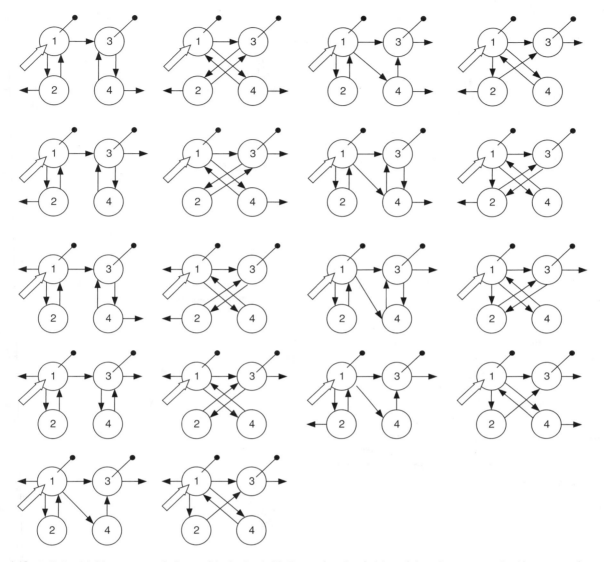

Figure 1.18 Indistinguishable parent-metabolite models for isoniazid. Parent drug is administered into Compartment 1 with parent and metabolite concentrations measured in Compartment 1 and 2, respectively. The models in the first column are pairwise symmetric to those in the second column by interchanging Compartments 2 and 4. The same is true for the third and fourth columns. All 18 of these models are kinetically indistinguishability and identifiable. Reprinted from Mathematical Biosciences, vol. 103, Zhang L-Q, Collins KC, and King PH: Indistinguishability and identifiability analysis of linear compartmental models, pp. 77–95. Copyright (1971) with permission of Elsevier.

some references for where to proceed should the simple techniques presented here be insufficient.

MODEL VALIDATION

Model validation is a contentious area. Modelers in the field cannot even agree to call it validation. One group uses the term "model qualification," instead of "model validation," the idea being that a model can never truly be validated so using the term 'validation' would be technically incorrect. Most books on modeling are strangely silent on this topic. Herein the term 'valid-

ation' will be used since both the Food and Drug Administration (FDA) guidance on population pharmacokinetic analysis (1999) and exposure-response analysis (2003) use the term "validation." This section will deal with general aspects of model validation. Much of what will be discussed will be drawn from Cobelli et al. (1984) and a 1981 workshop on Model Acceptance held by the Society for Computer Simulation (McLeod, 1982). The chapter on nonlinear mixed effect models will have more details on model validation for that class of models.

A fundamental principle of modeling is that a model can never be proven, only disproved. Thus, model validation attempts to disprove a model by applying a series of validity tests to a model and its predictions. The more validity tests a model passes, the greater credibility the model will have. If a model fails a test then the model is disproven and often times it is back to the drawing-board. Further, the degree of model validation will ultimately depend on the model objectives. If the objective is to simply characterize a set of data, model validation is usually minimal, but if the objective is prediction, then validation is usually more comprehensive.

One definition of model validation refers to the assessment and extent to which a model is founded and fulfills the purpose for which it was developed (Cobelli et al., 1984). First and foremost, a validated model must have a clearly stated purpose. Then, is the model credible and does the postulated model support its intended purpose? Models do not universally apply to all input conditions, but whether a model applies to a particular situation can be assessed. Thus, a model may be valid or useful in one situation, but invalid or useless in another. A model may also be valid for one set of data, but not for another. Lastly, a model may be valid for one set of assumptions but not valid for another set.

Many different tests of validation exist, few of which have a simple "pass/fail". Most validation tests are sliding subjective scales where on one end 'the model is valid' and on the other end 'the model is not valid'. The validity of a model under a test then lies somewhere between those two extremes. But, in order for model development to proceed iteratively, modelers need a "yes/no" answer to the question "is the model validated?" Hence, the outcome from a series of subjective tests that may vary from one modeler to another is transformed into a sometimes arbitrary binary outcome, a not very scientific process.

There is no universal, single statistical test or set of tests that will validate a model. Nothing can be done to allow us to say "if the model meets this, this, and this then the model is okay." McLeod (1982) reports that a valid model is based on the following properties:

- Degree to which the model duplicates past system behavior using historical data as an input,
- Degree to which model behavior conforms to existing theory,
- Degree to which the model accurately forecasts the future,
- Degree to which the model is found acceptable to other modelers,
- Degree to which the model is found acceptable to those who will use it, and the
- Degree to which the model yields opposite results when opposite values are assigned to the

values and opposite relationships are postulated and opposite assumptions are made.

As can be seen, validation is a holistic approach where the validity of the model is based on many difference aspects. The guidelines presented by McLeod (1982) can be generalized into the following validity checks:

- Face-validity,
- Credibility,
- Internal validity,
- External validity, and
- Pragmatic validity.

The more validity checks a model passes the more valid the model will be perceived.

Face validity refers to the model being appropriate on face value. For example, in a population pharmacokinetic analysis, creatinine clearance may seem a reasonable predictor of systemic clearance, but oral temperature may not. Hence, creatinine clearance has high face validity, but oral temperature does not. That is not to say that oral temperature cannot be a predictor. Oral temperature may be related to some unmeasured covariate that is directly related to systemic clearance, such that oral temperature is a surrogate for the unmeasured covariate. A second example would be if concentration-time data are multiphasic. In this instance, a multi-compartment model has high face validity, a single compartment model does not. Face validity examination should be done using common sense and without being afraid to challenge accepted beliefs.

Credibility goes beyond face-validity. A model with face validity seems to be a reasonable model. A credible model is one in which there is faith or belief in the validity of the model's predictions, outcomes, or conclusions. Credibility is not an attribute of the model but of the person's attitudes toward the model. Hence, credibility is person-specific. One person may believe the model has high credibility, but another may not. Rightly or wrongly, the credibility of a model is tied to the credibility of the modeler who developed the model. A modeler with little credibility will tend to create models with low credibility. Conversely, a modeler with high credibility will tend to have greater model acceptance. The simpler, more transparent the model, the more credibility it will have to outside reviewers, thus underscoring the need for effective communication and report writing. Lastly, models that produce predictions different than expected results (whether those expectations are correct or not) will have lower credibility than models that re-enforce currently held beliefs.

Internal criteria for validation refers to the model itself being judged without regards to external criteria. Are the data itself of sufficient quality to render a useful model? This is the old adage: "garbage in, garbage out." Are the model parameters globally identifiable? Does the model show reasonable goodness of fit? Are no systematic trends in the residuals apparent? Are the assumptions of the model reasonable? Are the model assumptions met, e.g., are the residuals normally distributed? Are no influential observations apparent? Are no observations discordant from their predicted value? Are the parameter estimates precise with small standard errors? Is the degree of unexplained variability small? What are the boundary conditions of the data and does the model predict those boundary conditions reasonable well? A valid model should answer all these questions in the affirmative. Quantitative measures of internal model validity, such as the coefficient of determination, are of limited value as a model with a high R^2 may be just as easily due to an overfit model as to a well fit, generalizable model. At most quantitative measures of validity are supportive evidence and should not be relied upon solely. A useful test for internal validity is the Turing test, in which the model predictions and observed data are shown to experts. If the experts cannot tell the difference, the model has passed its internal criteria check and will have a high degree of credibility later on.

External criteria for validation refers to aspects related to outside the model, specifically purpose, theory, and data. How does the model compare to other models? Does the model show empirical validity? In other words, do model predictions correspond to actual observed data with an appropriate level of accuracy? Is the model consistent? Does the model contain any mathematical or conceptual contradictions? Are the signs of the model parameters expected? For instance, is a parameter negative when it would be expected to be positive? Is the model consistent with theory? A valid model should answer 'yes' to all these questions.

Pragmatic validity refers to the model being able to meet its stated objective in a timely manner. For example, if the goal of the analysis was to develop a model to aid in dosing a drug in patients with renal impairment, one might ask "Does the model make predictions of suitable precision and accuracy to render its conclusions useful?" The model must also be testable. In other words, a testable model is one in which the components of the model can be tested to either confirm or reject the model. For example, if age is an important predictor in a model then an experimental study in young and elderly subjects can be used to confirm or reject the model. Lastly, the model must be done in a timely manner. An elegant solution to a problem that is presented past when it is needed is of little value.

How much validation must be done on a model depends on its purpose, whether the model is descriptive, predictive, or explanatory in nature. If the objective of

an analysis is to simply characterize a set of data, such as reporting the clearance and volume of distribution at steady state for a particular subject, model validation can be minimal—does the model predicted values match the actual observed data. If the objective is predictive then more stringent empirical validity is required. Not only should the model possess empirical validity, but the model should also be predictive of other data sets. This ability to predict external data sets has been previously called 'generalizability.' A model that is explanatory must have the highest degree of validity, embodying both descriptive and predictive models. The model must possess empirical validity, both to the model development data set as well to external data sets. The model structure must be plausible and reflect theoretical mechanisms. An explanatory model must also be testable. Empirical models, i.e., black-box models, such as low-order polynomials, may be able to adequately predict a model development data set, but may not be as accurate with external data sets.

The degree of validation can also depend on the consequences of using the model. If the model is used for internal discovery or synthesis of information, then a model that has low validity and poor predictability can still be acceptable. An example might be the fitting of receptor binding data to obtain binding constants with the idea being that lead selection in a drug discovery program will be based on the top candidates having high binding affinity. In this case, model validation would probably be minimal to none as the cost of choosing the wrong lead is assumed to be minimal. On the other side of the coin is a model whose use has high consequences, such as a model that is used as an aid for selecting a dosing recommendation. In this case, a poorly predictive model may lead to a sub-therapeutic response or worse, severe toxicity or death. In this case a great degree of model validation may be needed.

Sometimes when model validation is not needed, or to supplement already discussed validity checks, model stability is assessed. Model stability determines how robust the model parameters are to slight changes in the data and how robust the model predictions are to changes in the either the model parameters or input data. Collectively these tests are referred to as *sensitivity analysis*. If model outputs are particularly sensitive to some parameter then greater accuracy needs to be obtained in estimating that parameter. A stable model is one that is relatively robust to changes in the model parameters and the input data.

Early studies proposed that for models that can be expressed as an equation, the stability of the model to slight changes in the model parameters can be assessed using partial derivatives of the model parameters (see Nesterov (1980; 1999) for examples). Under this approach, a sensitivity index can be defined as the change in model response to change in model parameter. For example, for the 1-compartment model after intravenous administration

$$C = \frac{D}{V} \exp\left(-\frac{CL}{V}t\right) \qquad (1.90)$$

where C is concentration, t is time, D is dose, V is volume of distribution, and CL is clearance, the individual sensitivity indices are

$$\frac{\partial C}{\partial V} = \frac{D}{V^3} t(CL) \exp\left(-\frac{CL}{V}t\right) - \frac{D}{V^2} \exp\left(-\frac{CL}{V}t\right) \qquad (1.91)$$

$$\frac{\partial C}{\partial CL} = -\frac{Dt}{V^2} \exp\left(-\frac{CL}{V}t\right) \qquad (1.92)$$

while the joint sensitivity index is

$$\frac{\partial^2 C}{\partial V \partial CL} = \frac{2Dt}{V^3} \exp\left(-\frac{CL}{V}t\right) - \frac{Dt^2(CL)}{V^4} \exp\left(-\frac{CL}{V}t\right). \qquad (1.93)$$

The individual sensitivity indices measure how small changes in V or CL affect plasma concentrations. Sometimes the sensitivity indices are scaled, e.g., $(\delta C / \delta CL)/C$ or $(\delta C / C)/(\delta CL)/CL$, to obtain the fractional change in response to change in model parameter. The joint index measures the sensitivity of concentrations to small changes in both V and CL simultaneously. Individual sensitivities can be plotted on a surface plot to graphically examine how sensitivity changes over time, but such plots for joint sensitivity are more difficult because higher order graphics are required. So, usually these plots are evaluated at just a few points in time. While useful, however, these plots have not found widespread application in pharmacokinetics.

With the complexity of modern pharmacokinetic-pharmacodynamic models, analytical derivation of sensitivity indexes is rarely possible because rarely can these models be expressed as an equation. More often these models are written as a matrix of derivatives and the solution to finding the sensitivity index for these models requires a software package that can do symbolic differentiation of the Jacobian matrix. Hence, the current methodology for sensitivity analysis of complex models is empirical and done by systematically varying the model parameters one at a time and observing how the model outputs change. While easy to do, this approach cannot handle the case where there are interactions between model parameters. For example, two

model parameters alone may not have a large impact on the model outputs but when tested together have a much greater impact. There is also the issue of how to vary the parameters. One approach is to simply vary the parameters by plus or minus some percent, say $\pm$ 10%, or by plus or minus the standard error of the parameter estimate. Then using some summary measure of the data, the impact of the change in parameter value can be evaluated.

For example, Wu (2000) computed the AUC, AUMC, and MRT for a 1-compartment model and then showed what impact changing the volume of distribution and elimination rate constant by plus or minus their respective standard errors had on these derived parameters. The difference between the actual model outputs and results from the analysis can then be compared directly or expressed as a relative difference. Alternatively, instead of varying the parameters by some fixed percent, a Monte Carlo approach can be used where the model parameters are randomly sampled from some distribution. Obviously this approach is more complex. A more comprehensive approach is to explore the impact of changes in model parameters simultaneously, a much more computationally intensive problem, possibly using Latin hypercube sampling (Iman, Helton, and Campbell, 1981), although this approach is not often seen in pharmacokinetics.

Another type of model stability is influence analysis. It may be that a few observations are having an undue impact on the value of the parameter estimates. Such observations are said to be influential. In linear models much theory has been generated in identifying such observations, but for nonlinear models there is little theory and an empirical approach is taken. Usually, single subjects or groups of subjects are removed one at a time and the model is refit to the reduced data set. The resulting parameter estimates are then compared to the estimates obtained with all the data. A stable model should not show parameter estimates much different than the values obtained with all the data. But here again, what constitutes "much different" is usually based on subjective criteria. Although it is possible to take a quality control approach to the problem it has never been seen done in practice. More will be discussed on influence analysis in later chapters.

It may appear as though an unvalidated model is of limited value, but this is not necessarily true (Hodges, 1991). A model that is not valid shows what the model is not, which in itself can be a useful thing. For example, if a model of clearance against weight is a poor model then weight may not be a useful predictor. Sometimes a rough answer to a question is better than no answer at all. A bad model can also act as an aid to thinking and hypothesizing. In the previous example, if weight was not a predictor, well then what other variables could be? Or why wasn't weight a predictor? Perhaps the sample size was not large enough or the range of weights examined was too narrow? These thoughts may then lead to the next model or a different experiment. Lastly, good modelers become good through experience. Bad models may reveal what to do differently next time or maybe model development forced the modeler to learn some new modeling trick or technique, which is always a good thing.

THE IMPORTANCE OF EFFECTIVE COMMUNICATION

It is not enough for a modeler to build a useful model. The modeler must be able to convey the basis and results of the modeling exercise to others. Communication is defined as the transmittal of information between individuals and the acceptance of a good model can be hindered by poor communication techniques of either the presenter or the recipient. There is nothing that can be done to help the recipient communicate, but at least the modeler can learn something about what it takes to become a "model communicator" (pun intended). If at this point the reader is rolling their eyes and thinking "what does this have to do with modeling?" a good case for effective communication is the loss of the Mars Probe by the National Aeronautics and Space Administration (NASA) in 1999. The Mars Probe was sent to Mars to explore, collect samples, and send data back to Earth in preparation for future, possibly manned, Mars explorations. But before the probe could do this, NASA lost contact with the probe just prior to touch-down on the planet surface and the probe is believed to have crashed. NASA later admitted that "*simple confusion over whether measurements were metric [or English] led to the loss last week of the $125 million spacecraft as it approached Mars.*" So, this simple matter of the wrong units led to the loss of the craft, highlighting the importance of communication between parties. This is also an example of bad model validation.

Transmittal of information between parties is done using either written, verbal, or non-written means with the transmittal of scientific information usually conveyed by either written or verbal means. It is beyond the scope of this section to discuss in detail all the nuances that go into building an effective presentation or writing a scientific paper, but it is important to keep in mind a few points. First, who will be the recipient of the information? If the recipient is another modeler then detail is expected, but if it is a non-modeler then great detail is not expected and outcomes are expected instead. Look at the presentation or paper from the recipient's point of view because a recipient that does not understand what you did will remember little nor will they be swayed to accept your conclusions or be influenced by your ideas. Second, match the content of the material to the objective. You should know before you begin what you want as an outcome. The content should be based on the subject matter, the needs, values, and knowledge of the recipients, and your perceived credibility with the recipient. With published material the last item is not so important since peer review occurs prior to publication, but with verbal presentations, credibility is important.

Models are usually not accepted at face-value immediately by the recipient. Sometimes they are outright rejected as being useful or "the wrong model is chosen." Model acceptance occurs through four stages: awareness ("We have a model that explains how adverse events occur as plasma concentrations increase"), education ("The author understands how the model was developed and what the model does"), trial ("Using the model the FDA has accepted our recommendation that an additional study is not necessary because the change in exposure is such that a change in frequency of adverse events is not expected"), and retention ("We have successfully used models in the past and will use them again in the future as a regulatory strategy"). As the recipient moves through the process, model acceptance is facilitated when future models are presented. Hence, modelers themselves are frequently the least skeptical of models, whereas people with no experience with models may be highly skeptical.

Why models are rejected can be thought of as a pyramid. Models are rejected on one level by the recipient through a lack of understanding. At the next level, no emotional attachment is made to the model. And at the top of the pyramid is mistrust of the modeler, presenter, or the model itself. Overcoming resistance at each level is more difficult than the one below it. With a scientific paper there is no chance for feedback from the reader to the author, so the author has one chance at making an effective presentation of the material to the reader. But with oral presentations, there is a chance for interaction. Scientists often attempt to develop a presentation, write a paper, or answer questions that arise after a presentation from a lack of understanding point of view such that when a model is rejected by the audience we introspect what we could have presented differently to make them accept the model. Frequently some things could have been done better but more often an emotional connection is not made between the model and audience. If the audience wants the model to succeed and has positive feelings about it then model acceptance is facilitated. If the audience has negative emotions attached to a model or there is mistrust between the presenter and the audience then model acceptance will be low.

The features and benefits of the model must be presented whatever the means of communication. If the recipient understands the benefits that can be gained from the model, such as the model provides supporting evidence of efficacy such that a clinical trial is unnecessary or provides a rationale for changing dosage strength, then model acceptance will be facilitated. If the recipient does not understand why the model was done or what benefits the model offers, the model will not be as readily accepted.

If the concepts in this section appear to be fuzzy it is because they are. These are the concepts that are not usually discussed in graduate school. These concepts are not "hard" but "soft"; they are difficult to quantitate. But an understanding of the processes at work behind communicating between individuals is useful if one is to become a good communicator. There are a number of very good texts on presenting scientific data, including Chambers (2001) and D'Arcy (1998). The former deals more with scientific communication in general, whereas the latter deals more with oral presentations. Some of the more important points from the D'Arcy book are presented in Table 1.7. Maurer (2002) presents material on how to overcome resistance in the workplace. The ideas in that book can easily be applied to overcoming model resistance, something that every modeler experiences at some point in their career. The reader is referred to those texts for more details on this fascinating topic.

Good Plotting Practices

Graphs are central to pharmacokinetic and pharmacodynamic analysis. They allow the viewer to take in quantitative information, organize it, and detect patterns or structure that might not be readily noticed by other means. The problem is that there is no one best way to present data. When a graph is made, data are encoded in the figure through the use of symbols, position, size, and color. When a graph is read, the information is decoded by the reader. It is the decoding process that may lead to poor transfer of information because if the reader cannot decode the graph then they cannot decipher the point trying to be made. Everyone has probably experienced where poor choice of symbols on a scatter plot makes discrimination between other symbols difficult. Plotting of data is critical in the communication of scientific results, yet good plotting practices are rarely taught at any level in school. Many are sometimes surprised that there is actual scientific research studying how to best make simple plots to increase the ability of these plots to convey information. Also, there are many very good books on the use of graphics in scientific research. Some of this material will be presented here but the reader is urged to read the source material for a different view of presenting scientific data.

One of the leaders in conveying information through graphics, not necessarily scatter plots, is Edward Tufte, whose book "The Visual Display of Quantitative Information" (2001) was named one of the best 100 books of the 20th century by Amazon.com. One theme stressed throughout this book and by two accompanying volumes is "Above all else show the *data*" because too often the focus is on making pretty graphs. Tufte provides some general guidelines on how to best convey data to a reader and spends a little time with scatter plots (the usual plot seen in pharmacokinetics) in particular.

Good graphs have two main elements: simple in design and complex in data. Good graphs are devoid of decorations and integrate text and visuals to make an accessible display of detail that tells a story about the data. For this reason, many "graphics" packages, such as Microsoft Excel®, should be avoided because they tend to be heavy on design and light on complexity. Table 1.8 lists some other guidelines presented by Tufte on what constitutes good graphical excellence.

In the pharmacokinetic literature, three types of plots are most commonly seen: scatter plots, histograms, and bar charts. Good plotting practices for each of these graph types will be presented. Beyond these plots are others, like QQ plots, dot plots, and three-dimensional surface plots. It is beyond the scope of this chapter to cover every conceivable plot, but many of the good plotting practices that will be put forth should carry over into other plot types as well.

A common plot in pharmacokinetics is the scatter plot, e.g., Fig. 1.5. If x and Y are vectors of two continuous measurements, each observation pair is represented by a plotting symbol, such as a solid circle (●) or open circle (○), in an x-Y coordinate system. Sometimes the observations are categorized by strata, i.e., a third variable, such as treatment, in which case a unique symbol is used for each grouping variable. Vision appears to consist of two different processes. Rapid visual processing is the mechanical analysis of pictures to surfaces,

Table 1.7 Properties of a "model" communicator as presented by D'Arcy (1998).

- They are thoroughly prepared and and they plan their presentations
- They think about what they are doing from the audience's point of view.
- They take responsibility for the audience's ability to understand the topic.
- They personalize what they are doing.
- They illuminate and provide insight rather than dilute the science.
- They are comfortable with themselves, their material, and their situation.

Table 1.8 Guidelines on good graphics as presented by Tufte (2001).

- Using two-dimensional graphs to display one-dimensional data (such as three-dimensional histograms) is inefficient and often results in perceptual ambiguity. The corollary of this is that the number of dimensions in the plot should never exceed the number of dimensions in the data. See Fig. 1.19 for an example.
- Important events or data points of particular interest should be labeled on the graph and not just as some reference in the legend.
- Always use clear, concise, detailed labeling. Avoid computer labels, e.g., WGT for weight, which is a particular problem for the default labels used in graphics generated by S-Plus.
- Maximize the data-ink ratio, i.e., the proportion of a graph's ink that is devoted to the display of non-redundant information. See Fig. 1.19 for a poor example.
- If a grid is needed, do not make the grid color black or the line width the same width as other lines or symbols in the graph. Use a gray color instead to bring the data to the foreground. See Fig. 1.20 for an example.
- Avoid confusing legends. See Fig. 1.21 for an example.
- Plots should have greater length than height, the so-called golden rectangle, since our eye is naturally better at detecting trends on the horizontal than the vertical and it is easier to place labels in a wider graph than a thinner graph.
- Even though the eye is excellent at discriminating among colors, color can create "graphical puzzles" as the mind does not give a natural ordering to colors, except for red to reflect "hot spots" in the data. Using colors to identify data may result in verbal decoders, e.g., "now let's see, blue was the 10 mg/kg dose group and green is the 20 mg/kg dose group." If color must be used then shades of a single color are preferable to many different colors. If color must be used, never use the "Las Vegas" method of color coding where garish, clashing colors are chosen (Cleveland and McGill, 1984b). If the graph is to be published in a black and white format then color should be avoided entirely.

whereas Gestalt perception (in which the pattern of elements comprising the whole of something cannot merely be described as the sum of its parts — the whole is viewed in its entirety) synthesizes these surfaces into meaningful objects. Rapid visual processing is sensitive to brightness, line orientation, line endings[7], curvature, and possibly line crossings and closure (Tremmel, 1995). Effective plots are those that make use of these features.

Lewandowsky and Spence (1989) showed that when subjects were asked to identify groups of data from scatter plots with three strata, where each group was assigned a unique symbol, the most discriminable plots were those that utilized color symbols. Although it was recommended that color be used whenever possible the authors also point out that 8% of males and 1% of females have some form of difficulty distinguishing colors, usually a red-green indiscrimination, and that color may not always be best. In the absence of color, symbols should be as distinguishable as possible. They recommended letter symbols as a viable alternative to color using clearly separable letters (X, Q, and H) compared to poorly separable symbols (E, F, and H). The advantage of letter symbols is that the letters may be easily interpretable, e.g., 'M' for males and 'F' for females, and do not require look-up into a figure legend.

Tremmel (1995) later extended this study focusing on black/white symbol contrasts. The best symbols to use were those that were readily distinguishable.

Observations that had both shape and fill contrasts, such as (○, ■), were more easily discriminated than symbols with only fill contrast (●, ○) which were more readily discriminated than symbols with only shape contrast (○, □). Observations with both shape and fill contrasts make use of their brightness difference and curvature difference, two rapid processing properties. Symbols with fill contrasts make use of only brightness, while symbols with shape contrast make use of only curvature differences. The symbols ○ and ● are poor choices for symbols because, even though one symbol has a darker line than the other, they are difficult to distinguish except on close examination. The more rapid processing properties that are used the more easily the eye can discriminate between groups. Lewandowsky and Spence (1989) recommend that with two groups the symbol set (○, +) or (○, ∗) be used.

However, this recommendation does not take into account that graphs should be reproducible and be legible after reduction. A poor quality copier may not do a good job at reproducing the '+' or '∗' signs. Cleveland (1984b), another leader in the graphical presentation of data and one of the creators of the graphics portion of the language S developed at AT&T, presented many suggestions (shown in Table 1.9) for improving scatter plots, many of which are based on the principles already presented. presents some of those guidelines.

Many of Cleveland's guidelines are common sense, but when has that ever stopped someone from making a graph. Cleveland used extensive scientific research to determine what graph properties lead to efficient transfer of information to the reader.

In one study, Cleveland and McGill (1984a; 1985) described 10 elementary perceptual tasks viewers use to

---

[7] Asterisks∗ and plus signs (+) are examples of line endings or terminators. Asterisks contain eight line endings, whereas + symbols contain four line endings. The larger the number of terminators the greater the distinguish ability between symbols.

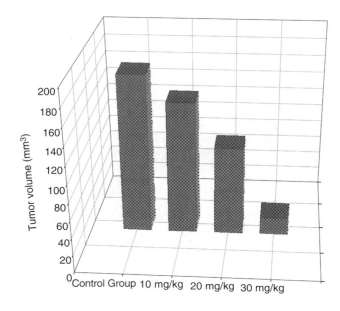

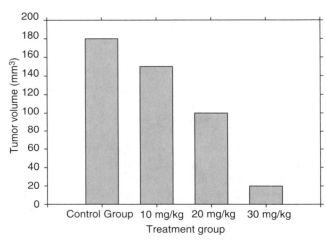

Figure 1.19 Example of a clunky plot (top). This plot uses three-dimensions to present one-dimensional data, makes poor use of color since the sides of the blocks are barely different than the grid, and uses Moire effects (the hatched lines in the blocks), which interact with the eye to produce vibration and movement thereby distracting the viewer from the data. The true difference between treatments is not as visually apparent as the simpler plot shown at the bottom.

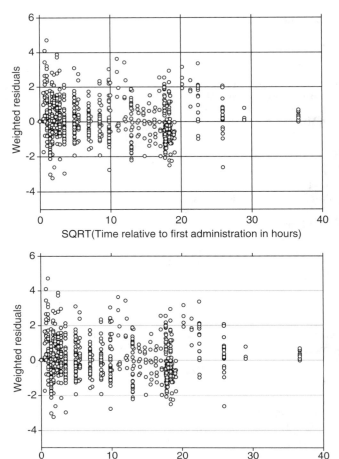

Figure 1.20 Example of how a grid can detract from a plot. The top plot shows an X-Y grid using a standard black line. The bottom plot shows a grid using a dotted line with light gray color. Notice how the grid traps the data in the top plot and actually forces the viewer to look at the grid instead of at the data. While in the bottom plot, the grid reinforces the message of the residual plot—that the residuals are centered around zero and that there are only two data points outside the boundaries ± 4.

extract quantitative information from graphs, which are shown in Fig. 1.22. This led the authors to order these tasks from the most to the least accurate in terms of readers being able to recover information from a graph:

1. Position along a common scale,
2. Position along non-aligned scales,
3. Length > direction > angle,
4. Area
5. Volume and curvature, and lastly,
6. Shading and color saturation.

Graphs should be made using elementary tasks as high in the ordering as possible. Hence, a bar chart is preferred to a pie chart. However, these tasks are not independent—there is much overlap between tasks, e.g., viewing positions along non-aligned scales could be considered making two length judgments. Interestingly, although color is important for discrimination, color was considered the least important property for conveyance of information, possibly because color is not a quantitative but a qualitative property. Humans cannot quantify one color against another.

Everyone has heard Benjamin Disraeli's famous quote, later popularized by Mark Twain, *"There are three kinds of lies: lies, damn lies, and statistics."* It is

Table 1.9 Guidelines on good graphics as presented by Cleveland (1984a).

- Graphs must be lucid, concise, and clearly described. The caption for the graph should explain everything that is on the graph. First describe what the graph is, then point out noticeable features, and then what is the importance of these findings.
- Graphs should be visually clear, capable of withstanding reduction and reproduction. Color tends not to reproduce well on black and white copiers, so avoid color if the text is to be printed in black and white.
- Make the data stand out and use visually distinctive graph elements.
- Avoid superfluous chart elements that detract from the data, such as putting too much writing on a graph. Remember that when everything is emphasized, nothing is emphasized.
- Put important conclusions to an analysis in a graph since some readers do not read the entire text.
- Proofread graphs, especially galley proofs.

very easy to deceive a reader using misleading statistics and graphics. Tufte (2001) writes extensively in his book that graphs often found in the lay press are misleading and poorly constructed. Even in the scientific arena, misleading graphs, created intentionally and unintentionally, are sometimes found (Cleveland, 1984a). The

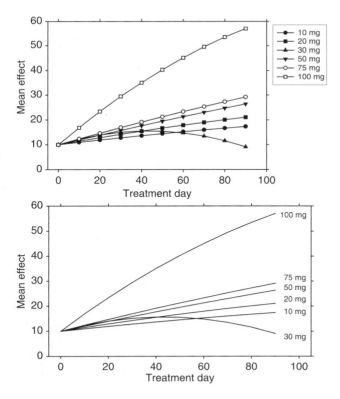

Figure 1.21 Avoid confusing legends. The top plot shows a typical plot in the scientific literature with legend on the side. The bottom plot shows a more efficient plot where the labels are placed to make immediately clear which series belongs to which treatment group. An even clunkier top plot would be the type where instead of actually labeling the treatments, e.g., 10 mg/kg, the label was 'Treatment A' and then in the legend Treatment A is defined as 10 mg/kg.

best way to spot a misleading plot or to avoid making one is through example. Figure 1.23 shows two graphs, one poorly created and intentionally designed to be misleading. At first glance in the top plot, the concordance between observed and predicted concentrations is high. But closer examination (bottom plot) shows that the range of the axes is slightly smaller than the other. When the axes are made the same range and a line of unity is added, the systematic underprediction of the model becomes more evident.

In Fig. 1.24 a scatter plot is shown with two different data rectangles. When the data rectangle is much smaller than the axes rectangle the apparent correlation between the variables is increased (Cleveland, Diaconis, and McGill, 1982). Darrell Huff (1954) in his best-selling book "How to Lie with Statistics" states that one way to mislead a reader is not to include zero on the ordinate. However, when large numbers are to be plotted this is clearly impractical. Figure 1.25 illustrates why Huff's suggestion should not be taken at dogma. There are many other examples of misleading data. An excellent review of how to show data badly is presented by Wainer (1984) and the reader is referred there for other amusing examples.

If X is a univariate random variable grouped by strata the bar chart summarizes some function of the data by groups using a series of bars, one for each group. Figure 1.26 shows for example, average clearance classified by race. The error bars show the standard deviation of the data. When making bar charts, avoid Moire effects (Fig. 1.19) which tend to make the bars wavy and visually disconcerting. Also avoid using three-dimensional bar charts (Fig. 1.19). Although three-dimensional bar charts may look pretty, they decrease the data to ink ratio[8] and lend nothing to ability to perceive differences between groups. Lastly, always clearly identify what the bars represent and what the error bars represent, if they are present.

Bar charts are limiting in the amount of data they present, usually only showing a measure of central tendency and some measure of variability. They are also misleading if the data are not normally distributed. A mean is often not a good measure of central tendency if the data are skewed, such as if the data were lognormal in distribution, and the error bars tend to be quite large (see Fig. 1.26). A better graph is the box and whisker plot (Tukey, 1977). In Fig. 1.26 the accompanying box and whisker plot is shown. The box represents the interquartile range (the 25th and 75th percentiles of the data). The line inside the box is usually

---

[8] The data to ink ratio is the ratio of the ink used to show data to the ink used to print the graphic.

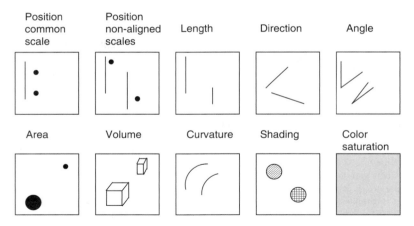

Figure 1.22 Elementary perceptual tasks identified by Cleveland and McGill (1984a). Reprinted with permission from The Journal of the American Statistical Association. Copyright 1984 by the American Statistical Association. All rights reserved.

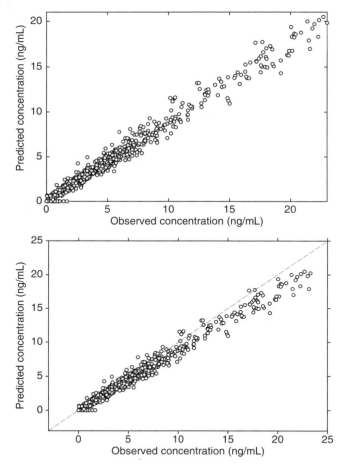

the mean, but could also be the median. The whiskers are the 5th and 95th percentiles. Observations outside the 5th and 95th percentiles are denoted by symbols, solid circles in this case. Box and whisker plots provide much more information than a bar chart and can also help in identifying possible outliers.

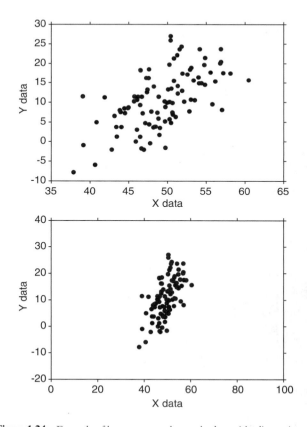

Figure 1.23 Example of poor and misleading graph construction. In the top plot the data rectangle is same in size as the axis length leading to symbols being plotted on top of axis lines. The tick marks pointing inwards further obscure the data. Lastly, the scale on the ordinate is smaller than the abscissa making the goodness of fit appear better than it truly is. In the bottom plot, the data rectangle is slightly smaller than the axis lengths and the tick marks point out, thus unobscuring the data. The axes are set to the same scale and a dashed line of unity is added. The systematic deviation of the predicted concentrations to observed concentrations as observed concentration increases is more clearly evident in the bottom plot.

Figure 1.24 Example of how a scatter plot can lead to misleading estimates of the correlation between two variables. When the data rectangle is small compared to the axes rectangle (bottom plot) the correlation appears larger than it really is. The same data are plotted in both plots and the correlation between variables is 0.5.

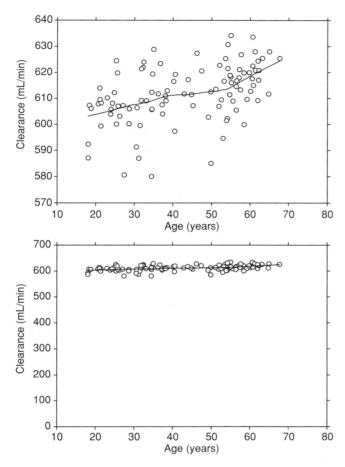

Figure 1.25 Do not always include zero in the axes. Use your best judgment. A best selling book on how statistics are used to "lie" states that zero should always be included in a plot showing magnitude (Huff, 1954). This should not be accepted as dogma. Here are two plots where zero is not included (top plot) and zero is included (bottom plot). The relationship between age and clearance is obscured when zero is included in the plot.

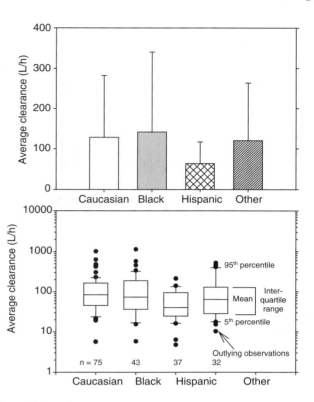

Figure 1.26 Example of a bar chart and box and whisker plot. The top plot is a bar chart showing average clearance for a drug classified by race. The error bars denote the standard deviation. Because pharmacokinetic parameters tend to be log-normal in distribution, the standard deviations tend to be large. The bars for the Hispanic and other groups show Moire effects. Tufte would argue that the only useful bar is the bar for Caucasians. The gray bar for Blacks decreases the data to ink ratio and is superfluous. The bottom plot shows the same data as a box plot on a log-scale. The important features of a box plot are noted. On the transformed scale the data appear normally distributed. Although the variability across groups appears the same, Hispanic subjects appear to have lower average clearance than the other groups. A useful modification is to print the sample size on the plot.

Related to the bar chart is the histogram, first reported by the famous statistician Karl Pearson (Stigler, 1986), which is used to plot continuous univariate data. If X is a continuous random variable the histogram breaks the data into series of ordered, adjacent, exhaustive intervals along the data range (called a bin) and plots the number of observations in the bin as a function of the midpoint of the bin using a bar chart. For example, if the range of data were 0 to 100 the bins might be 0 to 10, 10 to 20, 20 to 30, ..., 90 to 100. Often the distribution of residuals or weighted residuals are examined using histograms as a quick check for normality. Another use is to plot the distribution of some pharmacokinetic parameter and check for bimodality.

The histogram is notoriously insensitive, however, at detecting the thing it was designed to do—character-

ize the probability density function of the random sample. Too many bins may follow the distribution of the data but are influenced by random fluctuations in the data. Too few bins may lead to a distribution that does not approximate the true underlying distribution of the data. To illustrate this concept, 100 observations were drawn from a mixture of two normal distributions. 90 observations were drawn from a normal distribution having a mean of 18 and a standard deviation of 5, whereas the remaining 10 observations were drawn from a normal distribution having a mean of 35 and a standard deviation of 5. Figure 1.27 shows the resulting histogram when the number of bins is varied from 5 to 20. The bimodality of the distribution is not seen when the number of bins is small, whereas the distribution appears to consist of at least two normal distributions when the number of bins is too large.

In between these extremes, the bimodality of the data and approximate normality of each component appears to be captured.

So how does one choose a number of bins or bin width? Sturges (1926) first proposed the following rule of thumb for the number of bins (k) in a histogram

$$k = 1 + Ln(n) \qquad (1.94)$$

where n is the sample size, having a corresponding bin width of

$$h = \frac{\text{range of data}}{1 + Ln(n)}. \qquad (1.95)$$

Notice that by choosing the number of bins the bin width is chosen, and vice-versa. One can either choose the bin width and obtain the number of bins or choose the number of bins and obtain the bin width. Scott (1992) has shown that this choice of bin width leads to an oversmoothed histogram, especially when the sample size is large (~200 or more). Nevertheless, many software packages use this rule of thumb or modifications of it for their default bin width. Scott (1979) proposed using

$$h = \frac{3.49s}{\sqrt[3]{n}}, \qquad (1.96)$$

as the bin width, where s is the estimated standard deviation. Scott (1992) also proposed $\sqrt[3]{2n}$ for a lower bound on the number of bins and

$$\frac{(\text{range of data})\sqrt[3]{n}}{2.61(\text{Interquartile range})} \qquad (1.97)$$

as an upper bound on the number of bins. Wand (1997) expands on Scott's rule using kernel functions and although the new methods appear to be better at characterizing the underlying distribution of the data, many would not be able to implement such methodology easily. Freedman and Diaconis (2003) proposed

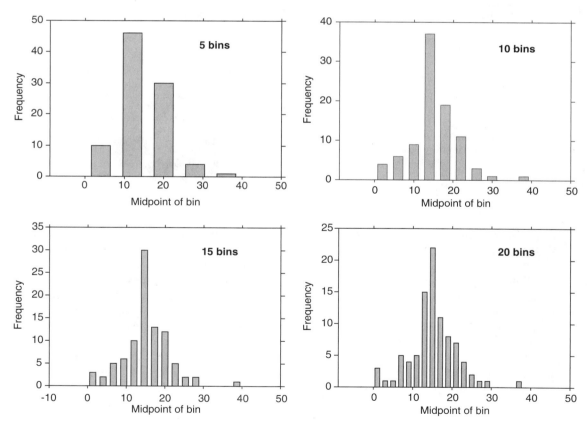

Figure 1.27 Example of how a histogram can miss the underlying distribution of the data if the number of bins is not chosen properly. A total of 90 observations were drawn from a normal distribution with mean 18 and standard deviation 5, while 10 observations were drawn from a normal distribution with mean 35 and standard deviation 5. The resulting histogram is plotted using 5 (upper left), 10 (upper right), 15 (bottom left), and 20 bins (bottom left). Using 5 bins would lead one to conclude the distribution consists of a single normal distribution, whereas with 20 bins one might conclude there were three underlying normal distributions.

$$h = \frac{2(\text{Interquartile range})}{\sqrt[3]{n}} \qquad (1.98)$$

as the bin width. Freedman and Diaconis' rule, which uses the interquartile range, instead of the standard deviation, is more robust to outliers and tends to choose smaller bins than Scott's rule. All the rules of thumb so far have some basis in assuming a normal distribution. For non-normal distributions more bins are needed. Doane (1976) proposed using

$$k = 1 + \text{Ln}(n) + \text{Ln}\left(1 + \gamma\sqrt{\frac{n}{6}}\right) \qquad (1.99)$$

in such cases, where γ is the estimated kurtosis of the distribution (Venables and Ripley, 1997).

For the example in Fig. 1.27 the standard deviation was 7.6, the kurtosis was 1.44, with an interquartile range of 7.0 and a range of 41.7. Under Sturges', Scott's, Freedman and Diaconis', and Doane's rule the number of bins should be 6, 7, 14, and 8, respectively. Scott's lower and upper bound on the number of bins are 6 and 11, respectively. Like others have shown, Sturges' and Scott's rule seem too conservative and do not detect the bimodality of the distribution. Freedman and Diaconis' rule seems a little too liberal. Doane's rule seems to be the better choice here. It should be clear to the reader by now that a histogram is not entirely telling in regards to the distribution of data because of the arbitrary nature of the number of bins. Whatever the graph, the variability in the data should always be shown, either as a range of observations, the standard deviation, or the standard error. This reminds the reader that all data have uncertainty and allows the reader to make their own conclusions regarding statistical tests or relationships between variables given the natural variability in the data. Hence, if an error bar is presented on a graph the caption should clearly state what that error bar represents. One way to misdirect the reader is to use standard error of the mean instead of the standard deviation, thus making the precision around some data point appear better than it is. Although some have argued that even a standard deviation bar is misleading because a point estimate showing plus or minus one standard deviation bar only shows 68% of the variability. Two standard deviations would be more representative of what the true distribution around that point estimate looks like.

To end, a graph is more than just a picture, and like the cliché says, it tells a story. Scientists need to learn how to make informative graphics that maximize the data to ink ratio without having a lot of clutter. It is only when graphs are made with the reader in mind that effective transfer of information to the reader will be made and, in so doing, make our point with force.

Writing a Modeling Report

The writing of a modeling report is extremely critical because it represents to a reviewer the process of model development and allows a reviewer to critique and adequately evaluate a reported model. Good documentation is the basis for model credibility. A model that is poorly documented will have poor credibility. As McLeod (1982) states, adequate and timely documentation is needed to:

- Ensure to all stakeholders the validity of the model under which it was designed,
- Ensure that the model and any simulation studies were properly designed and run,
- Indicate the manner in which the model should be used,
- Record the results of all analyses,
- Guard against the cumulative distortion of the information chain that exists between the modeler and end user,
- Call attention to any dead-ends and procedures that did not work so that others may learn from your mistakes,
- Permit peer evaluation,
- Facilitate model transfer, and
- Control against personnel turnover.

As most know, documentation is often done as an after thought once the modeling process is completed. This is unfortunate because by then the analyst must go back and review what was done and the exact reason why one path was chosen over another may not be clear at the time of writing. Good documentation should begin at the beginning and continue until the project is complete.

Two journals that have done an exemplary job with providing guidelines for model presentation in manuscripts are the *American Journal of Physiology (AJP)* and the *Annals of Biomedical Engineering (ABE)*, both of which use the same set of instructions. The FDA in their guidance on Exposure-Response Relationships (2003) also provides some guidelines on the reporting of pharmacokinetic-pharmacodynamic models. Surprisingly silent in this area are journals that actually publish pharmacokinetic modeling papers: Pharmaceutical Research, the Journal of Pharmaceutical Sciences, and the Journal of Pharmacokinetics and Pharmacodynamics.

Both AJP and ABE suggest that any mathematical details be written for the non-mathematician. All models should include a discussion of the model development strategy, the assumptions, and a summary of the meaning of the model (in this case a generic term for any model or equation) and its limitations. All parameter estimates should be presented with the precision of their estimates. How such parameter values were obtained, e.g., software, algorithms, should be indicated. Lengthy mathematical derivations can be saved for an appendix. Then there are common sense things that may not be so obvious, like be careful to distinguish between the number '1' and the letter 'l,' the number '0' and the letter 'o,' and the letter 'x' and the multiplication symbol '×.' Use variables that are simple, like y, and use subscripts whenever feasible and appropriate because they often simplify equations, e.g., ka could be denoted k_a. However, some people prefer not to use subscripts because the subscripted characters are hard to read and accurately reproduce when placed in a table with small font sizes. Use circles to denote compartments and arrows to denote flow from compartments. The journals also suggest denoting transfer from compartment i to compartment j as k_{ji}, unlike traditional pharmacokinetic texts where transfer from compartment i to compartment j as K_{ij} or k_{ij}. Be careful of this difference as it occurs in many other areas, as well.

Yates (1999), an editor of the American Journal of Physiology, also suggests that modeling papers contain the following characteristics:

- The model is shown with all equations, preferably expressed in mathematical notation conventional for the field.
- All variables are defined with defined units (dimensions) that are consistently maintained.
- All equations are dimensionally consistent.
- The justification for any initial assumptions or starting values are provided.

Yates also notes that most modeling papers present obscure models in that they fail to show how the model was developed or validated. In other words, the model is poorly documented. From a regulatory point of view, if something is not documented it never occurred. Someone once said that documentation is like chocolate: when it is good, it is very good, but when it is bad, its better than nothing. Good advice. A good modeling report should adequately document all models tested and the reason for their rejection so that a reviewer can follow the train of thought and if need be reproduce the entire modeling exercise.

Table 1.10 presents a sample table of contents for a modeling report used in support of a pharmacokinetic-pharmacodynamic analysis. The order of the report follows that of a scientific paper: introduction, methods, results, and discussion. Within each section, the relevant aspects related to the model are presented. For example, within the discussion section, how plausible the model is,

Table 1.10 Sample table of contents for a pharmacokinetic-pharmacodynamic modeling report.

1. Synopsis
2. Table of contents
3. Symbols and units defined
4. Abbreviations defined
5. Glossary
6. Introduction
   a. Introduction to the drug
   b. Review of previous published models
   c. Clear definition of problem
   d. Modeling objectives
7. Methods
   a. Experimental design
      i. Overall study design
      ii. Sampling scheme
      iii. Study populations
      iv. Procedures
      v. Bioanalytical methods
      vi. Pharmacodynamic measurement methods
      vii. Nature of data (response variables and all covariate information)
   b. Data preparation methods
      i. Data preparation methods
      ii. Data quality assurance
      iii. Handling of outliers and missing data
   c. Model development
      i. General overview
      ii. Initial parameter estimates
      iii. Assumptions
      iv. Physiological relevance
      v. Model limitations
      vi. Software used
   d. Model validation plan
8. Results
   a. Data accounting
      i. Subject accounting
      ii. Data manipulations (removal of outliers, etc.)
   b. Subject demographics
   c. Model description
      i. Final parameter values and precision
      ii. Goodness of fit plots
      iii. Model diagram and equations
   d. Model validation
      i. Model results vs. data
      ii. Sensitivity analysis
      iii. Cross-validation results
9. Discussion
10. Appendix
    a. Copy of protocol and amendments
    b. Bioanalytical reports
    c. Data validation documentation
    d. Imputed data
    e. Outliers deleted prior to analysis
    f. Raw data listing used for modeling
    g. Analysis code

References: Wastney, Wang, and Boston (1998), *American Journal of Physiology*, *Instructions to Authors* (http://www.the-aps.org/publications/journals/pub_-quick.htm), the *Annals of Biomedical Engineering* (http://www.ruf.rice. edu/~abme/instruct.html), and the Food and Drug Administration (United States Department of Health and Human Services et al., 2003).

how the model relates to other published models, how the model predicts the observed data, the strength and limitations of the model, and how realistic the model assumptions are may be discussed. While not meant as written in stone, this table is meant as an illustration.

ETHICS IN MODELING

The list of abuses in the name of medical science is long: the horrors of experimentation on Jewish prisoners during the Holocaust and the Tuskegee syphilis experiment to name just two. Within the pharmaceutical industry, abuses of this magnitude have not occurred but other abuses have. For example, in 1989 the House Committee on Oversight and Investigation, in cooperation with the U.S. Attorney General's Office, reported that some generic drug companies falsified data in support of Abbreviated New Drug Applications (ANDAs). Also reported was that some employees of the FDA's Office of Generic Drugs accepted bribes to expedite review of some generic drug companies ANDAs. In the most egregious example of wrong-doing, Bolar Pharmaceuticals submitted to the FDA as its own drug product, triameterene hydrochlorthiazide (the most profitable generic drug in the U.S. at the time), a sample that was actually the innovator's product (Ascione et al., 2001). The impact of these wrong-doings, and the resulting regulatory overhaul, is still being felt today.

The author personally ignored most of these abuses until he was involved with his own ethical "situation." Like many scientists, he never took a course in ethics in college. He thought that as scientists they were above all that ambiguity. He became more interested in ethics when he was hired as a consultant to develop a pharmacokinetic-pharmacodynamic model for a new drug. The sponsor was concerned that their drug prolonged QTc intervals on an electrocardiogram. Prolonged QTc intervals are believed to be a surrogate marker for Torsades de Pointes, an electrical abnormality in the heart, that may lead to sudden death. Many drugs have been removed from the market because of prolonged QTc intervals, including Seldane® and Cisapride®, and it would not be in the sponsor's best interest to develop a drug that prolonged QTc intervals.

The model did indeed confirm a positive linear relationship between drug concentrations and QTc intervals in patients with the disease being treated. However, upon receiving the report, the sponsor of the study was unhappy with the results. They were either hoping that the magnitude of effect would be less than observed or that no model could be developed, suggesting the drug

had no effect on QTc intervals. At this point, the sponsor rejected the final report and the analysis was scuttled. With no report there was no record of the analysis in the sponsor's subsequent New Drug Application. Later, at the FDA's advisory meeting on their drug, the sponsor presented numerous graphs trying to explain away the QTc interval effect of their drug and, to their credit, the advisory members rejected the analysis asking the sponsor to go back and do a more formal pharmacokinetic-pharmacodynamic analysis of the data, thus delaying approval of their drug.

Was it ethical for the sponsor to reject the report? The sponsor did make payment on the report, even though they rejected it. What was my ethical obligation? Before an attempt to answer these questions can be made, two questions must be answered. First, "What is ethics?" Merriam-Webster's online dictionary defines ethics as 1) a set, system, or theory of moral principles or values, 2) the principles of conduct governing an individual or group, and 3) a guiding philosophy. Thus, modelers are governed by the general set of conduct that relates to society as a whole and also to the groups in which the modeler associates.

The second question is how does ethics differ from values or morals? Morals refers to a person being able to choose between good and bad or right and wrong, something that in many simple cases is a matter of habit, and tends to have religious connotations (Seebauer and Barry, 2001). Ethics, which is a personal responsibility, is more of an attempt to follow societal or professional norms, about how people should act, based on ideal human character and morals. In contrast, values are personal judgments that determine how a person behaves and may have nothing to do with ethics. The importance of getting a higher education is a value that has nothing to do with ethics. Ethical values form principles that guide our behavior. Ethics puts ethical principles into actions. For example, honesty is a value and not stealing is a principle based on this value. Not publishing someone else's research is an ethical guideline based on the principle of not stealing.

Simply put, ethics is about doing the right thing. But what is the right thing? Obviously it is beyond the scope of this book to delve into all the issues regarding research ethics nor can the answers to many ethical problems be answered in a simple dichotomous response, yes/no or good/bad. However, in presenting this material it is hoped that the modeler will become sensitized to the ethical side of their profession and point the reader to further reading and introspection.

The first definition of ethics relates to conforming to universal norms, which are accepted behaviors that apply to all people. For example, the modeler should not knowingly make false statements in publications or reports since it is generally recognized that one should not lie. Another example would be the modeler who is employed on a contract basis and then steals the client's money giving nothing in return. In this case, universal norms dictate this as unethical behavior since it is wrong to steal. More subtly would be the modeler that knowingly does not do work they know to be of value because they have too much other work, possibly from other clients, and do not have the time. Some might consider this case to also be stealing from the client. Universal norms usually do not cause moral ambiguity (war and religious conflict being two current exceptions) and as such will not be discussed further.

The second definition of ethics relates to conduct—modelers should conform to professional standards of conduct. Obviously one code of conduct to which modelers should conform to are the norms related to responsibilities becoming a scientist. All scientists have a duty to ensure their work serves desirable ends (Shrader-Frechette, 1994). Hence, as a scientist one must strive to not harm the public, research subjects, democratic institutions, and the environment. To those ends, the foremost ethical goal in science is to not deceive, inveigle, or obfuscate the results of our research nor should others be allowed to do so. In other words, scientists must not commit fraud and neither should others be allowed to use our research to commit fraud.

Unfortunately, cases of scientific fraud, both intentional and unintentional, abound in the news, with perhaps the most famous being the controversy surrounding David Baltimore and Thereza Imanishi-Kari in the late 1980s. At issue was the whistle-blowing by Margot O'Toole, a post-doctoral fellow in Imanishi-Kari's laboratory who lost her job after raising questions about falsified data in a paper written by Imanishi-Kari and others, among them David Baltimore, former president of Rockefeller University and Nobel Laureate. After many internal reviews and staunch defense by Baltimore, both the Massachusetts Institute of Technology and the National Institutes of Health concluded Imanishi-Kari committed no wrong-doing. But O'Toole persisted and a congressional inquiry eventually occurred. The Secret Service concluded using forensic analysis that entire sets of data were forged between 1986 and 1989 and in 1991, two years later, Baltimore formally requested the paper in question to be retracted. In 1994, the Office of Research Integrity (ORI) issued 19 counts of scientific misconduct against Imanishi-Kari. By 1994, when Imanishi-Kari filed an appeal with the ORI, no fewer than five inquiries into the matter were made. In 1996, an appeals panel issued 6500 pages of transcripts into the matter and, despite finding the paper

to be *"rife with errors of all sorts,"* cleared Imanishi-Kari of all allegations of wrong-doing (Goodman, 1996). While not all cases of fraud will be of this magnitude, this case illustrates what could happen and should serve as an example to all scientists.

The second ethical goal in science is to strive to not let bias, both in our methods and interpretations, from entering our research. Some bias is blatant, but other types of bias are less so. For example, bias against a particular ethnic group is blatant. But at what point does outlier removal from a data set lead to data fudging? The line is not exactly clear. Bias does not necessarily have to be directed at a group of individuals, but can be a leaning towards using a particular methodology over another because we are more familiar with the former; the old adage "I have a hammer, everything is a nail." Both societal and personal bias' can also change over time. It wasn't that long ago that women of child-bearing age were excluded from Phase 1 clinical trials because of the feared impact should pregnancy occur and the misperceived impact that hormonal fluctuations may have on pharmacokinetic assessments.

Modelers that use data from clinical studies should also be careful to respect informed consent and the privacy of the patient information they have access to. With the Health Insurance Portability and Accounting Act of 2003, which was designed to ensure privacy of patient information, inappropriate disclosure of patient information can now lead to criminal charges and fines. Modelers who are also pharmacokineticists directly involved in clinical studies have an obligation to use minimally invasive sampling methods, e.g., saliva vs. plasma, with a minimum number of samples collected from each subject. If blood must be collected then a minimum amount of blood should be removed to protect the safety of the subjects (Svensson, 1989).

Other general responsibilities scientists have are appropriate giving and taking of credit for research work. In 1993, the University of Michigan was ordered to pay 1.2 million dollars to a researcher whose supervisor stole credit for her research after which the university failed to properly investigate the charges. The International Committee of Medical Journal Editors state that authorship on a manuscript requires *"(1) substantial contributions to conception and design, or acquisition of data, or analysis and interpretation of data; and (2) drafting the article or revising it critically for important intellectual content; and (3) final approval of the version to be published. Conditions 1, 2, and 3 must all be met."* A less obvious form of failing to give appropriate credit is with inadequate citation reference, i.e., failing to reference someone else's work.

One special item of note is conflict of interest. A conflict of interest arises when a certain circumstance compromises professional judgments. Pharmaceutical scientists employed in industry have an interesting conflict of interest between duty to the public and duty to the company. Hence, scientists in the pharmaceutical industry are constantly faced with conflicts of interest, though few would recognize them as such or admit them. Most scientists, which include modelers, want to present their experimental results objectively. But in the pharmaceutical industry there is constant pressure to present those results as positively as possible for fear that the "truth" will harm the drug's approval by regulatory authorities. This may be a legitimate concern. Modelers must then balance the needs of the employer against the needs of the physician and consumer since ultimately they are the ones who derive benefit from the model. More and more the results from a modeling exercise are included on the product label for a new drug, which are then used by physicians to make dosing recommendations. A model that is selectively developed, presented in a skewed manner to regulatory agencies, or misrepresented to the consumer (possibly by comparing one drug to another) may result in drug induced illness or death.

Pharmaceutical scientists employed as consultants are in an even more awkward position: duty to the public against duty to the hiring company against duty to one's self. The sponsor may put undue pressure on the consultant to interpret a result more positively or downplay negative aspects on some analysis. A particularly negative interpretation of some research finding and failure to make company suggested alterations to a report may lead to not being hired again by the drug company. Because of conflicts of interest, the integrity of data is always suspect. The only antidote for conflict of interest is full disclosure, thereby allowing the reviewer to judge for themselves whether the conflict is too severe. For this reason, many leading scientific journals now require financial disclosure related to a submitted manuscript and listing of any potential conflicts of interest.

Conflicts of interest present dilemmas as to who does the modeler ultimately owe the duty? Is it the company the modeler works for, the project team within the company who asked the modeler to perform the works, or, in the case of a contract research organization (CRO), the company that hires the modeler to do the work? Is it the regulatory agencies that review the model during the approval process? Is it the physician who prescribes the drug once the drug is approved for marketing? Or is it the consumer of the drug after filling the physician's prescription at the pharmacy? The answer lies with the objective of the modeling exercise. If the model is to be used internally for decision making, the client is the company in general and the project team in particular because it is the project team that is usually responsible for decisions regarding the development of the drug. If, however, the objective is to answer a regulatory issue or is directly related to the patient, the client is the physician. Some may argue, however, that the client is ultimately the consumer. But, since the consumer does not have the final say regarding which drug will be prescribed to them or the dose to be administered, I would argue the ultimate duty is owed to the physician. Data should be analyzed and interpreted to allow a physician to make an objective, unbiased decision regarding the best pharmacotherapy for a particular patient.

Not only should a modeler conform to the norms expected of a scientist in general, a modeler should also conform to the norms of other modelers in particular. However, there are no printed norms for modelers. The American Association of Pharmaceutical Scientists, the largest professional organization to which most pharmacokinetic modelers are members of, has a code of ethics, which is presented in Table 1.11. This code is very general and can be directed towards any typical scientist. Other professions have codes of conduct that may be relevant to modelers, one being the Ethical Guidelines for Statistical Practice developed by the American Statistical Association. Their guidelines are broken down into eight general topics: professionalism (the need for competence, judgment, and credibility), responsibilities to funders, clients, and employers, responsibilities in publications and testimony, responsibility to research subjects, responsibilities to research team colleagues, responsibilities to other statisticians and practitioners, responsibilities regarding allegations of misconduct, and responsibilities of employers employing statistical practitioners. Although there are some specifics in the guidelines related directly to statistical practice, in many aspects the remaining guidelines can be directly related to modeling.

A key component to setting any type of ethical guidelines for modelers must include the responsibilities owed the client and responsibilities owed the employer. Bayles (1989) presents various paradigms for the relationship between clients and modeler based on who has the power to make decisions. Responsibility then lies with the individual making the decisions and depends on the interaction between client and modeler. In one case, the client relinquishes control and input over the model, depending entirely on the modeler to make decisions. A second situation is where the modeler is expected to develop and present the model, but the client, such as a project team or perhaps small biotechnology company who has contracted an analysis to a consultant, has no modeling experience or basis to contribute to development of the model. Both situations can

Table 1.11 Code of ethics from The American Association of Pharmaceutical Scientists (AAPS).

AAPS member scientists recognize their special obligations to society and the public welfare. They utilize their integrity to advance the health and welfare of mankind. In their scientific pursuits they:

- Conduct their work in a manner that adheres to the highest principles of scientific research so as to merit the confidence and trust of peers and the public in particular regarding the rights of human subjects and concern for the proper use of animals involved and provision for suitable safeguards against environmental damage.
- Avoid scientific misconduct and expose it when encountered. AAPS uses the current federal definition of misconduct, 65 FR 76260–76264: Fabrication, falsification, and plagiarism in proposing, performing, or reviewing research or reporting research results.
- Recognize latitude for differences of scientific opinion in the interpretation of scientific data and that such differences of opinion do not constitute unethical conduct.
- Disclosure of sources of external financial support for, or significant financial interests in the context of, research reports/publications and avoid manipulation of the release of such information for illegal financial gain.
- Report results accurately, stating explicitly any known or suspected bias, opposing efforts to improperly modify data or conclusions and offering professional advice only on those subjects concerning which they regard themselves competent through scientific education, training, and research.
- Respect the known ownership rights of others in scientific research and seek prior authorization from the owner before disclosure or use of such information including comments of manuscripts submitted for pre-publication review.
- Support in their research and among their employers the participation and employment of all qualified persons regardless of race, gender, creed, or national origin.

Reprinted with permission from the American Association of Pharmaceutical Scientists (2002).

be viewed as paternalistic—the modeler acts in the best interests of the client. Ethical dilemmas arise when the client's interests and the modeler's best interest disagree.

At the other extreme is the agency model where the modeler acts as a hired gun carrying out the explicit wishes of the client. Model development, reporting, and interpretation are overseen and approved by the client at every step. Such a case may arise where the modeler is employed by a CRO and the client is employed by a pharmaceutical company. Under this paradigm, responsibility directly lies with the client, although they may fail to acknowledge this fact when things go awry. A number of ethical dilemmas may arise under this model. One situation may be that the client is not qualified to render decisions on model development although they may believe otherwise. The client may then lead the modeler down paths that, in the modelers opinion, should not be taken or may tell the modeler to perform tasks that are questionable, such as removing important covariates from a model because inclusion of the covariate has negative marketing implications. Another example might be when the client wishes to interpret a negative finding in a particularly positive light and the modeler, who recognizes the duplicitous nature of the interpretation, disagrees.

In between these two extremes is the fiduciary paradigm, where both parties are responsible but additional obligations are made because of the special knowledge of the modeler. Under this paradigm the client has more decision making authority than under the paternalistic paradigm and requires the client's consent and judgment as the modeler and client together participate in model development and interpreting the model's results. Clients then depend on the modeler to provide them with the information necessary to make an informed decision when problems arise. Hence, an implicit trust exists between client and modeler that the modeler will adequately convey the problem, perhaps present possible solutions, and then work honestly and loyally with the client in rendering a decision. Ethical dilemmas arise when the client is truly not competent to render an opinion and decisions are made contrary to what the modeler believes to be correct.

Of the two cases, paternalistic or fiduciary, the latter is the preferred relationship for modelers because responsibility is shared. Central to a fiduciary relationship is trust—the trust to fulfill what the client has asked the modeler to do in a timely manner with the client's best interests in mind. Only when the modeler has the client's trust can a fiduciary paradigm be achieved.

Bayles (1989) proposed seven obligations of modelers to clients: honesty, candor, competency, diligence, loyalty, fairness, and discretion. Each of these qualities will be briefly discussed. Honesty and candor go hand in hand. Modelers should be truthful with their clients, but candor goes beyond truthfulness requiring modelers to make full disclosure. Clients want a modeler to develop models. When equally plausible models exist, it is the modelers responsibility to present these alternatives to the client along with how these alternatives vary in cost, scope, and time to implementation. The modeler also has a responsibility to explain not only the strengths of a model, but also its inadequacies, in an objective manner without advocacy. Modelers must provide adequate documentation of the model assumptions and the development process in such a way that the model can be reproduced (Wallace, 1994).

Almost all ethical codes require that modelers take on only work they are competent to do and to remain current on new techniques and methodologies. Modelers should not present themselves to clients or employers as being able to do something they cannot do. But clearly not all modelers are at equal skill, so how is a modeler to learn something if they cannot do something new? The answer goes back to honesty and candor. If a modeler cannot do something, such as a Bayesian population pharmacokinetic model, this should be disclosed to the client and the client should be allowed the decision of allowing the modeler to do the work. More often than not, the client is understanding and willing to be a guinea pig, so to speak, for the modeler, perhaps at a substantial break in cost.

A modeler can be very competent but if the modeler is not diligent then an inadequate model or report can be developed. Conversely a modeler could be quite diligent but be incompetent. Diligence requires careful time management so that quality reports are presented to the client in a timely manner. Diligence is probably the biggest problem modelers face as they are often placed under tight timelines, with minimal financial support, and are faced with having to do other functions, perhaps for other clients, as well.

Loyalty goes directly to trust and is primarily affected by conflicts of interest. "Selling out" a client is definitely not in the client's best interest. Within the context of a modeler working for a CRO, giving one particular client priority over another client, perhaps because the latter client does not bring in as much revenue as the former client, is also a violation of the client's trust. If the client is the physician, misrepresentation of a model to regulatory agencies is a violation of that trust. Bayles (1989) believes that loyalty requires disclosing any conflicts of interest between two competing parties. This may be problematic in the context of a modeler employed by a CRO where there are two competing clients because this may require disclosure that both companies are clients of the CRO. For a modeler employed directly by a pharmaceutical company where two competing projects require attention, this may require going to management and identifying priorities. But in the case where the two clients are the pharmaceutical company and physician, disclosing conflicts of interest cannot occur.

Fairness requires that the modeler treat each client equally, not only in regards to loyalty and diligence, but also with the same degree of objectivity. In the case of a modeler employed by the pharmaceutical industry, the modeler should show neither bias towards the company nor the physician. Models should be developed and presented objectively. If the modeler is employed by a CRO, the modeler should not show favor to particular clients. All clients should receive services of equal quality.

Lastly, modelers should show discretion when discussing the results of their models. Confidentiality, which usually applies to specific facts, is included in discretion, but discretion is more broad. The results of a model can have a significant financial impact on a company or on the future of a new chemical entity within a pharmaceutical company. There is also a more pragmatic reason for discretion. A modeler showing a lack of discretion is often viewed negatively by the companies and persons around them.

Modelers also have an obligation to the consumers who may ultimately be prescribed the medication. Pharmacokinetic information may be presented at consumer group meetings, on the product label, or in direct-to-consumer advertising. As such, consumers have a right to know that particular dosing information may have been based on a model and what the results of the model were. Not all information need be shared with the public and one should also remember that failure to disclose important information is just as misleading as presenting false information. Another fundamental value to the consumer is protection from injury, which is more of a universal norm. Related to this is fairness. Modelers should be fair and not discriminate against specific classes on the basis of sex, race, etc. The modeler should not develop models that may lead to injury or discriminate.

Scientists in drug development have responsibilities to clients, be they project teams or hiring companies, and to physicians and consumers. Notice that regulatory authorities are not mentioned as a class pharmaceutical scientists have a responsibility to. That is because regulatory authorities are agents for the physicians and consumers—fulfilling one's obligation to physicians and consumer automatically fulfills the responsibility to the regulatory agency. Because of the joint obligation to clients, physicians, and consumers there is a delicate balance between what the client wants (data presented in the most positive manner) and what the physician and consumer wants (unbiased information).

There are many reasons for why ethics is important in modeling. One is that scientists have a duty to be honest and cause no harm. Another reason is that of model credibility—a model is credible as long as its modeler is credible. A modeler who gains the reputation for unethical behavior will not be trusted and as a result any model the modeler develops will also not be trusted. Lastly, and most importantly, withholding key information or biasing the interpretation of a particularly negative result may lead to harm and in extreme cases, where the modeler intentionally commits fraud, may result in delaying approval of a new drug by regulatory authorities, criminal or legal proceedings against the company, or all of the above.

CONCLUSIONS

Modeling is both an art and a science. While it is grounded in science and mathematics, often modelers make choices not involving science or mathematics, but based more on experience and intuition. Some have argued that that experience and intuition are what distinguish good modelers from mediocre ones (Cross and Moscardini, 1985). Take any two modelers and there is no guarantee that they will end up with the same model. In fact, it is likely they won't. This is the Rashomon effect, which does not necessarily mean that one model is wrong. Pharmacokineticists accept as dogma that all models are wrong, but it is still common to hear pharmacokineticists talk about the "wrong model" being used. As a profession we need to move away from this language and embrace the idea of a useful model or better model because non-modelers do not understand the nuances of modeling.

Model development in drug development is usually empirical or exploratory in nature. Models are developed using experimental data and then refined until a reasonable balance is obtained between overfitting and underfitting. This iterative process in model selection results in models that have overly optimistic inferential properties because the uncertainty in the model is not taken into account. No universally accepted solution to this problem has been found.

Once a reasonable model has been found, the results of the model must be interpreted in an objective manner, free of bias, and communicated to other scientists and non-technical managers. The ability to effectively communicate what the model is, its strengths and limitations, and how the model may be used to make decisions is critical. Poor communication will hamper the usefulness of a model more soundly than a weak model that is effectively communicated because at least the weak model will probably be used.

Lastly, the ethical component to modeling cannot be overemphasized. Many models are complex and it is easy to deceive a reader on model development, modeling results, and interpretation. Patients who are prescribed medication rely on the integrity of the pharmaceutical scientists involved in their medication's development. A breach of that trust may lead to deleterious consequences for the patient, the scientist involved, and for the company should any fraud be discovered afterwards. Beyond financial and safety reasons, ethical modeling leads to greater trust in the methodology and advances the profession.

Recommended Reading

Aarons, L., Karlson, M.O., Mentre, F., Rombout, F., Steimer, J.L., van Peer, A., and invited COST B Experts. Role of modelling and simulation in Phase I drug development. *European Journal of Pharmaceutical Sciences* 2001; 13: 115–122.

Balant, L.P., and Gex-Fabry, M. Modelling during drug and development. *European Journal of Pharmaceutical Sciences* 2000; 50: 13–26.

Breiman, L. Statistical modeling: The two cultures (with commentary). *Statistical Science* 2002; 16: 199–231.

Burnham, K.P., and Anderson, D.R. Model selection and multimodel inference: A practical information-theoretic approach. Springer-Verlag, New York, 2002.

Cobelli, C., Carson, E.R., Finkelstein, L., and Leaning, M.S. Validation of simple and complex models in physiology and medicine. *American Journal of Physiology* 1984; 246: R259–266.

Cobelli, C., and DiStefano, J.J. Parameter and structural identifiability concepts and ambiguities: A critical review and analysis. *American Journal of Physiology* 1980; 239: R7–24.

D'Arcy, J. Technically speaking: A guide for communication complex information. Battelle Press, Columbus, OH, 1998.

Tufte, E.R. The visual display of quantitative information. Graphics Press, Cheshire, CT, 2001.

Yamaoka, K., Nakagawa, T., and Uno, T. Application of Akaike's information criterion (AIC) in the evaluation of linear pharmacokinetic equations. *Journal of Pharmacokinetics and Biopharmaceutics* 1978; 6: 165–175.

Chapter 2

Linear Models and Regression

The purpose of models is not to fit the data, but to sharpen the questions

—Samuel Karlin (1924–), Evolutionary Geneticist

INTRODUCTION

A model is said to be linear if the partial derivatives with respect to any of the model parameters are independent of the other parameters. All models of the form

$$Y = \theta_0 + \sum_{k=1}^{p-1} \theta_k x_k \qquad (2.1)$$

where Y is a n × 1 vector of responses called the dependent variable, x is a n × 1 matrix of predictor or independent variables, n is the total number of observations, θ is a p × 1 vector of regression parameters, and p is the number of estimable parameters, are linear because

$$\frac{\partial Y}{\partial \theta_k} = x_k \qquad (2.2)$$

which does not depend on any other θ_j, $k \neq j$. Much has been written about linear regression models and little will be devoted towards it exposition herein, except for a few general properties of the linear model and a review

of some of its salient features. The reader is referred to Neter et al. (1996) or Myers (1986) for further details. The goal is to develop the concepts necessary for the exposition of the nonlinear model, the most common model type seen in pharmacokinetics.

The purpose of a model is to explain the behavior of a system and/or to predict current or future observations. Let

$$Y = \hat{\theta}_0 + \sum_{k=1}^{p-1} \hat{\theta}_k x_k + e_i \qquad (2.3)$$

and let the predicted value ($\hat{Y}_i$) be defined as

$$\hat{Y} = \hat{\theta}_0 + \sum_{k=1}^{p-1} \hat{\theta}_k x_k \qquad (2.4)$$

where $\hat{\theta}$ is the estimator for θ and e are independent, normally distributed residuals with mean 0 and variance σ^2. In general, the hat-notation, ∧, indicates that the value is estimated. By definition, the residuals are calculated as the difference between Eqs. (2.3) and (2.4), i.e.,

$$e = Y - \hat{Y}. \qquad (2.5)$$

It should be noted that for notation purposes, the symbol 'ε' will be used interchangeably with the symbol 'e,' although technically 'e' is an estimator of 'ε.'

The goal is to find the "best" line through the data and consequently find the "best" estimators for θ. One method is to find the set of $\hat{Y}'s$ that are closest to the observed Y based on some type of minimization criterion or objective function. Thus,

$$\hat{\theta}: \min [f(Y, \hat{Y})] \qquad (2.6)$$

where $f(Y, \hat{Y})$ is a specific function based on the observed and predicted values. It should be noted that many different types of objective functions exist. If

$$f(Y,\hat{Y}) = \sum_{i=1}^{n} (Y_i - \hat{Y}_i)^2 = \sum_{i=1}^{n} e_i^2 \qquad (2.7)$$

then the solution to the minimization problem is the method of ordinary least squares (OLS). The function defined in Eq. (2.7) is called the residual sum of squares or error sum of squares. The use of the word 'ordinary' is used to differentiate it from weighted least squares, which will be discussed in the chapter on Variance Models, Weighting, and Transformations. For weighted least-squares the objective function is

$$f(Y, \hat{Y}) = \sum_{i=1}^{n} w_i(Y_i - \hat{Y}_i)^2 = \sum_{i=1}^{n} w_i e_i^2 \qquad (2.8)$$

where w_i is the weight associated with the ith data point. A robust procedure for curve fitting is the least-absolute value criterion,

$$f(Y, \hat{Y}) = \sum_{i=1}^{n} |Y_i - \hat{Y}_i| \qquad (2.9)$$

sometimes called the L_1-norm criterion. Most often least squares is used as the minimization criterion because of its statistical properties. Since no pharmacokinetic software package provides alternative objective functions, like the L_1-norm, only least squares and its modifications will be discussed.

THE METHOD OF LEAST SQUARES AND SIMPLE LINEAR REGRESSION

The Concept of Ordinary Least Squares Applied to the Simple Linear Model

At the minimum of a function, the first derivative equals zero. In the case of the simple linear regression (SLR) model, $Y = \theta_0 + \theta_1 X + \varepsilon$, where the function being minimized is the residual sum of squares [Eq. (2.7)], the following equalities must hold

$$\frac{\partial}{\partial \theta_0} \sum_{i=1}^{n} [Y_i - (\theta_0 + \theta_1 x)]^2 = 0$$
$$\frac{\partial}{\partial \theta_1} \sum_{i=1}^{n} [Y_i - (\theta_0 + \theta_1 x)]^2 = 0 \qquad (2.10)$$

Applying the derivatives, the following pair of equations is obtained

$$n\theta_0 + \theta_1 \sum_{i=1}^{n} x_i = \sum_{i=1}^{n} Y_i \qquad (2.11)$$

$$\theta_0 \sum_{i=1}^{n} x_i + \theta_1 \sum_{i=1}^{n} x_i^2 = \sum_{i=1}^{n} x_i Y_i. \qquad (2.12)$$

These equations are referred to as the least squares normal equations. Solving Eqs. (2.11) and (2.12) simultaneously, θ_0 and θ_1 may be estimated by

$$\hat{\theta}_1 = \frac{S_{xy}}{S_{xx}} = \frac{\sum_{i=1}^{n} Y_i(x_i - \bar{x})}{\sum_{i=1}^{n} (x_i - \bar{x})^2}. \qquad (2.13)$$

$$\hat{\theta}_0 = \bar{Y} - \hat{\theta}_1 \bar{x} \qquad (2.14)$$

Intuitively, the concept of least squares makes sense since the predicted model attempts to minimize the squared deviations from the observed values (Fig. 2.1). Under OLS assumptions, every data point contributes equally to the estimate of the slope and intercept.

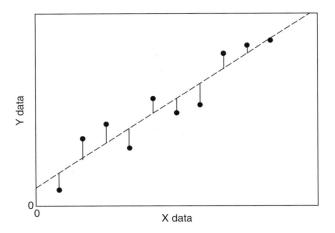

Figure 2.1 Illustration of the concept of least squares linear regression. The dashed line minimizes the squared deviation (indicated by solid lines) between the observed data and the predicted value.

The variance of the parameter estimates may then be obtained using the linear expectation rule

$$\begin{aligned}
\mathrm{Var}(\hat{\theta}_0) &= \mathrm{Var}(\overline{Y} - \hat{\theta}_1 \overline{x}) \\
&= \mathrm{Var}(\overline{Y}) + \overline{x}^2 \mathrm{Var}(\hat{\theta}_1) \\
&= \sigma^2 \left(\frac{1}{n} + \frac{\overline{x}^2}{S_{xx}} \right)
\end{aligned} \quad (2.15)$$

$$\begin{aligned}
\mathrm{Var}(\hat{\theta}_1) &= \mathrm{Var} \left(\frac{\sum_{i=1}^{n} Y_i(x_i - \overline{x})}{\sum_{i=1}^{n} (x_i - \overline{x})^2} \right) \\
&= \frac{1}{S_{xx}^2} \mathrm{Var} \left(\sum_{i=1}^{n} \sigma^2 (x_i - \overline{x})^2 \right). \\
&= \frac{\sigma^2}{S_{xx}}
\end{aligned} \quad (2.16)$$

The square roots of $\mathrm{Var}(\theta_0)$ and $\mathrm{Var}(\theta_1)$ are called the standard error of the parameter estimates denoted as $\mathrm{SE}(\theta_0)$ and $\mathrm{SE}(\theta_1)$, respectively. The residual variance estimator, σ^2, is estimated by

$$\hat{\sigma}^2 = \mathrm{MSE} = \frac{\sum_{i=1}^{n} (Y_i - \hat{Y}_i)^2}{n - p} \quad (2.17)$$

where MSE is referred to as the mean square error or residual mean square error. The numerator in Eq. (2.17) is called the residual sum of squares or sum of squares error, while the denominator is called the residual degrees of freedom or simply degrees of freedom. Degrees of freedom is a term that estimates the amount of known information (n) less the amount of unknown information (p). It can be shown that $E(\sigma^2) = \mathrm{MSE}$, which means that MSE is an unbiased estimate for the residual variance under the assumption that the model is correct. Actual estimation of Eqs. (2.15) and (2.16) is made using the MSE estimator for the residual variance.

The following assumptions are made with a linear model:

- The x's or independent variables are fixed and known with certainty.
- The residuals are independent with mean zero and constant variance.

When both X and Y are measured with error, this is called error-in-variables (EIV) regression, which will be dealt with in a later section. When x is not fixed, but random and X and Y have a joint random distribution, this is referred to as conditional regression, and will also be dealt with later in the chapter. When the residual's have non-constant variance, this is referred to as hetero-scedasticity, which will be dealt with in later chapters. Under OLS assumptions, the fitted regression line has the following properties:

1. The sum of the residuals equals zero.
2. The sum of the squared residuals is a minimum (hence least squares).
3. The sum of the observed Y values equals the sum of the predicted Y values.
4. The regression line always goes through the point $(\overline{x}, \overline{Y})$.

Also under OLS assumptions, the regression parameter estimates have a number of optimal properties. First, $\hat{\theta}$ is an unbiased estimator for θ. Second, the standard error of the estimates are at a minimum, i.e., the standard error of the estimates will be larger than the OLS estimates given any other assumptions. Third, assuming the errors to be normally distributed, the OLS estimates are also the maximum likelihood (ML) estimates for θ (see below). It is often stated that the OLS parameter estimates are BLUE (Best Linear Unbiased Predictors) in the sense that "best" means "minimum variance." Fourth, OLS estimates are consistent, which in simple terms means that as the sample size increases the standard error of the estimate decreases and the bias of the parameter estimates themselves decreases.

MAXIMUM LIKELIHOOD ESTIMATION OF PARAMETERS IN A SIMPLE LINEAR MODEL

Let $\hat{Y}(\hat{\theta}, x)$ be the vector of predicted values for Y. When the errors are normally distributed the likelihood function is given by

$$L(Y|\theta, \sigma) = \prod_{i=1}^{n} \frac{1}{\sqrt{2\pi\sigma^2}} \exp \left(-\frac{[Y_i - \hat{Y}_i]^2}{2\sigma^2} \right). \quad (2.18)$$

The log-likelihood function is the logarithm of the likelihood and is given by

$$\begin{aligned}
\mathrm{LL}(Y|\theta, \sigma) = &-\frac{n}{2} \mathrm{Ln}(2\pi) - \frac{n}{2} \mathrm{Ln}(\sigma^2) \\
&-\frac{1}{2\sigma^2} \sum_{i=1}^{n} [Y_i - \hat{Y}_i]^2.
\end{aligned} \quad (2.19)$$

To find the maximum likelihood estimates for θ and σ^2, the log-likelihood must be concentrated with respect to σ^2. After concentrating the log-likelihood, differentiate with respect to σ^2, set the derivative equal to zero, solve for σ^2, and substitute the result back into Eq. (2.19). The concentrated log-likelihood is then maximized with respect to θ.

Differentiating with respect to σ^2 and setting the derivative equal to zero leads to

$$\frac{dLL(Y|\theta, \sigma)}{d\sigma^2} = -\frac{n}{2\sigma^2} + \frac{1}{2\sigma^4}\sum_{i=1}^{n}[Y_i - \hat{Y}_i]^2 = 0. \quad (2.20)$$

Solving for σ^2 leads to

$$\sigma^2(\theta) = \frac{\sum_{i=1}^{n}[Y_i - \hat{Y}_i]^2}{n} \quad (2.21)$$

where $\sigma^2(\theta)$ denotes the dependence of σ^2 on θ. Substituting back into Eq. (2.19) leads to

$$LL(Y|\theta) = -\frac{n}{2}Ln(2\pi) - \frac{n}{2}Ln\left[\frac{\sum[Y_i - \hat{Y}_i]^2}{n}\right] - \frac{n}{2}. \quad (2.22)$$

The middle term in Eq. (2.22) is a function of the residual sum of squares. The first and last terms are constants. Only the middle term in the equation matters for maximization. By minimizing the negative of Eq. (2.22) (which is equivalent to maximizing the log-likelihood function) the maximum likelihood estimate of θ, which is equivalent to the OLS solution, is found. Once θ is found, the maximum likelihood estimate of σ^2 can be found, although the estimate is biased since the choice of denominator (n for maximum likelihood and n − p for least squares) is different. The same result can be obtained if the likelihood is concentrated with respect to θ first.

The fact that the same result was obtained with the OLS estimates is dependent on the assumption of normality and that the residual variance does not depend on the model parameters. Different assumptions or a variance model that depends on the value of the observation would lead to different ML estimates. Least squares estimates focus completely on the structural model in finding the best parameter estimates. However, ML estimates are a compromise between finding a good fit to both the structural model and the variance model. ML estimates are desirable because they have the following properties (among others):

1. They are asymptotically unbiased.
2. Asymptotically they have minimum variance.
3. They are scale invariant.

For more on the properties and derivation of likelihood functions, the reader is referred to the book appendix.

Precision and Inference of the Parameter Estimates for the Simple Linear Model

Under normal theory assumptions on the residuals, i.e., $\varepsilon \sim N(0, \sigma^2)$, a $(1-\alpha)100\%$ confidence interval for $\hat{\theta}_j$ can be computed from

$$\hat{\theta}_j \pm t_{\alpha/2, n-p}\sqrt{Var(\theta_j)} \quad (2.23)$$

where t is Student's two-tailed t-distribution with n − p degrees of freedom. A corresponding test for whether a model parameter equals zero (null hypothesis)

$$H_o: \theta_j = 0$$

vs. the alternative hypothesis that the parameter does not equal zero

$$H_a: \theta \neq 0$$

can be made from the $(1-\alpha)100\%$ confidence interval. If the $(1-\alpha)100\%$ confidence interval does not contain zero, the null hypothesis is rejected at level α. Similarly, an equivalent T-test can be developed where

$$T = \frac{ABS(\hat{\theta})}{SE(\hat{\theta})} \quad (2.24)$$

where ABS(.) is the absolute value function. If T is greater than Student's two-tailed t-distribution with n − p degrees of freedom, then the null hypothesis is rejected. Both the confidence interval approach and the T-test approach produce equivalent results. For larger sample sizes, the T-test is replaced by a Z-test based on the N(0,1) distribution. For this book, the T-test and Z-test will be used interchangeably.

If θ_j is the slope and the null hypothesis is rejected, then there is evidence to suggest that x affects Y in a linear manner. However, it is unwise to read too much into the rejection of the null hypothesis for the slope because rejection simply states that there is a trend in the data and speaks nothing to the quality of the fit. θ_j may be rejected but the quality of the regression line is poor, i.e., the model does a poor job at explaining the data. Also, rejection of the null hypothesis says nothing about the ability to predict future observations.

Regression Through the Origin

Sometimes the regression model is linear and is known to go through the origin at the point (0,0). An example may be the regression of dose against area under the curve (AUC). Obviously when the dose of the administered drug is zero then the AUC should be zero as well. In this case, x becomes a n×1 matrix of predictor variables with the column of ones removed and for the SLR model, the model reduces to $Y = \theta_1 x + \varepsilon$. The solution to the SLR model is

$$\hat{\theta}_1 = \frac{\sum_{i=1}^{n} x_i Y_i}{\sum_{i=1}^{n} x_i^2} \qquad (2.25)$$

with variance estimate

$$Var[\hat{\theta}_1] = \frac{MSE}{\sum_{i=1}^{n} x_i^2}. \qquad (2.26)$$

Regression through the origin is presented here because of a number of peculiarities to the model, some of which may be unfamiliar to pharmacokineticists. First, the residuals may not necessarily sum to zero and a residual plot may not fall around the zero line. But $\sum_{i=1}^{n} x_i e_i = 0$ and, thus, a residual plot using $x_i e_i$, instead of e_i, may be of more use. Second, it may be possible for the coefficient of determination to be negative because sometimes the residual sum of squares may be greater than the total sum of squares, an event that may occur if the data are curvilinear. Hence, the coefficient of determination is a meaningless statistic under this model. Third, confidence intervals for predicted values will increase in range as x_0, the value to be predicted, becomes removed from the origin, as opposed to the confidence intervals typically seen with SLR. Neter et al. (1996) suggest that using a regression through the origin model is not "safe practice," that an intercept model always be used. They argue that if the regression line does go through the origin, then θ_0 will be very close to zero using an intercept model, differing only by a small sampling error, and unless the sample size is small there will be no deleterious effects in using an intercept model. But if the regression line does not go through the origin and a no-intercept model is used, the resulting model may be quite biased.

Goodness of Fit Tests for the Simple Linear Model

As just mentioned, the T-test tests the significance of a particular parameter estimate. What is really needed is also a test of the overall significance of a model. To start, the total sum of squares of the observed data, SS_{total}, is partitioned into a component due to regression, $SS_{regression}$, and a component due to residual, unexplained error, SSE,

$$\sum_{i=1}^{n}(Y-\overline{Y})^2 = \sum_{i=1}^{n}(\hat{Y}-\overline{Y})^2 + \sum_{i=1}^{n}(Y-\hat{Y})^2. \qquad (2.27)$$
$$SS_{total} = SS_{regression} + SSE$$

Equation can be seen conceptually as

$$\begin{pmatrix} \text{Total Variability} \\ \text{of the Observations} \end{pmatrix} =$$
$$\begin{pmatrix} \text{Variability explained} \\ \text{by the model} \end{pmatrix} + \begin{pmatrix} \text{Unexplained} \\ \text{Variability} \end{pmatrix} \qquad (2.28)$$

Equally, terms on the right hand side of Eq. (2.27) can be viewed as variability due to the regression line and variability around the regression line. Clearly, a good model is one where $SS_{regression} \gg SSE$. Assuming that the residuals are independent and normally distributed with mean 0 and variance σ^2, an F-test can be computed to test the null hypothesis that $\theta = 0$,

$$F = \frac{[SS_{regression}/1]}{[SSE/(n-p)]} = \frac{SS_{regression}}{MSE}. \qquad (2.29)$$

Under the null hypothesis, F is distributed as an F-distribution with p, n−p degrees of freedom. If $F > F_{p, n-p, \alpha}$ the null hypothesis is rejected. This is called the analysis of variance approach to regression. The power of this approach comes in when multiple covariates are available (see Multiple Linear Regression later in the chapter). The F-test then becomes an overall test of the "significance" of the regression model.

One of the most commonly used yardsticks to evaluate the goodness of fit of the model, the coefficient of determination (R^2), develops from the analysis of variance of the regression model. If SS_{total} is the total sum of squares then

$$R^2 = \frac{SS_{regression}}{SS_{total}}. \qquad (2.30)$$

The correlation coefficient is the square root of R^2. These metrics have been discussed in greater detail in the previous chapter.

Prediction and Extrapolation in the Simple Linear Model

The goal of regression analysis is usually two-fold. First, a model is needed to explain the data. Second, using the model, predictions about mean responses or future observations may be needed. The distinction between mean responses and future observations must be clarified. Mean responses are based on already observed data. Future observations are unobserved. The confidence interval for a future observation should be wider than that of a mean response because of the additional uncertainty in future observations compared to the known observation. Now, let $\hat{Y}(x_0)$ be the estimated response (or expected value) given x_0 is

$$\hat{Y}(x_0) = \hat{\theta}_0 + \hat{\theta}_1 x_0. \qquad (2.31)$$

The standard error for $\hat{Y}(x_0)$ is interpreted as the standard error the mean response conditional on x_0. Thus, the variance of $\hat{Y}(x_0)$ is

$$\mathrm{Var}[\hat{Y}(x_0)] = \mathrm{Var}[\hat{\theta}_0 + \hat{\theta}_1 x_0] \qquad (2.32)$$

and using the estimate for σ^2, the estimated standard error of prediction is

$$SE[\hat{Y}(x_0)] = \sqrt{MSE\left[\frac{1}{n} + \frac{(x_0 - \bar{x})^2}{S_{xx}}\right]} \qquad (2.33)$$

with a corresponding $(1 - \alpha)100\%$ confidence interval given by

$$\hat{Y}(x_0) \pm t_{\alpha/2, n-p} \sqrt{MSE\left[\frac{1}{n} + \frac{(x_0 - \bar{x})^2}{S_{xx}}\right]}. \qquad (2.34)$$

Note that the standard error of prediction is not a constant for all values of x_0. but reflects where x_0 is collected in relation to the mean. Observations removed from the mean of x will have larger standard errors of prediction than values close to the mean. Equation (2.34) is developed as the confidence interval for a single observation measured at x_0. If more than one observation is made at x_0, the term 1/n in Eqs. (2.33) and (2.34) is substituted with the term m/n, where m is the number of observations at x_0. Note that m is contained within n. If the confidence interval is made for all points on the regression line, the result would be a confidence band.

The confidence interval for a future response, one not in the original data set, must be more variable due to the additional uncertainty in its measurement. Thus, Eq. (2.33) is modified to

$$SE[\hat{Y}(x_0)] = \sqrt{MSE\left[\frac{1}{m} + \frac{1}{n} + \frac{(x_0 - \bar{x})^2}{S_{xx}}\right]} \qquad (2.35)$$

where m is the number of future observations to be collected. The corresponding prediction interval is

$$\hat{Y}(x_0) \pm t_{\alpha/2, n-p} \sqrt{MSE\left[\frac{1}{m} + \frac{1}{n} + \frac{(x_0 - \bar{x})^2}{S_{xx}}\right]}. \qquad (2.36)$$

Clearly prediction intervals are wider than corresponding confidence intervals.

To illustrate further the distinction between confidence intervals for mean responses and prediction intervals for future observations, consider allometric scaling. In allometric scaling, the systemic clearance or volume of distribution is calculated for many different species, usually mouse, rat, and dog. A regression line of the log-transformed pharmacokinetic parameter is regressed again the log-transformed weight. One may then ask "What is the 95% confidence interval for clearance in the rat?" This is an example of confidence interval using Eq. (2.34). Next, someone may ask "If 10 rats were taken from the population, what is the 95% confidence interval for clearance in the rat?" This is another example of a confidence interval using Eq. (2.34) with the term 1/n replaced by 10/n. Then, someone may ask "What is the 95% prediction interval for clearance in a guinea pig?" This is an example of a prediction interval using Eq. (2.36) because guinea pigs were not in the original population. A similar question can be asked about humans—what is the clearance in humans given a dataset based entirely on animal data. This approach, called prospective allometric scaling, is often used in choosing the starting dose for a new drug in a first time in man study. Bonate and Howard (2000) argue that prospective allometric scaling can lead to unreasonably large confidence intervals because the extrapolation from animals to humans, based on body weight, is tremendous and that using this approach in practice should be done with great care. A further example of allometric scaling is presented in the chapter on Case Studies in Linear and Nonlinear Modeling.

Categorical Independent Variables

Up until now it has been assumed that x consists of continuous variables. OLS is not predicated on x being continuous, although this makes it convenient to explain the model. An extremely important data type is a categorical variable where the variable of interest takes on discrete values. These variables are also called factors or class variables. For instance, whether a person is considered a *smoker* can be coded as either 'yes' or 'no.' The variable *race* may take on the values: White, Black, Asian, or Hispanic. These variables must enter the model through what are called dummy variables or indicator variables which are themselves categorical variables that take on the value of either 0 or 1. If there are k levels in the categorical variable, then k−1 dummy variables are need to uniquely define that variable. For example, the variable *smoker* has two levels and thus needs a single dummy variable (0 or 1) to define that variable. Variable *race* has four levels and needs three dummy variables (D1–D3) to uniquely define that variable, as seen below:

Variable: Race	Dummy variables		
	D1	D2	D3
White	0	0	1
Black	0	1	0
Asian	1	0	0
Hispanic	0	0	0

The presence of a dummy variable results in a shift in the regression through its effect on the intercept (Fig. 2.2). The difference between the regression lines is an indication of the difference between the levels of the variable assuming that the regression coefficients for the continuous variables across classes remain constant among the factor levels. Also, note that the inferential statistics on the regression parameters, even the regression estimates themselves, are independent of how the factor levels are coded. For instance, with variable *sex* it makes no difference whether 'males' are coded as 0 or 1 as long as 'females' are coded 1 or 0, respectively.

MULTIPLE LINEAR REGRESSION

Rarely in a single experiment is one dependent variable and one independent variable collected. More often, many dependent variables and many independent variables are collected. Then, a scientist may wish to use the independent variables to explain a particular dependent variable. For example, suppose from a population pharmacokinetic analysis (which will be discussed in later chapters) total systemic clearance (CL) was estimated in a group of subjects. Also available were demographic information, such as age, weight, and smoking status. Of interest would be whether any of the demographic variables were related to clearance. It may be that smokers have higher clearance estimates than non-smokers and require more drug to achieve the same therapeutic effect.

In this case, multiple linear regression may be used to determine the significance of the demographic variables, which are often called covariates. The model may then be formulated as

$$CL = \theta_0 + \theta_1 Weight + \theta_2 Age + \theta_3 Smoker + \varepsilon. \quad (2.37)$$

As in simple linear regression, the same assumptions are made: ε_i is normally distributed, uncorrelated with each other and have mean zero with variance σ^2. In addition, the covariates are measured without error. In matrix notation then, the general linear model can be written as

$$Y = x\theta + \varepsilon \quad (2.38)$$

with solution

$$\hat{\theta} = (x^T x)^{-1} x^T Y. \quad (2.39)$$

In this case, x is a $n \times (k+1)$ matrix of independent variables where the first column of the matrix is a column of ones, which is necessary for inclusion of the intercept in the model, and k is the number of independent variables. An estimate of MSE is obtained by

$$MSE = \frac{(Y - x\hat{\theta})^T (Y - x\hat{\theta})}{n - p} = \frac{\sum_{i=1}^{n} (Y - x\hat{\theta})^2}{n - p} \quad (2.40)$$

which is exactly the same as Eq. (2.17), but written in matrix notation. The standard error of the parameter estimates is calculated by

$$SE(\hat{\theta}) = \sqrt{diag(x^T x)^{-1} MSE} \quad (2.41)$$

where diag(.) is the diagonal elements of $x^T x$. Similarly, T-tests and confidence intervals for the parameter estimates can be calculated using Eqs. (2.24) and (2.23), respectively. $(1 - \alpha)100\%$ confidence intervals for mean responses can be computed from

$$\hat{Y}(x_0) \pm t_{\alpha/2, n-p} \sqrt{MSE [x_o^T (x^T x)^{-1} x_0]} \quad (2.42)$$

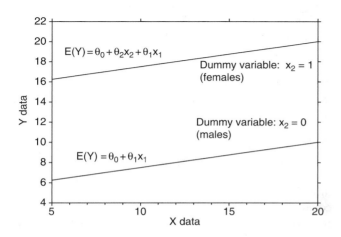

Figure 2.2 Plot of regression line for a single categorical covariate (sex) with two levels (males and females). The effect of the categorical variable is to shift the model intercept.

and $(1 - \alpha)100\%$ prediction intervals for future responses can be calculated from

$$\hat{Y}(x_0) \pm t_{\alpha/2, n-p}\sqrt{MSE[1 + x_0^T(x^Tx)^{-1}x_0]}. \quad (2.43)$$

Similarly, a $(1 - \alpha)100\%$ confidence band for the response function at any x can be developed using

$$x\hat{\theta} \pm \sqrt{MSE[1 + x^T(x^Tx)^{-1}x]}\sqrt{F_{p,n-p,\alpha}p}. \quad (2.44)$$

Confidence bands differ from confidence intervals in that they consider all the values of x simultaneously, as opposed to a single value x_0. Confidence bands are larger than confidence intervals.

Model Selection and Sequential Variable Selection

Procedures in Multiple Linear Regression

Even though many different covariates may be collected in an experiment, it may not be desirable to enter all these in a multiple regression model. First, not all covariates may be statistically significant—they have no predictive power. Second, a model with too many covariates produces models that have variances, e.g., standard errors, residual errors, etc., that are larger than simpler models. On the other hand, too few covariates lead to models with biased parameter estimates, mean square error, and predictive capabilities. As previously stated, model selection should follow Occam's razor, which basically states "the simpler model is always chosen over more complex models."

To strike the proper balance between an overparameterized model and an underparameterized model, one must strike a balance between a biased model and an overinflated variance model. Mallows (1973) proposed his C_p criterion which is defined as

$$C_p = \frac{SSE^*}{MSE} - (n - 2p^*), \quad (2.45)$$

where SSE^* is the sum of squares error from the model containing p^* parameters, where $p^* \leq p$. When $p^* = p$, then $C_p = p$. For example, if a model with four possible covariates is examined, the sub-model with covariates x_1, x_2 becomes

$$C_p = \frac{SSE(x_1, x_2)}{MSE} - (n - 6). \quad (2.46)$$

When there is no bias in the model, the expected value of C_p is p^*, the number of parameters in the model. Thus, when C_p is plotted against p^*, models with little bias will fall near the line $C_p \cong p^*$. Models with substantial bias will have C_p values greater than the line. In using Mallow C_p as a model selection criterion one chooses a C_p that is small and near p^*.

One way to identify important predictor variables in a multiple regression setting is to do all possible regressions and choose the model based on some criteria, usually the coefficient of determination, adjusted coefficient of determination, or Mallows C_p. With this approach, a few candidate models are identified and then further explored for residual analysis, collinearity diagnostics, leverage analysis, etc. While useful, this method is rarely seen in the literature and cannot be advocated because the method is a "dummy-ing down" of the modeling process—the method relies too much on blind usage of the computer to solve a problem that should be left up to the modeler to solve.

Related to all possible regressions, a variety of automated algorithms have been developed to screen a large number of covariates in a multiple regression setting and select the "best" model. Forward selection algorithms begin with no covariates in the model. Each covariate is then screened using simple linear regression. F-tests are then calculated reflecting each covariate's contribution to the model when that covariate is included in the model. These F-tests are then compared to a significance level criteria (F_{in}) set by the user a priori and if the F-tests meets F_{in} the covariate is included in the model. At each step only one covariate is added to the model—that covariate having the highest contribution to the F-test. For example, suppose $\{x_1, x_2, x_3, x_4\}$ were possible covariates and using simple linear regression x_3 was found to be the most significant covariate based on the F-test. The next step then compares the models $\{x_1, x_3\}$, $\{x_2, x_3\}$, and $\{x_3, x_4\}$. The contribution x_1, x_2, and x_4 make to their respective models is then compared and the covariate having the highest contribution is compared to F_{in}. The new variable is then added to the model if that F-test meets the entry criteria. If in this case, that variable was x_1, then the next models tested will be $\{x_1, x_3, x_2\}$ and $\{x_1, x_3, x_4\}$. This process repeats until no further variables are available or until the model with the highest contribution does not meet the entry criteria, at which point the algorithm stops.

Backwards elimination is similar to forward selection, except that the initial model contains all the covariates and removal from the model starts with the covariate of the least significance. Removal from the model then proceeds one variable at a time until no covariates meet the criteria for removal (F_{out}). Stepwise regression is a blend of both forward and backwards selection in that variables can be added or removed from the model at each stage. Thus, a variable may be added and a variable may be removed in the same step.

The algorithm quits when no additional covariates can be added on the basis of F_{in} and no covariates can be removed on the basis of F_{out}.

The problem with using all possible regressions or sequential methods is that they lead to the "dumbing down" of statistical analysis. The user plugs in some data and the computer spits out a "best model." Simply because a software manufacturer includes an algorithm in a package doesn't mean it should be used. Scientific judgment must play a role in covariate selection and model selection. Explanatory covariates should be based on physiological or physical sense. As an example, suppose volume of distribution were screened against clinical chemistry laboratories and inorganic phosphate was identified as a significant covariate. How does one interpret this? It is better to use a priori covariates that make sense in the model and then build on that model. As a rule, sequential variable selection procedures and all possible regressions should be used with caution. Harrell (http://www.pitt.edu/~wpilib/statfaq/regrfaq.html) presents some very valid criticisms of stepwise regression and all possible subsets regression. They are:

1. The coefficient of determination is often biased high.
2. The F- and chi-squared distribution next to each variable do not have the prescribed theoretical distribution.
3. Confidence intervals for effects and predicted values are too narrow.
4. p-values do not have the proper meaning anymore because of multiplicity.
5. The regression coefficients are biased.
6. The algorithm has problems with collinearity.
7. It is based on methods, i.e., F-tests for nested models, that were designed to test pre-specified hypotheses.
8. Increasing the sample size does not improve things.
9. It is too easy to use and causes people to quit thinking about their problem.
10. It uses a lot of paper.

In summary, automated techniques should not be used blindly, even though they often are.

COLLINEARITY AND ILL-CONDITIONING

When multiple covariates are included in the regression model, the possibility for collinearity, which is sometimes called multicollinearity or ill-conditioning, among the predictors arises. The term collinear implies that there is correlation or linear dependencies among the independent variable. Entire books (Belsley, Kuh, and Welsch, 1980) have been written o'n collinearity and all its nuances will not be discussed in its entirety here. Nevertheless, an analyst should at least understand what it is, how to detect it, and how to combat it.

Collinearity is actually simple to understand, although there are complex geometric reasons for its effect on parameter estimation. Consider two variables x_1 and x_2 that are regressed against Y. Now suppose x_1 and x_2 are correlated to the extent that they essentially are the same thing. Thus, x_2 does not provide any more information than x_1 and vice-versa. As the correlation between x_1 and x_2 increases, it becomes more and more difficult to isolate the effect due to x_1 from the effect due to x_2, such that the parameter estimates become unstable. The bottom line is that when collinearity exists among a set of predictors, the parameter estimates become extremely sensitive to small changes in the values of the predictors and are very much dependent on the particular data set that generated them. A new data set may generate completely different parameter estimates. Although collinearity is often due to correlation between variables, collinearity may be due to a few influential observations and not necessarily to the whole vector of data. Careful examination of the scatter plots between possible correlated variables should be done to rule out this cause of collinearity.

Collinearity manifests itself during the inversion of the matrix $x^T x$ in Eq. (2.39), such that small changes in x lead to large changes in the parameter estimates and their standard errors. When the predictors are uncorrelated, the values of the parameter estimates remain unchanged regardless of any other predictor variables included in the model. When the predictors are correlated, the value of a regression parameter depends on which other parameters are entered into the model and which others are not, i.e., collinearity destroys the uniqueness of the parameter estimate. Thus, when collinearity is present *"a regression coefficient does not reflect any inherent effect of the particular predictor variable on the response variable but only a marginal or partial effect, given whatever other correlated predictor variables are included in the model"* (Neter et al., 1996). Correlation between predictor variables in and of itself do not mean that a good fit cannot be obtained nor that predictions of new observations are poorly inferred, provided the inferences are made within the sample space of the data set upon which the model was derived. What it means is that the estimated regression coefficients tend to widely vary from one data set to the next.

There are a variety of methods to detect collinearity (Belsley, Kuh, and Welsch, 1980). First, examine the parameter estimates. A priori variables that are expected to be important which are not found to be statistically significant is a clue that collinearity may be present. If the values of the parameters change drastically if a row of x or column of x is deleted (such as a sign change), that is another clue. Second, examine the various collinearity diagnostics, of which there are many, some of which are better than others. Keep in mind, however, that there are no definitive cut-off values indicating whether collinearity is present.

The first simple diagnostic is to examine the correlation matrix of the covariates. High correlations, either positive or negative, are indicative of collinearity. However, the correlation matrix is sometimes unable to detect the situation where three or more covariates are collinear but no two correlations are high (Belsley, Kuh, and Welsch, 1980). Related to the inverse of the correlation matrix are variance inflation factors (VIF), calculated as

$$ \text{VIF} = \frac{1}{1 - R_i^2} \tag{2.47} $$

where R_i^2 is the coefficient of determination of x_i regressed against all other x. The higher the coefficient of determination, the higher the VIF, and the greater the collinearity. Possible collinearity is present when the VIF is greater than five and multicollinearity is almost certainly occurring when the VIF is greater than 10.

Another useful tool is to examine the eigenvalues of the $x^T x$ matrix, l_i. The number of eigenvalues near zero indicate the number of collinear covariates among the regressors. One of the most commonly used yardsticks to measure the degree of collinearity is the condition number (K), which can be calculated using many different methods. The first definition is simply the ratio of the largest to smallest eigenvalue

$$ K = \frac{l_1}{l_p} \tag{2.48} $$

where l_1 and l_p are the largest and smallest eigenvalues of the correlation matrix (Jackson, 1991). The second way is to define K as

$$ K = \sqrt{\frac{l_1}{l_p}}. \tag{2.49} $$

The latter method is often used simply because the conditions numbers are smaller. The user should be aware how a software package computes a condition number. For instance, SAS uses Eq. (2.49). For this book Eq. (2.48) will be used as the definition of the condition number. Condition numbers range from 1, which indicates perfect stability, to infinity, which indicates perfect

instability. As a rule of thumb, $\text{Log}_{10}(K)$ using Eq. (2.48) indicates the number of decimal places lost by a computer due to round-off errors due to matrix inversion. Most computers have about 16 decimal digits of accuracy and if the condition number is 10^4, then the result will be accurate to at most 12 (calculated as $16-4$) decimal places of accuracy.

It is difficult to find useful yardsticks in the literature about what constitutes a large condition number because many books have drastically different cut-offs. For this book, the following guidelines will be used. For a linear model, when the condition number is less than 10^4, no serious collinearity is present. When the condition number is between 10^4 and 10^6, moderate collinearity is present, and when the condition number exceeds 10^6, severe collinearity is present and the values of the parameter estimates are not to be trusted. The difficulty with the use of the condition number is that it fails to identify which columns are collinear and simply indicates that collinearity is present. If multicollinearity is present wherein a function of one or more columns is collinear with a function of one or more other columns, then the condition number will fail to identify that collinearity. See Belsley, Kuh, and Welsch (1980) for details on how to detect collinearity among sets of covariates.

Collinearity may also be caused by poor scaling and/or near singularity of the $x^T x$ matrix. If the collinearity is due to scaling, then one simple way to remove the collinearity is by centering. Centering creates a new variable x^* using

$$ x_{ij}^* = x_{ij} - \overline{x}_i \tag{2.50} $$

where x_{ij} is the value of the jth row of the ith variable and $\overline{x}_i$ is the mean of the ith variable. An expansion of centering is standardizing the covariates which is done using

$$ x_{ij}^* = \frac{x_{ij} - \overline{x}_i}{s_i} \tag{2.51} $$

where s_i is the standard deviation of the ith variable. After centering, x^* has zero mean with the same variance as the original data. After standardization, x^* has zero mean and variance 1, which forces approximate orthogonality between the covariates. A third method is scaling where each observation is divided by a column-dependent constant, such as the mean, making each column approximately the same scale.

For example, suppose with the linear model

$$ Y = \theta_0 + \theta_1 x_1 + \theta_2 x_2 \tag{2.52} $$

that

$$x^T x = \begin{bmatrix} 8 & 117 & 3607 \\ & 2251 & 58112 \\ & & 1861257 \end{bmatrix}. \quad (2.53)$$

The condition number of $x^T x$ is 1.92×10^5, which is quite ill-conditioned. The model could be centered on the mean of 15 and 450, respectively,

$$Y = \theta_0^* + \theta_1^*(x_1 - 15) + \theta_2^*(x_2 - 450) \quad (2.54)$$

with corresponding $x^T x$ matrix

$$x^T x = \begin{bmatrix} 8 & -3 & 7 \\ & 541 & 5357 \\ & & 234957 \end{bmatrix} \quad (2.55)$$

and condition number 29475, a 65-fold reduction over the original model. The '*' superscript in Eq. (2.54) denotes that the parameter estimates are not the same as those in Eq. (2.52). Or the model could be scaled to its mean

$$Y = \theta_0^* + \frac{\theta_1^* x_1}{15} + \frac{\theta_2^* x_2}{450}. \quad (2.56)$$

Then

$$x^T x = \begin{bmatrix} 8.0 & 7.8 & 8.0 \\ & 10.0 & 8.6 \\ & & 9.2 \end{bmatrix} \quad (2.57)$$

and the condition number becomes 47, a 40,000-fold reduction from the original condition number. In the original domain, inverting $x^T x$ would lead to a loss of about six decimals of precision on a double-precision computer, but inversion after transformation would lead to only a two decimal loss in precision. Lastly, the model could be standardized

$$Y = \theta_0^* + \frac{\theta_1^*(x_1 - 15)}{8.78} + \frac{\theta_2^*(x_2 - 450)}{183.21} \quad (2.58)$$

with $x^T x$ matrix

$$x^T x = \begin{bmatrix} 8.00 & -0.34 & 0.038 \\ & 7.02 & 3.33 \\ & & 7.00 \end{bmatrix} \quad (2.59)$$

and corresponding condition number of 2.83, a 682,000-fold reduction over the original condition number. Less than one decimal loss of precision would occur after

standardization. It makes little difference whether centering or standardizing with the mean or median, except that these estimates tend to be study specific. A more robust method of centering would be to use a consistent value across all studies and all drugs (Holford, 1996). For example, all BSA values would be centered by $1.7\,m^2$, weight by 70 kg, age by 40 years (70 years for elderly studies), 7.5 L/h for creatinine clearance, etc. In this manner parameter estimates can be compared across studies making them more relevant.

One advantage of centering over standardization or scaling is that the parameter estimates associated with x are the same as the original data. The only difference being the estimate of the intercept. However, since centering only transforms the data to have the same mean, the variance of the columns of x may still be of differing magnitudes. Even after centering, ill-conditioning may still be present. Scaling presents the opposite problem. After scaling, the variance of the columns of x may be of the same magnitude but the means may be vastly different. Hence, ill-conditioning may still be present after scaling. Only standardization transforms the data to the same mean and variance and from a purely numeric point of view is the method of choice. However, with standardization and scaling the parameter estimates obtained from the transformed data are not the same as the original data and must be transformed back to the original domain should one wish to interpret the parameter estimates. A disadvantage of transforming the predictor variables to the same scale is that the transformation does not always cure ill-conditioning. For example, centering will not prevent loss of numerical accuracy if any of the predictor variables are correlated with the model intercept (Simon and Lesage, 1988).

A fourth method to remove the collinearity is by transforming the collinear variables into another variable and use that variable as a surrogate. For example, height and weight are often highly correlated and can be combined into a composite variable called body surface area (BSA), which is a measure of the overall surface area on an individual. There are a number of different measures to compute BSA, but a common one is based on the height and weight on an individual

$$BSA = 0.0235(Weight)^{0.51456}(Height)^{0.42246} \quad (2.60)$$

where BSA is in m^2, weight is in kg, and height is in cm (Gehan and George, 1970). As an example, consider the data in Table 2.1. Apparent oral clearance was obtained from 65 individuals. Height and weight were collected on all subjects. Both height (Pearson's r: 0.2219, $p = 0.0757$) and weight (Pearson's r: 0.4684, $p < 0.0001$) were marginally correlated with clearance (see Fig. 2.3). Height

Table 2.1 Clearance, weight, and height estimates from 65 subjects.

Clearance (mL/min)	Weight (lb.)	Height (in.)	Clearance (mL/min)	Weight (lb.)	Height (in.)
62612	124.5	67.7	51530	117.2	66.4
54951	136.5	65.1	55333	142.4	65.1
54897	140.7	68.6	48292	115.0	66.5
55823	148.8	65.2	51453	143.9	69.5
68916	185.1	70.8	56779	122.5	70.2
74333	185.7	70.5	56346	145.6	71.1
62203	143.4	71.9	58239	168.9	72.6
40359	126.7	67.5	64677	182.0	67.9
51205	134.5	66.8	67045	167.8	71.1
57108	151.8	67.2	51764	140.0	71.7
51574	131.2	60.2	69917	165.1	74.6
49579	127.6	63.4	38738	107.4	63.7
62450	152.5	75.6	59912	132.2	66.3
49879	144.6	68.6	53475	134.4	67.6
53818	161.5	73.6	51197	154.2	72.4
53417	155.8	71.9	55603	149.6	72.4
65510	171.0	72.6	53013	123.0	70.7
45320	114.5	65.5	63697	155.0	76.4
53174	128.4	67.0	71911	137.8	65.8
56905	131.1	65.9	52606	138.2	71.1
67193	145.6	68.6	45523	153.3	73.9
48135	146.9	71.4	54643	157.6	72.6
53952	104.8	65.1	55699	135.7	65.9
51145	147.0	67.3	51787	132.1	73.6
58154	173.1	74.5	59247	140.9	69.8
51574	141.0	71.4	56044	141.9	68.7
59407	144.5	70.6	47898	134.8	72.9
69394	145.4	71.4	45694	152.0	70.2
60276	167.0	72.3	41664	116.2	66.3
50626	126.8	67.2	53827	130.6	70.2
37266	128.1	72.5	57166	141.7	74.2
52343	120.6	65.5	50248	147.1	70.5
43509	149.9	70.4			

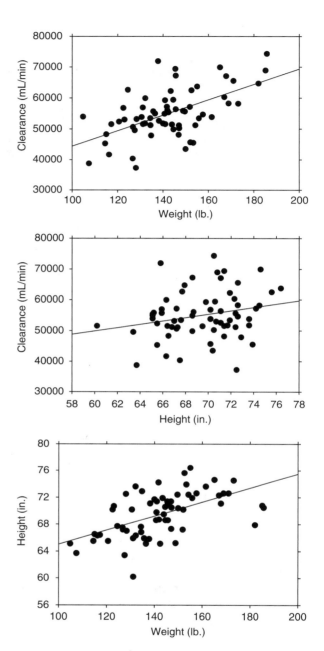

Figure 2.3 Correlation plot of data in Table 2.1. Solid line is least squares fit to the data.

and weight had a better correlation with each other (Pearson's r: 0.6038, p < 0.0001) than with clearance. The SAS output from the regression analysis is presented in Table 2.2.

When height and weight were included in the models alone, they were both positively related to clearance (p < 0.10). When both variables were included in the model, height showed a sign change and now has a negative relationship with clearance. This is the first warning sign that something is wrong. The eigenvalues of $x^T x$ were {2.99, 0.00854, 0.000939}. The condition number of the model with both covariates was 3185, which is not exceedingly large, but nevertheless indicated that that the resulting inverted matrix lost 3 to 4 decimal places during large. But, there were two eigenvalues near zero indicating that two variables were collinear. When BSA was used as the sole covariate, the coefficient of determination was slightly smaller than using weight alone, but far better than height. A further refinement in the model might be one where the intercept is removed

from the model since the 90% confidence interval for the intercept included zero. In summary, when the covariates were regressed alone they both were statistically significant as predictor variables for clearance. But when entered together, collinearity among predictors occurred and the effect of height became opposite what was expected.

Sometimes, even after rescaling, when the $x^T x$ matrix is still ill-conditioned, then either ridge regression or principal components regression may be necessary. Briefly, in ridge regression a small constant (k) is

Table 2.2 SAS output from regression analysis of Table 2.1 using clearance as the dependent variable.

			Both variables			
Variable	*DF*	*Parameter estimate*	*Standard error*	*T for H0: Parameter=0*	*Prob > |T|*	*Variance inflation*
Intercept	1	34810	17179.538954	2.026	0.0470	0.00000000
Height	1	−278.561305	290.86043976	−0.958	0.3419	1.44322425
Weight	1	277.806275	54.70976093	5.078	0.0001	1.44322425

			Collinearity diagnostics		
Number	*Eigenvalue*	*Condition index*[**]	*Var prop intercept*	*Var prop height*	*Var prop weight*
1	2.99052	1.00000	0.0002	0.0002	0.0012
2	0.00854	18.70927	0.0690	0.0152	0.7982
3	0.0009391	56.43213	0.9308	0.9846	0.2006

			Height only		
Variable	*DF*	*Parameter estimate*	*Standard error*	*T for H0: Parameter=0*	*Prob > |T|*
Intercept	1	17537	19877.615084	0.882	0.3810
Height	1	539.916181	285.79575217	1.889	0.0635

			Weight only		
Variable	*DF*	*Parameter estimate*	*Standard error*	*T for H0: Parameter=0*	*Prob > |T|*
Intercept	1	19595	6535.0993235	2.998	0.0039
Weight	1	248.769673	45.51058177	5.466	0.0001

			BSA only		
Variable	*DF*	*Parameter estimate*	*Standard error*	*t Value*	*Pr > |t|*
Intercept	1	1695.00446	10848	0.16	0.8763
BSA	1	30090	6100.33895	4.93	<.0001

[**]denotes that the condition index reported by SAS is calculated using Eq. (2.49) and is the square root of the condition number otherwise used throughout this book.

added to the x^Tx matrix prior to inversion so as to stabilize the matrix. Hence, the estimator for θ becomes

$$\hat{\theta} = x\left(x^Tx + kI\right)^{-1}x^TY \qquad (2.61)$$

where I is the identity matrix. The choice of the constant must be chosen with care because the resulting parameter estimates become biased to some degree. However, the reduction in the variance of the estimators may be greater than the resulting increase in bias such that the trade-off is of merit.

Principal components regression is another biased regression technique but when done successfully is superior to OLS in terms of prediction and estimation. Principal components (PC) are linear transformations of the original variables such that each PC is orthogonal or uncorrelated to the others (Jackson, 1991). There will be k principal components if there are k variables. Of these k principal components, j (j < k) components may contain most of the "information" contained in k. Thus, regression of the j principal components, instead of the original k variables, may be used for regression. The

predicted values can then be back-transformed to the original domain for prediction. The reader should see Neter et al. (1996) for further details of these algorithms.

INFLUENCE DIAGNOSTICS

Frequently data contain samples that are different than the bulk of the remaining data, i.e., these observations may be outliers. Outliers may arise from improper recording of data, assay error (both random and systematic), choice of an invalid model, or may not be outliers at all, but are in fact legitimate data points. Residual analysis is a tool to assess the fit of a model. Although useful, it fails to provide information on how individual observations may affect the parameter estimates or their standard errors. As most modelers have seen, a single observation may have a dramatic influence on estimation of the relationship between Y and x. Similarly, deleting a single observation in a nonlinear model may result in convergence, whereas inclusion of the data point may not. An observation which individually, or together with other observations, has a larger impact on a parameter estimate, such as the slope, its standard error, or associated T-test, than other observations is said to be *influential*. Influence diagnostics provide rational, objective measures to assess the impact individual data points have on the regression coefficients and their standard errors. Thus, by using influence diagnostics a modeler can have an impartial measure by which to either remove a data point from an analysis or weight that data point sufficiently so as to force it to have equal influence as other observations in the data set.

The purpose of this section is to provide a primer on influence diagnostics with the ultimate hope being that more rational decision making rules will be used before discarding data points from an analysis and greater use of influence diagnostics will result in their incorporation in pharmacokinetic software packages (something that is definitely lacking at this time). The reader is referred to Belsley, Kuh, and Welsch et al. (1980) or Neter et al. (1996) for further in-depth discussion on using influence diagnostics.

Influence in the x-direction

Although most are familiar with the influence a discordant observation in the Y-direction has on parameter estimation; the independent variables themselves also influence the parameter estimates. Recall that ordinary least squares minimizes the quantity

$$\sum_{i=1}^{n}\left(Y - \hat{Y}\right)^2 = \sum_{i=1}^{n}\left(Y - x\hat{\theta}\right)^2 \qquad (2.62)$$

which can be expanded to

$$\sum_{i=1}^{n}\left(Y - \hat{Y}\right)^2 = \sum_{i=1}^{n}\left(Y - x\left(x^T x\right)^{-1} x^T Y\right)^2. \qquad (2.63)$$

Let $h = x(x^T x)^{-1} x^T$ be called the HAT matrix. Then least squares minimizes

$$\sum_{i=1}^{n}(Y - hY)^2 \qquad (2.64)$$

and an alternative method for determining the predicted values of the dependent variable is

$$\hat{Y} = x\hat{\theta} = hY. \qquad (2.65)$$

The HAT matrix can be thought to map the observed values (Y) to the predicted values ($\hat{Y}$). One important aspect of the least squares model is that a better fit is

observed at remote observations than at observations near the middle of the data. By corollary, observations that have large HAT values will be better predicted because the method of least squares attempts to find parameter estimates that result in residuals near zero. Thus, it is said that observations with large HAT values have more influence than observations with small HAT values. Another term used to indicate influence in the x-direction is called *leverage*.[1] Observations with high leverage exert greater influence on parameter estimates than observations with low leverage.

Another way to look at the HAT matrix is as a distance measure—values with large HAT values are far from the mean of x. It can be shown that the HAT matrix has two useful properties: $0 \le h_i \le 1$ and $\Sigma h_i = p$ for i = 1 to n. The average size of h_i is then p/n. It is desirable to have all independent variables to have equal influence, i.e., each data point has $h_i \cong p/n$. As a rule of thumb, an independent variable has greater *leverage* than other observations when h_i is greater than 2p/n. Figure 2.4 presents an example of non-influential and influential x-values.

Consider the previous example where clearance was modeled as a function of BSA. There were 65 observations and two estimable parameters in the model. Hence, under the rule of thumb, observations with HAT values greater than 0.062 exerted greater leverage than other observations. Figure 2.5 presents the HAT values plotted against BSA. Four observations met the criteria for having high leverage.

This plot illustrates that observations with large HAT values in a model including an intercept are at the extremes of x. In the single predictor case, this corresponds to observations at the tails of the distribution of x. In the two-dimensional case this would correspond to observations near the ends of the ellipse. In the case where no intercept is in the model, only observations far removed from zero can have high leverage. It must be kept in mind that a large HAT value is not necessarily a bad thing. An observation with a large HAT value that is concordant with the rest of the data probably will not change the parameter estimates much. However, a large HAT value coupled with a large DFBETAS (see below) is a combination that spells trouble.

Influence in the Y-direction

Most pharmacokineticists are familiar with this case, when a single observation(s) is discordant from

---

[1] More formally, leverage is defined as the partial derivative of the predicted value with respect to the corresponding dependent variable, i.e., $h_i = \partial \hat{Y}_i / \partial Y_i$, which reduces to the HAT matrix for linear models.

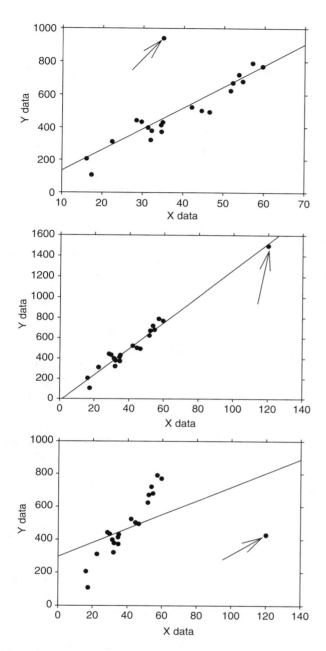

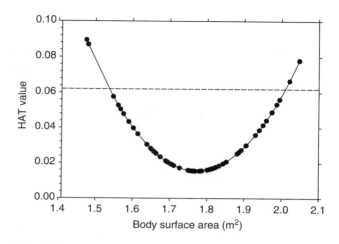

Figure 2.5 Plot of HAT values against body surface area under a simple linear model using the data in Table 2.1. The plot illustrates that HAT values are a function of the x-matrix and that observations with high HAT values are at the extremes in x. The dashed line is the yardstick for observations with high leverage, $2p/n$.

$$e_s = \frac{e_i}{\sqrt{MSE}}. \tag{2.66}$$

Under the assumption that the residuals are independent, normally distributed with mean 0 and constant variance, when the sample size is large, standardized residuals greater than ± 2 are often identified as suspect observations. Since asymptotically standardized residuals are normally distributed, one might think that they are bounded by $-\infty$ and $+\infty$, but in fact, a standardized residual can never exceed $\pm\sqrt{(n-p)(n-1)n^{-1}}$ (Gray and Woodall, 1994). For a simple linear model with 19 observations, it is impossible for any standardized residual to exceed ± 4. Standardized residuals suffer from the fact that they a prone to "ballooning" in which extreme cases of x tend to have smaller residuals than cases of x near the centroid of the data. To account for this, a more commonly used statistic, called studentized or internally studentized residuals, was developed

$$e_{si} = \frac{e_i}{\sqrt{MSE(1-h_i)}}. \tag{2.67}$$

Under the assumption that the residuals are independent, normally distributed with mean 0 and constant variance, when the sample size is large, studentized residuals greater than ± 2 are often identified as suspect observations. Like standardized residuals, studentized residuals are not bound by $-\infty$ and $+\infty$, but are bounded by $\pm\sqrt{(n-p)}$ (Gray and Woodall, 1994). An alternative statistic, one that is often erroneously interchanged with standardized residuals, are studentized deleted residuals, which are sometimes called jackknifed

Figure 2.4 Example of influential and non-influential observations. Top plot: Y-value is discordant from bulk of data but does not influence the estimate of the regression line. Middle plot: x-value is discordant from bulk of data but does not influence the estimate of the regression line. Bottom plot: x-value and Y-value are discordant from bulk of data and have a profound influence on the estimate of the regression line. Not all outlier observations are influential and not all influential observations are outliers.

the other observations in the Y-direction. Outliers in the Y-direction are often detected by visual examination or more formally by residual analysis. One common statistic is standardized residuals

residuals, externally studentized residuals, or R-student residuals

$$e_i^* = \frac{e_i}{\sqrt{MSE(i)(1 - h_i)}} \qquad (2.68)$$

where $MSE(i)$ is the square root of the mean square error with the ith data point removed. Fortunately a simple relationship exists between MSE and $MSE(i)$ so that e_i^* can be recalculated without having to fit a new regression after each data point is removed

$$MSE(i) = \frac{\left[(n - p)MSE - \dfrac{e_i^2}{1 - h_i}\right]}{n - p - 1} \qquad (2.69)$$

Upper bounds for externally studentized residuals have not been developed. Externally studentized residuals are distributed as a Student's t-distribution with $n - p - 1$ degrees of freedom. Thus in the case of a single outlier observation, a quick test would be to compare the value of the external studentized residual to the appropriate t-distribution value, although as Cook and Weisberg (1999) point out, because of issues with multiplicity a more appropriate comparison would be Student's t-distribution with α/n critical value and $n - p - 1$ degrees of freedom. In general, however, a yardstick of ± 2 or ± 2.5 is usually used as a critical value to flag suspect observations.

Identification of Influential Observations

Influential observations are ones that significantly affect the values of the parameter estimates, their standard errors, and the predicted values. One statistic used to detect influential observations has already been presented, the HAT matrix. An obvious way to detect these observations is to remove an observation one at a time and examine how the recalculated parameter estimates compare to their original values. This is the row deletion approach to influence diagnostics and on first glance it would appear that this process requires n-iterations—a numerically intensive procedure. Statisticians, however, have derived equations that directly reflect the influence of the ith observation without iteration. One useful diagnostic is DFFITS

$$DFFITS = \sqrt{\left[\frac{h_i}{1 - h_i}\right]}\left[\frac{e_i}{\sqrt{MSE(i)(1 - h_i)}}\right] \qquad (2.70)$$

which measures the impact of deleting the ith data point on predicted values and is the number of standard errors that the ith predicted value changes if that observation is

deleted from the data set. DFFITS are basically studentized deleted residuals scaled according to the leverage of the ith observation.

Another useful statistic that is used is called DFBETAS,

$$\begin{aligned} DFBETAS &= \frac{\beta - \beta(i)}{\sqrt{MSE(i)(x^Tx)^{-1}}} \\ &= \frac{(x^Tx)^{-1}x_i^Te_i}{(1 - h_i)\sqrt{MSE(i)(x^Tx)^{-1}}} \end{aligned} \qquad (2.71)$$

where $\beta(i)$ denotes the least squares parameter estimates with the ith data point removed. DFBETAS measures the number of standard errors that a parameter estimate changes with the ith observation deleted from the data set.

A large change in DFBETAS is indicative that the ith observation has a significant impact on the value of a regression coefficient. As a yardstick for small to moderate sample sizes, DFFITS and DFBETAS greater than ± 1 are indicative of influential observations. For larger sample sizes a smaller absolute value may be needed as a yardstick: one rule of thumb is $2n^{-0.5}$ for DFBETAS, and $2\sqrt{p}/n$ for DFFITS (Belsley, Kuh, and Welsch, 1980).

One problem with DFBETAS is that there will be $n \times p$ DFBETAS for the analyst to examine, which can be tedious to examine. Cook's distance, D_i, is a composite score that assesses the influence an observation has on the set of regression parameters and is computed by

$$D_i = \left(\frac{e_i^2}{(1 - h_i)^2}\right)\left(\frac{h_i}{p \times MSE}\right). \qquad (2.72)$$

As its name implies, Cook's distance is a distance measure that represents the standardized distance in p-dimensional space between β and $\beta(i)$. A large value of D_i indicates that the ith observation has undue influence on the *set* of regression parameters. Once an observation has been identified as exerting undue influence then DFBETAS can be examined to determine which regression parameters are affected. Interpreting Cook's distance and finding a yardstick is much more difficult than DFFITS or DFBETAS. Myers (1986) recommends interpreting a particular Cook's distance as follows: If Cook's D is about 50% of the F-value from an $F_{p, n-p}$ distribution then deletion of the ith observation moves the centroid of confidence region to the 50% confidence region.

Although DFFITS and DFBETAS provide a flag that the ith observation has an impact on the value of the jth regression coefficient, they do not give any indication of whether the influence that is exerted is positive or negative. Like the HAT matrix, a large DFFITS or DFBETAS is not necessarily a bad thing. It is the combination of a high leverage observation in the presence of large DFFITS or DFBETAS that results in erratic regression parameter estimates.

The variance-covariance of linear regression parameter estimates is given by $\sigma^2(x^Tx)^{-1}$ and a statistic that summarizes the properties of the variance/covariance matrix is the generalized variance of the regression parameters

$$GV = |Var(\beta)| = |MSE(x^Tx)^{-1}| \qquad (2.73)$$

where $|.|$ is the determinant function. Precise estimation of the regression parameters results in small determinants or GV. COVRATIO measures the ratio of the variance/covariance without and with the ith observation and is calculated using

$$COVRATIO = \frac{|MSE(i)(x_{(i)}^T x_{(i)})^{-1}|}{|MSE(x^Tx)^{-1}|} \qquad (2.74)$$

where $x_{(i)}$ denotes the x matrix without the ith observation. COVRATIOs greater than one are indicative that the ith observation improves the performance of the model over what would be seen without the observation in the data set. A combination of high leverage and a small residual results in an observation that improves the properties of the regression parameters. As a yardstick, observations with $COVRATIO > 1 + 3p/n$ or $COVRATIO < 1 - 3p/n$ (applies only when $n > 3p$) show undue influence on the generalized variance of the regression parameters.

Unless the number of observations is small, influence diagnostics are best examined graphically. Gray (1986) recommended for the linear model that a useful diagnostic plot is h_i against e_i^2/SSE, the normalized residual for the ith subject. Such a plot is called an L-R triangle for leverage and residual. Regardless of the data set, the L-R triangle data should show low leverage and small residuals such that the majority of the data cluster near $(p/n, 0)$. Cases will that have undue influence will be discordant from the bulk of the data. Obviously, plots of h_i against any influence diagnostics will find utility. Lastly, bubble plots having one of the other influence diagnostics, such as COVRATIO, may be used to gain a trivariable influence plot.

Belsley et al. (1980) present many more diagnostics, including ones for multiple row deletion, but most of the ones that have been presented herein are easily obtained using most, if not all, linear regression software. One last point is that these diagnostics are not independent of

each other, they are often correlated themselves and will show overlap in observations that are flagged.

So What Now?

Once an outlier or an influential observation is detected what can be done about it? Obviously an observation can be deleted, but clearly what is needed is a further examination of why that observation was flagged in the first place. If nothing of interest arises in re-examination of the data points, then there is no sound rationale for removal of the observation in question. One might then consider that the model itself is wrong. This is a very important concept because model misspecification is often discovered through outlier and influential observation analysis. Lastly, one might try a weighted linear regression model where the weights are proportional to the inverse of the HAT matrix. In other words, influential observations are given less weight in the model than uninfluential observations. Alternatively, all observations could have weights equal to '1,' except the data point(s) in question which is given a much smaller weight. In this manner the observation is not removed from the data set, but is simply given less weight in the modeling process.

Given the level of research activity devoted to identification of influential observations, considerably less effort has been devoted to what to do about them. Under guidelines (E9: Statistical Principles for Clinical Trials) developed by the International Conference on Harmonisation of Technical Requirements for Registration of Pharmaceuticals for Human Use (1997), more commonly called ICH, several principles for dealing with outliers or influential observations are presented. First, data analysis should be defined prior to analyzing the data, preferable before data collection even begins. The data analysis plan should specify in detail how outliers or influential observations will be handled. Second, in the absence of a plan for handling outliers or influential observations, the analyst should do two analyses, one with and the other without the points in question, and the differences between the results should be presented in the discussion of the results. Lastly, identification of outliers should be based on statistical, as well as scientific rationale, and that the context of the data point should dictate how to deal with it.

Example

Port et al. (1991) administered 5-fluorouracil (5-FU) treatments to 26 patients with advanced carcinomas of various origin under a variety of doses and treatment schedules. Monotherapy was given as 5-day courses weekly for 3 weeks, once weekly for three weeks, or once every 3 weeks. Combination therapy with methotrexate (MTX) was given once every 2 to 3 weeks. Serial blood samples for pharmacokinetic analysis were collected on Day 1 and 5-FU clearance was determined by noncompartmental methods. Some patients had multiple cycles of therapy and for those subjects only data from the first cycle was included in this analysis. The following covariates were available for analysis: sex, age, body surface area (BSA), 5-FU dose, and presence or absence of MTX. Scatter plots and box and whisker plots are shown in Fig. 2.6 with the data presented in Table 2.3.

Of interest was to determine whether a useful model relating 5-FU clearance and patient demographics could be developed for possible use in future individualized dosing regimens. Nonparametric correlation analysis between the covariates revealed that sex and BSA were correlated ($r = -0.4689$, $p = 0.0157$), a not surprising result since both males and females were enrolled in the study and males (which were coded as '1') would be expected to have higher BSA than females (which were coded as '0'). The sign of the correlation would change to positive had the coding been reversed. Also, 5-FU dose was correlated with presence or absence of MTX ($r = 0.4382$, $p = 0.0251$). This too was not surprising

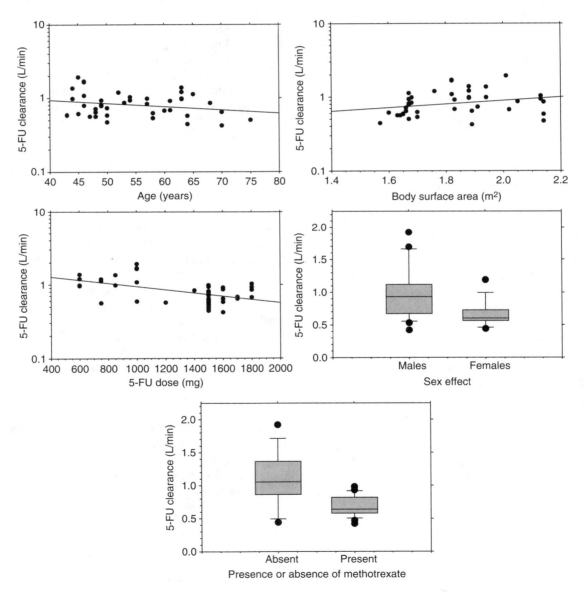

Figure 2.6 Scatter plots and box and whisker plots of 5-fluorouracil (5-FU) clearance as a function of patient demographics. Data presented in Table 2.3. Solid line is the least squares fit to the data. Note that some plots are shown on a log-scale.

Table 2.3 Treatment groups, patient demographics, and 5-FU clearance values from Port et al. (1991).

Subject	Sex	Age (Years)	BSA (m²)	Dose (mg)	MTX	5-FU CL (L/min)
1	1	43	1.65	1500	1	0.58
2	1	48	1.63	750	0	0.56
3	1	50	2.14	1500	1	0.47
4	0	68	2.14	1800	1	0.85
5	1	50	1.91	1500	1	0.73
6	1	48	1.66	1500	1	0.71
7	1	45	1.6	1500	1	0.61
8	0	53	2.05	1600	1	0.86
9	0	44	1.94	850	0	1.36
10	0	58	1.7	1500	1	0.53
11	1	61	1.83	1600	1	0.91
12	0	49	1.67	1500	1	0.81
13	0	70	1.89	1600	1	0.64
14	0	47	1.64	1500	1	0.56
15	0	63	1.88	600	0	0.98
16	1	46	1.67	1500	1	0.79
17	0	45	2.01	1000	0	1.92
18	0	46	1.82	1000	0	1.65
19	0	57	1.68	1400	1	0.83
20	1	52	1.76	750	0	1.19
21	1	64	1.27	1200	1	0.57
22	0	65	1.67	750	0	1.12
23	1	75	1.67	1500	0	0.5
24	1	64	1.57	1500	0	0.44
25	0	60	2.02	1800	0	0.67
26	0	54	2.13	1800	0	0.93

Legend: Sex: 0 = males, 1 = females; MTX: 0 = no methotrexate given, 1=methotrexate given; CL, clearance.

given the study design in that patients who were treated with MTX were also the ones who were treated with relatively high dose 5-FU. The magnitude of the correlations indicated that mild collinearity may be a problem during the analysis.

Examination of the univariate distribution of 5-FU clearance revealed it to be skewed and not normally distributed suggesting that any regression analysis based on least squares will be plagued by non-normally distributed residuals. Hence, Ln-transformed 5-FU clearance was used as the dependent variable in the analyses. Prior to analysis, age was standardized to 60 years old, BSA was standardized to $1.83 \, m^2$, and dose was standardized to 1000 mg. A p-value less than 0.05 was considered to be statistically significant. The results from the simple linear regressions of the data (Table 2.4) revealed that sex, 5-FU dose, and presence or absence of MTX were statistically significant.

Multiple regression of all covariates (Table 2.5) had a condition number of 1389, indicating that the model had little collinearity. Notice that presence or absence of MTX as a variable in the model was not statistically significant, possibly a result of the collinearity between presence or absence of MTX and 5-FU dose. Since with

Table 2.4 Results of simple linear regression analysis of the data in Table 2.3 using Ln-transformed 5-FU clearance as the dependent variable.

Variable	Intercept	SE(Intercept)	Slope	SE(Slope)	R2
Sex	−0.0922	0.0916	**−0.346**	0.135	0.2158
Age	0.366	0.453	−0.564	0.408	0.0738
BSA	**−1.416**	0.620	1.188	0.628	0.1297
Dose	0.428	0.264	**−0.505**	0.190	0.2278
MTX	−0.0763	0.107	**−0.305**	0.140	0.1640

Note: Bolded values were statistically significant at $p < 0.05$.

Table 2.5 Results of multivariate linear regression of data in Table 2.3 using Ln-transformed 5-FU clearance as the dependent variable.

Variable	Estimate	SE(Estimate)	t-value	p-value
Intercept	0.104	0.696	0.15	0.883
Sex	−0.247	0.123	−2.00	0.059
Age	−0.490	0.323	−1.51	0.146
BSA	0.995	0.589	1.69	0.106
Dose	−4.78	0.212	−2.26	0.035
MTX	−0.061	0.146	−0.42	0.681

Note: R^2 was 0.5750 with an adjusted coefficient of determination of 0.4688.

the univariate models, 5-FU dose had a higher coefficient of determination than presence or absence of MTX, a second multivariate model was examined where presence or absence of MTX was removed from the model. Table 2.6 presents the results. Now, age was not statistically significant. This variable was removed from the model and the reduced model's results are shown in Table 2.7. Sex was almost significant and it

Table 2.6 Results of multivariate linear regression of data in Table 2.3 using Ln-transformed 5-FU clearance as the dependent variable without MTX included in the model.

Variable	Estimate	SE(Estimate)	t-value	p-value
Intercept	0.025	0.656	0.04	0.971
Sex	−0.246	0.121	−2.04	0.054
Age	−0.452	0.305	−1.48	0.153
BSA	1.076	0.545	1.97	0.062
Dose	−0.535	0.160	−3.35	0.003

Note: R^2 was 0.5713 with an adjusted coefficient of determination of 0.4897.

Table 2.7 Results of multivariate linear regression of data in Table 2.3 using Ln-transformed 5-FU clearance as the dependent variable without MTX and age included in the model.

Variable	Estimate	SE(Estimate)	t-value	p-value
Intercept	0.522	0.558	0.04	0.971
Sex	−0.219	0.122	−1.79	0.087
BSA	1.176	0.556	2.12	0.046
Dose	−0.580	0.161	−3.60	0.002

Note: R^2 was 0.5263 with an adjusted coefficient of determination of 0.4617.

Table 2.8 Results of multivariate linear regression of data in Table 2.3 using Ln-transformed 5-FU clearance as the dependent variable without MTX, age, and sex included in the model.

Variable	Estimate	SE(Estimate)	t-value	p-value
Intercept	−1.004	0.512	1.96	0.062
BSA	1.622	0.520	3.12	0.005
Dose	−0.621	0.167	−3.73	0.001

Note: The coefficient of determination was 0.4574 with an adjusted coefficient of determination of 0.4102.

was decided to remove this variable from the model. The resulting model and influence diagnostics are shown in Table 2.8 and Table 2.9, respectively. Influence plots, including an L-R plot, are shown in Fig. 2.7. The condition number of this model was 451 indicating the new model had good parameter stability.

Examination of the collinearity diagnostics indicated that two of the observations had HAT values greater than the yardstick of $2 \times 3/26$ or 0.23. One studentized residual was greater than ± 2 (Subject 3). This subject also had a DFBETA of 1.023 for the intercept and −1.084 for the parameter associated with BSA, indicating that these parameters would change by more than 1 standard error should this subject be removed

from the data set. This subject had a COVRATIO of 0.444, much lower than the critical value of 0.65, and the largest absolute DFFITs in the data set. Clearly there was something unusual about this subject. At this point, one might then go back and examine what was unique about this subject. Although not the lowest clearance observed in the study, this subject did have the second lowest value. Why? Since this data set was taken from the literature this question cannot be answered. For purposes of this analysis, it was decided that Subject 3 would be removed from the data set. The resulting model after removal of Subject 3, as shown in Table 2.10 with influence diagnostics shown in Table 2.11, resulted in a model accounting for more than 59% of the total variance with all model parameters being statistically significant. The condition number of the final model was 481 indicating the model to be quite stable. Examination of the influence diagnostics showed that now possibly Subject 2 showed undue influence. Some modelers would indeed remove this subject from the model, but removal of Subject 2 is not advised given the sample size of the analysis. So, the final model was one where BSA positively affected 5-FU clearance and dose negatively affected 5-FU clearance, an indication of Michaelis–Menten elimination kinetics.

Table 2.9 Influence diagnostics for the regression model presented in Table 2.8.

Subject	Residual	R-Student	HAT	COV Ratio	DFFITS	DFBETAs Intercept	BSA	DOSE
1	−0.071	−0.247	0.071	1.220	−0.068	−0.033	0.041	−0.031
2	−0.555	−2.249	0.156	0.728	−0.967	−0.582	0.201	0.750
3	−0.716	**−3.130**	0.148	**0.444**	**−1.305**	**1.023**	**−1.084**	−0.041
4	0.064	0.237	0.182	1.386	0.112	−0.089	0.074	0.048
5	−0.071	−0.247	0.055	1.199	−0.059	0.025	−0.024	−0.016
6	0.123	0.428	0.068	1.196	0.116	0.053	−0.066	0.052
7	0.024	0.084	0.089	1.253	0.026	0.015	−0.018	0.012
8	0.031	0.109	0.107	1.277	0.038	−0.027	0.025	0.010
9	0.120	0.442	0.159	1.322	0.192	−0.022	0.100	−0.152
10	−0.205	−0.719	0.058	1.131	−0.178	−0.062	0.081	−0.080
11	0.282	0.999	0.059	1.063	0.249	−0.044	0.004	0.141
12	0.246	0.867	0.065	1.105	0.229	0.099	−0.125	0.103
13	−0.123	−0.428	0.063	1.189	−0.111	0.042	−0.028	−0.055
14	−0.097	−0.340	0.074	1.215	−0.096	−0.048	0.059	−0.043
15	−0.310	−1.239	**0.245**	1.236	−0.706	−0.054	−0.259	0.637
16	0.221	0.776	0.065	1.127	0.205	0.088	−0.112	0.092
17	0.496	1.948	0.142	0.826	0.792	−0.265	0.540	−0.517
18	0.513	1.946	0.081	0.772	0.578	0.082	0.145	−0.415
19	0.199	0.694	0.053	1.131	0.164	0.081	−0.083	0.040
20	0.084	0.307	0.151	1.329	0.130	0.041	0.015	−0.111
21	0.062	0.247	**0.286**	**1.588**	0.157	0.145	−0.144	0.009
22	0.103	0.377	0.151	1.321	0.159	0.083	−0.018	−0.129
23	−0.237	−0.836	0.065	1.113	−0.221	−0.095	0.120	−0.099
24	−0.276	−1.001	0.102	1.113	−0.337	−0.209	0.250	−0.144
25	−0.068	−0.245	0.130	1.302	−0.095	0.061	−0.043	−0.055
26	0.162	0.606	0.176	1.320	0.281	−0.220	0.181	0.125

Note: Bolded data indicate data that are questionable.

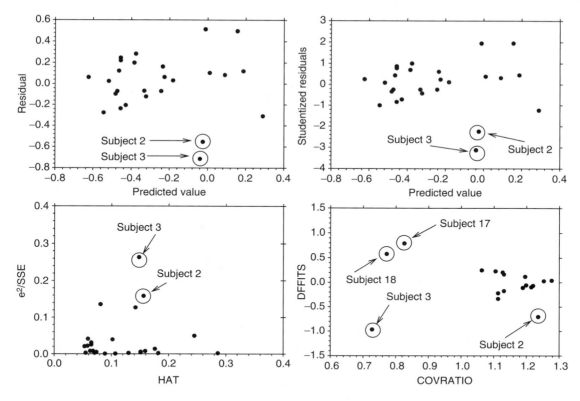

Figure 2.7   Residual plots and influence plots for final linear model shown in Table 2.8 using data presented in Table 2.3. Suspect values are noted in the plots.

CONDITIONAL MODELS

Up to now it has been assumed that x is fixed and under control of the experimenter, e.g., the dose of drug given to subjects or sex of subjects in a study, and it is of interest to make prediction models for some dependent variable Y or make inferences on the regression parameters. There are times when x is not fixed, but is a random variable, denoted X. An example would be a regression analysis of weight vs. total clearance, or age vs. volume of distribution. In both cases, it is possible for the experimenter to control age or weight, but more than likely these are samples randomly drawn from subjects in the population.

Table 2.10   Results of multivariate linear regression of data in Table 2.31 using Ln-transformed 5-FU clearance as the dependent variable using only BSA and 5-FU dose with subject 3 removed from the analysis.

Variable	Estimate	SE(Estimate)	t-value	p-value
Intercept	−1.445	0.458	−3.16	0.0045
BSA	2.102	0.468	4.49	0.0002
Dose	−0.616	0.142	−4.34	0.0003

Note: The coefficient of determination was 0.5950 with an adjusted coefficient of determination of 0.5581.

As subjects enroll in a study, the experimenter usually cannot control how old they are or what their weight is exactly. They are random. Still, in this case one may wish to either make inferences on the parameter estimates or predictions of future Y values. Begin by assuming that Y can be modeled using a simple linear model and that X and Y have a joint probability density function that is bivariate normal

$$f_{xy}(X,Y) =$$

$$\frac{1}{2\pi\sigma_X\sigma_Y\sqrt{1-\rho^2}} \exp\left\{-\frac{1}{2(1-\rho^2)}\left[\left(\frac{X-\mu_X}{\sigma_X}\right)^2\right.\right.$$

$$\left.\left. -2\rho\left(\frac{X-\mu_X}{\sigma_X}\right)\left(\frac{Y-\mu_Y}{\sigma_Y}\right) + \left(\frac{Y-\mu_Y}{\sigma_Y}\right)^2\right]\right\} \quad (2.75)$$

where μ_x and μ_y are the population means for X and Y, respectively, σ_x and σ_y are the standard deviations for X and Y, respectively, and ρ is the correlation between X and Y which can be expressed as

$$\rho = \frac{\sigma_{XY}}{\sigma_X\sigma_Y} \quad (2.76)$$

Table 2.11   Influence diagnostics for the model presented in Table 2.10.

Subject	Residual	R-Student	HAT	COV Ratio	DFFITS	DFBETAs Intercept	BSA	DOSE
1	−0.067	−0.274	0.071	1.225	−0.076	−0.035	0.043	−0.034
2	−0.541	**−2.696**	0.156	**0.559**	**−1.161**	−0.680	0.244	0.900
4	−0.062	−0.277	0.208	**1.436**	−0.142	0.116	−0.099	−0.058
5	−0.135	−0.555	0.062	1.173	−0.142	0.069	−0.067	−0.036
6	0.124	0.510	0.068	1.189	0.138	0.060	−0.075	0.062
7	0.041	0.170	0.089	1.257	0.053	0.030	−0.036	0.023
8	−0.071	−0.298	0.124	1.295	−0.112	0.084	−0.080	−0.029
9	0.052	0.225	0.166	1.369	0.100	−0.018	0.055	−0.078
10	−0.214	−0.888	0.058	1.093	−0.220	−0.069	0.091	−0.099
11	0.239	0.995	0.062	1.067	0.255	−0.060	0.023	0.142
12	0.244	1.022	0.065	1.063	0.270	0.110	−0.138	0.121
13	−0.182	−0.755	0.068	1.139	−0.205	0.089	−0.066	−0.098
14	−0.090	−0.372	0.074	1.218	−0.105	−0.051	0.063	−0.047
15	−0.361	−1.760	**0.249**	1.014	−1.015	−0.031	−0.392	0.906
16	0.219	0.913	0.065	1.095	0.241	0.098	−0.124	0.109
17	0.409	1.899	0.155	0.845	0.812	−0.319	0.578	−0.505
18	0.476	2.168	0.083	0.684	0.654	0.053	0.189	−0.461
19	0.196	0.805	0.053	1.108	0.190	0.088	−0.090	0.046
20	0.064	0.273	0.152	1.342	0.116	0.033	0.015	−0.099
21	0.168	0.805	**0.305**	**1.510**	0.533	0.497	−0.491	0.028
22	0.106	0.458	0.151	1.315	0.193	0.096	−0.021	−0.156
23	−0.238	−0.994	0.065	1.071	−0.263	−0.107	0.135	−0.118
24	−0.251	−1.075	0.103	1.092	−0.364	−0.224	0.266	−0.155
25	−0.163	−0.702	0.145	1.254	−0.288	0.197	−0.148	−0.161
26	0.039	0.172	0.202	1.434	0.087	−0.070	0.060	0.036

Note: Bolded data indicate data that were questionable.

where σ_{XY} is the covariance between X and Y. Further details regarding joint probability densities and conditional inference is presented in the book appendix. What is of interest is to find the conditional density function of Y given X. The probability density function for the conditional distribution of Y given X is

$$f_{XY}(Y|X) = \frac{f_{XY}(X,Y)}{f_X(X)}, \qquad (2.77)$$

where $f_X(X)$ is the marginal density of X, which is assumed normal in distribution. Hence, the conditional distribution of Y given X is the ratio of the bivariate normal density function to a univariate normal distribution function. After a little algebra then

$$f_{XY}(Y|X) = \frac{1}{\sigma_{XY}\sqrt{2\pi}} \exp\left[-\frac{1}{2}\left(\frac{Y - \theta_0 - \theta_1 X}{\sigma_{Y|X}}\right)^2\right] \qquad (2.78)$$

where

$$\theta_0 = \mu_Y - \mu_X \rho \frac{\sigma_Y}{\sigma_X}, \qquad (2.79)$$

$$\theta_1 = \rho \frac{\sigma_Y}{\sigma_X}, \qquad (2.80)$$

and

$$\sigma_{Y|X}^2 = \sigma_Y^2(1 - \rho^2). \qquad (2.81)$$

Notice that two assumptions have been made: normality of the responses and constant variance. The result is that the conditional distribution itself is normally distributed with mean $\hat{\theta}_0 + \hat{\theta}_1 x$ and variance $\sigma_{Y|X}^2$. Thus, the joint distribution function at any level of X can be "sliced" and still have a normal distribution. Also, any conditional probability distribution function of Y has the same standard deviation after scaling the resulting probability distribution function to have an area of 1.

If data are collected from a random population (X, Y) from a bivariate normal distribution and predictions about Y given X are desired, then from the previous paragraphs it may be apparent that the linear model assuming fixed x is applicable because the observations are independent, normally distributed, and have constant variance with mean $\theta_0 + \theta_1 X$. Similar arguments can be made if inferences are to be made on X given Y. Thus, if X and Y are random, all calculations and inferential methods remain the same as if X were fixed.

ERROR-IN-VARIABLES REGRESSION

One assumption until now has been that the dependent and independent variables are measured without error. The impact of measurement error on the regression parameter estimates depends on whether the error affects the dependent or independent variable. When Y has measurement error, the effect on the regression model is not problematic if the measurement errors are uncorrelated and unbiased. In this case the linear model becomes

$$Y = \theta_0 + \sum_{k=1}^{p-1} \theta_k x_k + \varepsilon + \kappa \qquad (2.82)$$

where κ is the measurement error in Y. This model can be rewritten as

$$Y = \theta_0 + \sum_{k=1}^{p-1} \theta_k x_k + \varepsilon^* \qquad (2.83)$$

where ε^* is the sum of the measurement error and model error. Equation (2.83) is functionally equivalent to Eq. (2.5). Thus, measurement error in Y is absorbed by the model error term and standard OLS techniques may be used.

Before proceeding, a distinction needs to be made between X being simply a random variable and X being random due to random measurement error. This distinction is important and the question is sometimes asked, what's the difference? If X is random but measured accurately, the experimenter has no control over its measurement, and its value may vary from study to study. An example of this might be the weight of subjects in a clinical study. If this random variable X is measured without error, then an exact, accurate measurement of X can be obtained only for *that* study. If, however, X is random due to measurement error, then repeated measurement of X within the same study will result in differing values of X each time X is measured and a misleading relationship between X and Y will be obtained.

One other distinction needs to be made between random X and X with random measurement error. Neither implies that X is biased. Bias implies a constant effect across all measurements. For example, if a weight scale is not calibrated properly and when no one is standing on it, the scale records a measure of 1 kg, then when any person is measured the weight will be biased high by 1 kg. This is not the type of measurement error that is being discussed here because any constant bias in a measuring instrument will be reflected in the estimate of the intercept. Random measurement error means that repeated measuring of a variable will vary from measurement to measurement even though its value has not changed. An example of this might be when a patient goes to the doctor's office and his weight is measured at 180 lbs. The nurse forgets to write down the value and so the patient is weighed again. This time the weight is 179 lbs. That patient hasn't lost a pound in the few moments between measurements; they are still the same weight. But due to random measurement error, their weight changed from one reading to the next.

If both X and Y are random variables and X is measured without random error, then all the theory presented for the case of fixed x is still applicable if the following conditions are true:

1. The conditional distribution for each of the Y_i given X_i is independent and normally distributed with conditional mean $\theta_0 + \theta_1 X_i$ and conditional variance σ^2, and
2. The X_i are independent random variables whose distribution does not depend on the model parameters θ or σ^2.

This was discussed in the previous section. In contrast, when the independent variable has measurement error, then the analyst observes

$$X_k = x_k + \delta_k \qquad (2.84)$$

where X_k is the observed value of x_k and δ_k is the vector of measurement errors for x_k. It is usual to assume that $\delta \sim N(0, \sigma_k^2)$ with independent measurement errors. The model is then

$$Y = \theta_0 + \sum_{k=1}^{p-1} \theta_k x_k + \varepsilon. \qquad (2.85)$$

Since X_k is observed, not the true value of x_k, the true value must be replaced with the observed value. Then the linear model becomes

$$Y = \theta_0 + \sum_{k=1}^{p-1} \theta_k (X - \delta)_k + \varepsilon \qquad (2.86)$$

which can be expanded to

$$Y = \theta_0 + \sum_{k=1}^{p-1} \theta_k X_k + (\varepsilon - \theta_k \delta_k). \qquad (2.87)$$

Equation (2.87) looks like an ordinary regression model with predictor variable X and model error term $(\varepsilon - \hat{\theta}_k \delta_k)$

$$Y = \theta_0 + \sum_{k-1}^{p-1} \theta_k X_k + \varepsilon^*. \tag{2.88}$$

However, the expected value of ε^* is zero with variance $\sigma^2 + \sum_{k=1}^{p-1} \theta_k^2 \sigma_k^2$. Thus the variance of the measurement errors are propagated to the error variance term, thereby inflating it. An increase in the residual variance is not the only effect on the OLS model. If X is a random variable due to measurement error such that when there is a linear relationship between x_k and Y, then X is negatively correlated with the model error term. If OLS estimation procedures are then used, the regression parameter estimates are both biased and inconsistent (Neter et al., 1996).

Obtaining unbiased and consistent parameter estimates under these conditions using OLS is difficult. Measurement error in x is traditionally handled by two types of models:

- Classical error models and calibration models, where the relationship between X given x is modeled, and
- Regression calibration models, where the relationship between x given X is modeled.

Alternative models may be developed to include additional covariates which are not measured with error, e.g., $X = f(R,Z)$. The classical model is used when an attempt to measure x is made but cannot be done so due to various measurement errors. An example of this is the measurement of blood pressure. There is only one true blood pressure reading for a subject at a particular point in time, but due to minor calibration errors in the instrument, transient increases in blood pressure due to diet, etc., possible recording errors and reading errors by the nurse, etc., blood pressure is a composite variable that can vary substantially both within and between days. In this case it makes sense to try and model the observed blood pressure using Eq. (2.84). Under this model, the expected value of X is x. In regression calibration problems, the focus is on the distribution of x given X. For purposes herein, the focus will be on the classical error model. The reader is referred to Fuller (1987) and Carroll et al. (1995) for a more complete exposition of the problem.

In the pharmacokinetic arena, there are many cases where the independent variable is measured with error and a classical measurement model is needed. Some examples include in vitro–in vivo correlations, such as the relationship between Log P and volume of distribution (Kaul and Ritschel, 1990), in vivo clearance estimates based on in vitro microsomal enzyme studies

(Iwatsubo et al., 1996; Iwatsubo et al., 1997), or the estimation of drug clearance based on creatinine clearance (Bazunga et al., 1998; Lefevre et al., 1997). In these three examples, log P, in vitro clearance, and creatinine clearance, all have some measurement error associated with them that may be large enough to produce significantly biased regression parameter estimates.

Before a solution to the problem is presented, it is necessary to examine what happens when the measurement error in x is ignored and the SLR model applies. When a classical error model applies, the effect of measurement error in x is attenuation of the slope and corresponding inflation of the intercept. To illustrate this, consider the linear model $Y = x + 10$, where x is a set of triplicate measurements at {50, 100, 250, 500, 750, 1000}. Y is not measured with error, only x has error. Figure 2.8 plots the resulting least squares fit with increasing measurement error in x. As the measurement error variance increases, the slope of the line decreases with increasing intercept. Sometimes the attenuation is so severe that bias correction techniques must be used in place of OLS estimates.

Let's assume the SLR model applies, where x has mean μ_x and variance σ_{x^2} and $\varepsilon \sim N(0, \sigma^2)$. The predictor x cannot be observed, but X can, where $X = x + \delta$ with δ being the difference between the observed and true values having mean 0 and variance σ_k^2. Thus, the total variance of X is $\sigma_{x^2+\sigma_k^2}$. Then the OLS estimate of the slope of Y on X is not $\hat{\theta}_1$, but

$$\hat{\theta}_1^* = \lambda \hat{\theta}_1 \tag{2.89}$$

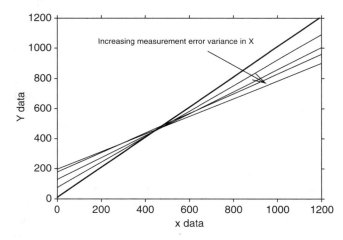

Figure 2.8 Effect of increasing measurement error in X on least squares fit. Heavy line is the true least squares fit to model $Y = x + 10$. Y has no measurement error associated with it. x has increasing degrees of measurement error as indicated by the direction of the arrow, the result being the slope is attenuated and the intercept is inflated.

where

$$\lambda = \frac{\sigma_x^2}{\sigma_x^2 + \sigma_k^2} < 1 \qquad (2.90)$$

The denominator in Eq. (2.90) represents the total variability of X, whereas the numerator is the variability in x, the true values. λ is sometimes called the attenuation factor or reliability factor and represents the proportion of variation in x found in X. The net effect of measurement variance of the predicted values is greater than when x has error in x is that $\hat{\theta}_1$ is attenuated towards zero and the no measurement error. Corresponding to this is that as the slope decreases, the intercept increases in response.

Measurement error causes double-trouble: attenuation of the slope and increased error about the regression line. However, when more complex error structures are assumed, such as when X is not an unbiased estimate of x or the variance of δ depends on x, then it is possible for the opposite effect to occur, e.g., $\hat{\theta}_1$ is inflated (Carroll, Ruppert, and Stefanski, 1995). Rarely are these alternative measurement error models examined, however. The bottom line is that measurement error in the predictors leads to biased estimates of the regression parameters, an effect that is dependent on the degree of measurement error relative to the distribution of the predictors.

Hodges and Moore (1972) showed for the linear model, the maximum bias introduced by measurement error in the predictors, assuming an additive error model, can be estimated by

$$\text{bias} = \hat{\theta} - (n-p-1)(x^T x)^{-1} U\hat{\theta}, \qquad (2.91)$$

where

$$U = \begin{bmatrix} \sigma_1^2 & & & 0 \\ & \sigma_2^2 & & \\ & & \ldots & \\ 0 & & & \sigma_k^2 \end{bmatrix} \qquad (2.92)$$

with the diagonal elements of U being the measurement error variance for the kth predictor variable. Bias estimates can be transformed to relative bias estimates by

$$\text{relative bias} = \frac{\text{bias}}{\hat{\theta}} \times 100\% \qquad (2.93)$$

If Eq. (2.93) indicates that severe bias is present in the parameter estimates, then the parameter estimates need to be bias-corrected. It should be mentioned, however, that correcting for bias is not without its downside.

There is a trade-off involved, the bias vs. variance trade-off, which states that by correcting for bias in measurement error models, the variance of the unbiased estimator increases relative to the biased estimator leading to larger confidence intervals. In general, for large sample sizes and for moderate attenuation correction, bias correction is beneficial. The reader is referred to Fuller (1987) for further details.

In the case of simple linear regression when λ is known, an unbiased estimate of the slope can be obtained by rearrangement of Eq. (2.89), i.e.,

$$\hat{\theta}_1 = \frac{\hat{\theta}_1^*}{\lambda}. \qquad (2.94)$$

Stefanski et al. (Carroll et al., 1996; Carroll, Ruppert, and Stefanski, 1995; Cook and Stefanski, 1994; Stefanski and Cook, 1995) present a "remeasurement method" called simulation-extrapolation (SIMEX), which is a Monte Carlo approach to estimating and reducing measurement error bias, in the same vein as the bootstrap is used to estimate sampling error. The advantage of the SIMEX algorithm is that it is valid for linear and nonlinear models and for complex measurement error structures, included heteroscedastic variance models. The method assumes that σ_{k^2}, the variance of the measurement error, is known to some degree of certainty. If σ_{k^2} is not known, then it must be estimated. If no estimate of σ_{k^2} can be obtained, then no method can be used to obtain unbiased parameter estimates.

The basic idea is to add random measurement error to the predictor variables using Monte Carlo and develop the relationship between measurement error and parameter estimates. Using this relationship, the parameter estimates for the case of no measurement error can then be extrapolated. When asked what does SIMEX offer over other methods in reducing the bias of parameter estimates in regression models, Stefanski (personal communication) responds by asking "does the bootstrap offer any advantage for computing the standard error of the sample mean?" Thus, SIMEX is analogous to bootstrap methods, i.e., it may be over-kill for simple problems or it may be the only solution but for complex problems.

SIMEX is easiest to understand in the linear regression case and its exposition will be as described by Carroll et al (1995). Begin by assuming the simple linear model. Recall that σ_x^2 represents the variance in x with no error and σ_k^2 is the measurement variance of X. Now suppose that there are m − 1 additional data sets in addition to the original data with each of these additional data sets having successively larger measurement error variances, i.e., $(1 + \lambda_m)\sigma_{k^2}$ where $0 = \lambda_1 > \lambda_2 > \lambda_3 > \ldots \lambda_M$. Then for each of these datasets the slope of the mth data set, $\hat{\theta}_{1,m}^*$, does not consistently estimate $\theta_{1,m}$ but instead estimates

$$\hat{\theta}_m^* = \frac{\theta_k \sigma_x^2}{\sigma_x^2 + (1 + \lambda_m)\sigma_k^2}. \qquad (2.95)$$

This problem can now be thought of as a nonlinear regression problem where $\hat{\theta}_m^*$ is regressed against λ_m. The regression parameters in the absence of measurement error can be obtained by extrapolating λ to -1. However, modeling Eq. (2.95) is not practical since σ_k^2 and σ_x^2 may not be known. Carroll et al. (1995) suggest that in their experience it is much easier to regress λ_m against $\hat{\theta}_{1,m}^*$ using a quadratic polynomial

$$\hat{\theta}_{1,m}^* = \gamma_0 + \gamma_1 \lambda_m + \gamma_2 \lambda_m^2 \qquad (2.96)$$

evaluated over the equally spaced interval $0 < \lambda_m \leq 2$. Estimation of the standard error of SIMEX parameter estimates can be calculated using the bootstrap or jackknife, a process which should not increase computing time to prohibitive levels given the current processor speed of most personal computers.

Therefore, the SIMEX algorithm is as follows. First a simulation step is performed:

1. Define $X(\lambda_m) = X_i + \sqrt{\lambda_m}\sigma_k Z$ where Z are independent, random variates with mean zero and variance 1.
2. For each data set, regression is done and the parameter estimates saved.
3. Repeat steps 1 and 2 many times (>100).
4. Calculate the average parameter estimate.
5. Following the extrapolation step regress the average parameter estimates vs. λ using a quadratic polynomial.
6. Extrapolate to $\lambda = -1$.

If the variance model is not homoscedastic, a suitable transformation needs to be found prior to performing the algorithm. Carroll et al. (1995) stress that the "*extrapolation step should be approached as any other modeling problem, with attention paid to the adequacy of the extrapolant based on theoretical considerations, residual analysis, and possible use of linearizing transformations*" and that "*extrapolation is risky in general even when model diagnostics fail to indicate problems.*"

As an example, consider the data presented by Lefevre et al. (1997). In that study, eight healthy subjects with normal renal function and fifteen patients with varying degrees of renal impairment were given an infusion of desirudin, the recombinant form of the naturally occurring anticoagulant hirudin, found in the European leech *Hirudo medicinalis*, with doses ranging from 0.125 to 0.5 mg/kg infused over a 30 min period. Serial blood samples were collected and the clearance of hirudin was calculated using noncompartmental methods. The raw data values were not reported in the publication, but the data were presented as a plot. This plot was re-analyzed by taking the X-Y coordinates for each data point and determining the associated X-Y value. The reanalyzed data are presented in Table 2.12 and plotted in Figure 2.9. Lefevre et al. (1997) reported that plasma clearance (CL) of hirudin could be related to creatinine clearance (CrCL) by the equation: $CL = 1.73 \times CrCL - 17.5$. The reanalyzed model gave OLS estimates of 1.71 $\pm$ 0.13 for the parameter associated with CrCL and -15.1 ± 9.3 mL/min for the intercept ($R^2 = 0.9058$, MSE = 442.9). Ignore for the moment that a better model might be a no-intercept model. Residual analysis suggested that the residuals were homoscedastic and that data weighting was unnecessary.

In order to use the SIMEX algorithm on this data, an estimate of the measurement variance for creatinine clearance must be obtained. In discussions with clinical chemists, the upper limit of measurement error associated with measuring serum or urine creatinine using the Jaffe Reaction is 5%. Assuming mean 24 hour values for urinary volume, urinary daily creatinine excretion, and serum creatinine of 1000 mL, 1.5 g, and 1.1 mg/dL, respectively, an approximate measurement error variance for creatinine clearance was found to be 60 $(mL/min)^2$.

Table 2.12 Desirudin clearance as a function of creatinine clearance.

Creatinine CL (mL/min)	Desirudin CL (mL/min)
8.22	13.61
9.79	17.33
25.07	16.09
24.28	19.80
25.07	23.51
27.42	27.23
36.19	29.21
44.41	47.03
44.26	56.93
58.75	70.54
63.45	133.66
76.37	105.20
82.25	134.90
82.64	141.09
93.21	102.72
96.34	170.79
107.70	148.51
105.74	170.79
106.14	199.26
111.23	195.54
125.72	170.79

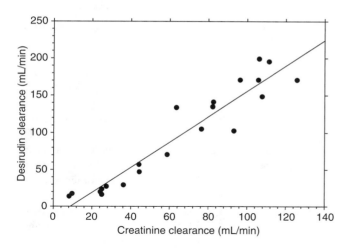

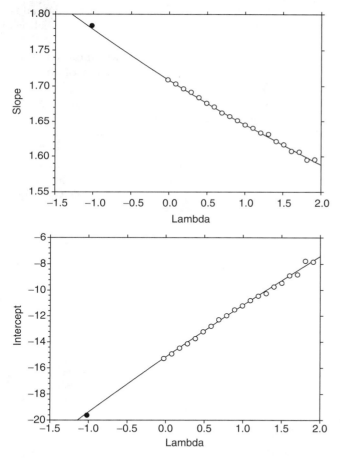

Figure 2.9 Plot of desirudin clearance as a function of creatinine clearance. Data redrawn from Lefevre et al. (1997). Solid line is the ordinary least squares fit.

Figure 2.10 Plot of SIMEX extrapolation to desirudin data show in Figure 2.9. Legend, • extrapolated value for slope (top) and intercept (bottom) at $\lambda = -1$; o, mean regression parameter using 100 iterations for each value of λ; solid line is the second order polynomial fit.

With this as an estimate of the assay measurement variance, the SIMEX algorithm was applied. Figure 2.10 plots the mean regression parameter against varying values of λ using 1000 iterations for each value of λ. Extrapolation of λ to -1 for both the slope and intercept leads to a SIMEX equation of

$$Cl = -19.4 + 1.78 \times CrCl, \qquad (2.97)$$

values not too different from the OLS estimates. The bias of the OLS estimates for slope and intercept using Eq. (2.91) was 0.06 and -4.1 mL/min, respectively, with a relative error of 23% and 4%, respectively. The jackknife SIMEX estimates for slope and intercept were 1.90 ± 0.43 (mean $\pm$ standard error of mean) and -21.0 ± 4.9 mL/min, respectively. Hence, the OLS estimates in this case were relatively unbiased.

Surprisingly, even though the parameter estimates obtained from regression of independent variables with measurement errors are biased, one can still obtain unbiased prediction estimates and corresponding confidence intervals. The reason is that even though X has measurement error, the model still applies to the data set on hand. The problem arises when one wishes to make predictions in another population or data set. In this case, three options are available (Buonaccorsi, 1995). First, carry out the regression of Y on X and calculate the predicted response ignoring the measurement error. Second, regress Y on X, recognizing that X is measured with error, but obtain a modified estimate of σ^2, and calculate a modified prediction interval. Third, correct for the measurement error of X and regress Y against the corrected X. The prediction interval then uses the parameters obtained from the corrected regression. Options 1 and 2 are reasonable assuming that the value to be predicted has the same measurement error distribution as the current data.

Buonaccorsi (1995) present equations for using Option 2 or 3 for the simple linear regression model. In summary, measurement error is not a problem if the goal of the model is prediction, but keep in mind the assumption that the predictor data set must have the same measurement error distribution as the modeling data set. The problem with using option 2 is that there are three variance terms to deal with: the residual variance of the model, σ^2, the uncertainty in θ, and the measurement error in the sample to be predicted. For complex models, the estimation of a corrected σ^2 may be difficult to obtain.

POLYNOMIAL REGRESSION

Sometimes one sees in the literature models of the form

$$Y = \theta_0 + \sum_{k=1}^{m} \theta_k x_k + \sum_{l=m+1}^{p-1} \theta_l x_1^q + \varepsilon \qquad (2.98)$$

where q is the power term, being described as 'nonlinear models.' This is in error because this model is still linear in the parameters. Even for the terms of degree higher than 1,

$$\frac{\partial}{\partial \theta_1} = q x_1^{q-1} \qquad (2.99)$$

which means that the parameters are independent of other model parameters. What may confuse some people is that polynomial models allow for curvature in the model, which may be interpreted as nonlinearity. Since polynomial models are only special cases of the linear model, their fitting requires no special algorithms or presents no new problems.

Often a polynomial may be substituted as a function if the true model is unknown. For example, a quadratic model may be substituted for an E_{max} model in a pharmacodynamic analysis or a quadratic or cubic function may be used in place of a power function

$$Y = \theta_1 X^{\theta_2} \qquad (2.100)$$

as shown in Fig. 2.11. It is almost impossible to distinguish the general *shape* of the quadratic model and power model. The change in intercept was added to differentiate the models graphically. Also note that an increase in the number of degrees of freedom in the model increases its flexibility in describing curvature as evidenced from the cubic model in Fig. 2.11.

Polynomial model development proceeds the same as model development when the degree of the equation is 1. However, model development generally proceeds first from simpler models and then terms of higher order are added later. Hence, if a quadratic term is added to a model, one should keep the linear term as well. The function of the linear term is to provide information about the basic shape of the curve, while the function of the quadratic term is to provide refinements to the model. The LRT or information criteria can be used to see if the additional terms improves the goodness of fit. Extreme caution should be made in extrapolating a polynomial function as the function may deviate significantly from the interval of data being studied. Also, higher order models (>2) are usually avoided because, even though they often provide good fits to the data, it is difficult to interpret their coefficients and the predictions they make are often erratic.

When two or more predictors are modeled using quadratic polynomials, responses surfaces of the type shown in Fig. 2.12 can be generated. These are extremely useful in examining how two variables interact to generate the response variable. They are also very useful for detecting and characterizing antagonism or synergy between drug combinations. Although not used commonly clinically, response surfaces are useful both *in vitro* and *in vivo*. models. See Greco et al. (1995) for details and Carter et al. (1985), Rockhold and Goldberg (1996), and Stewart (1996) for examples.

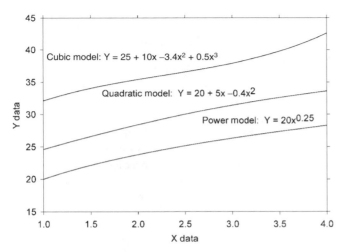

Figure 2.11 Plot of a cubic, quadratic, and power function.

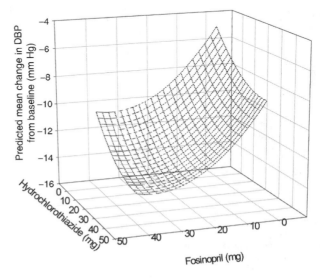

Figure 2.12 Quadratic response surface of predicted mean change from baseline in diastolic blood pressure following 8 weeks of randomized therapy to fosinopril and/or hydrochlorthiazide). Data presented in Pool et al. (1997).

HANDLING MISSING DATA

Anyone who does data analysis will eventually run into the problem of missing data, either the dependent variable is missing or one or more of the independent variables is missing. The problem of handling missing data is far too complex to cover it in its entirety within this book and many excellent books are available on the subject for readers who wish greater detail. These include books by Allison (2002), Little and Rubin (2002), and Schafer (1997).

It is worthwhile to consider the regulatory opinion on missing data, keeping in mind that these guidances were written with an eye toward formal statistical analysis, such as hypothesis testing, and not with an eye toward pharmacokinetic or pharmacodynamic modeling per se. Having said that, more and more modeling is done to support New Drug Applications and that in the future it is likely that increased scrutiny will be paid towards these issues. ICH E9 (1998) states that missing data is a potential source of bias and as such every effort should be done to collect the data in the first place. The guidance also recognizes that despite best efforts, missing data is a fact of life in clinical studies. Also, trial results are valid "*provided the methods for dealing with missing data are sensible, . . . particularly those pre-defined in the protocol.*" Unfortunately no recommendations are made in the guideline on what those "methods" are. The guideline does state that no universal method for handling missing data is available and that any analysis based on data containing missing values should also have a corresponding sensitivity analysis to see what effect the method of data handling has on the analysis results.

The Committee for Proprietary Medicinal Products (CPMP) (2001) has also issued a points to consider document related to missing data that expands on the ICH E9 guideline. The CPMP document is mainly concerned with the issue of bias and how missing data affects detecting and estimating treatment effects. The CPMP does not generally accept analyses where all missing data is deleted and only data with complete cases is analyzed. They recommend that all efforts be directed at avoiding missing data in the first place, something that seems intuitively obvious but needs to be restated for its importance. The CPMP also recommends that whatever method used to handle missing data be stated a priori, before seeing the data, in a data analysis plan or the statistical methods section of the study protocol. The final report should include documentation on any deviations from the analysis plan and defend the use of the pre-specified method for handling missing data. Lastly, a sensitivity analysis should be included in the final report indicating the impact of the missing data

handling procedure on treatment outcomes. This may be as simple as a complete case analysis versus imputed data analysis (which will be discussed later).

Types of Missing Data and Definitions

Little and Rubin (2002) define three types of missing data mechanisms. The first and most restrictive is missing completely at random (MCAR) in which cases that are missing are indistinguishable from cases that have complete data. For example, if a sample for drug analysis was broken in the centrifuge after collection and could not be analyzed, then this sample would be MCAR. If the data are MCAR then missing data techniques such as casewise deletion are valid. Unfortunately, data are rarely MCAR.

Missing at random (MAR), which is a weaker assumption than MCAR, is where cases of missing data differ from cases with complete data but the pattern of missingness is predictable from other variables in the dataset. For example, suppose in a Phase 3 study all patients at a particular site failed to have their weight collected at study entry. This data would be MAR because the missingness is conditional on whether the data were collected at a particular site or not. When data are MAR, the missing data mechanism is said to be 'ignorable' because the missing data mechanism or model is independent of the parameters to be estimated in the model under consideration. Most data sets consist of a mixture of MCAR and MAR.

If data are missing because the value was not collected then that value is truly missing. In more statistical terms, if the data are missing independent of the actual value of the missing data then the missing data mechanism is said to be *ignorable*. If, however, data are missing because their value is above or below some level at which obtaining quantifiable measurements is not possible then this type of missing data is an entirely different problem. In this case, the data are missing because of the actual value of the observation and the missing data mechanism is said to be *non-ignorable*. These last type of data are extremely tricky to handle properly and will not be discussed in any great detail herein. The reader is referred to Little (1995) and Diggle and Kenward (1994) for details.

Last, is the pattern of missingness as it relates to missing covariates. Figure 2.13 presents a schematic of the general pattern of missingness. Some covariates have missing data; others do not. There may be gaps in the covariates. But if the covariates can be rearranged and reordered $x_1, x_2, . . . x_p$, such that the degree of missingness within each covariate is less than the preceding covariate then such a pattern of missingness is montonic

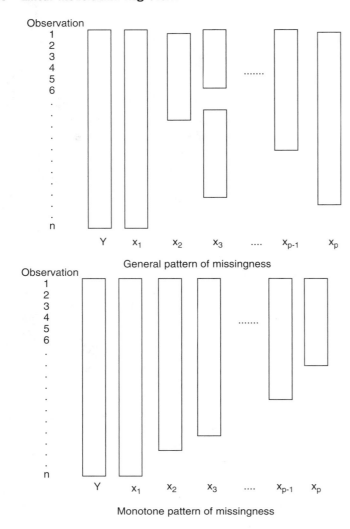

Figure 2.13 General (top) and monotonic (bottom) pattern of missingness in the covariates.

or nested. Monotonic missingness is useful because there are specific ways to impute monotonic missing data.

Methods for Handling Missing Data: Missing Dependent Variables

If the missing data are the dependent variable and the reason for missingness is not non-ignorable, then the missing, data should be deleted from the analysis. If however, the missing dependent variable is missing because it is below or above some threshold value then more complicated methods to analyze the data are needed. For instance, the dependent variable may be missing because its value was below the lower limit of quantification (LLOQ) of the method used to measure it. For example, white blood cell count may be near zero after chemotherapy and may not be measurable using current technologies. In this case the value may be

reported as $< 0.1 \times 10^9/\text{L}$. In such a case, the true value for white blood cell count lies between 0 and the LLOQ of the assay. Such data are said to be *censored*. Another instance might be when the value exceeds some threshold beyond which an accurate and quantifiable measurement cannot be made, such as determining the weight of a super-obese individual whose weight exceeds the limit of the scale in a doctor's office. In this case only that the subject's weight was larger than c, the upper limit of the scale is known. A value is said to be censored from below if the value is less than some threshold or censored from above if the value exceeds some constant. With censored data, the usual likelihood function does not apply and parameter estimates obtained using maximum likelihood will be biased.

For data where the dependent variable is censored, the log-likelihood function is the sum of the log-likelihoods for observations not censored plus the sum of the log-likelihoods for censored observations. To obtain parameter estimates, one needs access to an optimization package that can fit a general likelihood function, like MATLAB (The MathWorks Inc., Natick, MA). A simpler more pragmatic (but certainly more biased) approach in the case where observations are censored from below, imputation is usually done by setting the value equal to zero, equal to some fraction of the constant, such as one-half the LLOQ of the assay, or randomly assigning the data point a value based on a probability distribution. For instance, a sample may be randomly drawn from the interval [0, LLOQ] based on a uniform distribution. Observations censored from above are more problematic because there may be no theoretical upper limit and in such cases, imputation is usually done by setting the missing value equal to the upper threshold. Whatever the imputation method used, the usual caveats apply. The reader is referred to Breen (1996) for a good exposition to the problem. Unfortunately at this time, no major statistical package, such as SAS or S-Plus, or pharmacokinetic software package can handle the censored data case using the correct log-likelihood equations.

Methods for Handling Missing Data: Missing Independent Variables

There are many different ways for handling missing data including ignore the missing data (complete case analysis), mean or median substitution, hot deck methods, regression methods, and maximum likelihood and its variants. The simplest method, called listwise deletion or complete case analysis, is to ignore the missing data and model only the data that have no missing data. The advantages of this method are that it can be applied to any type of statistical model and is easy to do.

Hence, casewise deletion is the method of choice for handling missing data in most statistical software packages. A disadvantage of this method is that it may lead to biased results, especially if the data are not MCAR, but are MAR, such as if the data were more likely to be missing because of assignment to a particular treatment arm. If the data are MCAR, then the model parameters will be unbiased but the standard errors will be larger due to a reduced sample size. Hence, power will be decreased at detecting significant treatment effects. The CPMP does not generally accept listwise deletion analysis because it violates the intent to treat principle[2]. The Points to Consider document does state, however, that listwise deletion may be useful in certain circumstances, such as in exploratory data analysis and confirmatory trials as a secondary endpoint, to illustrate the robustness of other conclusions.

Imputation, which is basically making up data, substitutes the made-up data into the missing data and treats the imputed data as if it were real. Imputation is generally recognized as the preferred approach to handling missing data and there are many different ways to impute missing data. The first approach is naïve substitution wherein the mean or median value is substituted for all missing values. For example, if a person's weight was missing from a data set then the mean weight, perhaps stratified by sex, would be substituted. While preserving the mean of the marginal distribution of the missing variable, it biases the distribution of the variable. The result is that if the variable is indeed related to the dependent variable and the proportion of missing data is large, then naïve substitution may distort the relationship between variables. It is generally recognized that this approach does more harm than good, unless the proportion of missing data is small (less than a few percent), where at best the substitution adds no information.

If the missing value is one of the independent variables then naïve substitution ignores any correlations that may be present among predictor variables. To account for any correlations between variables, conditional mean imputation may be used wherein for cases with complete data the variable with missing data is regressed against the other predictor variables and then the predicted value is substituted for the missing value. In general, all variables are used in the analysis and no attempt is made to reduce the imputation model to its simplest form.

---

[2] The intent to treat principle essentially states that all patients are analyzed according to the treatment they were randomized to, irrespective of the treatment they actually received. Hence, a patient is included in the analysis even if that patient never received the treatment.

A variant of naïve substitution is to use random substitution wherein an observation is randomly sampled from the observed values and substituted for the missing value. This approach too tends to maintain the mean on-average but may obscure real relationships among the variables. Another variant of naïve substitution is hot-deck imputation, which requires pretty large data sets to be useful and has been used for many years by the U.S. Census Bureau. The basic idea is that each missing value is randomly replaced from other subjects having similar covariates. Suppose the weight of a 67 year old male was missing, but weight was collected on three other 67 year old males in the study, then the weight of the missing value is randomly drawn from one of the three observable weights. The advantage of the method is that it imputes realistic values since the imputed value is itself actual data and is conceptually simple. But what if there were no other 67 year old males in the study. How would the imputation work? This is where hot deck is often criticized, in the choice of the "donor" cases since one then must set up "similarity" criterion to find matching donors. Also, besides SOLAS (Statistical Solutions, Saugus MA), no other software package has a built-in hot deck imputation algorithm. The user must program their own filters and similarity measures which makes the method data-specific and difficult to implement.

Regression-based methods impute the missing values using least-squares regression of the missing covariate against the observed covariates (Little, 1992). In other words, the missing covariate becomes the dependent variable and the other covariates with no missing data become the independent variables. Ordinary least-squares, or sometimes weighted least-squares that down-weights incomplete cases, is then used to obtain the regression model and the missing value is imputed based on the predicted value. A modification of this approach is to add random error to the predicted value based on the residual mean square error to account for unexplained variability. Little (1992) suggests that when the partial correlation between Y and the observed x's is high then a better imputation can be had by including Y, as well as the observed x's, in the imputation process. This may seem like cheating but if Y is not included in the imputation then biased parameter estimates may result using the filled-in data.

If the covariates show a monotone pattern of missingness (Fig. 2.13) then the imputation procedure can be done sequentially. For instance, suppose that x_1, x_2, x_3, and x_4 are the covariates that exhibit monotone missingness and that x_1 and x_2 have no missing data. In the first step, x_3 would be imputed based on the regression of x_3 against Y, x_1, and x_2. Then given imputed values for x_3, x_4 would be imputed using the regression of Y, x_1, x_2, and x_3 against x_4. In this manner all the covariates can be imputed. One problem that may arise using regression based methods is that the covariates may show collinearity. The covariate design matrix used in the imputation may be near singular with the resulting parameter estimates showing instability. A check of the correlation matrix prior to imputation may be useful to detect which covariates show collinearity. Collinearity could also arise if one or more of the covariates show excessive skewness. In which case, a transformation to normality may be useful prior to imputation.

A parametric method for handling missing data is maximum likelihood. Recall that in linear regression maximum likelihood maximizes the likelihood function L(.)

$$L(Y|\theta,\sigma) = \prod_{i=1}^{n} f(Y|\theta) \qquad (2.101)$$

where f is the probability density function. In the case where missing data are present the likelihood function becomes the entire sample

$$L(Y|\theta,\sigma) = \prod_{i=1}^{m} f(x_i, Y_i|\theta) \prod_{i=m+1}^{n} g(Y_i|\theta) \qquad (2.102)$$

where g is the probability density function for the missing data and there are m cases with observed data and n-m cases of missing data. The problem then becomes to find the set of θ that maximizes the likelihood. In order to maximize the likelihood certain distributional assumptions must be made, the most common being a multivariate normal distribution. Although direct maximization of the likelihood is possible, the software to do such maximization is not readily available.

Two alternatives to direct maximization of the likelihood are available: the EM algorithm, which is the default multiple imputation (MI) algorithm in SAS, and Markov chain data augmentation. The expectation-maximization (EM) is difficult to explain in lay terms, but in brief, the EM approach to missing data proceeds in two steps. In the first step, the expectation step, the algorithm essentially computes a regression based imputation to the missing values using all available variables. After the expectation step, the maximization step computes new estimates of the likelihood as if the variable had no missing data. Then the E-step is repeated, etc., until stability of the estimates is obtained.

Data augmentation using Markov Chain Monte Carlo (MCMC), which has its basis in Bayesian statistics, is much like the EM algorithm except that two random draws are made during the process. Markov chains are a sequence of random variables where the current value depends on the value of the previous step. In the first step, starting values are made. For a multivariate normal model, the starting values are the means and covariance matrix or the means and covariances obtained using the EM algorithm. For each missing variable, given the estimates of the mean and covariance, estimates of the regression parameters relating the variable with missing data to the other variables are obtained. Using the regression estimates the predicted values for all missing data are calculated. Then (and this is the first random, stochastic step in the process) normally distributed random variability is added to the predicted values and substituted for the missing data. The means and covariances for the imputed data set are then computed. Based on these updated means and covariances (and this is the second random stochastic step in the process) a random draw from the posterior distribution of the means and covariances is made. Using the randomly drawn means and covariances, the entire process is repeated until convergence is achieved. The imputations obtained at the final step in the process are those that are used in the statistical analysis.

Related to MCMC are two fundamental issues: how many iterations are needed before convergence is achieved and what posterior distribution should be used. There is no satisfactory answer for whether or not convergence (or stationarity) has been achieved. The default in SAS is to use 50 burn-in iterations before the first imputation is available for use. Schaffer (1997) used anywhere from 50 to 1000 iterations in examples used in his book. Of course the more iterations the better, but increasing the number of iterations also increases the computation time, which may become prohibitive. Allison (2002) suggests that as the proportion of missing data increases the number of iterations should increase. If only 5% of the data are missing then fewer iterations are needed, although typically 500 to 1000 iterations is usually seen in the literature for most realistic data sets. The reader is referred to Gelman et al. (1995) for further details on MCMC and convergence. The second fundamental issue related to MCMC is the choice of the posterior distribution. In order to obtain the posterior distribution, one needs a prior distribution, which is a probability distribution associated with the prior beliefs of the data before actual collection of any data. An uninformative prior is often used in the absence of any prior knowledge, which is what SAS does as a default.

The problem with any imputation method wherein a single value is substituted for the missing data and then the data set is analyzed as if it were all complete cases is that the standard errors of the model parameters are underestimated because the sampling variability of the imputed values is not taken into account. For this reason multiple imputation arose. With multiple imputation many different datasets are generated, each with their own set of imputed values, and each imputed data set is analyzed as if complete. The parameter estimates across data sets are then combined to generate improved estimates of the standard errors. Multiple imputation, when done correctly, can provide consistent, asymptotically normally distributed, unbiased estimates of model parameters given the data are MAR. Problems with multiple imputation include generation of different parameter estimates every time it is used, is difficult to implement if not built into a statistical package, and is easy to do the wrong way (Allison, 2002).

Rubin (1987) proposed that if m-imputed data sets are analyzed that have generated m-different sets of parameter estimates then these m-sets of parameter estimates need to be combined to generate a set of parameter estimates that takes into account the added variability from the imputed values. He proposed that if θ_i and $SE(\theta_i)$ are the parameter estimates and standard errors of the parameter estimates, respectively, from the ith imputed data set, then the point estimate for the m-multiple imputation data sets is

$$\theta_{MI} = \frac{1}{m} \sum_{i=i}^{m} \theta_i. \tag{2.103}$$

So the multiple imputation parameter estimate is the mean across all m-imputed data sets. Let $\overline{U}(\theta_i)$ be the variance of θ_i, i.e., the standard error squared, averaged across all m-data sets

$$\overline{U}(\theta_i) = \frac{1}{m} \sum_{i=1}^{m} [SE(\theta_i)]^2 \tag{2.104}$$

and let $\overline{B}(\theta_i)$ be the variance of the point estimates across imputations

$$\overline{B}(\theta_i) = \frac{1}{m-1} \sum_{i=1}^{m} (\theta_i - \overline{\theta}_i)^2. \tag{2.105}$$

Then the variance associated with θ_i is

$$Var(\theta_i) = \overline{U}(\theta_i) + \left(1 + \frac{1}{m}\right) \overline{B}(\theta_i). \tag{2.106}$$

The multiple imputation standard error of the parameter estimate θ_i is then the square root of Eq. (2.106). Examination of Eq. (2.106) shows that the multiple imputation standard error is a weighted sum of the within- and between-data set standard errors. As m increases to infinity the variance of the parameter estimate becomes the average of the parameter estimate variances.

Rubin (1987) also showed that the relative increase in variability (RIV) due to missing data is a simple function

$$RIV = \frac{\left(1 + \frac{1}{m}\right) \overline{B}(\theta_i)}{\overline{U}(\theta_i)} \tag{2.107}$$

and that the overall fraction of "missing data" can be calculated as

$$\zeta = \frac{\left[\dfrac{RIV + 2}{(m-1)\left(1 + \frac{1}{RIV}\right)^2}\right]}{RIV + 1}. \tag{2.108}$$

Given an estimate of RIV the relative efficiency of a parameter estimate based on m imputations to the estimate based on an infinite number of imputations can be calculated by $(1 + \xi/m)^{-1}$. For example, with 5 imputations and 40% missing data the relative efficiency is 93%. With 10 imputations the relative efficiency is only 96%. Thus, the difference between 5 and 10 imputations is not that large and so the increase in relative efficiency with the larger number of imputation sets may not be worth the computational price. Typically, the gain in efficiency is not very large when more imputation data sets are used and it is for this reason that when multiple imputation is used and reported in the literature the number of imputed data sets is usually five or less.

There are two additional twists related to multiple imputation using MCMC. Obviously multiple imputation creates multiple datasets. For a fixed amount of computing time, one can either increase the number of iterations in the Markov chain generating a fixed number of imputed data sets or one can increase the number of imputed data sets to be analyzed using a smaller number of iterations in the Markov chain. Allison (2002) suggests that more imputation data sets be generated instead of spending more time on increasing the number of iterations in the Markov chain. The second twist is that several different data sets need to be generated. To do this, independent Markov chains are generated, one for each data set, using perhaps different starting values; this is called the parallel approach. Care must be taken with this approach that convergence has been achieved with each individual Markov chain. Alternatively one very long Markov chain can be generated and then the data sets generated every k iterations are chosen. For example, a Markov chain of 3000 iterations could be generated with the first 500 iterations used for burn-in and then every 500th data set thereafter used for the imputed data sets. With this method the question of independence must be raised—are the imputed data sets truly independent if they are run from the same Markov chain? As k decreases the issue of correlated data sets becomes more and more important, but when k is very large, the correlation is negligible. For example, the issue of correlation would be valid if the imputed data every 10 iterations were used, but becomes a non-issue when k is in the hundreds. In general, either method is acceptable, however.

To illustrate these concepts a modification of the simulation suggested by Allison (2000) will be analyzed. In this simulation 10,000 observations of three variables were simulated: Y, x_1, and x_2. Such a large sample size was used to ensure that sampling variability was small. x_1 and x_2 were bivariate normally distributed random variables with mean 0 and variance 1 having a correlation of 0.5. Y was then generated using

$$Y = 1 + x_1 + x_2 + Z \qquad (2.109)$$

where Z was normally distributed random error having mean 0 and variance 1. Four missing data mechanisms were then examined:

1. Missing completely at random: x_2 was missing with probability 0.5 independent of Y or x_1;
2. Missing at random, dependent on x_1: x_2 was missing if $x_1 < 0$;
3. Missing at random, dependent on Y: x_2 was missing if $Y < 0$; and
4. Non-ignorable: x_2 was missing if $x_2 < 0$.

The data were then fit using linear regression of (x_1, x_2) against Y. The results are presented in Table 2.13. Listwise deletion resulted in parameter estimates that were unbiased, except when the data were MAR and dependent on the value of Y in which case all three parameter estimates were severely biased. Surprisingly, even when the missing data mechanism was non-ignorable the parameter estimates were unbiased and precise. The standard errors for all models with missing data were about 25% to 200% larger than the data set with no missing data because of the smaller sample sizes. MI tended to decrease the estimates of the standard errors compared to their original values. When the data were MAR or MCAR, the parameter estimates remained unbiased using MI with MCMC, even when the data were MAR and dependent on Y. The bias that was observed was now removed. But when the missing data were non-ignorable, the parameter estimates obtained by MI became biased because MI assumes the data MAR.

So how is MI incorporated in the context of exploratory data analysis since obviously one would not wish to analyze m different data sets. A simple method would be to impute m + 1 data sets, perform the exploratory analysis on one of the imputed data sets, and obtain the final model of interest. Then using the remaining m-data sets compute the imputed parameter estimates and standard errors of the final model. It should be kept in mind, however, that with the imputed data set being used to develop the model, the standard errors will be smaller than they actually are since this data set fails to take into account the sampling variability in the missing values. Hence, a more conservative test of statistical significance for either model entry or removal should be considered during model development.

Table 2.13 Parameter Estimates and standard errors from simulated multiple imputation data set.

Missing data mechanism	Parameter	Number of observations without missing data	Listwise deletion mean (Standard deviation)	MCMC mean (Standard deviation)
No missing data	Intercept	10,000	1.005 (0.0101)	.
	x_1		0.987 (0.0116)	.
	x_2		0.998 (0.0117)	.
MCAR	Intercept	4982	1.000 (0.0141)	0.993 (0.0101)
	x_1		0.986 (0.0162)	0.978 (0.0118)
	x_2		0.996 (0.0164)	1.012 (0.0133)
MAR on x_1	Intercept	5023	0.998 (0.0234)	1.001 (0.0284)
	x_1		0.996 (0.0250)	0.994 (0.0126)
	x_2		0.992 (0.0166)	0.993 (0.0142)
MAR on Y	Intercept	6942	1.419 (0.0123)	1.000 (0.0122)
	x_1		0.779 (0.0133)	0.988 (0.0162)
	x_2		0.789 (0.0136)	0.996 (0.0150)
Nonignorable on x_2	Intercept	5016	1.017 (0.0234)	1.66 (0.0187)
	x_1		0.973 (0.0166)	1.13 (0.0148)
	x_2		1.016 (0.0254)	1.22 (0.0300)

Note: True values are 1.000 for intercept, 1.000 for x_1, and 1.000 for x_2. Results based on 10,000 simulated observations. MI was based on 5 imputed data sets having a burn-in of 500 iterations.

A totally different situation arises when covariates are missing because of the value of the observation, not because the covariate wasn't measured. In such a case the value is censored, which means that the value is below or above some critical threshold for measurement. On the other hand, a covariate may be censored from above where the covariate reported as greater than upper limit of quantification (ULOQ) of the method used to measure it. In such a case the covariate is reported as >ULOQ, but its true value may lie theoretically between ULOQ and infinity. The issue of censored covariates has not received as much attention as the issue of censored dependent variables. Typical solutions include any of the substitution or imputation methods described for imputed missing covariates that are not censored.

In summary, case-deletion is easy but can lead to biased parameter estimates and is not generally recommended by regulatory authorities. In contrast, multiple imputation, although computationally more difficult, is generally recognized as the preferred method to handling missing data and like any statistical analysis requires certain assumptions be met for validity. The analyst is especially warned in the case of censored data and the effects of case-deletion or multiple imputation on parameter estimation. This section has presented a high-level overview of MI and handling missing data that is far from complete. The reader is strongly encouraged to read more specialized texts on the topic prior to actually implementing their use in practice. Before closing this section, the best advice for missing data is to have none – do everything possible to obtain the data in the first place!

SOFTWARE

Every statistical package, and even spreadsheet programs like Microsoft Excel®, has the capability to perform linear regression. SAS (SAS Institute, Cary, NC, www.sas.com) has the REG procedure, while S-Plus (Insightful Corp., Seattle, WA, www.insightful.com) has available its lm function. Statistical packages are far more powerful than the spreadsheet packages, but spreadsheet packages are more ubiquitous. The choice of either S-Plus or SAS is a difficult one. S-Plus has better graphics, but SAS is an industry standard—a workhorse of proven capability. S-Plus is largely seen in the pharmacokinetic community as a tool for exploratory data analysis, while SAS is viewed as the de facto standard for statistical analysis in pharmaceutical development. All the examples in this book were analyzed using SAS (version 8) for Windows.

Using statistical reference data sets (certified to 16 significant digits in the model parameters) available from the National Institute of Standards and Technology (NIST) Information Technology Department (http://www.itl.nist.gov/div898/strd), McCullough (1999) compared the accuracy of SAS (version 6.12) and S-Plus (version 4.5), both of which are older versions than are currently available, in fitting a variety of linear models with varying levels of difficulty. Data sets of low difficult should be easily fit by most algorithms, whereas data sets of high difficult, which are highly collinear, may produce quite biased parameter estimates because different software may use different matrix inversion algorithms. McCullough found that SAS and S-Plus both demonstrate reliability in their linear regression results. However, for analysis of variance problems, which should use the same linear regression algorithms, the results were quite variable. Neither SAS or S-Plus passed average difficulty problems. When the linear regression data sets were analyzed using Microsoft's Excel 97 (Microsoft Corp., Seattle, WA, *www.microsoft.com*) built-in data analysis tools, most performed reasonable well, but failed on a problem that was ill-conditioned, leading the authors to conclude that Excel 97 is "inadequate" for linear regression problems (McCullough and Wilson, 1999). Further, when Excel 97 analyzed the analysis of variance data sets, the software delivered acceptable performance on only low-level difficulty problems and was deemed inadequate. In conclusion, for linear regression problems using SAS's REG procedure or S-Plus's lm function, both perform adequately with reasonable accuracy. Microsoft Excel 97 cannot be recommended for linear regression models.

SUMMARY

Linear regression is one of the most important tools in a modelers toolbox, yet surprisingly its foundations and assumptions are often glossed over at the graduate level. Few books published on pharmacokinetics cover the principles of linear regression modeling. Most books start at nonlinear modeling and proceed from there. But, a thorough understanding of linear modeling is needed before one can understand nonlinear models. In this chapter, the basics of linear regression have been presented, although not every topic in linear regression has been presented—the topic is too vast to do that in one chapter of a book. What has been presented are the essentials relevant to pharmacokinetic and pharmacodynamic modeling. Later chapters will expand on these concepts and present new ones with an eye towards developing a unified exposition of pharmacostatistical modeling.

Recommended Reading

Allison, P.D. *Missing data*. Sage Publications, Inc., Thousand Oaks, CA, 2002.

Belsley, D.A., Kuh, E. and Welsch, R.E. *Regression diagnostics: Identifying influential data and sources of collinearity*. John Wiley and Sons, Inc., New York, 1980.

Cook, J.R. and Stefanski, L.A. Simulation-extrapolation estimation in parametric measurement error models. *Journal of the American Statistical Association* 1994; 89: 1314–1328.

International Conference on Harmonisation of Technical Requirements for Registration of Pharmaceuticals for Human Use. Statistical Principles for Clinical Trials (E9). 1998.

Myers, R.H. *Classical and modern regression with applications*. Duxbury Press, Boston, 1986.

Neter, J., Kutner, M.H. Nachtsheim, C.J. and Wasserman, W. *Applied linear statistical models*. Irwin, Chicago, 1996.

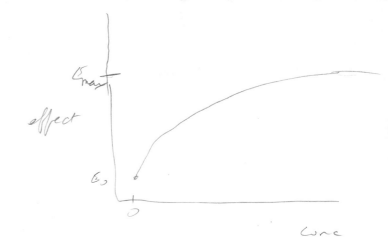

Chapter 3

Nonlinear Models and Regression

Do not worry about your difficulties in mathematics. I can assure you mine are still greater.

—Albert Einstein (1879–1955), Physicist and Nobel Laureate

INTRODUCTION

A model is nonlinear if any of the partial derivatives with respect to any of the model parameters are dependent on any other model parameter or if any of the derivatives do not exist or are discontinuous. For example, the E_{max} pharmacodynamic model,

$$E = \frac{E_{max}C}{EC_{50} + C} \tag{3.1}$$

where E is the observed effect, E_{max} the maximal effect, EC_{50} the concentration that produces 50% of the maximal effect, and C the concentration having two parameters, E_{max} and EC_{50}, with partial derivatives

$$\frac{\partial E}{\partial E_{max}} = \frac{C}{EC_{50} + C} \tag{3.2}$$

and

$$\frac{\partial E}{\partial EC_{50}} = \frac{-E_{max}C}{(EC_{50} + C)^2}. \tag{3.3}$$

Since both the partial derivatives with respect to the model parameters are a function of either itself or the other parameter, the model is nonlinear in the parameters. Because E_{max} is dependent only on EC_{50}, it is said to be *conditionally linear* on EC_{50}.

However, in the model

$$Y = \begin{cases} \theta_0 + \theta_1 x & x \le x_0 \\ \theta_2 + \theta_3 x & x > x_0 \end{cases} \tag{3.4}$$

the regression parameters themselves are not dependent on any other model parameter, i.e., $\delta Y/\delta\theta_1$ is independent of θ_0, but the estimates are dependent on the value of x_0. Such models are called segmented, threshold, or change-point models and take the general form

$$Y = \begin{cases} f(x; \theta) & x \le x_0 \\ f(x; \theta^*) & x > x_0 \end{cases} \tag{3.5}$$

However, for this model, the derivative is not continuous at $x = x_0$ and nonlinear least squares algorithms, ones that do not require derivatives, such as the Nelder–Mead algorithm (which is discussed later in the chapter), are generally required to estimate the model parameters (Bartholomew, 2000).

Models that are transformed in predictor variables to some inherently nonlinear function are not nonlinear. For example, the model

$$Y = \theta_0 + \theta_1\sqrt{x_1} + \theta_2\sin(x_2), \tag{3.6}$$

is not nonlinear because the partial derivatives are not dependent on any other model parameter. This may be easier seen by rewriting Eq. (3.6) as

$$Y = \theta_0 + \theta_1 x_1^* + \theta_2 x_2^*, \tag{3.7}$$

93

where

$$x_1^* = \sqrt{x_1} \tag{3.8}$$

and

$$x_2^* = \sin(x_2), \tag{3.9}$$

which can been seen in the form of a linear model. Also, as has been shown in the previous chapter on Linear Models and Regression, the quadratic model, which is curvilinear, is not nonlinear because the partial derivatives are independent of the model parameters.

Unlike linear regression where the user has little or no control over how the parameter estimates are obtained, the analyst has many variables to control in nonlinear regression. These are listed in Table 3.1. It must be recognized up-front that different combinations of these variables will lead to different parameter estimates—sometimes dramatically different.

NONLINEAR LEAST SQUARES

A general nonlinear model can be expressed as

$$Y = f(\theta; x) + \varepsilon \tag{3.10}$$

where Y is an $n \times 1$ vector of responses, f is the expectation function or structural model, θ is a $p \times 1$ vector of model parameters, x is an $n \times q$ matrix of predictor variables, and ε is an $n \times 1$ vector of independent, normally distributed residuals. For example, for Eq. (3.1), the predictor variable x is concentration, $\theta = \{E_{max}, EC_{50}\}$, and the response Y is effect. It is generally assumed that x is measured with certainty and has no measurement error in its value. If x is not measured with certainty, the assumption is made that the variance of the predictor variable is small relative

Table 3.1 Variables the analyst has control over in nonlinear regression.

- Algorithm
- Maximum number of iterations
- Variance model
- Convergence criteria
- Parameter bounds
- Tolerance criteria
- Gradient calculations
- Increments for partial derivatives
- Bayesian terms

to the response variable. If this assumption is not true, then an error-in-variables approach must be used. In Eq. (3.1), drug concentrations are not measured with certainty and an error-in-variables approach should always be considered, although this is rarely done in practice.

Using the method of least squares, $\hat{\theta}$, the estimator for θ, minimizes the residual sum of squares

$$S(\theta) = \sum_{i=1}^{n} [Y_i - f(\theta; x_i)]^2. \tag{3.11}$$

Equation (3.11) is sometimes called the objective function, although it should be stressed that there are many different types of objective functions, such as extended least squares. For purposes of this book, an objective function will be defined as any quadratic function that must be minimized to obtain a set of parameter estimates. For this chapter the focus will be on the residual sum of squares as the objective function, although in later chapters more complex objective functions may be considered.

Like the linear least squares case, it can be shown that if $\varepsilon \sim N(0, \sigma^2)$ then the least squares estimate of θ is also the maximum likelihood estimate of θ. This is because the likelihood function is

$$L(x; \theta) = \prod_{i=1}^{n} \frac{1}{(2\pi\sigma^2)^{\frac{n}{2}}} \exp\left(\frac{-(Y - \hat{Y})}{2\sigma^2}\right) \tag{3.12}$$

so that if σ^2 is known, maximizing $L(x; \theta)$ with respect to θ is the same as minimizing $S(\theta)$ with respect to θ. However, the problem of finding the value of θ which minimizes the residual sum of squares is more complicated than linear models because the parameters in the model are correlated. Once Eq. (3.11) is differentiated with respect to the model parameters and set equal to zero, no single explicit solution can be obtained using linear algebra. For example, in the E_{max} model in Eq. (3.1) above

$$S(\theta) = \sum_{i=1}^{n} \left[Y_i - \frac{E_{max}C_i}{EC_{50} + C_i}\right]^2, \tag{3.13}$$

which after obtaining the partial derivatives and setting them equal to zero yields the following equations

$$0 = 2 \sum_{i=1}^{n} \left[\left(Y_i - \frac{E_{max}C_i}{EC_{50} + C_i}\right)\left(\frac{C_i}{EC_{50} + C_i}\right)\right] \tag{3.14}$$

$$0 = 2 \sum_{i=1}^{n} \left[\left(Y_i - \frac{E_{max}C_i}{EC_{50} + C_i} \right) \left(\frac{-E_{max}C_i}{(EC_{50} + C_i)^2} \right) \right]. \quad (3.15)$$

Unlike linear models where normal equations can be solved explicitly in terms of the model parameters, Eqs. (3.14) and (3.15) are nonlinear in the parameter estimates and must be solved iteratively, usually using the method of nonlinear least squares or some modification thereof. The focus of this chapter will be on nonlinear least squares while the problem of weighted least squares, data transformations, and variance models will be dealt with in another chapter.

The basic problem in nonlinear least squares is finding the values of θ that minimizes the residual sum of squares which is essentially a problem in optimization. Because the objective functions used in pharmacokinetic–pharmacodynamic modeling are of a quadratic nature (notice that Eq. (3.13) is raised to the power 2), they have a convex or curved structure that can be exploited to find an estimate of θ. For example, consider the data shown in Fig. 3.1. Using a 1-compartment model with parameters θ = {V, CL}, volume of distribution (V) can be systematically varied from 100 to 200 L and clearance (CL) can be systematically varied from 2 to 60 L/h. With each parameter combination, the residual sum of squares can be calculated and plotted as a function of the variables V and CL, as shown in Fig. 3.1.

Using this crude grid, the minimum residual sum of squares can be found at a volume of distribution of 126 L and a clearance of 18 L/h, which was very near the theoretical values of 125 L and 19 L/h, respectively, used to simulate the data. Often a grid search, such as the one done here, is a good way to obtain initial parameter estimates. In fact, some software offer a grid search option if initial parameter estimates are unavailable.

Specific algorithms have been developed to take advantage of the nature of the objective function surface. Most state of the art software is currently designed so the user needs to do as little as possible. They are designed to be as robust as possible and to converge if convergence can be achieved. Nevertheless, it is important for users to be able to recognize the advantages and disadvantages of each method and when one method might be favored over another. The common iterative methods found in pharmacokinetic software packages include the Gauss–Newton, Gauss Newton with Levenberg and Hartley modification, Gauss Newton with Hartley modification, and Nelder–Mead algorithms. Each of these algorithms will be discussed below.

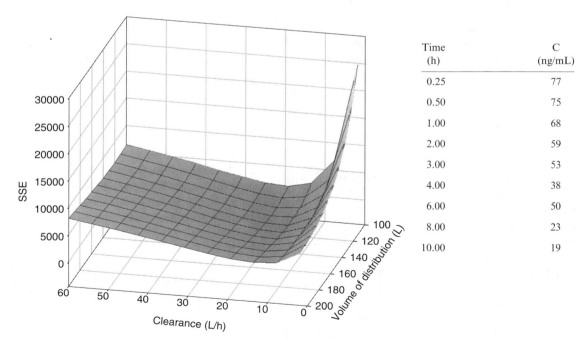

Time (h)	C (ng/mL)
0.25	77
0.50	75
1.00	68
2.00	59
3.00	53
4.00	38
6.00	50
8.00	23
10.00	19

Figure 3.1 Surface plot of residual sum of squares (SSE) for data shown to the right of the figure fit to a 1-compartment model with intravenous administration. The volume of distribution was varied from 0 to 100 L and clearance was varied from 2 to 60 L/h.

FUNCTIONS WITH ONE VARIABLE

Nonlinear regression is essentially a problem in optimization—maximizing the log-likelihood function. Since it is easier to find the minimum of a function, the negative of the log-likelihood function must be found. In order to understand the algorithms used in nonlinear regression, some background and terminology with regards to a linear model will first be introduced. As an example, consider the linear model reported by Reklaitis, Ravindran, and Ragsdell (1983)

$$Y = 5x^6 - 36x^5 + \frac{165}{2}x^4 - 60x^3 + 36. \quad (3.16)$$

The first derivative and second derivatives, respectively, are

$$\frac{dY}{dx} = Y'(x) = 30x^5 - 180x^4 + 330x^3 - 180x^2 \quad (3.17)$$

$$\frac{d^2Y}{dx^2} = Y''(x) = 150x^4 - 720x^3 + 990x^2 - 360x. \quad (3.18)$$

Recall from calculus that the derivative is the rate of change of a single-value function. The first derivative is useful mathematically because points where the first derivative are zero indicate the function's inflection points, which can either be a maxima or a minima. The sign of the second derivative where the first derivative equals zero tells whether the function is maximal (negative second derivative) or minimal (positive second derivative). Hence, necessary conditions for x^* to be a local minima (maxima) of f(x) on the interval $a \le x \le b$ are that f(x) is twice differentiable, i.e., a second derivative exists,

$$\left.\frac{dY}{dx}\right|_{x=x^*} = 0$$

$$\left.\frac{d^2Y}{dx^2}\right|_{x=x^*} \ge 0 \ (\le 0 \text{ for maxima}).$$

The term "necessary conditions" implies that if any of these conditions are not met, then x^* is not a local minimum (maximum). On the other hand, if these conditions are met, this is no guarantee that x^* is a global minimum. A function f(x) defined on the interval {a, b} attains its global minimum at the point x^{**} if and only if $f(x^{**}) \le f(x)$ for all x in the interval {a, b}. In other words, the global minimum is obtained at the smallest value of Y for all x in the interval {a, b}.

When a function is not unimodal, many local minima may be present. The global minimum is then obtained by identifying all local minima and selecting the local minima with the smallest value. The same pro-

cedure is used to find the global maximum except that the largest local maxima is found instead. This process is not a trivial task sometimes. Returning to Eq. (3.16), the function Y and its first derivative over the range 0–3.3 are plotted in Fig. 3.2. The points where the first derivative cross the zero axis are 1, 2, and 3. The second derivatives at 1, 2, and 3 are 60, −120, and 540, indicating that x = 1 and x = 3 are minima, but that x = 2 is a maxima. Also indicated on the plot is that x = 1 is a local minima, x = 3 is the global minimum, and x = 2 is the global maximum over the interval {0, 3.3}.

One method to finding the minimum of a function is to search over all possible values of x and find the minimum based on the corresponding values of Y. These algorithms include region elimination methods, such as the Golden Search algorithm or point-estimation methods, such as Powell's method, neither of which require calculation of the derivatives. However, these types of methods often assume unimodality, and in some cases, continuity of the function. The reader is referred to Reklaitis Ravindran, and Ragsdell (1983) or Rao (1996) for details.

Another method for finding the minimum of a function, one that requires the function to be twice differentiable and that its derivatives can be calculated, is the Newton–Raphson algorithm. The algorithm begins with an initial estimate, x_1, of the minimum, x^*. The goal is to find the value of x where the first derivative equals zero and the second derivative is a positive value. Taking a first-order Taylor series approximation to the first derivative (dY/dx) evaluated at x_1

$$\frac{dY}{dx} = \frac{dY}{dx_1} + \frac{d^2Y}{dx_1^2}(x - x_1), \quad (3.19)$$

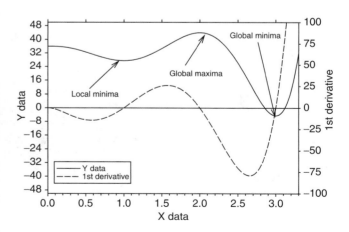

Figure 3.2 Plot of the sixth-order polynomial function $Y = 5x^6 - 36x^5 + \frac{165}{2}x^4 - 60x^3 + 36$ and its first derivative. The plot indicates that a complex function that is not unimodal will have many local minima and maxima, but there will be only one global minima and global maxima.

setting it equal to zero, and rearranging for x yields

$$x = x_1 - \left(\frac{d^2Y}{dx_1^2}\right)^{-1}\left(\frac{dY}{dx_1}\right), \qquad (3.20)$$
$$= x_1 - h$$

where h is called the step length. The value of x then becomes the next value in the sequence, i.e., x_2. In geometric terms, using the first derivative, a tangent line is extended from x_1. The point where the tangent line crosses the x-axis where the first derivative equals zero is usually an improved estimate of x^* and is taken as the next estimate, x_2. Thus using the first and second derivative a step of length h is taken to a new point. This is illustrated in Fig. 3.3. Unfortunately, the Newton–Raphson algorithm does not guarantee convergence and may in fact diverge depending on the function and the starting points in the algorithm. Table 3.2 presents an example of the Newton–Raphson algorithm finding the minimum for Eq. (3.16) using starting values of 0.7 and 1.60. In both cases, a minimum is identified in a few function calls. Choosing 0.7 as the starting value leads to a value of 1.0 as the minimum, whereas 1.6 leads to a

Table 3.2 Newton–Raphson solution to finding the local minima of Eq. (3.16).

i	x_i	dY/dx_i	dY/d^2x_i	x_{i+1}
Starting value: 0.70				
1	0.70	−13.19	22.16	1.30
2	1.30	17.85	52.24	0.95
3	0.95	−2.72	56.64	1.00
4	1.00	0.09	60.09	1.00
Starting value: 1.60				
1	1.60	25.80	−7.68	4.96
2	4.96	16956.16	25498.56	4.30
3	4.30	5419.61	10714.92	3.79
4	3.79	1696.52	4601.51	3.42
5	3.42	507.53	2070.60	3.18
6	3.18	135.68	1036.75	3.04
7	3.04	26.45	649.51	3.00
8	3.00	2.08	548.97	3.00
9	3.00	0.02	540.07	3.00
10	3.00	0.00	540.00	3.00
11	3.00	0.00	540.00	3.00

value of 3.0. Hence, different starting values may lead to different optima, none of which may in fact be the global minimum, although in this example one of the local minima is the global minimum.

Till now only minimization of a linear model function has been considered. In nonlinear regression, the function to minimize is more complex as it involves squaring the differences between observed and predicted model values and then summing these over all observations. Other types of objective functions may involve more complex calculations, such as finding the determinant of the covariance matrix. Still, as will be shown, the methods used to find the minimum of a one variable linear model can be extended to minimizing a negative log-likelihood function quite easily. Indeed, because of the special nature of the sum of squares surface (quadratic in nature), this information can be used to develop special, more efficient algorithms at finding the minimum residual sum of squares.

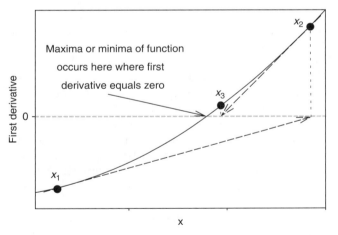

Figure 3.3 Line plot demonstrating convergence with the Newton–Raphson algorithm with one variable, x. A function is at a minima when the first derivative equals zero and the second derivative is positive. The algorithm starts at x_1. A tangent line (dashed arrow) is drawn from x_1 and extended to the x-axis where the first derivative equals zero. A perpendicular line (dotted line) is then drawn to the first derivative function, which becomes the second step in the sequence, x_2. The process is then repeated. A tangent line (dashed arrow) is drawn from x_2 and extended to the x-axis where the first derivative equals zero. A perpendicular line (dotted line) is then drawn to the first derivative, which becomes the third step in the sequence, x_3. Notice that in this case as the algorithm proceeds the value of the first derivative gets closer and closer to where the first derivative equals zero. It should be stressed that the Newton–Raphson algorithm does not guarantee convergence. The function may diverge from the global minimum if there are many local minima and the starting value is far removed from the global minimum.

FUNCTIONS OF SEVERAL VARIABLES: THE GRADIENT AND HESSIAN

Optimizing a univariate function is rarely seen in pharmacokinetics. Multivariate optimization is more the norm. For example, in pharmacokinetics one often wishes to identify many different rate constants and volume terms. One solution to a multivariate problem can be done either directly using direct search (Khorasheh, Ahmadi, and Gerayeli, 1999) or random search algorithms (Schrack and Borowski, 1972), both of which are basically brute force algorithms that repeatedly evaluate the function at selected values under the assumption that if enough combinations of variables are examined, the minimum or maximum will eventually be identified. The advantages of direct search methods are that a global maximum or minimum will always be identified, can work with either continuous or discontinuous functions, and do not require evaluation of the first and second derivatives.

Direct search methods have a disadvantage in that as the number of variables increases, so does the length of time to solve the problem, sometimes leading to exceedingly long search times. They also fail to take into account the information contained by evaluating the derivatives at the point under evaluation. For example if the first derivative is positive, the function is increasing and viceversa. This is useful information when one wants to find the maximum or minimum.

Analogous to the first and second derivatives in the univariate case are the gradient, denoted ∇, and the Hessian, denoted ∇^2, respectively. The gradient is used to define inflection points in multivariate problems much like the derivative can be used in univariate problems. Similarly, the Hessian can be used to identify whether a point on the gradient is at a maximum or minimum. The role of the gradient in multidimensional optimization can easily be understood using an example provided by Chapra and Canale (1998). Suppose you are at a specific location on a mountain and wanted to find the top of the mountain. Obviously you would look for the top and then start walking towards it. Unless you were really lucky would this approach work. More often, you would have to walk a short direction, reevaluate where you are, and walk toward another point. This process is repeated until you were at the top of the mountain. At each point, when you stop and look-up, this is equivalent to evaluating the gradient. When you walk to a new point, this is the equivalent of the step length. This process, while effective, is not very efficient because of all the stopping and looking you must do. A better way would be to walk until the path stops increasing and then reevaluate where you are at. Each time the path length may be different before you stop. This is basically the method of steepest ascent, which is illustrated in Fig. 3.4. The same concept applies to finding the minimum of a function, but in the opposite manner.

GRADIENT ALGORITHMS

Nonlinear least squares requires an iterative solution starting from set of initial value progressing to a different set of parameters which (hopefully) minimizes some objective function. As the name implies, gradient algorithms use the information contained in the gradient

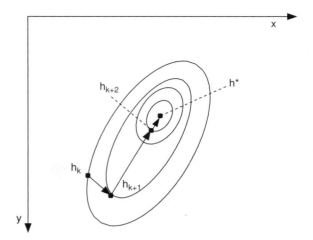

Figure 3.4   Graph showing the method of steepest ascent. The method starts at h_k, moves to h_{k+1}, then h_{k+2}, and finishes at h^*.

of the objective function for estimating where and how far to make the next step in the iterative process. In the parameter space, the objective function response surface can be represented as a surface plot as in Fig. 3.1 or a contour surface. For a linear model, the contours of the objective function response surface are perfectly elliptical with a single global minimum at $(x^Tx)^{-1}x^TY$. For a nonlinear model, the contours are not elliptical and may be quite "banana shaped" with perhaps many local minima; this concept is illustrated in Fig. 3.5. Although the objective function contour surface is often bowl shaped at the minimum, $\hat{\theta}$, the exact shape is a function of θ, which can vary, and the data, which are fixed. If the ellipse at the minimum, $S(\hat{\theta})$, is elongated in the sense that values removed from $\hat{\theta}$ are nearly as good as $\hat{\theta}$ or if the contours are banana shaped, the problem is said to be ill conditioned, which will be discussed later at greater length. Because in a nonlinear model the contours are not perfectly elliptical, different algorithms may reach a different set of final parameter estimates.

All the algorithms that will be presented assume that the objective function, its gradient, and Hessian exist and are continuous functions. They also all use a similar iteration function, namely

$$\theta^{(i+1)} = \theta^{(i)} + \alpha h \qquad (3.21)$$

where $\theta^{(i+1)}$ is the next iteration of parameter estimates, $\theta^{(i)}$ is the current set of parameter estimates, α is the step-length parameter, and h is the search direction from $\theta^{(i)}$. Note that the current iteration is denoted as $\theta^{(i)}$ to differentiate it from θ^i, which suggests that θ is being raised to the power i. The difference between the methods is how α and h are chosen.

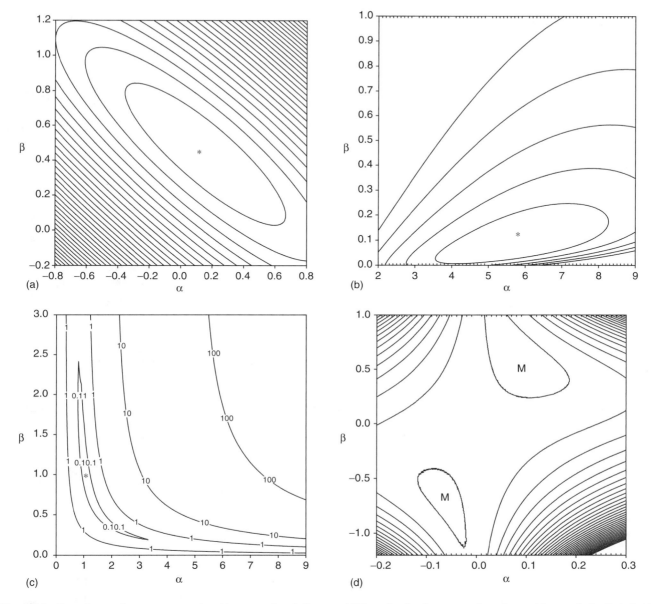

Figure 3.5 Example sum of squares contour plots. (a) contour plot of a linear model illustrating that the contours for such a model are perfectly elliptical with the global minimum at the center. (b) example of a well defined nonlinear model having a single global minimum and nearly elliptical contours. (c) contour plot of a nonlinear model showing "banana"-shaped contours indicative of ill conditioning. (d) contour plot of a nonlinear model with multiple solutions. All nonlinear models were parameterized in terms of α and β. Upper right and bottom left examples were suggested by Seber and Wild (1989). The symbol (*) indicates global minimum. M indicates local minimum.

Newton or Newton–Raphson Based Methods

Begin by assuming a function, called the objective function and denoted as $S(\theta)$, must be minimized. For notation, let $\theta^{(i)}$ be the ith estimate of the least squares estimator $\hat{\theta}$, which minimizes the objective function.

Further, let ∇ denote the gradient and ∇^2 denote the Hessian *of the objective function* evaluated at the current parameter estimates $\theta^{(i)}$. A first-order Taylor series approximation to $S(\theta)$ about $\theta^{(i)}$ can be written as

$$S(\theta) \cong S(\theta^{(i)}) + \nabla(\theta^{(i+1)} - \theta^{(i)}) \qquad (3.22)$$

ignoring higher order terms. The second term in Eq. (3.22) will dictate whether $S(\theta)$ increases or decreases since $S(\theta^{(i)})$ is a constant. The greatest decrease in $S(\theta)$ occurs when the search direction in Eq. (3.21) is the greatest negative scalar product of the second term. Hence, setting

$$h = -\nabla \qquad (3.23)$$

and substituting into Eq. (3.21) leads to

$$\theta^{(i+1)} = \theta^{(i)} - \alpha \nabla \qquad (3.24)$$

where α is chosen so that $S(\theta^{(i+1)}) < S(\theta)$. This method is often referred to as the method of steepest descent or Cauchy's method and is the best local gradient strategy to find a minimum. It may not, however, be a good global direction strategy because since the method is based on evaluating the gradient when it equals zero, which can occur at either a maxima or minima, the method will converge to a maxima just as easily as a minima.

A more efficient strategy would be to control both direction and distance. Consider a second-order Taylor series approximation to $S(\theta)$ expanded around $\theta^{(i)}$

$$S(\theta) \cong S(\theta^{(i)} + \nabla(\theta^{(i+1)} - \theta^{(i)}) + \frac{1}{2}\nabla^2(\theta^{(i+1)} - \theta^{(i)})^2 \quad (3.25)$$

ignoring higher order terms. The gradient of this approximation is

$$\frac{d}{d\theta^{(i)}} S(\theta) = \nabla + \nabla^2(\theta^{(i+1)} - \theta^{(i)}). \qquad (3.26)$$

The next point in the sequence is where the gradient of the approximation is zero

$$\frac{d}{d\theta^{(i)}} S(\theta) = \nabla + \nabla^2(\theta^{(i+1)} - \theta^{(i)}) = 0 \qquad (3.27)$$

and so the next point in the sequence is

$$\theta^{(i+1)} = \theta^{(i)} - \frac{\nabla}{\nabla^2}. \qquad (3.28)$$

This method is referred to as Newton's method and has reliable convergence properties for the types of objective functions typically found in pharmacokinetics. For non-quadratic objective functions, however, sometimes, convergence will not be achieved. To this end, then, Eq. (3.28) is modified to include a step length

$$\theta^{(i+1)} = \theta^{(i)} - \alpha^{(i)} \frac{\nabla}{\nabla^2} \qquad (3.29)$$

such that $S(\theta^{(i+1)}) < S(\theta^{(i)})$ and $0 < \alpha^{(i)} < 1$. As might be surmised, this approach is referred to as Newton's modified method. The major difficulty, however, with Newton-based methods is that calculation of the gradient and Hessian is required, which may be difficult. The method also has poor convergence when the starting values are far removed from the final estimates.

One condition for a minimum is that the Hessian be positive definite. Marquardt (1963) proposed adding a small constant to the Hessian, called λ, such that the Hessian remains positive definite

$$\theta^{(i+1)} = \theta^{(i)} - [\nabla^2 + \lambda I]^{-1} \nabla \qquad (3.30)$$

where I is the identity matrix. It is possible to choose λ so that $S(\theta^{(i+1)}) < S(\theta^{(i)})$ and then decrease λ to zero as the algorithm converges to the minimum. Marquardt's method is useful when the model parameters have a high degree of correlation.

Gauss–Newton Methods and Its Modifications

One problem with Newton methods is the calculation of the Hessian, which can be computationally burdensome. In such cases it may be easier to compute

$$\theta^{(i+1)} = \theta^{(i)} - H^{-1} \nabla \qquad (3.31)$$

where H is an approximation to the Hessian. These methods are called quasi-Newton methods, the most popular of which is the Gauss–Newton algorithm (also called the Fisher method of scoring). Instead of linearizing the objective function like Newton methods, the algorithm begins by making a first-order Taylor series approximation to the expectation function $f(\theta; x)$ about $\theta^{(i)}$

$$f(x; \theta) \cong f(x; \theta^{(i)}) + \frac{\partial f(x; \theta)}{\theta_1}(\theta_1 - \theta_1^{(i)}) + \\ \dots + \frac{\partial f(x; \theta)}{\theta_p}(\theta_p - \theta_p^{(i)}) \qquad (3.32)$$

which may be rewritten as

$$f(x;\theta) - f(x;\theta^{(i)}) = \frac{\partial f(x;\theta)}{\theta_1}(\theta_1 - \theta_1^{(i)}) + \dots + \frac{\partial f(x;\theta)}{\theta_p}(\theta_p - \theta_p^{(i)})$$
$$\varepsilon^{(i)} = \frac{\partial f(x;\theta)}{\theta_1}h_1^{(i)} + \dots + \frac{\partial f(x;\theta)}{\theta_p}h_p^{(i)}.$$
$$\varepsilon^{(i)} = J^{(i)}h^{(i)}$$
$$(3.33)$$

where $J^{(i)}$ is an $n \times p$ matrix of partial derivatives of the expectation function evaluated at the current parameter estimates (called the Jacobian) and $h^{(i)}$ is the difference between generic estimates and the set of current estimates. The left hand side of Eq. (3.33) is the residual between the observed value and linear approximation to the observed values evaluated at the current estimates $\theta^{(i)}$. Notice that the right hand side of Eq.

(3.33) consists of a linear function with the partial derivatives serving as the predictor variables and $h^{(i)}$ serving as the parameters to be estimated. The Gauss–Newton algorithm builds on this linear model structure by solving for $h^{(i)}$ using a standard ordinary least-squares solution

$$h^{(i)} = \left[J^{(i)T}J^{(i)}\right]^{-1}J^{(i)T}\varepsilon^{(i)} \qquad (3.34)$$

where J and ε are evaluated at the current parameter estimates. Equation (3.34) is functionally equivalent to the solution of a linear regression problem

$$\hat{\beta} = (x^Tx)^{-1}x^TY \qquad (3.35)$$

where $x = J^{(i)}$ and $Y = \varepsilon^{(i)}$. The next estimate of θ is then

$$\begin{aligned} \theta^{(i)} &= \theta^{(i)} - \alpha h^{(i)} \\ &= \theta^{(i)} - \alpha[J_T J]^{-1}J^T\varepsilon^{(i)} \end{aligned} \qquad (3.36)$$

Hence, the Gauss–Newton algorithm solves the solution to h through a series of linear regressions. For the base algorithm α is set equal to 1. This iterative process is repeated until there is little change in the parameter values between iterations. When this point is achieved, convergence is said to have occurred. Ideally, at each iteration, $f(x; \theta^{(i+1)})$ should be closer to Y than $f(x; \theta^{(i)})$.

What linearization does is convert a nonlinear expectation function into a series of linear functions and replaces the irregular bowl of the objective function response surface into an elliptical one that "looks about right" and has the same first derivatives as the nonlinear model at $\hat{\theta}$. At each step of the iteration process, starting at some point $\theta^{(i)}$, the parameter values move to the bottom of the linearized bowl around $\theta^{(i)}$ and that is then taken as the next point. Hopefully, this process converges to the global minimum, rather than diverge.

The Gauss–Newton algorithm has many advantages. First, it has been shown that the algorithm is consistent, i.e., that $\theta \rightarrow \hat{\theta}$ as $n \rightarrow \infty$, provided that the initial values are close enough to $\hat{\theta}$ to start and n is large enough. Second, only the matrix of first derivatives of the expectation function, J, needs to be calculated. No calculation of the Hessian is needed. The disadvantages with the basic Gauss–Newton algorithm are that the parameter values can oscillate wildly, often reversing direction. Also, there is no guarantee that at each step the residual sum of squares decreases. The residual sum of squares may increase when the linear approximation is at a point in space where the linearizing approximation is invalid. To avoid this situation, some software

programs use a process known as "step halving" wherein initially $\alpha = 1$ to start, then α is halved until

$$S(\theta^{(i+1)}) < S(\theta^{(i)}). \qquad (3.37)$$

Hartley (1961) proposed setting α equal to 1, 0.5, and 0 and computing the residual sum of squares for each value of α, denoted these as SSE(1), SSE(0.5), and SSE(0), respectively. $\alpha^{(i)}$ is then chosen by

$$\alpha^{(i)} = 0.5 + 0.25 \times SSE(0) \\ - \frac{SSE(1)}{SSE(1) - 2 \times SSE(0.5) + SSE(0)}. \qquad (3.38)$$

This is one of three algorithms that WinNonlin uses for nonlinear regression.

Up to now, the Gauss–Newton algorithm as described is a line-search strategy in that the algorithm chooses a direction and searches along this line from the current parameter values to a new set of parameter values that have a lower objective function value. In other words, a line search algorithm fixes the direction and looks for a distance to travel in which the objective function is lower than the current set of parameter values. The Levenberg–Marquardt algorithm is a trust region modification of the Gauss–Newton algorithm in the sense that both the direction and distance of the next step are variable. The algorithm begins by fixing a maximum distance and then seeks a direction to obtain the best solution given this constraint. If the step is unsatisfactory, the distance is reduced and the step is tried again (Nocedal and Wright, 1999). Specifically, Marquardt proposed modifying the Levenberg algorithm [Eq. (3.30)] such that h, the search direction at the ith step, be computed by

$$h^{(i)} = \left[J^{(i)T}J^{(i)} + \lambda \text{diag}(J^{(i)T}J^{(i)})\right]^{-1}J^{(i)T}\varepsilon^{(i)} \qquad (3.39)$$

where diag(.) is the diagonal of the matrix and λ is called Marquardt's parameter (Marquardt, 1963). Marquardt's contribution was to suggest using the diagonal of the Jacobian instead of the identity matrix (I) in Eq. (3.30). As $\lambda \rightarrow 0$, the Levenberg–Marquardt compromise approaches the Gauss–Newton algorithm and as $\lambda \rightarrow \infty$, it approaches Cauchy's method of steepest descent. For some programs, λ is predefined to start at some value, then change "on the fly" as the iterations proceed. For example, PROC NLIN in SAS starts with $\lambda = 0.001$ by default. If at any iteration the objective function decreases, then at the next iteration λ is changed to $1/10\lambda$. If not, λ is changed to 10λ. If the sum of squares is reduced at each iteration, then $\lambda \rightarrow 0$ and the algorithm is essentially pure Gauss–Newton. The advantage of the Levenberg–Marquardt compromise is that it works best when the parameter estimates are highly correlated. Win-Nonlin (1997) uses a modified form the Levenberg–Marquardt compromise that the designers indicate has better convergence properties than the original Levenberg–Marquardt algorithm and may be of use with a badly distorted sum of squares surface where convergence is necessary at the expense of speed and number of iterations (Davies and Whitting, 1972).

If the objective function is defined as in Eq. (3.11), the estimate of h then minimizes the objective function

$$S(\hat{\theta}) = \sum_{i=1}^{n} \left[Y_i - f(x; \theta^{(i)}) \quad - \frac{\partial f(x; \theta)}{\theta_1} (\theta_1 - \theta_1^{(i)}) - \\ .. \frac{\partial f(x; \theta)}{\theta_p} (\theta_p - \theta_p^{(i)}) \right]^2 . \quad (3.40)$$

Notice that Eq. (3.40) is not the same as Eq. (3.11). The two objective functions are different and the magnitude of the difference will depend on how good the linearizing approximation is to the expectation function. In practice, the approximation is valid when the residuals are "small." If the expectation function is inadequate, the starting values are poor, or if outliers are in the dataset, any of these may lead to a situation where "large" residuals are present, possibly leading to a situation called the "large residual problem." The basic Gauss–Newton algorithm will fail in most cases of the large residual problem. The Levenberg–Marquardt algorithm, although it is fairly robust and works well on most problems, will converge slowly and may not at all in some large residual problems. Quasi-Newton methods that take into account the poor approximation to the Hessian by either adding back in the missing term into the Hessian equation, or by approximating the Hessian directly, have been developed, but to the author's knowledge, no pharmacokinetic software package, SAS or S-Plus for that matter, has this option. If a model fails to converge or if particular residuals are larger than the bulk of the residuals, the analyst should examine the validity of the assumptions made in the fitting and either remove a particular data point or reexamine the choice of model or starting values.

Lastly, in order to estimate the search direction, an estimate of the Jacobian must be available. Although the most precise estimates of the Jacobian are when it is calculated analytically using the partial derivatives of the expectation function, these are often prone to typographical errors when they are manually typed into a software program. Almost every software package evaluates their derivatives numerically using forward, backwards, or central differences. Forward difference uses data at the ith and (ith+1) data points to estimate the derivative. Backward difference uses data at (ith−1) and ith data points, whereas central difference uses values that are more evenly spaced around the point of

interest. It is possible to improve the accuracy of the gradient approximations with higher order Taylor series approximations, although few software programs do so. Between the three methods, the central difference method provides better approximation to the true gradient since the truncation term in the central difference method is smaller (Chapra and Canale, 1998). The disadvantage of having to evaluate the derivatives numerically is speed and precision; analytical evaluation of derivatives is much faster and more precise.

In summary, the differences between the various modifications of the Gauss–Newton algorithms are largely in the choice of h, the search direction, and α, the step length. Cauchy's algorithm is based on direction only, whereas Levenberg–Marquardt's algorithm is based on direction and distance. Cauchy's is more of a brute force algorithm, whereas Levenberg–Marquardt is more subtle and makes more use of the information at hand. Ideally, an algorithm could start using one method, say Cauchy's method, and then switch to a more efficient algorithm after a few iterations. No pharmacokinetic software package takes this approach, however.

DERIVATIVE FREE ALGORITHMS

The methods discussed so far are called gradient-based optimization methods because the basis for convergence is dependent on the computation of the gradient. However, gradient methods may not converge or converge very slowly. Hence, there is a need for other types of optimization methods that do not utilize the gradient. Another class of optimization methods called *direct search* methods require only that the objective function exist and be a smooth continuous function. In the case of nonlinear least squares, the objective function response surface meets all these requirements. The basic idea behind direct search algorithms is to choose a base point in the response surface and to examine around the base point until a point lower on the surface is found. This new point then becomes the base point and the process is repeated until the minimum point on the surface is achieved. The difference in the various direct search algorithms is how they "examine" the response surface around the base point.

The classic example of a direct search algorithm is the *simplex* method of Nelder and Mead (1965), who utilized a method originally devised by Spendley et al. (1962). In p-dimensional space, a simplex is a polyhedron of p + 1 equidistant points forming the vertices. For a two-dimensional problem, the simplex is an equilateral triangle. For three-dimensions, the simplex is a tetrahedron. This algorithm, which has no relation to the simplex algorithm in linear programming and is one of three algorithms used by WinNonlin for nonlinear regression, is based on the fact that a new simplex can be generated from any face of the current simplex by projecting any vertex an appropriate distance through the centroid of the remaining two vertices. Given this, the basic idea is to find the extreme of a function by considering the worst points on the simplex and then projecting a vertex through its opposite face forming a symmetrical image (Fig. 3.6). Once the reflection is made, the simplex can either contract or expand to form a new simplex (this is Nelder and Mead's (1965) contribution to the algorithm). The process is repeated until convergence is achieved. The advantage of the algorithm is that it will always converge and is often able to find quite reasonable estimates. The disadvantage is that the method is slow[1] relative to the gradient methods. Still with modern computing speeds, the Nelder–Mead algorithm may not be so slow anymore.

CONVERGENCE

As mentioned earlier, convergence occurs when there is no useful change in the objective function from one iteration to the next. By comparing the observed difference in objective function from one iteration to the next against a set value defined a priori, an algorithm can decide whether convergence is achieved. This set value is called the convergence criteria and is usually small, less than 0.0001. A modification of the convergence criteria is a relative change criteria where convergence is achieved if the difference in the objective function from one iteration to the next changes less

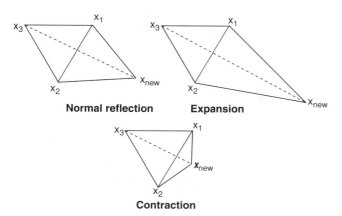

Normal reflection   **Expansion**

Contraction

Figure 3.6 Expansion and contraction of a simplex.

---

[1] The Nelder–Mead algorithm used to be called the Amoeba algorithm, but given the speed of today's computer processors this is probably an outdated criticism.

than a fixed percentage. Given a set of starting parameters, it may take many iterations to reach the convergence criteria and sometimes the convergence criteria may never be reached. Thus, balanced against the convergence criteria is a criteria for the maximum number of iterations an algorithm may go through before the program "gives up" and says that convergence cannot be achieved. Usually 50 iterations is the default value for most programs.

Often convergence is not initially achieved with a given set of initial parameter estimates. Most software packages, as part of their standard output, list the values of the parameter estimates at each iteration and their corresponding objective function. From this the analyst can determine how close the starting values were to the final estimates or whether the estimates were bouncing around from one value to another without honing in on a single value.

If convergence is not achieved, a number of questions should be asked and some corrective measures should be taken. First, is the model correctly specified? Are all the parameters identifiable? Are the derivatives correctly specified (not needed for programs that compute the derivatives numerically)? Do the starting values have the correct values and units? Do the starting values correspond to the right parameters? Do the starting values have the right signs? Are the right predictor variables and dependent variables defined? If the answer is yes to all these questions, then examine the output at each iteration. Do some parameter combinations move in the same direction? If so, the model may be over-parameterized and these parameters may be collinear. A useful plot is to plot one parameter against the others from all the iterations. Parameters that are correlated may lead to ill-conditioned problems and poor parameter estimation. Do any of the parameters become unreasonably large or small? This could be an indication that the derivatives are being computed incorrectly. Try changing the starting parameter estimates and see if this helps. It may be that there is not enough data to fit the chosen model. For example, in an E_{max} model, Eq. (3.1), an estimate of E_{max} may not be possible if plasma concentrations are not larger than the EC_{50} (Dutta, Matsumoto, and Ebling, 1996). If all other solutions fail, try increasing the convergence criterion, increasing the maximal number of iterations, or using a different algorithm.

Sometimes failure to achieve convergence is due to exchangeability. Consider the model

$$Y = \theta_1 e^{-\theta_2 t} + \theta_3 e^{-\theta_4 t}. \qquad (3.41)$$

The first and second term in Eq. (3.41) can be switched to produce the exact same estimate of Y. Hence, the pairs (θ_1, θ_2) and (θ_3, θ_4) are exchangeable. Sometimes an optimization program will switch θ_1 and θ_3 back and forth and back and forth *ad infinitum* never achieving convergence. One could remove the exchangeability by enforcing the restriction $0 \le \theta_2 \le \theta_4$ with the following model

$$Y = \theta_1 e^{-\theta_2 t} + \theta_3 e^{-(\theta_2 + \theta_4)t}. \qquad (3.42)$$

Since θ_1 and θ_3 depend on θ_2 and θ_4 no other restrictions are forced on θ_1 and θ_3.

Sometimes standardizing, centering, or scaling the independent variables may help the optimization process and further facilitate convergence. Large differences in the magnitude in the columns of the Jacobian matrix can result in unstable parameter estimates. This is the same problem in the linear case when the columns of $x^T x$ are of differing scales. Also, such large differences may lead to convergence problems. In centering, each column of the independent variables matrix has the mean (x) of the column subtracted from each observation in the column

$$x_c^* = x - x. \qquad (3.43)$$

After centering, each observation has zero mean but different variances. In scaling, each observations is divided by a column-specific constant, usually the standard deviation (s)

$$x_{scaling}^* = \frac{x}{s}. \qquad (3.44)$$

After scaling, each observation has unit variance but different means. Standardization involves both centering and scaling. Each observations has the mean subtracted and is then divided by the column standard deviation,

$$x_{st}^* = \frac{x - x}{s}. \qquad (3.45)$$

After standardization, each observation has zero mean and unit variance. Typically, centering is tried first because the estimates and the units of the parameter associated with x remain the same, whereas with scaling or standardization the units and the parameter estimates themselves are different. If centering fails, usually standardization is tried next.

It is important to remember that convergence criteria are really just stopping criteria and that these criteria do not guarantee that true convergence has been achieved (Bates and Watts, 1988). Some good indicators that convergence has been achieved are if the rate of convergence is fast, for if the objective function surface is well behaved, most algorithms will reach the minimum quickly. Further, every user of optimization software must be aware of local minima, which is a point on the objective function surface that appears to be the function minimum, but is not. Unfortunately, even for what appear to be relatively simple compartmental models, such as a 2-compartment model with intravenous administration where there are only four estimable parameters, local minima occur quite frequently and should be guarded against (see Purves (1996) and Liang and Derendorf (1998) for example).

INFERENCES ON THE PARAMETER ESTIMATES

With linear models, exact inferential procedures are available for any sample size. The reason is that as a result of the linearity of the model parameters, the parameter estimates are unbiased with minimum variance when the assumption of independent, normally distributed residuals with constant variance holds. The same is not true with nonlinear models because even if the residuals assumption is true, the parameter estimates do not necessarily have minimum variance or are unbiased. Thus, inferences about the model parameter estimates are usually based on large sample sizes because the properties of these estimators are asymptotic, i.e., are true as $n \to \infty$. Thus, when n is large and the residuals assumption is true, only then will nonlinear regression parameter estimates have estimates that are normally distributed and almost unbiased with minimum variance. As n increases, the degree of unbiasedness and estimation variability will increase.

In order to make inferences about the parameter estimates, an estimate of the error variance (the mean square error), σ^2, is needed. The estimator for σ^2 is same as for linear regression

$$\hat{\sigma}^2 = MSE = \frac{SSE}{n - p}$$
$$= \frac{\sum_{i=i}^{n} (Y_i - \hat{Y}_i)^2}{n - p} \qquad (3.46)$$
$$= \frac{\sum_{i=i}^{n} [Y_i - f(x;\hat{\theta})]^2}{n - p}$$

where $\hat{\theta}$ is the vector of final parameter estimates. For nonlinear regression, MSE is a biased estimator for σ^2, but the bias is small for large n. For reasonably large sample sizes, when the residuals are independent and normally distributed with mean zero and variance σ^2, and the sample size is large, the sampling distribution of $\hat{\theta}$ is normally distributed with mean θ and variance–covariance matrix

$$Var(\hat{\theta}) = \Sigma = MSE(J^TJ)^{-1} \qquad (3.47)$$

where J is the Jacobian evaluated at $\hat{\theta}$ and Σ is a p × p matrix whose diagonal elements, denoted Σ_{ii}, are the variances of the parameter estimates. There are other methods used to estimate Σ. One method is based on the Hessian,

$$\Sigma = MSE(\nabla^2) \qquad (3.48)$$

where ∇^2 is the Hessian matrix evaluated at the final model parameter estimates. Another method, sometimes called the heteroscedastic consistent variance estimator, is

$$\Sigma = MSE[\nabla^2]^{-1}(J^TJ)[\nabla^2]^{-1}. \qquad (3.49)$$

Most software packages use Eq. (3.47) as the default variance estimator. The standard error of the parameter estimates are computed as the square root of the diagonal elements of the variance–covariance matrix

$$SE(\theta) = \sqrt{\Sigma_{ii}}. \qquad (3.50)$$

Note that the form of Eq. (3.47) is the same as for the variance of the estimators in a linear model with x^Tx replaced by J^TJ.

Donaldson and Schnabel (1987) used Monte Carlo simulation to determine which of the variance estimators was best in constructing approximate confidence intervals. They conclude that Eq. (3.47) is best because it is easy to compute, and it gives results that are never worse and sometimes better than the other two, and is more stable numerically than the other methods. However, their simulations also show that confidence intervals obtained using even the best methods have poor coverage probabilities, as low as 75% for a 95% confidence interval. They go so far as to state *"confidence intervals constructed using the linearization method can be essentially meaningless"* (Donaldson and Schnabel, 1987). Based on their results, it is wise not to put much emphasis on confidence intervals constructed from nonlinear models.

Inferences on the parameter estimates are made the same as for a linear model, but the inferences are approximate. Therefore, using a T-test in nonlinear regression to test for some parameter being equal to zero or some other value is risky and should be discouraged (Myers, 1986). However, that is not to say that the standard errors of the parameter estimates cannot be used as a model discrimination criterion. Indeed, a model with small standard errors is a better model than a model with large standard errors, all other factors being equal. Once the variance of θ is determined, a coefficient of variation (CV) for the parameter estimates can be determined to assess the relative precision of the estimate

$$CV(\%) = \sqrt{\frac{\Sigma_{ii}}{\theta}} \times 100\%. \qquad (3.51)$$

Models with CVs less than 25% are usually deemed to be precise parameter estimates.

If $\hat{\theta} \sim N(\theta, \Sigma_{ii})$, then an approximate $(1 - \alpha)100\%$ confidence interval, sometimes called a univariate, planar, or linear confidence interval, can then be constructed from

$$\hat{\theta} \pm t_{n-p}, 1 - \frac{\alpha}{2}\sqrt{\Sigma_{ii}} \qquad (3.52)$$

where $1 - \alpha$ is the desired level of confidence and t is Student's two-tailed t-value with n-p degrees of freedom. Jacobian-based $(1 - \alpha)100\%$ joint confidence intervals, sometimes called confidence regions, consider all the parameters simultaneously such that

$$(\theta - \hat{\theta})^T(J^TJ)(\theta - \hat{\theta}) \le MSE \times p \times F_{p,n-p-1,1-\alpha} \quad (3.53)$$

where F is the value from an F-distribution with p and $n-p-1$ degrees of freedom. In the case where p = 2, the confidence region forms an ellipse and in three dimensions forms a football-shaped region. Bates and Watts (1987) do not recommend joint confidence intervals because of their undesirable coverage properties.

The question, when does asymptotic theory not hold for a particular data set always lingers in a nonlinear regression model. There are no simple rules to tell when to trust the variance estimates and when not to, but there are some useful guidelines that can be used (Bates and Watts, 1988). First, quick convergence of the model to the final parameter estimates is a good indication that the linear approximation to the model is a good one and that the variance estimators are appropriate. Bates and Watts (1980) provide curvature measures of nonlinearity that appear to be quite useful in measuring the adequacy of the linear approximation. But, no software manufacturer has implemented their use and so their use will not be discussed here. An alternative is to use the bootstrap to directly estimate the variance or confidence intervals of the parameter estimates. By examination of the distribution of the bootstrapped parameter estimates, one can determine how close the distribution is to normality and whether the degree of bias in the parameter estimates is small. One difficulty with this approach, however, is that some of the bootstrap iterations may not converge or may be wildly different from the original parameter estimates. For these reasons, it is often built into the algorithm that bootstrap iterations that fail for whatever reason are discarded and a new dataset created. Another difficulty is that bootstrap standard errors cannot be computed using the current state of pharmacokinetic software.

FUNCTIONS OF MODEL PARAMETERS

Standard errors and confidence intervals for functions of model parameters can be found using expectation theory, in the case of a linear function, or using the delta method (which is also sometimes called propagation of errors), in the case of a nonlinear function (Rice, 1988). Begin by assuming that $\hat{\theta}$ is the estimator for θ and Σ is the variance–covariance matrix for $\hat{\theta}$. For a linear combination of observed model parameters

$$g(\hat{\theta}) = a + \sum_{i=1}^{k} b_i \hat{\theta}_i \qquad (3.54)$$

the expected value [E(.)] and variance [Var(.)] is given by

$$
\begin{aligned}
E[g(\hat{\theta})] &= a + \sum_{i=1}^{k} b_i E[\hat{\theta}_i] \\
&= a + \sum_{i=1}^{k} b_i \theta_i
\end{aligned} \qquad (3.55)
$$

$$
\begin{aligned}
\text{Var}[g(\hat{\theta})] &= \sum_{i=1}^{k} b_i \text{Var}(\hat{\theta}_i) + \\
&\sum_{j=1}^{k} b_j \text{Var}(\hat{\theta}_j) + \sum_{i=1}^{k}\sum_{j=1}^{k} 2b_i b_j \text{Cov}(\hat{\theta}_i, \hat{\theta}_j), \ i \neq j, \\
&= \sum_{i=1}^{k} b_i \Sigma_{ii} + \sum_{j=1}^{k} b_j \Sigma_{jj} + \sum_{i=1}^{k}\sum_{j=1}^{k} 2b_i b_j \Sigma_{ij}, \ i \neq j \quad (3.56)
\end{aligned}
$$

which can be written in matrix notation as

$$E[g(\hat{\theta})] = b^T \theta \qquad (3.57)$$

$$\text{Var}[g(\hat{\theta})] = b^T \Sigma b, \qquad (3.58)$$

respectively, where b is the vector of b_is. In practice, θ and Σ are replaced by their OLS or maximum likelihood estimates. Suppose, e.g., a 2-compartment model is fit and one wishes to estimate V_{ss}, the steady-state volume of distribution, which can be calculated as the sum

of the volume of the central compartment (V_c) and peripheral compartment (V_p). If

$$
\begin{bmatrix} V_c \\ V_p \end{bmatrix} \sim \left[\begin{pmatrix} 80\,\text{L} \\ 200\,\text{L} \end{pmatrix}, \begin{pmatrix} 100 & 75 \\ 75 & 200 \end{pmatrix} \right]. \qquad (3.59)
$$

The expected value of V_{ss} is 280 L with variance

$$
\begin{aligned}
\text{Var}(V_{ss}) &= \text{Var}(V_c) + \text{Var}(V_p) + 2\text{Cov}(V_c, V_p) \\
&= 100 + 200 + 2 \times 75 \qquad (3.60) \\
&= 450\,\text{L}^2
\end{aligned}
$$

Up to this point normality has not been assumed. Equations (3.55) and (3.56) do not depend on normality for their validity. But, if $\hat{\theta}$ was normally distributed then $g(\hat{\theta})$ will also be normally distributed. So returning to the example, since V_c and V_p were normally distributed, then V_{ss} will be normally distributed.

If $g(\hat{\theta})$, be it univariate or multivariate, is a nonlinear function then an approach repeatedly seen throughout this book will be used—the function will first be linearized using a first-order Taylor series and then the expected value and variance will be found using Eqs. (3.55) and (3.56), respectively. This is the so-called delta method. If $g(\hat{\theta})$ is a univariate, nonlinear function then to a first-order Taylor series approximation about θ would be

$$g(\hat{\theta}) \approx g(\theta) - (\hat{\theta} - \theta)\frac{\partial g}{\partial \theta}. \qquad (3.61)$$

The expected value can now be found through a linear combination of random variables

$$E[g(\hat{\theta})] \approx g(\theta) \qquad (3.62)$$

since $E(\hat{\theta} - \theta) = 0$. The variance is given by

$$\text{Var}[g(\hat{\theta})] \approx \sum_{ii} \left(\frac{\partial g}{\partial \theta}\right)^2. \qquad (3.63)$$

For example, suppose the terminal elimination rate constant (λ_z,) was estimated using four observations. If the mean and variance of λ_z was 0.154 per hour and $6.35E - 4$ (per hour)^2, respectively. Then the mean and variance for half life ($t_{1/2}$) defined as $\text{Ln}(2)/\lambda_z$, would be 4.5 h and

$$
\begin{aligned}
\text{Var}(t_{1/2}) &= \text{Var}(\lambda_z)\left(\frac{\text{Ln}(2)}{\lambda_z^2}\right)^2 \\
&= 6.35E - 4(29.22)^2, \qquad (3.64) \\
&= 0.542\,\text{h}^2
\end{aligned}
$$

respectively. If λ_z were normally distributed then an approximate 95% confidence interval for half life would be

$$4.5 \pm 4.303\sqrt{0.542} \qquad (3.65)$$

or (1.3, 7.7 h).

If $g(\theta)$ is a nonlinear function of two or more model parameters then the multivariate delta method can be used. For a function of two variables a first-order Taylor series approximation around θ_i and θ_j can be written as

$$g(\hat{\theta}_i, \hat{\theta}_j) = g(\theta_i, \theta_j) + (\hat{\theta}_i - \theta_i)\frac{\partial g}{\partial \theta_i} + (\hat{\theta}_j - \theta_j)\frac{\partial g}{\partial \theta_j} \qquad (3.66)$$

with expected value and variance

$$E[g(\hat{\theta}_i, \hat{\theta}_j)] = g(\theta_i, \theta_j) \qquad (3.66)$$

$$\begin{aligned} \text{Var}[g(\hat{\theta}_i, \hat{\theta}_j)] = & \sum_{ii}\left(\frac{\partial g}{\partial \theta_i}\right)^2 + \sum_{jj}\left(\frac{\partial g}{\partial \theta_j}\right)^2 \\ & + 2\left(\frac{\partial g}{\partial \theta_i}\right)\left(\frac{\partial g}{\partial \theta_j}\right)\sum_{ij} \end{aligned} \qquad (3.68)$$

In matrix notation,

$$\text{Var}[g(\hat{\theta})] = h^T\sum h \qquad (3.69)$$

where h is the matrix of first derivative with respect to θ. As an example, suppose that a 1-compartment model with intravenous administration was parameterized in terms of the primary pharmacokinetic parameters {CL, V}. If clearance had a mean of 50 L/h, V had a mean of 150 L, and the variance–covariance matrix of {CL, V} was

$$\sum = \begin{bmatrix} CL & V \\ 55 & 20 \\ 20 & 225 \end{bmatrix} \qquad (3.70)$$

then the mean half life would be

$$t_{1/2} = \frac{\text{Ln}(2)V}{CL} = \frac{\text{Ln}(2)150\,L}{50\,L/h} = 2.1\,h, \qquad (3.71)$$

with variance

$$\begin{aligned} \text{Var}(t_{1/2}) &= \left(\frac{\partial g}{\partial CL} \ \frac{\partial g}{\partial V}\right)\sum\begin{pmatrix}\frac{\partial g}{\partial CL} \\ \frac{\partial g}{\partial V}\end{pmatrix} \\ &= \left(\frac{-\text{Ln}(2)V}{CL^2} \ \frac{\text{Ln}(2)}{CL}\right)\sum\begin{pmatrix}\frac{-\text{Ln}(2)V}{CL^2} \\ \frac{\text{Ln}(2)}{CL}\end{pmatrix} \end{aligned}$$

$$\text{Var}(t_{1/2}) = (-0.04158 \ \ 0.01386)\begin{bmatrix} 55 & 20 \\ 20 & 225 \end{bmatrix}\begin{pmatrix} -0.04158 \\ .01386 \end{pmatrix}$$

$$= 0.115\,h^2, \qquad (3.72)$$

respectively. For nonlinear functions, even if all the input parameters are normally distributed, the transformed parameter does not necessarily follow a normal distribution and, hence, development of confidence intervals based on a normal or Student's t-distribution may not be appropriate.

Sometimes the transformation function $g(\hat{\theta})$ is so complex that the partial derivatives are not easily calculated or, in the case above, while the variance of $g(\hat{\theta})$ can be calculated, the distribution of $g(\hat{\theta})$ may not be determinable. For such cases, a simulation approach may be used. With this approach, each model parameter in $g(\hat{\theta})$ is stochastically simulated assuming the distribution of the parameter and then $g(\theta^*)$ is calculated and stored as $g(\theta_i^*)$. This process is repeated B times, usually more than 1000. The variance is then calculated as

$$\text{Var}[g(\hat{\theta})] = \frac{\sum_{i=1}^{n}[g(\theta_i^*) - g(\theta^*)]^2}{B - 1}. \qquad (3.73)$$

where

$$\bar{g}(\theta^*) = \frac{\sum_{i=1}^{n} g(\theta_i^*)}{B}. \qquad (3.74)$$

Approximate $(1 - \alpha)100\%$ confidence intervals can be developed using any of the methods presented in the bootstrapping section of the book appendix. Using the previous example, CL was simulated 1,000 times from a normal distribution with mean 50 L/h and variance $55\,(L/h)^2$ while V was simulated 10,000 times with a mean of 150 L and variance $225\,L^2$. The correlation between V and CL was fixed at 0.18 given the covariance matrix in Eq. (3.70). The simulated mean and variance of CL was 49.9 L/h and $55.5\,(L/h)^2$, while the simulated mean and variance of V was 149.8 L with variance $227\,L^2$. The simulated correlation between CL and V was 0.174. The mean estimated half life was 2.12 h with a variance of $0.137\,h^2$, which was very close to the Taylor series approximation to the variance. The Shapiro–Wilk test for normality indicated that the distribution of half life was not normally distributed ($p < 0.01$). Hence, even though CL and V were normally distributed the resulting distribution for half life was not. Based on the 5 and 95% percentiles of the simulated half life values, a 90% confidence interval for half life was estimated to be (1.6, 2.8 h).

It is important to remember that for nonlinear functions the function is first linearized using a Taylor series approximation and then the mean and variance are calculated based on the *approximation*. How good the approximation is depends on how nonlinear g is around θ and on the size of the variance of $\hat{\theta}$. Better approximations to $g(\theta)$ can be found through higher order approximations. For example, a second order Taylor series about θ leads to

$$E\left[g(\hat{\theta})\right] \approx g(\theta) + \frac{1}{2} \text{Var}(\hat{\theta}) \left(\frac{\partial g}{\partial^2 \theta}\right). \qquad (3.75)$$

since $E\left[(\hat{\theta} - \theta)\right]^2 = \text{Var}(\hat{\theta})$. This makes it clear that although for first order approximations, the expected value of the function is a function of the expected values, this is not the case with higher order approximations. In general, for nonlinear functions, $E[g(\hat{\theta})] \neq g[E(\theta)]$, although it is often assumed so. And of course, the method for two variables can be expanded for more than two variables.

OBTAINING INITIAL PARAMETER ESTIMATES

Some optimization algorithms are so good that if convergence is going to be achieved then poor initial estimates will not matter. Similarly if the model is not very nonlinear, but behaves in a more linear fashion, then poor initial estimates will not matter so much. But, if the model is highly nonlinear then good initial parameter estimates are crucial. Obviously, convergence problems will be slight and convergence will be rapid the closer the starting values are to the true parameters (unless the system is unidentifiable). Often the analyst has an idea what the values should be beforehand based on knowledge of the system, e.g., rate constants must be greater than zero, or based on prior knowledge, e.g., the half life of the drug is about 12 h from previous studies. A good source for starting values in a pharmacokinetic system is to perform noncompartmental analysis on the data first.

One method to obtain initial estimates is linearization of the problem. For example, the 1-compartment model with bolus intravenous administration can be reformulated to a linear problem by taking the log-transform on both sides of the equation. This is a trivial example, but is often reported in texts on nonlinear regression. Another commonly used method is by "eyeballing" the data. For example, in an E_{max} model, E_{max} can be started at the maximal of all the observed effect values. EC_{50} can be started at the middle of the range of concentration values. Alternatively, the data can be plot-

ted, log (concentration) versus effect, with EC_{50} being the concentration that produces an effect midway between the baseline and E_{max}. One last method may be to use historical data and prior knowledge. For example, for 1- and 2-compartment models without lag-times having time to maximal drug concentrations in the range of 2–6 h, an absorption rate constant (k_a) of 0.7 per hour seems to work as a reasonable starting value. Still another method to obtain initial estimates is to reduce the model by looking at the limits. For example, if the model is

$$Y = \theta_1 + \theta_2 e^{-\theta_3 t} \qquad (3.76)$$

then at $t = 0$, $Y = \theta_1 + \theta_2$. As $t \to \infty$, $Y \to \theta_1$. Hence, θ_2 can be obtained by difference $Y(0) - \theta_1$. Once θ_1 and θ_2 are found, Eq. (3.76) can be solved for $\theta_3 t$ obtaining

$$\text{Ln}\left(\frac{Y - \theta_1}{\theta_2}\right) = Y^* = -\theta_3 t. \qquad (3.77)$$

Hence, regressing Y^* against t (without intercept) an estimate of θ_3 can be obtained.

Peeling, curve stripping, or the method of residuals is an old technique advocated in some of the classic textbooks on pharmacokinetics (Gibaldi and Perrier, 1982) as a method to obtain initial estimates. The method will not be described in detail; the reader is referred to the references for details. Its use will be briefly illustrated. Consider the biexponential model

$$Y = \theta_1 e^{-\theta_2 t} + \theta_3 e^{-\theta_4 t}, \qquad (3.78)$$

where θ_2 and θ_4 are the fast and slow disposition rate constants such that $\theta_2 > \theta_4$. Since θ_2 is greater than θ_4, the first term of Eq. (3.78) will reach zero faster than the second term. Hence, Eq. (3.78) reduces to

$$Y = \theta_3 e^{-\theta_4 t} \qquad (3.79)$$

for large t. Let the breakpoint for large t be defined as t^*. Taking the natural log of both sides of Eq. (3.79) gives

$$\text{Ln}(Y) = \text{Ln}(\theta_3) - \theta_4 t, \quad t \geq t^*. \qquad (3.80)$$

For values of t greater than or equal to t^*, linear regression of $\text{Ln}(Y)$ versus t will give an estimate of θ_3 and θ_4. The next step is to use Eq. (3.80) to predict Y for the values of t not included in the estimation of θ_3 and θ_4 ($t < t^*$) and then calculate the residuals, $\tilde{Y}$,

$$\tilde{Y} = Y - \theta_3 e^{-\theta_4 t}, \, t < t^*. \qquad (3.81)$$

The residuals can then be used to estimate the first term in Eq. (3.78), which after taking the natural log becomes

$$Ln(\tilde{Y}) = Ln(\theta_1) - \theta_2 t, \quad t < t^*. \quad (3.82)$$

This process can be continued for models with more than two exponents, though rarely successful due to propagation of errors from one strip to the next. Curve stripping is usually quite successful when the values of the rate constants in the exponents differ by an order of magnitude. The only decision that the analyst must make is what is the breakpoint t^* and how many exponents the model contains. Some programs curve strip automatically (WinNonlin) to obtain starting values or alternatively there are programs specifically designed to automate this process (RSTRIP).

Given the speed of modern computers, one method for obtaining initial estimates is by a grid search, which was illustrated earlier in the chapter (Fig. 3.1). In a grid search, the parameter space for each parameter is broken down into an upper and lower range and into k discrete parameter values within the upper and lower bound. For each combination of parameter estimates, the objective function is calculated. The parameter combination with the smallest objective function is used as the starting values for the model. This approach may be slow for multi-parameter models such that most algorithms use a limited number of points in the parameter space to decrease the time to generate the grid. For example, WinNonlin uses three points for each parameter, the upper limit, lower limit, and mid-range, so that if there are four parameters to be estimated there will be 3^4 or 81 possible combinations. A modification of the grid search approach is to randomly sample in the parameter space many, many times and use the combination with the smallest objective function as the starting parameters. Ultimately, the best method to choose initial values depends on the "cost" of computing the objective function, the step size, and the number of estimable parameters.

ILL CONDITIONING AND NEAR SINGULARITY

Recall that ill conditioning was discussed in the previous chapter on linear models and regression as a major source of parameter instability when the matrix $x^T x$ was near singular. Ill conditioning arises in nonlinear regression through inversion of the $J^T J$ matrix. Like linear models, the condition number of the $J^T J$ matrix (calculated as the ratio of the largest to smallest eigenvalue) can be used to assess the degree of instability in the inversion process. But, for most pharmacokinetic studies where 10–15 samples are collected per subject,

large condition numbers will be observed even in the best of situations.

Every user in a software package should learn how that condition number is calculated, as it has direct bearing on its interpretation. For instance, WinNonlin Pro (Version 4.0) reports the condition number as the square root of the largest to smallest eigenvalue in the transformed parameter space (see Section on Constrained Optimization for details). SAAM II (Heatherington, Vicini, and Golde, 1998) and this book use the ratio of largest to smallest eigenvalue in the original parameter space as the condition number because $_{10}$ of the condition number, calculated in this manner, indicates the number of decimal places lost by a computer due to round-off errors during matrix inversion. SAS's NLIN procedure does not report a condition number.

For individual pharmacokinetic data, there are no hard and fast rules for what constitutes a "large" condition number. Different books report different values depending on how they calculate the condition number. For example, Gabrielsson and Weiner (2000), who calculate the condition number using the square root method in the transformed parameter space, report 10^p as a large condition number, where p is the number of estimable model parameters. Niedwiecki and Simonoff (1990) suggest that condition numbers be calculated in the original parameter space as the natural log of the largest to smallest eigenvalues, and that values greater than 5.3 are harmful. Heatherington, Vicini, and Golde (1998) indicate that a condition number greater than 10^7 is indicative of ill conditioning. In this book, for routine pharmacokinetic data from a single subject (10–15 observations per subject), condition numbers less 10^6 in the original parameter space will be considered acceptable and that condition numbers calculated within WinNonlin of less than 10^p are acceptable.

Ill-conditioned matrices can be due to either insufficient data to fit a model or a poor model. A model-driven situation where ill conditioning is a problem is when the model parameter estimates themselves are highly correlated (correlations greater than 0.95). An example of the latter situation using logarithms of thermometer resistance (Y) as a function of temperature (x) was reported by Simonoff and Tsai (1989) and Meyer and Roth (1972) (Table 3.3).

The following nonlinear model was fit to the data

$$Y = \theta_1 + \frac{\theta_2}{\theta_3 + x} + \varepsilon. \quad (3.83)$$

Table 3.4 presents the results of the model fits to the data and Fig. 3.7 plots the observed and predicted model fits for the data. The model was an excellent fit to the data. The residual sum of squares was less than 1E-5 and the

Table 3.3 Thermometer resistance (Y) as a function of temperature (x).

x	Y	x	Y
50	10.457	90	9.019
55	10.262	95	8.858
60	10.071	100	8.700
65	9.885	105	8.546
70	9.703	110	8.395
75	9.527	115	8.248
80	9.354	120	8.104
85	9.184	125	7.963

Table 3.4 Nonlinear regression analysis of log-thermometer resistance as a function of temperature using Eq. (3.83) with x = 50 and x = 49.5.

Parameter	x = 50 (original data)		x = 49.5 (modified data)	
θ_1	−5.103	(0.0397)	−6.076	(0.449)
θ_2	6112	(34.03)	6993	(412)
θ_3	342.8	(1.190)	373.2	(13.48)
SSE	2.15E-6		2.13E-4	

Note: Starting values for $\{\theta_1, \theta_2, and\ \theta_3\}$ were $\{-5, 6000, and\ 344\}$. Values are reported as estimate (standard error of estimate). Legend: SSE, residual sum of squares.

standard error of the parameter estimates (which will be discussed later in the chapter) were precise. Based on these criteria alone, this model would be deemed highly successful. However, the correlations between parameter estimates was greater than 0.99 for all pairwise correlations and the condition number of the model was 3.17×10^{21} (the smallest eigenvalue was $\sim 5.04 \times 10^{-21}$). Table 3.4 also presents the results of the fit when x_1 was changed from 50 to 49.5, a change of 1% in a single

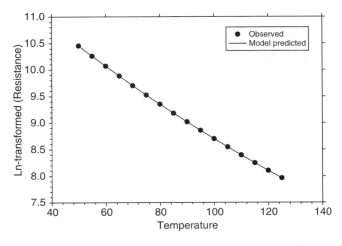

Figure 3.7 Scatter plot of log-thermometer resistance as a function of temperature and model predicted fit using Eq. (3.83). Starting values were $\theta_1 = -5$, $\theta_2 = 6000$, $\theta_3 = 344$. Model was fit using the Gauss–Newton method within the NLIN procedure in SAS.

observation. Although there was a small change in x_1, there was a large change in the parameter estimates, by as much as 19%. The standard errors were also much larger making the 95% confidence intervals much larger than the original model. These results show that despite an excellent goodness of fit the model was unstable.

If the model parameters are highly correlated, one option is to reparameterize the model into a more stable form, which is often of a more simpler form. Simonoff and Tsai (1989), and later Niedzwiecki and Simonoff (1990), call these model transformations "guided transformations" and the idea is as follows. Since collinearity implies that at least one column of J is close to or nearly a linear combination of the other columns, i.e., using Column 1 as an example,

$$\frac{\partial f(x;\theta)}{\partial \theta_1}\bigg|_{\theta=\hat{\theta}} \approx a_2\left(\frac{\partial f(x;\theta)}{\partial \theta_2}\bigg|_{\theta=\hat{\theta}}\right) + \dots a_p\left(\frac{\partial f(x;\theta)}{\partial \theta_p}\bigg|_{\theta=\hat{\theta}}\right) \quad (3.84)$$

then

$$\frac{\partial f(x;\theta)}{\partial \theta_1} = a_2\frac{\partial f(x;\theta)}{\partial \theta_2} + \dots + a_p\frac{\partial f(x;\theta)}{\partial \theta_p}. \quad (3.85)$$

Equation (3.85) is called a guiding equation. Once the appropriate guiding equation is found (there may be many for a model with many parameters), solve the guiding equations for one of the model parameters, substitute the result into the original equation, and simplify. The reformulated model is then fit to the data.

In the Simonoff and Tsai example, the matrix of partial derivatives had a correlation coefficient of 0.99998 between θ_2 and θ_3. Hence θ_2 was highly collinear with θ_3 and would imply that

$$\frac{\partial}{\partial \theta_2}\bigg|_{\theta=\hat{\theta}} \approx a_2\frac{\partial}{\partial \theta_3}\bigg|_{\theta=\hat{\theta}} \quad (3.86)$$

In this case (dropping the hat notation),

$$\frac{\partial}{\partial \theta_2} = \frac{1}{\theta_3 + x}, \text{ and} \quad (3.87)$$

$$\frac{\partial}{\partial \theta_3} = -\frac{\theta_2}{(\theta_3 + x)^2}. \quad (3.88)$$

Hence the guiding equation would be

$$\frac{1}{\theta_3 + x} = -\frac{a_2\theta_2}{(\theta_3 + x)^2}. \quad (3.89)$$

Solving for θ_2 yields

$$\theta_2 = -\frac{(\theta_3 + x)}{a_2}. \qquad (3.90)$$

Substituting Eq. (3.90) into Eq. (3.83) yields

$$Y^* = \theta_1 - \frac{(\theta_3 + x)}{a_2} \frac{x}{(\theta_3 + x)}, \qquad (3.91)$$

which after simplifying yields

$$Y^* = \theta_1 - \frac{1}{a_2} x = \theta_1 + \theta_2^* x. \qquad (3.92)$$

Hence, the reformulated model was a linear model over the interval [50, 125], which was evident from a plot of the data. However, the authors point out that a quadratic model might be more appropriate since there was some curvature in the data. Since the original model and reformulated model clearly diverged as $x \to \infty$ using the reformulated model for extrapolation would not be wise.

Another interesting example is when the model is

$$Y = \theta_1(1 - e^{-\theta_2 x}) \qquad (3.93)$$

and θ_1 and θ_2 are collinear. When expressed graphically the plot could easily be mistaken for an E_{max} model. In this case, the guiding equation is

$$1 - e^{-\theta_2 x} = a_1 \theta_1 x e^{-\theta_2 x}. \qquad (3.94)$$

Solving for $\exp(-\theta_2 x)$ yields

$$e^{-\theta_2 x} = (1 + a\theta_1 x)^{-1}. \qquad (3.95)$$

Substituting Eq. (3.95) into Eq. (3.93) yields

$$Y^* = \frac{\theta_1 x}{\theta_2^* + x}, \qquad (3.96)$$

which shows that the reformulated model is the E_{max} model most are familiar with. It should be noted that not all models can be reformulated, that reformulated models may still exhibit high collinearity (in which maybe the process should be repeated), that the reformulated model is not necessarily a simpler model than the original model, and that the reformulated model may lack any physical or mechanistic meaning that may have been associated with the previous model. Still, a reformulated model often leads to more stable and less biased parameter estimates and standard errors,

and better coverage properties of the confidence interval around the predicted values.

Another example that leads to ill conditioning is when the data do not support the model, even the data generating model. A simpler model may provide an adequate fit even though it is not the true model. Consider the data presented in Fig. 3.8. The data values were generated using the model

$$C = 10e^{-0.66t} + 10e^{-0.25t} + 18e^{-0.071t}. \qquad (3.97)$$

Notice that there is no error term in Eq. (3.97). The data perfectly fit the model. However, the solid line was fit using the model

$$C = 16.54e^{-0.498t} + 21.41e^{-0.0796t}, \qquad (3.98)$$

which would also appear to be an accurate fit to the data. The reason these two models fit the data equally well is that the data were *parameter redundant* over the range of sample times (Reich, 1981). It is interesting to compare the condition numbers between these two models. The condition number for the triexponential model used to generate the data was 6.32×10^8, whereas the condition number for the fitted biexponential model was 1.77×10^6, a value considerably less. Thus, the results for the biexponential equation were more stable than the triexponential equation *over the range of data examined.*

Sometimes collecting more data will improve the stability of the model. Unfortunately, this is not an option for a study that is already completed. For

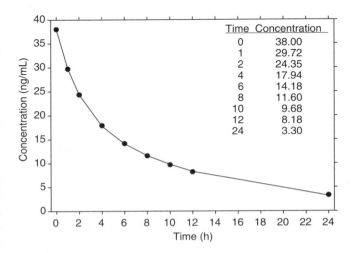

Figure 3.8 Example of parameter redundancy in nonlinear models. Symbols were generated using the model given by Eq. (3.97). Solid line is the predicted fit using Eq. (3.98). The biexponential model predicted values cannot be distinguished from data generated using a triexponential equation. Starting values were {10, 1, 10, and 0.25}. Model was fit using the Levenberg–Marquardt method within the NLIN procedure in SAS.

example, Eq. (3.97) can be distinguished from Eq. (3.98) only if samples are collected longer than 24 h. In Fig. 3.9, samples were collected out to 96 h. As time progressed the inadequacy of the biexponential model became more and more apparent. With the additional sampling times, the condition number for the triexponential equation decreased to 2.63×10^8 and the condition number of the biexponential equation decreased to 1.63×10^6. Notice that the condition number for the biexponential equation barely changed, but there was a large decrease in the condition number for the triexponential equation. The large change in condition number indicated the instability of the parameter estimates of the triexponential model. However, this was an ideal situation. If in reality the assay error was moderate to large, these models may never be distinguishable.

The last example of where ill conditioning may arise is when the columns of J are of differing magnitudes or scale, similar to linear models when the columns of x are of different scale. At the simplest level, for a pharmacokinetic model where time is the independent variable, simply changing the units of time can have a dramatic effect on the condition number and ill conditioning depending on the algorithm and software package. For example, suppose samples for pharmacokinetic analysis are collected at 0, 0.5, 1, 1.5, 2, 3, 4, 6, 8, 12, 18, and 24 h after intravenous drug administration with values of 39.4, 33.3, 29.2, 29.8, 24.3, 20.7, 17.8, 10.7, 6.8, 3.4, 1.0, and 0.3, respectively. Assume a 1-compartment model

with bolus intravenous administration is appropriate to model the data

$$C = C(0)e^{-\theta t}, \qquad (3.99)$$

where C is the concentration, C(0) and θ are the estimable model parameters, and t is the time. The first derivatives for the model are

$$\frac{\partial}{\partial C(0)} = e^{-\theta t} \qquad (3.100)$$

$$\frac{\partial}{\partial C(0)} = -t \times C(0)e^{-\theta t} \qquad (3.101)$$

with Jacobian matrix

$$J = \begin{bmatrix} \dfrac{\partial}{\partial C(0)} & \dfrac{\partial}{\partial \theta} \end{bmatrix}. \qquad (3.102)$$

Using starting values of 35 for C(0) and 0.01 for θ, only six iterations were required for convergence using the Gauss–Newton algorithm within Proc NLIN in SAS. The model parameter estimates were $C(0) = 38.11 \pm 0.72$ and $\theta = 0.2066 \pm 0.009449$ per hour. The matrix $J^T J$ was

$$J^T J = \begin{bmatrix} 4.06 & -201.21 \\ -201.21 & 23{,}388 \end{bmatrix} \qquad (3.103)$$

with eigenvalues of 2.33 and 23,390 and a corresponding condition number of 10,043. Now consider what happens at one end of the time scale when time is transformed from hours to seconds. Under the transformation, the model parameter estimates were $C(0) = 38.12 \pm 0.72$ and $\theta = 5.738E-5 \pm 2.625E-6$ per second. Notice that the only change was in θ and that the new estimate of θ in s was exactly 1/3600th (the conversion factor of hours to seconds) the estimate of θ in hours. The matrix $J^T J$ was

$$J^T J = \begin{bmatrix} 4.06 & -724326 \\ -724326 & 303{,}088{,}318{,}806 \end{bmatrix} \qquad (3.104)$$

with eigenvalues of 2.33 and 303,088,318,808 and corresponding condition number of 1.30×10^{11}. At the other end of the time scale, when time was transformed from hours to days, the model parameter estimates were $C(0) = 38.12 \pm 0.72$ and $\theta = 4.96 \pm 0.227$ per day. The matrix $J^T J$ was

$$J^T J = \begin{bmatrix} 4.06 & -8.38 \\ -8.38 & 40.60 \end{bmatrix} \qquad (3.105)$$

with eigenvalues of 2.23 and 42.44 and corresponding condition of 19.0. Again, the only change was in θ and

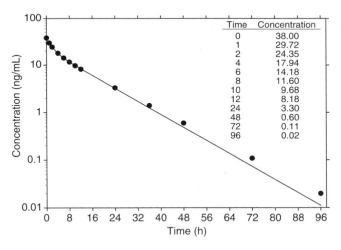

Time	Concentration
0	38.00
1	29.72
2	24.35
4	17.94
6	14.18
8	11.60
10	9.68
12	8.18
24	3.30
48	0.60
72	0.11
96	0.02

Figure 3.9 Example of parameter redundancy resolution through the collection of more samples. Data were generated using the triexponential model given in Eq. (3.97). Solid line is the predicted fit using the model $C = 16.73 \times \exp(-0.492\,t) + 21.21 \times \exp(-0.0787\,t)$. This figure is the same as Fig. 3.8 with the exception that samples were collected out to 96 h. Model predicted values based on a biexponential equation can now be distinguished from data generated using a triexponential equation. Starting values were {10, 1, 10, and 0.25}. Model was fit using the Levenberg–Marquardt method within the NLIN procedure in SAS.

that the new estimate of θ in days was exactly 24-times (the conversion factor of hours to days) the estimate of θ in hours. Inverting $J^T J$ in Eq. (3.104) resulted in a highly unstable matrix, whereas inverting $J^T J$ in Eqs. (3.103) and (3.105) resulted in a more stable matrix. But note that in all cases, the parameter estimate for α remained the same, the mean square error remained the same, as did the CV of the parameter estimates. Changing the scale did not affect the model precision or parameter precision and hence, any statistical inference on the model parameters. The only thing that changed was the estimate of θ.

So why all the fuss? First, a large condition number is indicative that a model is sensitive to the data used to fit the model. Small changes in the data may lead to large changes in the parameter estimates (see the Simonoff and Tsai example presented previously in this section). Second, some optimization algorithms are sensitive to scale, whereas others are not (Nocedal and Wright, 1999). The algorithm used in the example above to estimate the model parameters was the Gauss–Newton algorithm in the NLIN procedure in SAS, which is relatively insensitive to scaling. However, the gradient method in SAS, which uses the method of Steepest Descent, is sensitive to scale. When the model was fit to the seconds data set using the gradient algorithm, the iterative process did not show any improvement in the step size at the initial evaluation of the parameter estimates and failed to converge, i.e., the algorithm was unable to move beyond the initial parameter estimates. Obviously, algorithms that are not sensitive to scale are preferable to algorithms that are. But, by forcing the parameter estimates to be approximately the same, less ill-conditioning results, thereby easing the convergence process.

The algorithms within WinNonlin are also relatively insensitive to large differences in scale among the parameters because WinNonlin first transforms the parameters to a new domain where each parameter has approximately the same mean and range. Fitting is then done within this transformed domain and then back-transformed to the original domain for reporting of parameter values. When the example above was fit using the Gauss–Newton algorithm with Levenberg and Hartley modification within WinNonlin (Version 4.0), all three data sets had a condition number of 3.49, indicating that each model was quite stable to small changes in the data set.

Because of the possibility for unstable matrix inversion, even after centering, most software programs use one of two different matrix inversion algorithms that result in more stable inverses. These are the QR decomposition and singular value (SV) decomposition. In the QR decomposition, let $J = QR$, where Q is an

$n \times k$ matrix $[k = \min(n, p)]$ and R is a $k \times p$ upper triangular matrix. Note that $R \neq r$ from the Gauss–Newton algorithm. The step size in the Gauss–Newton algorithm can be calculated as $h_i = I^1 Q^T \varepsilon$, where ε is the vector of residuals. The next iteration of parameter estimates is calculated using Eq. (3.36). In the singular value decomposition, let $A = J^T J$ be an $n \times n$ matrix at the ith iteration in the fitting process and $|\lambda_1| \geq |\lambda_2| \geq \ldots |\lambda_n|$ be the eigenvalues associated with A. A can, then be decomposed to $A = UDV$, where

$$D = \begin{bmatrix} \sqrt{\lambda_1} & 0 & 0 & 0 \\ 0 & \sqrt{\lambda_2} & 0 & 0 \\ 0 & .. & .. & 0 \\ 0 & 0 & 0 & \sqrt{\lambda_p} \end{bmatrix} \quad (3.106)$$

and U and V are the $n \times n$ matrices whose columns are the eigenvectors associated with AA^T and $A^T A$, respectively. The diagonal elements of D are called the singular values of A. The Moore–Penrose generalized inverse of A, often denoted A^-, is then

$$A^- = UD^{-1}V. \quad (3.107)$$

Since D is a block diagonal matrix, the inverse is easily calculated as a block diagonal matrix with diagonal elements $\left(\sqrt{\lambda_i}\right)^{-1}$.

Both the QR and SV decomposition attempt to do the same thing—invert an unstable matrix to a more stable form and both methods produce exactly the same result. The difference between the inversion algorithms is speed and memory. The QR decomposition is about 250% faster than the SV decomposition, but for normal pharmacokinetic applications, the difference will be negligible. The SV decomposition also requires more memory as it must store three matrices. Despite its slowness and memory demands, many researchers advocate the use of SV decomposition for matrix inversion in linear and nonlinear models (Belsley, Kuh, and Welsch, 1980; Dennis, 1977; Eubank and Webster, 1985; Mandel, 1982), although Bates and Watts (1988) recommend using QR decomposition for nonlinear models. Win-Nonlin uses the SV decomposition for its matrix inversion, whereas ADAPT II uses the QR decomposition. SAS provides SV decomposition as an option, but not as the default in PROC NLIN.

CONSTRAINED OPTIMIZATION

To date now it has been assumed that there are no constraints on the values the model parameters can assume, i.e., the range of parameter values can be from $-\infty$ to $+\infty$. For some parameters in a model this may not be valid. For example, in pharmacokinetic models it is impossible to have negative rate constants. Hence, their range takes on values $[0, \infty)$. Therefore, it becomes imperative to be able to take these constraints into account during the fitting process. Unfortunately, it is not as simple as an if–then statement that bounces an illegal parameter value back into a valid parameter space because doing so would make the objective function response surface become discontinuous.

Constraints in nonlinear regression are handled in many different ways, depending on the software. One method is to add a penalty function, $c(\theta)$, to the objective function,

$$P(\theta) = S(\theta) + c(\theta) \qquad (3.108)$$

thereby generating a new objective function that increases in value should the parameter estimates go outside their valid parameter space. For example, using the log penalty function

$$P(x; \theta) = S(x; \theta) - cLn(\theta), \qquad (3.109)$$

where c is a positive-value dampening constant, a positive penalty is imposed if θ is within the interval $[0, 1)$ and a negative penalty is imposed if $\theta > 1$. In this manner, values of θ away from zero are favored over values of θ near zero. Unfortunately, this method fails if θ becomes negative during the search process so a recovery procedure must be added to test for positivity before calculating the natural logarithm of θ. If more than one parameter needs to be constrained more penalty terms can be added to the penalty function, one for each parameter that needs to be constrained.

Another method to add constraints to a model is to transform the model parameters themselves or to reformulate the model such that the constraints always hold. For example, suppose in Eq. (3.99) that the rate constant θ always must be a positive value, then the model can be reformulated as

$$Y = A \exp(-\exp(\theta^*)t) \qquad (3.110)$$

where $\theta = \exp(\theta^*)$ and θ^* can take on any real value. Similarly if E_{max} in Eq. (3.1) was required to be a positive value then Eq. (3.1) could be reformulated as

$$E = \frac{\exp(E_{max}^*)C}{EC_{50} + C} \qquad (3.111)$$

where $E_{max} = \exp(E_{max}^*)$.

Prior to any optimization, WinNonlin takes a double transformation of the parameter values. First, suppose θ is constrained to be between a and b, i.e., $a < \theta < b$, WinNonlin then transforms θ to the unit hypercube

$$\theta^* = \frac{\theta - a}{b - a} \qquad (3.112)$$

so that $0 < \theta^* < 1$. Then Eq. (3.112) is transformed using the inverse normal transform (normit)

$$\theta^* = \int_{-\infty}^{\beta} \Phi(x)dx \qquad (3.113)$$

so the range of θ goes from $-\infty$ to ∞. β is then used for the analysis such that $-\infty < \beta < \infty$. Hence, the constrained problem is transformed to an unconstrained optimization problem and makes it easy to deal with situations where the parameter values differ by orders of magnitude.

Another method is to treat the constraints as either active or inactive. The constraints are inactive when the current value is within the valid parameter space, in which case the current value is treated as a parameter. Should the current value be outside the valid parameter space and the objective function shows improvement, the current value is then set equal to the bound upon which the parameter has crossed, at which the parameter is treated as a constant. Hence, there is no penalty for crossing outside the valid parameter space. This is the approach taken by SAAM II.

Constraints should have no impact on the value of the parameter estimates themselves nor should they affect the fitting process, unless the parameter is near a boundary. A parameter may bounce into an invalid parameter space causing the algorithm to either "crash," in which case widening the bounds may be necessary, or to finish the optimization process and report the parameter estimate as a boundary value. In no instance when the final parameter estimates fall on a boundary should these be considered "optimal" values.

INFLUENCE DIAGNOSTICS

Research and development of influence diagnostics for nonlinear models have not received as much attention as for the linear model. One obvious approach to determine the influence an observation has on the data would be to delete the ith observation, refit the model, and recompute the parameter estimates. One can then compare the refit parameter estimates with the original estimate and see their degree of similarity. In the case where all observations are deleted one at a time, this is the jackknife approach to influence diagnostics. The problem with this approach is that it is computer intensive and may take long hours to complete. The advantage of this approach is that one can not only determine the influence a particular case has on parameter estimates, but one can develop nonparametric estimates of the standard error of the parameter estimates. The basic theory for the jackknife has been extensively discussed by Efron (1998) and Ritschel and Kearns (1994) and is presented in the Appendix of the book.

Alternatively, a nonlinear analogy to the HAT matrix in a linear model can be developed using the Jacobian matrix, instead of x. In this case,

$$HAT_{tpl} = J(J^T J)^{-1} J^{-1} \qquad (3.114)$$

and the diagonal elements are used as the leverage estimates. HAT_{tpl} is called the tangent plane leverage (tpl) matrix and the appropriateness of its use depends on the adequacy of the Taylor series approximation to $S(\theta)$ evaluated at $\hat{\theta}$ (St Laurent and Cook, 1993). The difficulty in its use is that one first needs access to the Jacobian, something that cannot be done except with WinNonlin, and then needs a software package that does matrix calculations, such as MATLAB or GAUSS, to do the actual calculation. HAT_{tpl} is not calculated by any current pharmacokinetic software package. Another influence measure sometimes seen in the statistical literature is the Jacobian leverage matrix (St Laurent and Cook, 1992), which is more sensitive than HAT_{tpl}, but for this measure not only does one need access to the Jacobian, but one also needs access to the Hessian, which cannot be obtained from any standard statistical software package. Thus, its use will not be discussed here.

Gray (1986) presented a useful influence diagnostic for linear models that can be applied to nonlinear regression models. He recommended that HAT_{tpl} for each subject be plotted against e^2/SSE, the normalized residual for the ith subject. Such a plot is called an L–R triangle for leverage and residual. For models to fit using equal weights, the L–R triangle data should show low leverage and small residuals such that the majority of the data cluster near $(p/n, 0)$. These limits will change if the model is fit using a variance model of unequal weights. Cases that have undue influence will be discordant from the bulk of the data.

As an example, consider the oral administration data in Table 3.5 and which is plotted in Fig. 3.10. One observation in the data set, at 12-h post dose, was questionable. A 1-compartment model with first-order absorption

$$Y = \frac{D}{V_d}\left[\frac{k_a}{k_a - k_{10}}\right][\exp(-k_{10}t) - \exp(-k_a t)] + \varepsilon \quad (3.115)$$

Table 3.5 Example of jackknifing a nonlinear regression problem.

Time (h)	Concentration (ng/ml)	V_d (mL)	k_a (per hour)	k_{10} (per hour)	V_d (mL) 109679[*]	k_a (per hour) 0.0606[*]	k_{10} (per hour) 0.8485[*]
	Jackknife parameter estimates				Pseudovalues		
0.5	296	110079	0.8646	0.0602	105280	0.6713	0.0651
1	500	109760	0.8536	0.0605	108792	0.7920	0.0616
1.5	599	109581	0.8685	0.0606	110762	0.6286	0.0605
2	696	109845	0.8463	0.0605	107859	0.8728	0.0620
3	785	112407	0.8690	0.0585	79671	0.6231	0.0839
4	763	111752	0.8735	0.0591	86882	0.5731	0.0771
6	671	109292	0.8426	0.0608	113938	0.9127	0.0586
8	622	110358	0.8606	0.0608	102212	0.7150	0.0582
12	*350*	109931	0.8337	0.0531	106911	1.0107	0.1431
24	275	103718	0.7759	0.0727	175250	1.6473	−0.0726
36	168	105536	0.7961	0.0683	155255	1.4248	−0.0245
48	57	109532	0.8466	0.0608	111296	0.8696	0.0578
				Mean	113675	0.8951	0.0526
				Std Dev	26482	0.3307	0.0538
				SEM	7645	0.0955	0.0155

Concentration data obtained after oral administration of 100 mg of drug.
[*] Estimates based on all data values.
Bolded values were questionable after examination of the scatter plot.
Starting values were 100000 mL for V_d, 1 per hour for k_a, and 0.05 per hour for k_{10}. Model was a 1-compartment model with absorption and was fit using Levenberg–Marquardt algorithm within Proc NLIN in SAS. The administered dose was 100 mg.
Legend: SEM, standard error of mean; Std Dev, standard deviation.

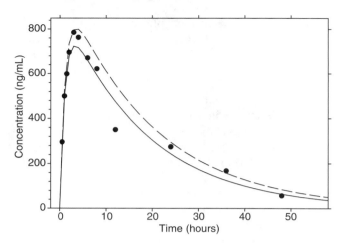

Figure 3.10 Eq. (3.115) was fit to the data in Table 3.5 using the Levenberg–Marquardt algorithm. Starting values were 100 L, 1.0 per hour, and 0.05 per hour for V_d, k_a, and k_{10}, respectively. The solid line is the least squares fit to the data with all data. The data point at 12 h is of questionable influence. The dashed line is the least squares fit to the data with the 12 h time point removed from the data set.

was fit to the data with the Levenberg–Marquardt algorithm within SAS with equal weights using all available data and the dose was fixed to 100 mg. The following parameter estimates (± standard errors) were obtained: $V_d = 110 \pm 6.71$ L, $k_a = 0.849 \pm 0.124$ per hour, and $k_{10} = 0.0606 \pm 8.42\text{E-3}$ per hour. The sum of squares error was 24521.7. The leverage-residual (L–R) plot is shown in Fig. 3.11. The 12-h time point was clearly discordant from the rest of the data.

To see how this data point impacted the parameter estimates, the n-1 jackknife procedure was performed on the data. The parameter estimates after removal of this observation from the data set were: $V_d = 110 \pm 2.7$ L, $k_a = 0.834 \pm 0.124$ per hour, and $k_{10} = 0.0531 \pm 3.09\text{E-3}$

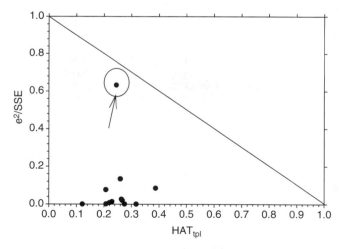

Figure 3.11 L–R plot for the data in Fig. 10. The questionable 12-h time point is indicated. Solid line is the boundary condition.

per hour. Although there was practically no difference in the parameter estimates with and without the observation, the goodness of fit with the subject removed dramatically improved (Fig. 3.10). The jackknife estimates were 114 ± 7.65 L for V_d, $0.0526 \pm \text{rm } 0.0155$ per hour for k_{10}, and 0.895 ± 0.0955 per hour for k_a indicating that the data point in question unduly influenced the estimates of the model parameters and should either be removed from the data set or differentially weighted to provide less impact than other observations.

CONFIDENCE INTERVALS FOR THE PREDICTED RESPONSE

Confidence intervals for predicted responses in nonlinear models are exceedingly difficult to calculate with the current state of statistical software. The reason being that the calculation requires decomposition of the Jacobian using the QR decomposition with further matrix manipulations. For simple models with p-estimable parameters and n observations, an approximate $(1 - \alpha)100\%$ confidence interval for a single predicted response, x_0, can be developed from

$$f(x_0; \hat{\theta}) \pm \sqrt{\text{MSE}} \| J_{x_0}^T R_x^{-1} \| t_{n-p, \alpha/2} \qquad (3.116)$$

where $f(x_0; \hat{\theta})$ is the predicted response at x_0 given the final parameter estimates $\hat{\theta}$, J_{x_0} is $p \times 1$ Jacobian matrix of partial derivatives evaluated at x_0, R is the R matrix from the QR decomposition of the $n \times p$ matrix of partial derivatives evaluated at, $x \| . \|$ is the norm of the argument,[2] MSE is the mean square error of the fit, and t is Student's t having $n-p$ degrees of freedom and $\alpha/2$ critical value. Similarly a $(1 - \alpha)100\%$ confidence band for a matrix of predicted responses can be developed from

$$f(x; \hat{\theta}) \pm \sqrt{\text{MSE}} \| J_x^T R_x^{-1} \| \sqrt{p F_{p, n-p, \alpha}} \qquad (3.117)$$

where J_x denotes the matrix of partial derivatives evaluated at x, as opposed to x_0, and F is the value from a F-distribution with p, $n-p$ degrees of freedom. The terms to the right of the $\pm$ sign in Eqs. (3.116) and (3.117) are collectively referred to as the standard error of prediction. Confidence intervals in this case deal with the expected response at a single point x_0, whereas confidence bands consider all the values of x simult-

---

[2] *Note*: The p-norm of a matrix is defined as $\left(\sum_{i=1}^{n} |x|^p \right)^{1/p}$. Unless p is explicitly defined, p is assumed to equal 2.

aneously. Confidence bands are larger than confidence intervals.

As an example, consider the data in Table 3.5 wherein a 1-compartment model with absorption [Eq. (3.115)] was fit to the data. The model has partial derivatives

$$\frac{\partial Y}{\partial V_d} = \frac{-D}{V_d^2}\left[\frac{k_a}{k_a - k_{10}}\right][\Delta EXP] \tag{3.118}$$

$$\frac{\partial Y}{\partial k_a} = \frac{D \times \Delta EXP}{V_d(k_a - k_{10})} - \frac{D \times \Delta EXP}{V_d}\left[\frac{k_a}{(k_a - k_{10})^2}\right]$$
$$+ \frac{Dt}{V_d}\left[\frac{k_a}{(k_a - k_{10})}\right]e^{-k_a t} \tag{3.119}$$

$$\frac{\partial Y}{\partial k_{10}} = \frac{D \times \Delta EXP}{V_d}\left[\frac{k_a}{(k_a - k_{10})^2}\right]$$
$$- \frac{Dt}{V_d}\left[\frac{k_a}{(k_a - k_{10})}\right]e^{-k_{10} t} \tag{3.120}$$

where D is dose and $\Delta EXP = e^{-k_{10}t} - \exp^{-k_a t}$. The Jacobian of the model evaluated at the final parameter estimates was

$$J = \begin{bmatrix} -0.002822 & 292.504 & -82.631 \\ -0.004483 & 373.588 & -284.669 \\ -0.005653 & 354.864 & -555.893 \\ -0.006274 & 295.988 & -863.866 \\ -0.006743 & 162.805 & -1514.322 \\ -0.006706 & 64.435 & -2145.423 \\ -0.006152 & -25.037 & -3236.166 \\ -0.005490 & -45.588 & -4071.155 \\ -0.004319 & -42.287 & -5094.003 \\ -0.002092 & -20.691 & -5222.899 \\ -0.001013 & -10.020 & -3892.945 \\ -0.000490 & -4.852 & -2516.063 \end{bmatrix}. \tag{3.121}$$

The R matrix using QR decomposition of the Jacobian is

$$R = \begin{bmatrix} 0.0016874 & -432.65 & 6830.4 \\ 0 & -534.61 & -4917.2 \\ 0 & 0 & -6211.3 \end{bmatrix}. \tag{3.122}$$

The F-value using 3, 9 degrees of freedom was 3.86, Student's two-tailed t-distribution with 9 degrees of freedom was 2.262, and the mean square error was 2427.8. Suppose the 95% confidence interval for the predicted value at T_{max} was needed. At a T_{max} of 3 h, the predicted value was 740.03 ng/mL. The Jacobian matrix evaluated at 3 h under the final parameter estimates was

$$J_{x_0} = \{-0.0067275 \quad 162.64 \quad -1512.1\} \tag{3.123}$$

and

$$J_{x_0}R_x^{-1} = \{-0.40082 \quad 0.020154 \quad -0.21329\}. \tag{3.124}$$

The norm of $J_{x_0}R_x^{-1}$ was 0.45449. Hence the 95% confidence interval at T_{max} was {689.37 ng/mL, 790.68 ng/mL}. A 95% confidence band across all predicted responses is shown in Fig. 3.12. As can be seen, the standard error of prediction was not a constant, but varied from 0 ng/mL at t = 0 h to about 104.6 ng/mL at t = 22.8 h. At no point along the curve was the standard error of prediction constant.

INCORPORATING PRIOR INFORMATION INTO THE LIKELIHOOD

Science is rarely done in a vacuum. When an experiment is conducted, the scientist often has some notion about what the outcome will be. In modeling, the analyst may have some idea of what the model parameters will be. For example, at the very least, one can make the assumption that the rate constants in a compartmental model are all positive—that the rate constants cannot be negative. The section on Constrained Optimization in this chapter illustrated how such constraints can be incorporated into the fitting process. However, sometimes the analyst has even more knowledge about the value of a model parameter, such as the distribution of the parameter. Such a distribution is referred to as the prior distribution. For example, suppose in a previous study clearance was estimated to be normally distributed with a mean of 45 L/h and a standard deviation of 5 L/h.

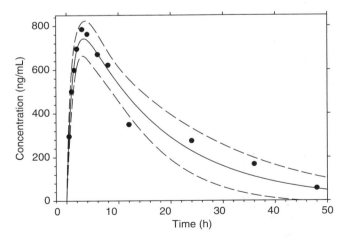

Figure 3.12 Model predicted fit and 95% confidence band for data presented in Table 3.5. A 1-compartment model with absorption was fit to the data using the Levenberg Marquardt algorithm within the NLIN procedure in SAS. Starting values were 100 L, 1.0 per hour, and 0.05 per hour for V_d, k_a, and k_{10}, respectively.

Now, in a different study with the same drug, clearance needs to be estimated. All the methodology presented until this section totally ignores such prior information—all parameter estimates are based on the observed data and not on any other, independently collected data. However, shouldn't other, independent data be incorporated in the current estimates of the model parameters? Bayesians answer this question with an affirmative. Frequentists say 'no.' Bayesian modeling is beyond the scope of this chapter and the reader is referred to Congdon (2001) and Gelman et al. (1995) for further details. Nevertheless, some software packages, such as SAAM II and Adapt II, allow such prior information to be included in the fitting process through the likelihood function and the details of how such information are included in the likelihood will be discussed.

Bayesian statistics has at its heart the following fundamental equality

$$p(\theta|Y) = p(\theta)p(Y|\theta) \quad (3.125)$$

which is more often referred to as Bayes theorem, so that the probability of θ given a set of observed data (Y) equals the probability of observing θ times the probability of observing the data given θ. $p(\theta)$ represents our prior beliefs about the parameters θ, while $p(Y|\theta)$ is the probability of observing the data given θ, which is the likelihood of the data, i.e., $L(\theta|Y) = p(Y|\theta)$. A more simple mnemonic is

$$\text{posterior} \propto \text{prior} \times \text{likelihood}.$$

In other words, the product of the likelihood of the observed data [e.g., Eq. (3.12)] and the prior distribution is proportional to the probability of the posterior distribution, or the distribution of the model parameters taking into account the observed data and prior knowledge. Suppose the prior distribution is p-dimensional multivariate normal with mean θ and variance Ω, then the prior can be written as

$$f(\theta) = \frac{1}{(\sqrt{2\pi})^n \sqrt{\det(\Omega)}} \exp\left(-\frac{1}{2}(\theta - \theta)^T \Omega^{-1}(\theta - \theta)\right) \quad (3.126)$$

where $\det(\Omega)$ is the determinant of the variance–covariance matrix of the prior distribution. Since the parameters of the prior are uncorrelated, the prior distribution can be simplified to

$$f(\theta) = \prod_{j=1}^{p} \frac{1}{\sqrt{2\pi\Omega_j}} \exp\left(-\frac{(\theta - \theta)^2}{2\Omega_j}\right). \quad (3.127)$$

Recall that the likelihood function for a model with Gaussian random errors (the observed data) can be written as

$$L(x;\theta) = \prod_{i=1}^{n} \frac{1}{(2\pi\sigma^2)^{\frac{n}{2}}} \exp\left(\frac{-(Y - \hat{Y})^2}{2\sigma^2}\right). \quad (3.128)$$

Combining Eqs. (3.127) and (3.128) gives the posterior distribution

$$L_{\text{posterior}} = \left\{\prod_{i=1}^{n} \frac{1}{(2\pi\sigma^2)^{\frac{n}{2}}} \exp\left(\frac{-(Y - \hat{Y})^2}{2\sigma^2}\right)\right\} \times \left\{\prod_{j=1}^{p} \frac{1}{\sqrt{2\pi\Omega_j}} \exp\left(-\frac{(\theta - \theta)^2}{2\Omega_j}\right)\right\}, \quad (3.129)$$

assuming that the prior and the observed likelihood are independent. Taking the negative logarithm (excluding constants) then leads to the objective function

$$LL_{\text{posterior}} = \sum_{i=1}^{n} \text{Ln}(\sigma^2) + \sum_{i=1}^{n} \frac{1}{2}\left(\frac{Y - \hat{Y}}{\sigma}\right)^2 + \sum_{j=1}^{p} \text{Ln}(\Omega_j) + \frac{1}{2}\sum_{j=1}^{p}\left(\frac{\theta - \theta}{\Omega_j}\right)^2. \quad (3.130)$$

Minimizing Eq. (3.130) with respect to θ then produces an estimate of θ that incorporates prior knowledge about θ into the estimate combined with the observed data likelihood, thereby reflecting all the information that is relevant to θ. SAAM II forces the user to assume a normal prior distribution, while Adapt II allows for normal and log-normal prior distributions. But, if access can be made to general optimization software, such as within MATLAB, then an analyst is not limited to specific prior distributions, or indeed, normal likelihood functions. The reader is referred to Lindsey (2000; 2001) for such examples.

In many cases, if the prior knowledge of θ is vague, such a prior is said to be *diffuse* or *uninformative*, and the Bayesian estimates for the model parameters simplify to the frequentist estimate of the model parameters. In other words, as the standard deviation of the prior distribution increases, the posterior parameter estimates will tend to converge to the parameter estimates in the absence of such prior knowledge. For example, a 1-compartment model with absorption was fit to the data in Table 3.5 using SAAM II where the model was now reparameterized in terms of clearance and not k_{10}. Equal weights were assumed and starting values of 5000 mL/h, 110 L, and 1.0 per hour for Cl, V_d, and k_a, respectively, were used.

Figure 3.13 presents a plot of the model parameter estimates as a function of the prior standard deviation for clearance and a fixed mean of 4500 mL/h. As the standard deviation becomes smaller and smaller, i.e., as the prior distribution becomes more and more concentrated around its mean, the estimate for clearance converges to the mean of the prior distribution. However, as the standard deviation becomes larger and larger, i.e., as the prior becomes uninformative, the estimates converge to the clearance values used to generate the data. Further, as the standard deviation becomes smaller so does the standard error of the parameter estimate associated with clearance. However, using Bayesian estimation does not come without a price. Because with clearance changes, the other parameters in the model change in response and become more biased. Also, the standard error of the estimates associated with V_d and k_a increase with decreasing prior standard deviation on clearance (data not shown) as their values become more and more biased and uncertain.

One major limitation of SAAM II is that it forces the user to assume a normal prior distribution, which for pharmacokinetic problems is not realistic as most pharmacokinetic parameters are log-normal in distribution and their values will always be positive. Adapt II is not limited to normal prior distributions, but also allows for log-normal prior distributions. Hence, Adapt II may be preferred to SAAM II for some Bayesian problems. Nevertheless, using prior information can be useful to solve a problem with a near singular solution or if it is important to include such prior information in the model.

ERROR-IN-VARIABLES NONLINEAR REGRESSION

The same caveats that apply to linear models when the predictor variables are measured with error apply to nonlinear models. When the predictor variables are measured with error, the parameter estimates may become biased, depending on the nonlinear model. Simulation may be used as a quick test to examine the dependency of parameter estimates within a particular model on measurement error (Fig. 3.14). The SIMEX algorithm, as introduced in the chapter on Linear Models and Regression, can easily be extended to nonlinear models, although the computation time will increase by orders of magnitude.

SUMMARIZING THE RESULTS: THE TWO-STAGE METHOD

Often in pharmacokinetics the analyst has data on more than one individual. In a typical Phase 1 clinical trial, there might 12–18 subjects who have pharmacokinetic data collected. Applying a compartmental model to each individual's data generates a vector of parameter estimates, each row of which represents a realization from some probability distribution. For example,

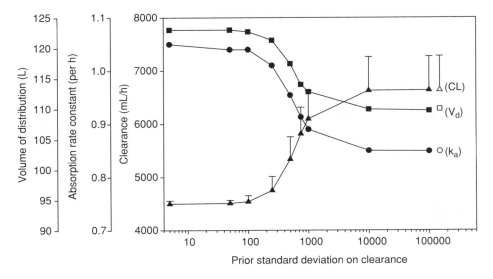

Figure 3.13 Model parameter estimates as a function of the prior standard deviation for clearance. A 1-compartment model with absorption was fit to the data in Table 3.5 using a proportional error model and the SAAM II software system. Starting values were 5000 mL/h, 110 L, and 1.0 per hour for clearance (CL), volume of distribution (V_d), and absorption rate constant (k_a), respectively. The Bayesian prior mean for clearance was fixed at 4500 mL/h while the standard deviation was systematically varied. The error bars represent the standard error of the parameter estimate. The open symbols are the parameter estimates when prior information is not included in the model.

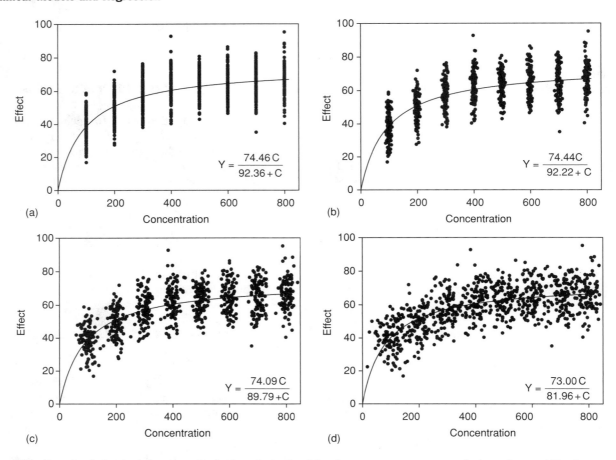

Figure 3.14 Example of using simulation to examine the dependency of model parameters on measurement error in the predictor variables. Concentration-effect data were simulated using an E_{max} model [Eq. (3.1)] with $E_{max} = 75$ and $EC_{50} = 100$. The standard deviation in the observed effect was set equal to 10. A design matrix at {100, 200, 300, 400, 500, 600, 700, and 800} was used with 100 data points simulated at each design point (a). Concentration data were then randomly perturbed using a measurement error standard deviation of 5 (b), 15 (c), and 30 (d). Each data set was then fit the E_{max} model using the Levenberg–Marquardt algorithm within the NLIN procedure in SAS. The initial values were the true values used to simulate the data. The resulting models are printed within each individual scatter plot. Despite increasing measurement error, estimates of E_{max} appear relatively insensitive to measurement error, although EC_{50} appears to decrease from the true values as measurement error increases, suggesting that EC_{50} is more sensitive to measurement error than E_{max}.

pharmacokinetic data might be available on 18 subjects. If the same model is applied to each subject then the analyst will generate 18 unique, independent estimates of clearance or volume of distribution. It is natural then to want to estimate the population mean and variance of the distribution.

Given a vector of parameter estimates, $\theta = \{\hat{\theta}_1, \hat{\theta}_2, \ldots \hat{\theta}_n\}$, one estimator for the population mean (θ) is the arithmetic mean, which is calculated using the well-known equation

$$\bar{\theta} = \frac{\sum_{i=1}^{n} \hat{\theta}_i}{n}. \tag{1.131}$$

However, most pharmacokinetic parameters tend to be skewed in a log-normal manner since their lower bound

can never decrease below zero. The arithmetic mean is useful for symmetric distributions, but not for skewed distributions. A better estimator might be the geometric mean, which is calculated by

$$\bar{\theta}_g = \sqrt[n]{\prod_{i=1}^{n} \hat{\theta}_i} = \left(\prod_{i=1}^{n} \hat{\theta}_i \right)^{\frac{1}{n}} \tag{1.132}$$

and is related to the log-normal distribution as follows

$$Ln[\bar{\theta}_g] = Ln \left[\left(\prod_{i=1}^{n} \hat{\theta}_i \right)^{\frac{1}{n}} \right] \tag{1.133}$$

$$Ln[\bar{\theta}_g] = \frac{\sum_{i=1}^{n} Ln(\hat{\theta}_i)}{n} \tag{1.134}$$

$$\bar{\theta}_g = \exp\left[\frac{\sum_{i=1}^{n} Ln(\hat{\theta}_i)}{n}\right]. \qquad (1.135)$$

Hence, the geometric mean is the exponentiated arithmetic mean of the log-transformed values. Once the mean is calculated, an estimate of the variance of the parameter Ω is usually estimated by

$$\Omega = \frac{(\hat{\theta} - \bar{\theta})^T(\hat{\theta} - \bar{\theta})}{n - 1}. \qquad (3.136)$$

This approach has been called the two-stage approach because in the first stage each individual's parameter of interest is determined. In the second stage, the individual parameter estimates are pooled to yield estimates of the population moments. It is generally recognized that mean estimates calculated in this manner are usually unbiased when the number of subjects is large. The problem with the two-stage approach comes in estimating the variance of the population. Ω assumes that $\hat{\theta}$ is known with certainty, which is not the case. $\hat{\theta}$ is an estimate of some individual's parameter and has some measure of bias associated with it. For example, if few samples are collected during the absorption phase of a concentration-time profile then the bias in the estimate of the absorption rate constant may be large and may be estimated with poor precision. Hence, the two-stage approach fails to take into account the variability in the estimation of $\hat{\theta}$ and any variance based on these estimates tends to be inflated (Beal and Sheiner, 1985).

Mixed-effects models, which will be described in later chapters, do not suffer from this flaw and tend to produce both unbiased mean and variance estimates. As an example, Sheiner and Beal (1980) used Monte Carlo simulation to study the accuracy of the two-stage approach and mixed effects model approach in fitting an E_{max} model with parameters $\{V_{max}, K_m\}$. Data from 49 individuals were simulated. The relative deviation from the mean estimated value to the true simulated value for V_{max} and K_m was 3.7% and −4.9%, respectively, for the two-stage method and −0.9 and 8.3%, respectively, for the mixed effects model approach. Hence, both methods were relatively unbiased in their estimation of the population means. However, the relative deviation from the mean estimated variance to the true simulated variance for V_{max} and K_m was 70 and 82%, respectively, for the two-stage method and −2.6 and 4.1%, respectively, for the mixed effects model approach. Hence, the variance components were significantly overestimated with the two-stage approach. Further, the precision of the estimates across simulations tended to be more variable with the two-stage approach than with the mixed effects

model approach. Because of results like this, the two-stage approach is recognized as not being optimal in estimating population model parameter estimates.

Numerous approaches have been developed over the years to correct for the bias in the estimation of the variance using the two-stage approach, but these are not easily implemented nor do they always succeed in producing unbiased estimates of the variance components. The reader is referred to Steimer et al. (1984) and Racine-Poon and Wakefield (1998) for details on these alternative measures.

MISSING AND CENSORED DATA

Missing and censored data should be handled exactly as in the case of linear regression. The analyst can use complete case analysis, naïve substitution, conditional mean substitution, maximum likelihood, or multiple imputation. The same advantages and disadvantages for these techniques that were present with linear regression apply to nonlinear regression.

FITTING DISCORDANT MODELS AMONG INDIVIDUALS

A not uncommon problem when fitting concentration-time data for each individual among a group of individuals is that some individuals may have data consistent with a 3-compartment model while others are more consistent with a 2-compartment model or some may better fit a 2-compartment model while others fit just a 1-compartment model. This reason for this phenomenon is usually due to the analytical assay. Think of the lower limit of quantification (LLOQ) of an assay acting as filter; anything above the LLOQ is observable but anything below the LLOQ is missing. If each subject does follow the more complex model but the data are such that the concentrations in the last phase of the concentration-time profile are below the LLOQ then the data will appear to have fewer phases in the concentration-time profile, even though the model does in fact follow the more complex model.

The question is what to do? Report the data as is? Try to fit all the individuals to the model with more compartments? This last option is not an option. Trying to fit the more complex model will, if convergence can even be achieved, usually result in a model with highly unstable parameter estimates showing large standard errors. The solution to this problem is to use a population approach through nonlinear mixed effects modeling using the more complex model, wherein individuals without data in the last phase of profile "borrow" information from individuals having data consistent with the more complex model (Schoemaker and Cohen, 1996). But in this case, when individual data are modeled, reporting the data as is may be the only option. The question though is, are these parameters accurate?

Deterministic simulation will be used to illustrate the effect of fitting a less complex to model to data arising from a more complex model. Concentration-time data were simulated from a 3-compartment model with the following parameters: CL = 1.5; Q2 = 0.15; Q3 = 0.015; V1 = 1, V2 = 0.5; V3 = 0.25. A bolus unit dose of 100 was injected into the central compartment (V1). A total of 50 samples were collected equally spaced for 48-time units. The data are shown in Fig. 3.15 and clearly demonstrate triphasic elimination kinetics. Now suppose the LLOQ of the assay was 0.01. Data above this line are consistent with biphasic elimination kinetics. What hap-

pens when a 2-compartment model is fit to data above the LLOQ? Using OLS the parameter estimates for the 2-compartment model were CL = 1.5; V1 = 1.0; Q2 = 0.16; and V2 = 0.57. The standard errors in all cases were <0.0001. The estimates related to the central compartment under the 2-compartment model were the same as the true values, but the estimates related to the peripheral compartment were biased. In this case, the deviation from a 2-compartment model is apparent at later time periods, but in an experimental situation having fewer data points this deviation might not be apparent. Now suppose the LLOQ was 0.1 units. In this case, the data are clearly biphasic. Fitting a 2-compartment model to this data gave the following results: CL = 1.5; V1 = 1.0; Q2 = 0.16; and V2 = 0.56. The standard errors in all cases was <0.0001. The same results occurred with a lower LLOQ. Parameters related to the central compartment were unbiased whereas parameters related to the peripheral compartment were biased.

This simple simulation can be expanded to different combinations of parameters, using a 1-compartment model to fit data simulated through a 2-compartment model, or even expanding the model to include an absorption compartment. The end result is the same—all parameters related to the central compartment will be unbiased estimates of the true values, whereas parameters related to the peripheral compartments will be biased. In going back to the original problem, it is okay to report data from individuals having fewer compartments but the limitations of the results and the interpretation of the results must be kept in mind.

SOFTWARE

As has been alluded to, there are many different software packages that can perform nonlinear regression. If the model can be expressed as an explicit function of {Y, x} then the NLIN procedure in SAS (SAS Institute, Cary, NC, www.sas.com) can be used as can the NLS2 algorithm within S-Plus (Insightful Corp., Seattle, WA, www.insightful.com). The most common software packages to fit pharmacokinetic data based on compartmental models are WinNonlin (Pharsight Corp., Mountain View, CA, www.pharsight.com), SAAM II (SAAM Institute, Seattle, WA, www.saam.com), and Adapt II (Biomedical Simulations Resource at the University of Southern California, bmsrs.usc.edu). All are designed to handle individual pharmacokinetic data, although Adapt II and SAAM II can handle multiple input-output experiments easier than WinNonlin. On

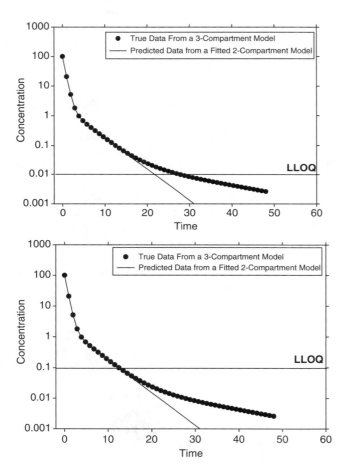

Figure 3.15 Scatter plot of a 2-compartment model fit to data simulated from a 3-compartment model. Data above the lower limit of quantification (LLOQ) were censored prior to fitting. Regardless of the LLOQ, the resulting fit using the less complex model will result in unbiased estimates of parameters related to the central compartment but biased estimates of parameters related to the peripheral compartments.

the other hand, WinNonlin does batch processing of multiple subjects, whereas SAAM II and Adapt II does not. Adapt II has the advantage that it is free,[3] but has poor graphics capabilities compared to WinNonlin and SAAM II. Of all the packages, SAAM II has the easiest and best simulation capability. There are many other subtle differences between the three pharmacokinetic packages and generally the one a person chooses is a matter of personality, economics, and regulatory requirements.

McCullough (1998; 1999) compared the accuracy of SAS's NLIN procedure and the nls and nlregb functions in S-Plus using the NIST nonlinear regression reference data sets, which are accurate to 11 decimal places. In each case, he used the program's default algorithm. For both SAS and S-Plus, in many instances with problems of average and high-level difficulty, convergence could not be obtained and, when convergence was obtained, the results were not accurate to a single decimal point. Problems of low-level difficulty were reliably solved using both SAS and S-Plus. In contrast, Microsoft's Excel 97 produced zero digit accuracy on most problems, even ones considered to be of low-level difficulty (McCullough and Wilson, 1999). McCullough concluded that whenever possible, the analytical derivatives should be specified by the analyst and included in the model. Also, the defaults used by each of the packages are unreliable and each problem should be approached on a case by case basis.

Heatherington, Vicini, and Golde (1998) compared 88 nonlinear models using SAAM II (version 1) and WinNonlin (1995) and found good agreement between the programs, despite many subtle algorithmic differences. Both programs required different numbers of iterations to achieve convergence, but after convergence was achieved, a less than 1% difference in the parameter estimates was observed, largely due to differences in the standard error estimates. The only real differences observed between the programs was in data sets with multiple outputs. The reported parameter estimates began to diverge when the number of data sets fit simultaneously increased.

The choice of computer processor may also have an impact on the results of fitting a nonlinear regression model. Wakelkamp solved an indirect response model described by three differential equations on four computers with different central processing units using the

same version of PCNONLIN, a precursor version to WinNonlin: a 66 MHz Intel DX2 80486, a 166 MHz Pentium, a 200 MHz Pentium Pro, and a Cyrix $6x86$ 150. Differences were observed both in the number of iterations for convergence and in the model parameters. For example, K_{in} was reported to be 715, 1010, 1010, and 681 mL/(hr min) on an Intel 66 MHz DX2 80486, Intel 166 MHz Pentium, Intel 200 MHz Pentium Pro, and Cyrix 6x 86 150 processor, respectively. It should be noted that none of these processors are available any longer, but still they highlight that differences may exist in the results generated by a Pentium or AMD computer processor. Proost (1999) later criticized these results and noted that the difference may be more a reflection of software/hardware/operating system interactions, rather than simply hardware differences. Nevertheless, this example illustrates that naïve use of an software package may lead to differences when others attempt to fit the model.

SUMMARY

Nonlinear regression is a standard topic taught in graduate level pharmacokinetics since it is required for almost every pharmacokinetic problem encountered. Like linear regression, a complete exposition of the topic is out of the question due to space constraints. The reader is referred to Seber and Wild (1989), Bates and Watts (1988), and Ross (1990) for more complete exposition of nonlinear modeling and applications. With nonlinear regression, the user must make choices (algorithm, convergence criteria, weights, parameter bounds, etc.) and the choices the user makes will have an impact on the final estimates for the model parameters. Understanding how these choices interact and what to do when convergence does not occur is essential for a pharmacokinetic modeler to understand.

Pharmacokinetic and pharmacodynamic modeling is not something that is taught, but something that is caught, and while this chapter is a didactic presentation of nonlinear modeling, only through practical experience and trial and error will the real nuances of how these variables interact will be understood.

RECOMMENDED READING

Bates, D.M. and Watts, D.G. Nonlinear regression analysis and its applications. New York: John Wiley & Sons, 1988.

Donaldson, J.R. and Schnabel, R.B. Computation experience with confidence regions and confidence intervals for nonlinear least squares. *Technometrics* 1987; 29:67–82.

---

[3] Although Adapt II is free, in order to use the program, a Fortran compiler must be available to compile the Adapt II source code. All the supported compilers for the most recent version (Version 4), however, are commercial and must be bought for a fee.

Gabrielsson, J. and Weiner, D. Pharmacokinetic and pharmacodynamic data analysis: Concepts and applications, 3rd edition. Swedish Pharmaceutical Press, Stockholm, Sweden, 2000.

Niedzwiecki, D. and Simonoff, J.S. Estimation and inference in pharmacokinetic models: The effectiveness of model reformulation and resampling methods for functions of parameters. *Journal of Pharmacokinetics and Biopharmaceutics* 1990; 18: 361–377.

Chapter 4

Variance Models, Weighting, and Transformations

That which is static and repetitive is boring. That which is dynamic and random is confusing. In between lies art.

—John A. Locke (1632–1704), British philosopher and medical researcher

INTRODUCTION

In the previous chapters it was assumed that the model relating an n-size matrix of predictor variables x to an n-size vector of paired responses Y was of the functional form

$$Y = f(\theta; x) + \varepsilon \tag{4.1}$$

where θ is the vector of model parameters that are estimated by $\hat{\theta}$, and ε is a vector of independent residuals with mean 0 and constant variance. The right hand side of Eq. (4.1) is composed of two parts: a structural model $f(\theta; x)$ and a stochastic error term. In this particular case, the stochastic part of the model is additive and independent of x and θ. Under this model

$$\mathrm{Var}\,(\varepsilon) = \sigma^2. \tag{4.2}$$

Equation (4.2) is called a residual variance model, but it is not a very general one. In this case, the model states that random, unexplained variability is a constant. Two methods are usually used to estimate θ: least-squares (LS) and maximum likelihood (ML). In the case where $\varepsilon \sim N(0, \sigma^2)$, the LS estimates are equivalent to the ML estimates. This chapter will deal with the case for more general variance models when a constant variance does not apply. Unfortunately, most of the statistical literature deals with estimation and model selection theory for the structural model and there is far less theory regarding choice and model selection for residual variance models.

So why not assume an additive error model and always use OLS estimation anyway? First, there is no guarantee in reality that an additive error term is even valid. Indeed, for some response measures, an additive error model may lead to nonsensical values. For example, suppose one were modeling drug concentrations, if $f(\theta; x)$ was small and the error term was large and negative, such as might happen on the tail of the left side of the normal distribution, then *theoretically* it is possible for concentrations to be negative. In reality, drug concentrations cannot be negative so that clearly the stochastic term in Eq. (4.2) is incorrect. Thus, a stochastic error term that constrains drug concentrations to be positive or zero would be more appropriate. Second, the estimates for the structural terms in the model are dependent on the choice of residual variance model and can vary depending on which variance model is chosen. Third, hypothesis tests for parameters and confidence intervals usually assume constant variance. Therefore, one must develop alternate algorithms for fitting data when heteroscedasticity, or nonconstant variance, is present.

RESIDUAL VARIANCE MODELS

When dealing with pharmacokinetic data, it is actually quite rare for the assumption of constant variance to be met. When the observations exhibit nonconstant variance, the data are heteroscedastic and the basic model needs to be modified to

$$Y = f(\theta; x) + g(\Phi; z; \theta; x)\varepsilon \qquad (4.3)$$

where g(.) is a variance function that relates the covariates x and z, the structural model parameters θ, and residual variance model parameters Φ to the variance of Y. All other variables are the same as before. Since g(.) is a constant and ε is assumed to be independent, with mean zero and variance σ^2, then by the variance of a linear combination of random variables, the variance of Y is given by

$$Var(Y) = \sigma^2[g(\Phi; z; \theta; x)]^2. \qquad (4.4)$$

Equation (4.4) is a residual variance model like Eq. (4.2) but far more flexible. Most often the residual variance model is simply a function of the structural model $f(\theta; x)$ in which case Eq. (4.4) is simplified to

$$Var(Y) = \sigma^2[g(f(\theta; x))]^2. \qquad (4.5)$$

Notice that nothing beyond the first two moments of Y is being assumed, i.e., only the mean and variance of the data are being defined and no distributional assumptions, such as normality, are being made. In residual variance model estimation, the goal is to understand the variance structure as a function of a set of predictors, which may not necessarily be the same as the set of predictors in the structural model (Davidian and Carroll, 1987). Common, heteroscedastic error models are shown in Table 4.1. Under all these models, generic ε is assumed to be independent, having zero mean and constant variance.

Table 4.1 Representative variance models seen in pharmacokinetic and pharmacokinetic-pharmacodynamic models.

Variance model	Functional form
Unweighted *additive*	$Y = f(\theta; x) + \varepsilon$
Constant coefficient of variation (CV) or proportional error	$Y = f(\theta; x)(1 + \varepsilon)$
Exponential error	$Y = f(\theta; x)\exp(\varepsilon)$
Error as a function of the mean	$Y = f(\theta, x) + g[f(\theta; x)]\varepsilon$
Additive on another scale, e.g., Ln	$h(Y) = h[f(\theta; x)] + \varepsilon$
Combined additive and proportional	$Y = f(\theta; x)(1 + \varepsilon_1) + \varepsilon_2$

Usually, variability increases as a systematic function of the mean response $f(\theta; x)$ in which case a common choice of residual variance model is the power of the mean model

$$Var(Y) = \sigma^2[f(\theta; x)]^{\Phi} \qquad (4.6)$$

where if $\Phi = 0$ then the variance is a constant, i.e., the data are homoscedastic, and if $\Phi = 2$ then the variance is gamma or log-normal. Figure 4.1 plots the variance of a hypothetical response as a function of the mean response for each of the residual variance models in Eq. (4.6). Notice that as Φ increases the variance of the response increases at a faster rate.

To illustrate how different error variance structures may influence observed values, concentrations (C) were simulated from a 1-compartment model with first-order absorption

$$C = \frac{D}{V}\left(\frac{k_a}{k_a - CL/V}\right)\left[\exp\left(-\frac{CL}{V}t\right) - \exp(-k_at)\right]$$
$$(4.7)$$

where D was a dose equal to 1 mg, V volume of distribution equal to 10 L, CL clearance equal to 1.5 L/h, and k_a the absorption rate constant equal to 0.7 per h. A total of 1000 equally spaced data points were simulated over the time interval of 0–24-h post dose. Three residual variance models were simulated: constant standard deviation equal to 2 ng/mL, proportional error equal to 15% coefficient of variation (CV), and constant standard deviation equal to 2 ng/mL plus proportional error (15% CV). The data are presented in Fig. 4.2. Constant variance results in approximately the same spread of data

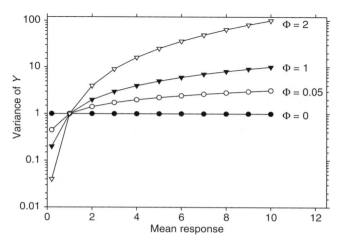

Figure 4.1 Variance of Y as a function of the mean response assuming a power of the mean residual variance model.

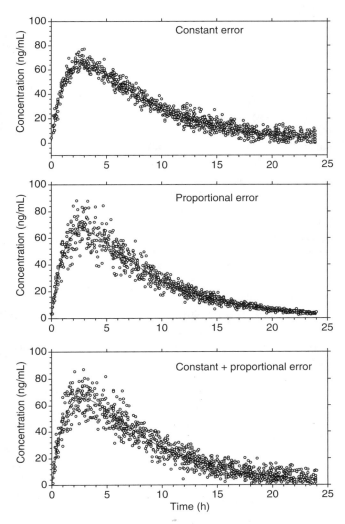

Figure 4.2 Examples of how different variance structures can influence observed concentrations. A total of 1000 concentrations were simulated from a 1-compartment model with the following parameters: clearance = 1.5 L h, volume of distribution = 10 L, absorption rate constant = 0.7 per h, dose = 1 mg. Three error structures were simulated: constant standard deviation of 2 ng/mL, 15% proportional error, and constant standard deviation of 2 ng/mL plus 15% proportional error.

regardless of the location of the x variable and can result in negative values. In contrast, for proportional error structures, the range of observed concentrations is larger when mean concentrations are larger. When the error consists of constant variance and proportional variance, the range of observed concentrations is larger when the mean concentration is large, but it is also quite large at lower concentrations and may become negative in value.

To choose an appropriate variance function, the analyst must consider all sources of variation (Davidian and Carroll, 1987; Davidian and Haaland, 1990). As an example, consider an analytical assay where the variance of the response increases as a function of the analyte concentration. Also, suppose there is some minimum

level of variation observed when no analyte is present. Then, an appropriate residual variance model may be

$$g(x; \theta; \Phi) = \Phi_1 + f(x; \theta)^{\Phi_2} \qquad (4.8)$$

so that

$$\text{Var}(Y) = \sigma^2 \left(\Phi_1 + f(x; \theta)^{\Phi_2} \right)^2. \qquad (4.9)$$

Davidian and Haaland (1990) call this a "components of variance" model because Φ_1 is the variance component from the detector when no analyte is present and $f(x; \theta)^{\Phi_2}$ is the variance component from the analyte response. Residual variance models can be empirically determined by trial and error, and indeed most are chosen in this manner, but hopefully they will be selected based on the scientist's knowledge of the process. A full description of variance model estimation is made in Davidian and Carroll (1987) and Carroll et al. (1988).

TESTING FOR HETEROSCEDASTICITY

In order to find an appropriate residual variance model, one must first determine whether the assumption of homoscedasticity is violated. But, before undertaking anything, the question of whether it is worth the effort to find a residual variance model must be answered. One rule of thumb for a designed experiment where the independent variables are fixed is that weighting offers little benefit when the ratio of the largest to smallest standard deviation is less than 1.5 but will generally be called for when the ratio exceeds 3 (Carroll and Ruppert, 1988). If this rule of thumb is passed, one proceeds in determining whether heteroscedasticity is present, keeping in mind that an incorrect model may be disguised as heteroscedasticity.

Diagnosis of heteroscedasticity is often done using a residual plot, whereby the residuals from an OLS fit are plotted against their predicted values. A fan or megaphone shaped pattern of residuals is indicative of nonconstant variance. For small sample sizes this plot may be insensitive or ambiguous. Cook and Weisberg (Johnston, 1972) propose plotting e^2/MSE versus predicted values as a test for heteroscedasticity, where e is the OLS residuals defined previously and MSE is the mean square error from the OLS fit to the data. An equivalent plot is to plot squared residuals versus predicted values since the use of MSE is to scale the squared residuals. They argue that often with positive and negative residuals, the usual residual plots are difficult to interpret, but by squaring the residuals, the sample size is effectively doubled. They also suggest that squared standardized residuals be plotted against log predicted values so as to remove the influence of influential observations from the residual plot.

Carroll and Ruppert (1988) suggest plotting the absolute value of residuals against predicted values and that when the range of squared values is large it might be more useful to plot log squared residuals[1] or residuals to the two-thirds power instead. In all cases, nonconstant variance will have a megaphone shaped pattern. Carroll and Ruppert (1988) have shown that if the power of the mean model holds (Eq. (4.6) is valid), plotting the log of the absolute value of the residuals versus the log of the predicted values will show a linear relationship with slope approximately equal to Φ. In practice, however, the slope tends to underestimate the true value of Φ.

Another quick and dirty test for heteroscedasticity suggested by Carroll and Ruppert (1988) is to compute the Spearman rank correlation coefficient between absolute studentized residuals and predicted values. If Spearman's correlation coefficient is statistically significant, this is indicative of increasing variance, but in no manner should the degree of correlation be taken as a measure of the degree of heteroscedasticity. They also suggest that a further refinement to any residual plot would be to overlay a nonparametric smoothed curve, such as a LOESS or kernel fit.

As a more formal test for heteroscedasticity for linear models, Goldfeld and Quandt (1965) proposed the following method:

1. Rank the (x, Y) observations in ascending x;
2. Omit c observations where c is specified a priori and divide the remaining n-c observations into two groups of (n-c)/2;
3. Fit separate OLS fits to the two datasets and compute the residual sum of squares for each group; and
4. Compute $\lambda = SSE_2/SSE_1$.

Under the null hypothesis, λ is distributed as a random variable having an F-distribution with {(n-c-2p)/2, (n-c-2p)/2} degrees of freedom. This method was shown to have good power at small sample sizes for detecting heteroscedasticity. Goldfeld and Quandt (1965) suggest that c = 8 for n = 30 observations and c = 16 if n = 60 observations. Using Monte Carlo simulation, Judge et al. (1982) suggest that c = 4 if n = 30 and c = 10 if n = 60. Unfortunately, these tests cannot be applied to a nonlinear model.

---

[1] Caution should be used when plotting the log of the squared residuals because small squared residuals near zero will result in inflated log squared residuals. For this reason it may be useful to trim the smallest squared residuals prior to plotting.

There are a number of other more formal tests for heteroscedasticity, all of which are part of a general class of statistics called *Score tests*. At this time, score tests have not found general acceptance among pharmacokineticists and are largely advocated by the econometrics community. A number of conjectures may be raised regarding why these tests have not permeated the pharmacokinetics community. One reason might be that since these tests were developed by econometricians, most pharmacokineticists are unfamiliar with that body of work. Second, even classic texts on regression models, such as Myers (1986), fail to discuss score tests in their sections on handling heteroscedasticity. Third, their implementation is not included in most statistical/pharmacokinetic software packages and their routine calculation becomes problematic. Despite these problems, score tests may be useful in the future. First, these tests have been shown to be quite robust to residual variance model misspecification (Breusch and Pagan, 1979). Second, Hall (1979) used Monte Carlo simulation to show that most score tests have good power even at small sample sizes. Lastly, despite the fact that these tests were designed to formally test for the presence of heteroscedasticity assuming a linear structural model, they may also be used for nonlinear models. The reader is referred to the following references for further details: Belanger, Davidian, and Giltinan (1979), Goldfield and Quandt (1996; 1965), Harrison and McCabe (1966), and Parks (1972).

IMPACT OF HETEROSCEDASTICITY ON OLS ESTIMATES

One method for dealing with heteroscedastic data is to ignore the variability in Y and use unweighted OLS estimates of θ. Consider the data shown in Fig. 4.2 having a constant variance plus proportional error model. The true values were volume of distribution = 10 L, clearance = 1.5 L/h, and absorption rate constant = 0.7 per/h. The OLS estimates from fitting a 1-compartment model to the data were as follows: volume of distribution = 10.3 ± 0.15 L, clearance = 1.49 ± 0.01 L/h, and absorption rate constant = 0.75 ± 0.03 per h. The parameter estimates themselves were quite well estimated, despite the fact that the assumption of constant variance was violated. Figure 4.3 presents the residual plots discussed in the previous section. The top plot, raw residuals versus predicted values, shows that as the predicted values increase so do the variance of the residuals. This is confirmed by the bottom two plots of Fig. 4.3 which indicate that both the range of the absolute value of the residuals and squared residuals increase as the predicted values increase.

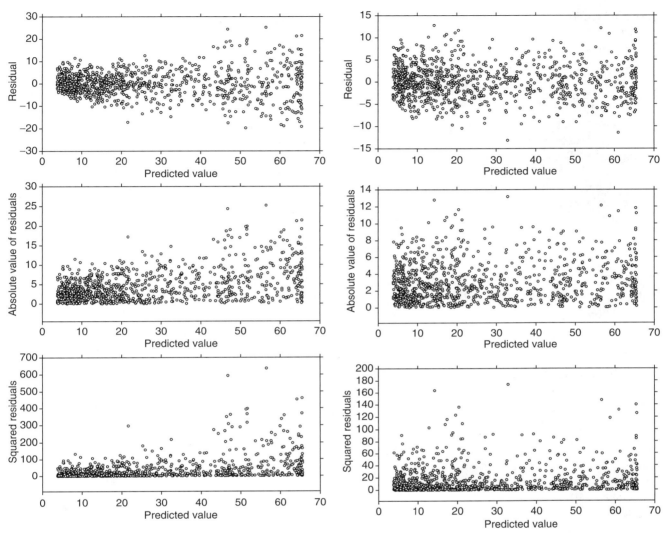

Figure 4.3 Residual plots from fitting a 1-compartment model using OLS to the data shown in the bottom plot of Fig. 4.2 having a constant plus proportional error variance structure.

Figure 4.4 Residual plots from fitting a 1-compartment model with first-order absorption using OLS to the data in the top plot in Fig. 4.2, which as a constant variance structure.

In contrast, the data in the top plot of Fig. 4.2 using a constant residual variance model led to the following parameter estimates after fitting the same model: volume of distribution $= 10.2 \pm 0.10$ L, clearance $= 1.49 \pm 0.008$ L/h, and absorption rate constant $= 0.71 \pm 0.02$ per h. Note that this model is the data generating model with no regression assumption violations. The residual plots from this analysis are shown in Fig. 4.4. None of the residual plots show any trend or increasing variance with increasing predicted value. Notice that the parameter estimates are less biased and have smaller standard errors than the estimates obtained from the constant variance plus proportional error model.

This is the effect of violating the assumptions of OLS: the parameter estimates have decreased precision when the incorrect residual variance model is used. The precision of the predicted values is also sacrificed. In general, confidence intervals generated around the mean predicted values will be reliable near the midrange of the function, but will be severely inflated near the extremities (Garden, Mitchell, and Mills, 1980).

IMPACT OF HETEROSCEDASTICITY ON PARAMETER INFERENCE

Not only does the choice of the variance function influence the structural parameters themselves, the variance function also influences the precision of the estimates. Also, although OLS estimates are unbiased in the presence of heteroscedasticity, the usual tests of significance are generally inappropriate and their use can lead to invalid inferences. In the case of heteroscedasticity, the usually reported variance–covariance estimator for the parameter estimates is

$$\Sigma = \sigma^2 (x^T V^{-1} x)^{-1} \qquad (4.10)$$

where $V = E(\varepsilon\varepsilon')$ is the variance of Y which in this case is a diagonal matrix whose elements are σ^2. Equation (4.10) is the default method used for most software packages (like SAS). However, this estimator does not produce consistent estimates of the variance–covariance matrix. A heteroscedastic consistent estimate of the variance–covariance matrix (sometimes called the sandwich estimator) for $\hat{\theta}$ is

$$\Sigma = (x^T x)^{-1} x^T V x (x^T x)^{-1}. \qquad (4.11)$$

If the errors are homoscedastic and V is a diagonal matrix whose elements are σ^2, then Eqs. (4.10) and (4.11) reduce to

$$\Sigma = \sigma^2 (x^T x)^{-1} \qquad (4.12)$$

the variance–covariance estimate for $\hat{\theta}$ under OLS. In practice, V is replaced by a diagonal matrix whose diagonal elements are given by the squared residuals since V is often unknown and σ^2 is replaced by the mean square error. For the nonlinear model, x is replaced by J, the Jacobian matrix of first derivatives of $f(.)$ with respect to θ evaluated at the final parameter estimates $\hat{\theta}$. So for the homoscedastic nonlinear model, the variance–covariance matrix is given by

$$\Sigma = \sigma^2 (J^T J)^{-1}. \qquad (4.13)$$

Three additional heteroscedastic consistent estimators for Σ have been reported over the years. The simplest was reported by Hinkley (1977)

$$\Sigma = \frac{n}{n-p} (x^T x)^{-1} x^T V x (x^T x)^{-1}. \qquad (4.14)$$

MacKinnon and White (1985) suggested that the influence a residual has on the parameter estimates needs to be considered and that two other estimates of Σ might be

$$\Sigma = (x^T x)^{-1} x^T \mathrm{diag}\left(\frac{V}{1 - h_{ii}}\right) x (x^T x)^{-1} \qquad (4.15)$$

$$\Sigma = (x^T x)^{-1} x^T \mathrm{diag}\left(\frac{V}{(1 - h_{ii})^2}\right) x (x^T x)^{-1} \qquad (4.16)$$

where h_{ii} is the HAT matrix, $x(x^T x)^{-1} x^T$. As before, x is replaced by J in the nonlinear case. Whatever

the method, the standard error of the parameter estimates is

$$SE(\theta_i) = \sqrt{\Sigma_{ii}}. \qquad (4.17)$$

Hence, the precision of the parameter estimates is influenced by both the variability in x and Y.

Long and Ervin (2000) used Monte Carlo simulation to compare the four estimators under a homoscedastic and heteroscedastic linear model. The usually reported standard error estimator [Eq. (4.10)] was not studied. All heteroscedastic estimators of Σ performed well even when heteroscedasticity was not present. When heteroscedasticity was present, Eq. (4.11) resulted in incorrect inferences when the sample size was less than 250 and was also more likely to result in a Type I error than the other estimators. When more than 250 observations were present, all estimators performed equally. Long and Ervin suggest that when the sample size is less than 250 that Eq. (4.16) be used to estimate Σ. Unfortunately no pharmacokinetic and most statistical software packages use these heteroscedastic-consistent standard error estimators.

To further illustrate these concepts, data were simulated using an E_{max} model where E_{max} was the maximal effect set equal to 75, EC_{50} was the concentration that produces 50% of the maximal effect set equal to 25, and C was concentration randomly sampled from the interval [0, 500]. Normally distributed random error with a constant coefficient of variation set equal to 20% of the mean of Y was added to each observation. The data are shown in Fig. 4.5 and were fit using a number of different weighting schemes. The results are presented in Table 4.2. Notice that as the weights become greater

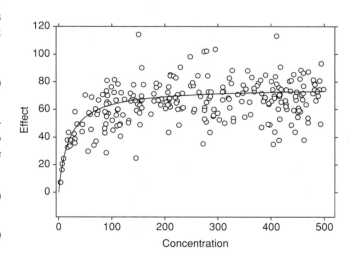

Figure 4.5 Scatter plot of simulated data from an E_{max} model with 20% constant coefficient of variation, where $E_{max} = 75$ and $EC_{50} = 25$. Legend: Solid line is weighted least-squares fit with weights $1/Y$.

Table 4.2 Parameter estimates and their standard errors for data in Fig. 4.5.

| Weight | Maximal effect (E_{max}): True value = 75 Standard error based on covariance matrix given in equation | | | | | | EC$_{50}$: True value = 25 Standard error based on covariance matrix given in equation | | | | | |
	Est.	(4.10)	(4.11)	(4.14)	(4.15)	(4.16)	Est.	(4.10)	(4.11)	(4.14)	(4.15)	(4.16)
1 (OLS)	73.11	1.51	1.41	1.41	1.41	1.41	20.44	3.54	2.70	2.72	2.72	2.72
$1/(0.1Y)$	69.95	1.46	1.46	1.46	1.46	1.46	21.16	2.99	2.99	3.00	3.00	3.00
$1/(0.2Y)$	69.95	1.46	1.46	1.46	1.46	1.46	21.16	3.11	2.99	3.00	3.00	3.00
$1/Y$	69.95	1.46	1.46	1.46	1.46	1.46	21.16	3.11	2.99	3.00	3.00	3.00
$1/(2Y)$	69.95	1.46	1.43	1.44	1.43	1.43	21.16	3.11	2.99	3.00	3.00	3.00
$1/Y^2$	66.52	1.42	1.62	1.63	1.63	1.63	22.80	2.52	3.73	3.75	3.74	3.75
$1/(2{*}Y^2)$	66.52	1.42	1.62	1.63	1.63	1.63	22.80	2.52	3.73	3.75	3.74	3.75
$1/Y^3$	62.44	1.43	1.92	1.93	1.93	1.93	24.60	1.74	5.02	5.04	5.03	5.04
$1/(4Y^3)$	62.44	1.43	1.92	1.93	1.93	1.93	24.60	1.74	5.02	5.04	5.03	5.04

Note: Est, estimate.

and greater, the estimate of E_{max} becomes more and more biased but the estimate of EC_{50} becomes less and less biased. This is because the weights tend to give more and more emphasis to smaller concentrations than larger concentrations, which tends to drive the estimate of EC_{50} smaller and smaller. As the weights become larger and larger, the usually reported standard errors become smaller and smaller. In contrast, the heteroscedastic-consistent standard errors, which were originally smaller than the usually reported standard errors, become larger when the weights were increased. Little difference was observed between the various heteroscedastic-consistent standard errors.

Also, notice in Table 4.2 that multiples of $f(Y)^{-1}$, e.g., Y, $2Y^{-1}$, $3Y^{-1}$, etc., all lead to the same set of parameter estimates and standard errors. It is only when the power of the weights (Φ) change do the parameter estimates themselves change. The reason for this is that the multiplier is a constant value that has no effect on the minimization process. In other words, if the global minimum is obtained with one set of weights, then using the same set of weights, but multiplied by some constant value, will have no effect on the distribution space of the sum of squares. Consider the data in Fig. 4.5 where there are two parameters. The parameter space and objective function can be conveniently viewed in XYZ space, where XY are the parameters and Z is the objective function. When the global minimum is found with one set of weights, the global minimum will always be at the same set of parameter estimates in XY space, but its absolute value in Z space will be different depending on the multiplier used. This is illustrated in Fig. 4.6. This figure shows the sum of squares surface for weighting scheme Y^{-1} (top) and $2Y^{-1}$ (bottom). The surfaces are identical except with regard to the position of the objective function, in which the weighting scheme $2Y^{-1}$ has its minimum at one-half that of weighting scheme Y^{-1}. So regardless of whether Y was weighted by Y^{-1} or

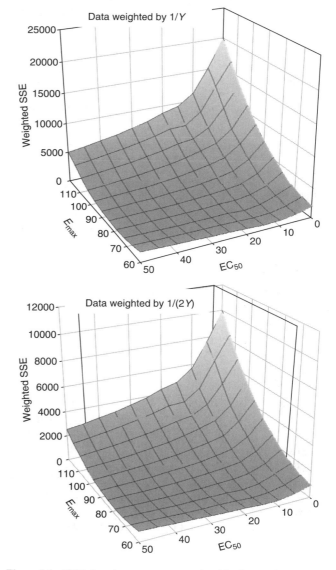

Figure 4.6 XYZ plot of parameter space and weighted sum of squares for data in Fig. 4.5 for varying parameter values and weighting schemes.

some more specific residual variance model of Y, by using an estimate of the coefficient of variation, e.g., $0.1\,Y^{-1}$, the resulting parameter estimates were similar.

RESIDUAL VARIANCE MODEL PARAMETER ESTIMATION USING WEIGHTED LEAST-SQUARES

Carroll and Ruppert (1988) and Davidian and Giltinan (1995) present comprehensive overviews of parameter estimation in the face of heteroscedasticity. In general, three methods are used to provide precise, unbiased parameter estimates: weighted least-squares (WLS), maximum likelihood, and data and/or model transformations. Johnston (1972) has shown that as the departure from constant variance increases, the benefit from using methods that deal with heteroscedasticity increases. The difficulty in using WLS or variations of WLS is that additional burdens on the model are made in that the method makes the additional assumption that the variance of the observations is either known or can be estimated. In WLS, the goal is not to minimize the OLS objective function, i.e., the residual sum of squares,

$$O_{OLS} = \min \sum_{i=1}^{n} [Y_i - f(x_i; \theta)]^2 \qquad (4.18)$$

but to minimize the weighted sum of squares

$$O_{WLS} = \min \sum_{i=1}^{n} w_i [Y_i - f(x_i; \theta)]^2 \qquad (4.19)$$

where w_i is explicitly known and defined as inverse variance of the ith observation,

$$w_i = \frac{1}{Var(Y_i)}. \qquad (4.20)$$

When the variance of an observation is large, less weight is given to that observation. Conversely, when an observation is precisely measured with small variance, more weight is given to that observation, a beneficial property. Obviously, ordinary least-squares is a special case of weighted least-squares in that all the observations have weights equal to one.

The choice of weights in WLS is based on either the observed data or on a residual variance model. If the variances are known and they are not a function of the mean, then the model can be redefined as

$$Y_i^* = Y_i \sqrt{w_i} \qquad (4.21)$$

$$f^*(w_i; x_i; \theta) = f(x_i; \theta) \sqrt{w_i} \qquad (4.22)$$

where the transformed responses now have constant variance σ^2 with means given by the transformed function f^*. θ can then be estimated by the method of ordinary least-squares. Unfortunately, this situation is uncommon.

If replicate measurements are taken at each level of the predictors, then one simple approach to estimation of the weights is to calculate the sample variance at each level i of the predictors (σ_i^2) and use these to form the weights as

$$w_i = \frac{1}{\sigma_i^2}. \qquad (4.23)$$

However, when the number of replicates is small, as is usually the case, the estimated variance can be quite erroneous and unstable. Nonlinear regression estimates using this approach are more variable than their unweighted least-squares counterparts, unless the number of replicates at each level is 10 or more. For this reason, this method cannot be supported and the danger of unstable variance estimates can be avoided if a parametric residual variance model can be found.

When no replicates are available, common weights that use the observed data include $1/Y$ or $1/Y^2$. These two weighting schemes in essence assume that the variance model is proportional to the mean or mean squared, respectively, and then crudely use the observation itself to estimate the mean. Although using observed data has a tremendous history behind it, using observed data as weights is problematic in that observed data are measured with error. A better estimate might be $1/\hat{Y}$ or $1/\hat{Y}^2$ where the predicted values are used instead. In this manner, any measurement error or random variability in the data are controlled.

The particular choice of a residual variance model should be based on the nature of the response function. Sometimes Φ is unknown and must be estimated from the data. Once a structural model and residual variance model is chosen, the choice then becomes how to estimate θ, the structural model parameters, and Φ, the residual variance model parameters. One commonly advocated method is the method of generalized least-squares (GLS). First it will be assumed that Φ is known and then that assumption will be relaxed. In the simplest case, assume that θ is known, in which case the weights are given by

$$w = \frac{1}{[g(f(x; \theta); z; \Phi)]^2}. \qquad (4.24)$$

When θ is known exactly then the weights can be formed directly from Eq. (4.24), but when θ is not known exactly (and it is estimated by $\hat{\theta}$) then the weights are estimated by

$$\hat{w} = \frac{1}{\left[g(\ f(x; \hat{\theta}); z; \Phi) \right]^2}. \qquad (4.25)$$

Notice that in Eqs. (4.24) and (4.25) that the weights are based on the predicted value for a particular combination of x and z, not an observed value. Hence, the method of GLS is as follows:

1. If θ is not known with certainty, estimate θ by $\hat{\theta}$ from an initial unweighted regression.
2. Form estimated weights using Eq. (4.25).
3. Use the weights from Step 2 and reestimate θ by WLS.

The new estimate of θ is a more efficient estimator since it makes use of the variability in the data. A modification of this process is to combine Steps 2 and 3 into a single step and iterate until the GLS parameter estimates stabilize. This modification is referred to as iteratively reweighted least-squares (IRWLS) and is an option available in both WinNonlin and SAS. Early versions of WinNonlin were limited in that g(.) was limited to the form in Eq. (4.6) where Φ is specified by the user. For example, specifying $\Phi = 0.5$, forces weights

$$w = \frac{1}{\sqrt{f(x; \theta)}}. \qquad (4.26)$$

Later versions of WinNonlin offer the option of having the user define the weights using more complex functions, provided that Φ is specified and known by the user.

Simulations have shown that only two or three iterations are needed for convergence of GLS and that at least two iterations should be done to "wash out" the effect of the OLS estimates on θ (Carroll and Ruppert, 1988). One advantage of GLS is that the estimate of θ will still be consistent even if an incorrect residual variance model is used. If a wrong variance model is used, the precision of the estimator may be not be precise, because the variance is misrepresented. If the residual variance model used is not too far from the true residual variance model, the loss of precision is usually minor, however (Davidian, personal communication). It should be noted that WinNonlin further scales the weights such that the sum of the weights for each function is equal to the number of data values (with nonzero weights). The WinNonlin User's Manual states that this process has no effect on the fitting process but provides enhanced numerical stability through stabilization of the matrix inversion process (Pharsight Corporation, 2002). However, Heatherington, Vicini, and Golde (1998)

reported examples where this statement may not be true and final parameter estimates may significantly differ depending on whether the weights were scaled or unscaled.

Having forced the user to define Φ is problematic because often the value of Φ is not known a priori and must be estimated from the data. Hence the GSL algorithm may be modified to

1. If θ is not known with certainty, estimate θ by $\hat{\theta}$ from an initial unweighted regression.
2. Estimate Φ by $\hat{\Phi}$ based on the estimate of $\hat{\theta}$.
3. Form the weights using Eq. (4.25).
4. Use the weights from Step 3 and reestimate θ by WLS.
5. Iterate if needed.

While Step 2 seems simple enough, estimating Φ is not trivial. One method is to use a general optimization routine to estimate Φ by pseudolikelihood (PL), wherein the predicted responses are treated as fixed variables and Φ and σ are minimized with respect to

$$O_{PL} = \sum_{i=1}^{n} \left[\frac{[Y_i - f(x_i; \theta^r)]^2}{[g(f(x; \theta^f), z, \Phi)]^2} + Ln\left\{ [g(\ f(x; \theta^f), z, \Phi)]^2 \right\} \right]$$

$$(4.27)$$

where the superscript f refers to θ^f being fixed. In essence, the user now does two optimizations: the first being the optimization to obtain $\hat{\theta}$, the second to obtain an estimate of Φ and σ. In the case where the residual variance model is a power of the mean, Eq. (4.27) is modified to

$$O_{PL} = \sum_{i=1}^{n} \left[\frac{[Y_i - f(x_i; \theta^f)]^2}{\sigma^2 f(x_i; \theta^f)^\Phi} + [\sigma^2 f(x_i; \theta^f)^\Phi] \right]. \qquad (4.28)$$

$\hat{\sigma}^2$ is estimated by the weighted residual sum of squares

$$\hat{\sigma}^2 = \sum_{i=1}^{n} w_i [Y_i - f(x_i; \hat{\theta}^f)]^2 \qquad (4.29)$$

and can be thought of as a proportionality constant in the fitting process. Minimizing Eq. (4.27) is equivalent to maximizing the normal log-likelihood evaluated at $\hat{\theta}^f$. The advantage of PL is that it does not depend on the distribution of the data (Davidian and Giltinan, 1995), but only depends on being able to specify the first two moments, i.e., mean and variance of the residuals.

One criticism of PL is that it does not take into account the loss of degrees of freedom in estimating $\hat{\theta}^f$, which leads to a modification of the PL objective function called restricted maximum likelihood (REML)

$$O_{REML} = O_{PL} - p\, Ln\, (\sigma^2) + Ln\, (J^T WJ), \qquad (4.30)$$

where J is the matrix of first derivatives of f(.) with respect to θ evaluated at the final parameter estimates and W is a diagonal matrix whose diagonal elements are given by Eq. (4.25).

Both PL and REML are based on squared residuals and thus may be sensitive to outliers and nonnormality. Davidian and Carroll (1987) suggest in this case to use a modification of Eq. (4.27) wherein the objective function is based on absolute residuals, instead of squared residuals. See Davidian and Carroll (1987) or Davidian and Giltinan (1995) for details. Huber (1981) showed that if just two outlier observations are included in a dataset of 1000 observations, this is sufficient for the absolute residual method to have greater efficiency in estimating the variance function than squared residuals. Despite the advantages of PL or REML over WLS with fixed Φ, no pharmacokinetic software package has implemented them into routine use.

Another common fitting algorithm found in the pharmacokinetic literature is extended least-squares (ELS) wherein θ, the structural model parameters, and Φ, the residual variance model parameters, are estimated simultaneously (Sheiner and Beal, 1985). The objective function in ELS is the same as the objective function in PL

$$O_{ELS} = \sum_{i=1}^{n} \left[\frac{[Y_i - f(x_i; \theta)]^2}{[g(f(x; \theta); z; \Phi)]^2} + Ln\{[g(\, f(x; \theta); z; \Phi)]^2\} \right]$$
$$(4.31)$$

the difference being θ and Φ are minimized simultaneously rather than iteratively (hence $\hat{\theta}$ is not fixed during the process). ELS is maximum likelihood estimation under the assumption of normality. Sheiner and Beal (1988) originally advocated its routine use in pharmacokinetic analysis and have implemented its use in the NONMEM population pharmacokinetic analysis software package (Boeckmann, Sheiner, and Beal, 1994). Also, SAAM II utilizes ELS as its objective function, except that Eq. (4.31) is divided by the total number of observations in the data set.

Building on work done earlier, Beal and Sheiner (1988) used Monte Carlo simulation to compare the parameter estimates obtained from ELS, GLS, WLS, OLS, and a few other modifications thereof. The models studied were the 1-compartment model, 1-compartment model with absorption, and E_{max} model. Each model was evaluated under five different residual variance models. All the methods used to deal with heteroscedasticity were superior to OLS estimates. There was little difference between estimates obtained using GLS and

ELS and that "earlier enthusiasm expressed for ELS must be tempered." Two other notable observations were made. First, if the residual variance model was incorrectly specified with ELS, this adversely affected the ELS parameter estimates. Belanger et al. (1971) indicated that this should not be a problem with GLS. Second, considerable advantage was gained when Φ was treated as an estimable parameter, rather than a fixed value as in IRWLS or WLS, as estimable residual variance models are more robust to residual variance model misspecification than fixed residual variance models.

However, not everyone agrees with the superiority of ELS in parameter estimation (van Houwelingen, 1988), while others criticize that standard nonlinear regression software is not equipped for ELS. Giltinan and Ruppert (1989) present a variant of ELS (technically it is GLS with PL estimation of Φ, which is asymptotically equivalent to ELS when $\sigma \to 0$) that can be used on standard statistical software packages and demonstrate their method using a polyexponential equation analyzed by SAS. Their method replaces simultaneous estimation of σ and Φ by breaking it down into stages, i.e., they use a GLS approach. Their algorithm is as follows:

1. Estimate θ from an initial unweighted regression and call this value $\hat{\theta}$.
2. Substitute and fix $\hat{\theta}$ for θ in Eq. (4.28) and minimize Eq. (4.28) in σ and Φ.
3. Form estimated weights proportional to $f(\hat{\theta}, x_i)^{-\hat{\Phi}}$.
4. Use the weights from Step 3 and reestimate θ by weighted least-squares.
5. Return to Step 2 and iterate until convergence.

It may be unclear how σ and Φ can be estimated simultaneously using Eq. (4.28). Using a little algebra, they show that by fixing θ, minimizing Eq. (4.28) in σ and Φ is equivalent to minimizing

$$\min \left[\sum_{i=1}^{n} \frac{\tilde{\hat{Y}}^{0.5\Phi}(Y_i - \hat{Y}_i)}{\hat{Y}_i^{0.5\Phi}} \right]^2 \qquad (4.32)$$

in Φ, where $\tilde{\hat{Y}}$ is the geometric mean predicted value

$$\tilde{\hat{Y}} = \left[\prod_{i=1}^{n} \hat{Y}_i \right]^{\frac{1}{n}}. \qquad (4.33)$$

Now if a new response variable, $U_i = 0$ is created for all i and a new predictor variable, V, is created

$$V_i = \left(\frac{\tilde{\hat{Y}}_i}{\hat{Y}_i} \right)^{0.5\Phi} (Y_i - \hat{Y}_i),\ i = 1, 2, \ldots n, \qquad (4.34)$$

then regressing U on V will choose the value of Φ that minimizes

$$\min\left[\sum_{i=1}^{n}(U_i - V_i)^2\right], \qquad (4.35)$$

which is easily seen to be a standard least-squares problem. Giltinan and Ruppert (1989) indicate that the method they propose is not true ELS, though in most instances the difference is likely to be insignificant. It should be noted that in the appendix presented in that paper there were two typographical errors. This chapter's appendix presents the corrected SAS code.

ELS also produces inconsistent estimates of θ when the wrong variance model is used, whereas GLS does not. The difference is because GLS estimates θ by an estimating equation linear in Y, whereas ELS solves one that is quadratic in Y. For most pharmacokinetic data, however, where the variance is small relative to the range of the mean responses, ELS and GLS produce essentially equivalent results and the danger of the inconsistency vanishes. If, however, the variance is large relative to the range of responses, the two estimation methods may produce divergent results (Davidian, personal communication).

As a last comment, caution should be exercised when fitting small sets of data to both structural and residual variance models. It is commonplace in the literature to fit individual data and then apply a residual variance model to the data. Residual variance models based on small samples are not very robust, which can easily be seen if the data are jackknifed or bootstrapped. One way to overcome this is to assume a common residual variance model for all observations, instead of a residual variance model for each subject. This assumption is not such a leap of faith. For GLS, first fit each subject and then pool the residuals. Use the pooled residuals to estimate the residual variance model parameters and then iterate in this manner until convergence. For ELS, things are a bit trickier but are still doable.

Monte Carlo Comparison of the Methods

A Monte Carlo experiment was conducted comparing the different algorithms. Dose–effect data were simulated using an E_{max} model with intercept where E_0 was set equal to 200, E_{max} was set equal to -100, ED_{50} was set equal to 25, and dose was fixed at the following levels: 0, 10, 20, 40, 80, 160, and 320. A total of 25 subjects were simulated per dose level. The only source of error in this simulation was random error, which was added to each observation under the following residual variance models:

1. Normally distributed homoscedastic random error with a standard deviation of 10.
2. Normally distributed random error with a constant coefficient of variation set equal to 15% of the mean of Y.
3. Normally distributed random error with additive and proportional error term. The proportional component was a coefficient of variation set equal to 10% of the mean of Y. The additive component had a constant standard deviation equal to 10.
4. Uniformly distributed random error on the interval $[-25, 25]$.
5. Heavy-tailed normal distribution where 80% of the deviations from true values were normally distributed with a standard deviation of 10 and the remainder were normally distributed with a standard deviation of 20.
6. Mixture of normal distributions where 30% of the observations had a shift in their baseline (E_0) of 100 and all observations had a standard deviation of 10.

Each of these residual error models resulted in data sets with approximately the same mean and range of simulated data; the difference being in the shape of the distributions. 250 data sets were generated with 175 observations per data set. The E_{max} model was fit to each data set using the Marquardt–Levenberg algorithm within the NLIN procedure in SAS. The following weighting algorithms were examined:

1. Ordinary least-squares, denoted as OLS,
2. Weighted least-squares with weights equal to $1/Y$, denoted as WLS(1),
3. Weighted least-squares with weights $1/Y^2$, denoted as WLS(2),
4. Generalized least-squares with weights equal to $1/\hat{Y}$, denoted as GLS(1),
5. Generalized least-squares with weights equal to $1/\hat{Y}^2$, denoted as GLS(2), and
6. Extended least-squares with estimated Φ and weights equal to $1/Y^{\Phi}$, denoted as ELS.

After the 250 data sets were fit, the mean parameter estimate and coefficient of variation for the distribution of estimates was calculated.

The results are shown in Table 4.3. When the error was homoscedastic, all algorithms produce unbiased estimates of the parameters. Hence, weighting data unnecessarily had no detrimental impact on parameter estimation. Little difference was observed between the fitting algorithms when the error was proportional or constant plus proportional, except for both the WLS algorithms which had slightly more bias than the others in estimating E_0 and E_{max}. Surprisingly, when the error was uniformly distributed, which violates the assumption

Table 4.3 Results of Monte Carlo simulation testing the effect of residual variance model misspecification on nonlinear regression parameter estimates.

True residual variance model: Homoscedastic

	Mean value			Between simulation CV(%) of parameter estimates		
Algorithm	E_0	E_{max}	ED_{50}	E_0	E_{max}	ED_{50}
OLS	200.0	−100.1	25.1	1.0	2.7	8.5
WLS(1)	199.5	−101.6	25.2	1.0	2.7	8.6
WLS(2)	199.0	−100.1	25.3	1.1	2.7	9.1
GLS(1)	200.0	−100.1	25.1	1.0	2.7	8.6
GLS(2)	200.0	−100.1	25.1	1.0	2.7	8.8
ELS	200.0	−100.1	25.1	1.0	2.7	8.6

True residual variance model: Constant CV (15%)

	Mean value			Between simulation CV(%) of parameter estimates		
Algorithm	E_0	E_{max}	ED_{50}	E_0	E_{max}	ED_{50}
OLS	200.2	−100.5	25.7	2.8	5.6	23.1
WLS(1)	195.7	−98.3	25.7	3.0	6.2	24.4
WLS(2)	190.9	−96.1	25.9	3.4	7.1	28.7
GLS(1)	200.2	−100.5	25.8	2.8	5.6	23.8
GLS(2)	200.2	−100.5	25.8	2.9	5.6	24.5
ELS	200.2	−100.4	25.7	2.7	5.6	21.9

True residual variance model: Additive with constant CV (15%)

	Mean value			Between simulation CV(%) of parameter estimates		
Algorithm	E_0	E_{max}	ED_{50}	E_0	E_{max}	ED_{50}
OLS	200.4	−100.8	25.8	2.9	6.5	23.3
WLS(1)	195.2	−99.0	25.9	3.2	7.0	26.0
WLS(2)	189.8	−97.3	26.6	3.8	8.2	36.2
GLS(1)	200.4	−100.8	25.8	2.9	6.5	23.8
GLS(2)	200.3	−100.8	25.9	2.9	6.5	24.4
ELS	200.4	−100.7	25.7	2.9	6.5	23.1

True residual variance model: Uniform (−25, +25)

	Mean value			Between simulation CV(%) of parameter estimates		
Algorithm	E_0	E_{max}	ED_{50}	E_0	E_{max}	ED_{50}
OLS	200.0	−100.4	25.4	1.5	3.3	14.4
WLS(1)	199.0	−101.4	25.5	1.5	3.3	14.5
WLS(2)	198.0	−102.4	25.7	1.5	3.3	14.9
GLS(1)	200.0	−100.4	25.4	1.5	3.3	14.4
GLS(2)	200.0	−100.4	25.4	1.5	3.3	14.5
ELS	200.0	−100.4	25.4	1.5	3.3	14.4

True residual variance model: Heavy-tailed normal

	Mean value			Between simulation CV(%) of parameter estimates		
Algorithm	E_0	E_{max}	ED_{50}	E_0	E_{max}	ED_{50}
OLS	200.0	−101.1	25.2	1.6	3.9	14.6
WLS(1)	198.5	−102.0	25.9	1.8	5.0	18.3
WLS(2)	197.7	−107.2	30.9	2.8	18.7	93.2
GLS(1)	200.0	−101.1	25.2	1.6	3.9	14.5
GLS(2)	200.0	−101.1	25.2	1.6	3.9	14.6
ELS	200.0	−101.1	25.2	1.6	3.9	14.7

Table 4.3 (*Continued*)   Results of Monte Carlo simulation testing the effect of residual variance model misspecification on nonlinear regression parameter estimates.

True residual variance model: Mixture distribution

Algorithm	Mean value			Between simulation CV(%) of parameter estimates		
	E_0	E_{max}	ED_{50}	E_0	E_{max}	ED_{50}
OLS	230.5	−101.6	27.4	3.8	11.5	48.8
WLS(1)	222.3	−106.1	26.9	3.3	8.6	33.3
WLS(2)	215.5	−108.2	26.5	2.8	6.5	24.0
GLS(1)	230.5	−101.6	27.4	3.8	11.5	47.5
GLS(2)	230.5	−101.6	27.4	3.8	11.5	47.4
ELS	230.5	−101.6	27.5	3.7	11.6	49.5

Note: True values were $E_0 = 200$, $E_{max} = -100$, and $ED_{50} = 25$. Number of simulations was 250 with 100% completed successfully.

of normality, all methods gave precise estimates on average and no discernible difference was observed between the algorithms. When the error was heavy-tailed normal, all methods produced roughly equivalent parameter estimates, except for WLS(2). All methods overestimated E_0, although WLS did less so. Also, E_{max} and EC_{50} were precisely estimated, except with WLS. Further, considerably more variability was observed across simulations with WLS(2) than with the other estimation methods. Only when the error was decidedly nonnormal, a mixture distribution did the parameter estimates to diverge from their true values. But, even with a mixture distribution, little difference was observed between OLS and GLS or ELS. Again, it was only with the WLS methods was a slight difference noticed in the estimation of E_{max} and E_0.

In summary, in this example, which was not very complex, little difference among the algorithms was observed when the error structure was normally distributed or slightly non-normal. WLS(2) did appear to have problems in unbiased parameter estimation under certain conditions. All algorithms did surprisingly well when the error was uniform in distribution. Only when the error was decidedly nonnormal, a mixture of normal distributions, were biased parameter estimates produced. Clearly, there will be situations where one algorithm produces more precise and less biased parameter estimates compared to other algorithms, but this can only be known through Monte Carlo simulation. These results indicate that there was very little difference in ELS and GLS estimates. WLS estimation where the weights are proportional to the *observed* data cannot be recommended.

RESIDUAL VARIANCE MODEL PARAMETER ESTIMATION USING MAXIMUM LIKELIHOOD

Besides a least-squares approach to variance model estimation, model parameters may be estimated by ML. In contrast to LS, which only makes assumptions about the first two moments of the data, ML makes the additional assumption regarding the distribution of the data, e.g., normal, log-normal, etc., the advantage being that inferences about θ can easily be made. If the heteroscedastic data are normally distributed, the LS estimators are the ML estimators, just like in the homoscedastic case. Carroll and Ruppert (1999; 1988) have shown, both theoretically and through simulation, that ML estimators in a heteroscedastic model are sensitive to the assumption of normality and to small errors in defining the variance model. GLS estimators, while sensitive to the normality assumption in theory, are more robust to variance model misspecification. If, however, the data are in fact normally distributed, the ML estimators are more efficient than GLS estimators and will produce improved estimates, but the improvement will usually not be large, typically less than 25%. Even if the data appear to be normally distributed, small degrees of skewness or kurtosis will lead to less efficient estimators than GLS estimates. Hence, ML estimation in the case of heteroscedastic residuals is not recommended unless the residual variance model is correctly specified.

MODEL AND/OR DATA TRANSFORMATIONS TO NORMALITY OR LINEARITY

Introduction

Heteroscedasticity is often accompanied with lack of normality in the distribution of the residuals. This is problematic because, as was shown in previous sections, some fitting algorithms like ELS are sensitive to deviations from normality. Handling heteroscedasticity alone can often be done using residual variance models and weighted least-squares, but weighted least-squares alone do not handle deviations from normality. There are two general approaches to handling nonnormality (assuming homoscedasticity). The first approach is to actually model the distribution of the residuals as a skewed probability density, such as the gamma distribution. This leads to a class of models known as generalized linear or generalized nonlinear models. The reader is referred to McCullagh and Nelder (1989) and Lindsey et al. (2000) for details on this class of models. The second approach, one that is more often used in pharmacokinetics and the one that will be discussed herein, is to transform the data and/or model such that the transformed residuals are normally distributed. While a great deal of effort has been spent by the statistical community on correcting for nonnormality in regression models, all the research has been predicated on having an appropriate structural model. Nonnormality may not be an artifact of the data, but may be due entirely to having a poor structural model. So before anything is done, acceptance of the model must be made.

A second problem is that sometimes a nonlinear function cannot be found that adequately fits the response data. In this case, it may be possible to transform the independent variable such that the model becomes linear and a suitable regression function can easily be found. Another often used approach is to transform the dependent variable such that the model becomes linear. This approach cannot be advocated any longer since often times the transformation, while creating a linear regression model, often leads to heteroscedasticity and non-normality in the residual. In a sense, the analyst is robbing Peter to pay Paul, so to speak.

Testing for Normality

Before undertaking a transformation of the data, one must first ascertain whether the residuals are non-normally distributed. As a first step, one should do a normal probability plot, which is a scatter plot of the observed residuals against their expected values assuming normality. A plot that is nearly a straight line is consistent with normality, whereas a plot that deviates from linearity is consistent with an error distribution that is not normally distributed. Looney and Gulledge (1985) suggest calculating the correlation coefficient as an adjunct to the normal probability plot with a high correlation coefficient being consistent with normality. Looney and Gulledge (1985) present a table of critical correlation coefficients under the normal distribution. If the observed correlation coefficient is greater than the tabulated value for a given α, then the null hypothesis of a normal distribution is not rejected. However, the pitfalls of using a correlation coefficient to assess goodness of fit were presented in earlier chapters, so use of this statistic is the analyst's discretion.

Second, a univariate test for normality is usually conducted. Many software packages have these built-in to their procedures, e.g., Shapiro–Wilks test in the Uni-variate Procedure within SAS. If the analyst does not have access to a program that provides these tests, a useful test for normality is the so-called "omnibus test for normality" (D'Agostino, 1971; D'Agostino, Belanger, and D'Agostino JR, 1990). Given the residuals (e), calculate the skewness, γ_1, and kurtosis, γ_2, as

$$\gamma_1 = \frac{m_3}{\sqrt{m_2^3}} \tag{4.36}$$

$$\gamma_2 = \frac{m_4}{m_2^2} \tag{4.37}$$

where

$$m_k = \frac{\sum_{i=1}^{n} (e_i - e)^k}{n} \tag{4.38}$$

and n is the sample size. Compute

$$J = \gamma_1 \sqrt{\frac{(n+1)(n+3)}{6(n-2)}} \tag{4.39}$$

$$\beta_2 = \frac{3(n^2 + 27n - 70)(n+1)(n+3)}{(n-2)(n+5)(n+7)(n+9)} \tag{4.40}$$

$$W^2 = -1 + \sqrt{2\beta_2 - 1} \tag{4.41}$$

$$\delta = \sqrt{\frac{2}{W^2 - 1}} \tag{4.42}$$

$$Z_1 = \left(\frac{1}{\sqrt{Ln(W)}}\right) \cdot Ln\left[\frac{J}{\delta} + \sqrt{\left(\frac{J}{\delta}\right)^2 + 1}\right]. \tag{4.43}$$

Under the null hypothesis that the sample comes from a normal distribution, Z_1 is approximately normally distributed. Eqs. (4.39)–(4.43) to are based on the skewness of the samples. The other half of the omnibus test is based on the kurtosis. Compute

$$E(\gamma_2) = \frac{3(n-1)}{n+1} \tag{4.44}$$

$$Var(\gamma_2) = \frac{24n(n-2)(n-3)}{(n+1)^2(n+3)(n+5)} \tag{4.45}$$

$$q = \frac{\gamma_2 - E(\gamma_2)}{\sqrt{Var(\gamma_2)}} \tag{4.46}$$

$$\beta_2 = \frac{6(n^2 - 5n + 2)}{(n+7)(n+9)} \sqrt{\frac{6(n+3)(n+5)}{n(n-2)(n-3)}} \tag{4.47}$$

$$A = 6 + \frac{8}{\beta_2}\left[\frac{2}{\beta_2} + \sqrt{1 + \frac{4}{\beta_2^2}}\right] \tag{4.48}$$

$$Z_2 = \frac{\left[\left(1 - \frac{2}{9A}\right) - \sqrt[3]{\frac{1 - \frac{2}{A}}{1 + q\sqrt{\frac{2}{A-4}}}}\right]}{\sqrt{\frac{2}{9A}}} \qquad (4.49)$$

Under the null hypothesis that the residuals come from a normal distribution, Z_2 is approximately normally distributed. The omnibus test statistic is then calculated as

$$K^2 = Z_1^2 + Z_2^2. \qquad (4.50)$$

Under the null hypothesis, K^2 has a chi-squared distribution with 2 degrees of freedom. If K^2 is greater than the critical value, the null hypothesis of a normal distribution is rejected. While these are a lot of equations, they can easily be calculated within a spreadsheet program.

Transformations of the Independent Variable

Sometimes it is useful to transform a nonlinear model into a linear one when the distribution of error terms is approximately normal and homoscedastic. Such a case might be when a suitable nonlinear function cannot be found to model the data. One might then try to change the relationship between x and Y so that a model can be found. One way to do this is to change the model

and dependent variable simultaneously, the so-called transform-both-sides approach. This will be discussed later. Another method is to transform the independent variable alone. When the error terms are homoscedastic normal, it is perfectly valid to transform the independent variables to force model linearity since this change will not affect the error structure of the model. Figure 4.7 presents sample nonlinear regression patterns assuming constant error variance with along with some simple transformations of x. Notice that a simple transform, such as 1/x, can have dramatic effects on the shape of the relationship between x and Y. Also note that the error pattern does not change either, which is important, because if the error pattern did change then one problem would be created (heteroscedasticity or skewness) by solving another (nonlinearity). Many times the appropriate transform needs to be found through exploratory data analysis, i.e., trial and error.

Transformations of the Dependent Variable

There is a great body of literature on transformations of the dependent variable since these type of transformations are often used to account for unequal error variances and/or nonnormality of the error distribution. Useful references for this type of transformation are Carroll and Ruppert (1988, 1984).

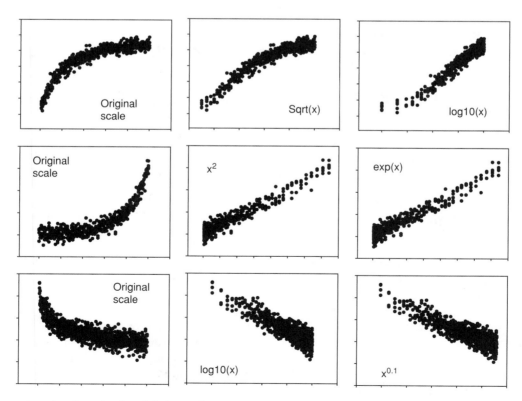

Figure 4.7 Scatter plots of nonlinear functions (left plots) and transformations in the x-variable (right two plots) that lead to approximate linearity.

One of the most common transformations is the natural logarithmic transformation of multiplicative models. Many pharmacokinetic parameters, such as area under the curve (AUC) and maximal concentration, are log-normal in distribution (Lacey et al., 1997), and hence, using the Ln-transformation results in approximate normality. The rationale is as follows (Westlake, 1988). For a drug that has linear kinetics and elimination occurs from the central compartment (the usual assumptions for a noncompartmental analysis) then

$$AUC = \frac{D}{CL/F} \exp(\varepsilon) \qquad (4.51)$$

where D is dose and CL/F is apparent oral clearance. Taking the log of Eq. (4.51) leads to

$$Ln(AUC) = Ln(D) - Ln(CL) + Ln(F) + \varepsilon \qquad (4.52)$$

which leads to an additive model with homoscedastic error. A similar argument may be made for maximal concentration. Many of the guidances issued by the Food and Drug Administration (FDA) require Ln-transformation prior to statistical analysis (United States Department of Health and Human Services et al., 2001).

At times, particularly if Y is negative, such as may be the case when modeling percent change from baseline as the dependent variable, it may necessary to add a constant c to the data. Berry (1987) presents a method that may be used to define the optimal value of c while still ensuring a symmetrical distribution. The method makes use of skewness and kurtosis, which characterize the degree of asymmetry of a distribution. These statistics will be used to identify a transformation constant c such that the new data set will have better normality properties than the original scores. Let γ_1 and γ_2 be the skewness and kurtosis of the distribution as defined by Eqs. (4.36) and (4.37), respectively, substituting $Ln(Y + c)$ for the variable e in Eq. (4.38). If g is defined as

$$g = |\gamma_1| + |\gamma_2| \qquad (4.53)$$

then the optimal value of c is the value of c which minimizes g, which can be found using either a numerical optimization routine or a one dimensional grid search.

The log transformation is actually a specific case of a more general class of transformations known as Box–Cox (1964) transformations. Box and Cox proposed that the following transformation be used

$$h(Y; \lambda) = \begin{cases} \dfrac{Y^\lambda - 1}{\lambda} & \text{if } \lambda \neq 0 \\ Ln(Y) & \text{if } \lambda = 0 \end{cases} \qquad (4.54)$$

creating a new model

$$h(Y; \lambda) = f(x; \theta^*) + \varepsilon. \qquad (4.55)$$

Equation (4.55) includes a new parameter λ in the model. Most often λ is specified a priori because most software packages do not allow the dependent variable to depend on an estimated parameter. However, as given by Neter et al. (2000), λ can be estimated using a grid search on the interval $-2, -1.8, -1.6, \ldots 2$. Ideally one would then find the value of λ that minimizes the residual sum of squares (SSE). But, by allowing λ to vary, the magnitude of SSE will vary as well and direct comparison of the SSE for each value on the grid is not appropriate. Hence, by standardizing the $h(Y; \lambda)$ values so that the residual sum of squares does not depend on λ, one can choose that value of λ that minimizes the SSE. Thus, the procedure is as follows:

1. Transform $h(Y; \lambda)$ to $h(Y; \lambda)^*$ using

$$h(Y; \lambda)^* = \begin{cases} \dfrac{(Y_i^\lambda - 1)}{\lambda [\bar{Y}_{geo}]^{\lambda - 1}} & \text{if } \lambda \neq 0 \\ Ln(Y_i) \bar{Y}_{geo} & \text{if } \lambda = 0 \end{cases}. \qquad (4.56)$$

where

$$\bar{Y}_{geo} = \left(\prod_{i=1}^{n} Y_i \right)^{\frac{1}{n}} \qquad (4.57)$$

is the geometric mean of Y.

2. Regress $h(Y; \lambda)^*$ against x and compute the residual sum of squares (SSE).
3. Do Steps 1 and 2 for all values of λ on the grid $\{-2, 2\}$.
4. The maximum likelihood estimate of λ is the value of λ with the smallest SSE.

An alternative method to estimating λ is as follows:

1. Regress $h(Y; \lambda)$ against x.
2. Calculate the normal probability plot for the residuals and compute the correlation coefficient.
3. Do Steps 1 and 2 for all values of λ on the grid $\{-2, 2\}$.
4. The value of λ is the value with the highest correlation coefficient.

Ordinarily λ does not have to be known to very fine precision, but a rough ballpark, say one place behind the decimal is sufficient. If greater precision in the estimation of λ is needed, once a value of λ on the interval $\{-2, 2\}$ is identified, e.g., 0.5, then the grid can be refined and the process repeated, e.g., $\{0.4–0.6$ by

0.01}. On the other hand, once λ is identified, often one chooses a value near λ that lends greater interpretation. For example, if the identified value of λ was 0.7, the one might reset λ to 0.5 which is the square root transformation. Also, if λ is near 1, then no transformation is needed. Still one might want to examine how the SSE surface around λ varies to determine whether resetting the value of λ to a more interpretable value is indeed a valid action.

Box–Cox is not the only transform that is used, although it is the most commonly used one. One limitation of the Box–Cox transformation is that it is valid only for positive values of Y greater than zero. For zero and negative values, Box and Cox proposed a shifted power transform of the form

$$h(Y; \lambda_1, \lambda_2) = \begin{cases} \dfrac{(Y + \lambda_2)^{\lambda_1} - 1}{\lambda_1} & \text{if } \lambda \neq 0 \\ \text{Ln}(Y + \lambda_2) & \text{if } \lambda = 0 \end{cases} \quad (4.58)$$

where λ_2 is a constant such that $Y > -\lambda_2$. Frame (personal communication) proposed a slight modification of the Box–Cox transformation

$$h(Y; \lambda) = \begin{cases} \dfrac{\exp(Y^{\lambda}) - 1}{\lambda} & \text{if } \lambda \neq 0 \\ \text{Ln}(Y) & \text{if } \lambda = 0 \end{cases} \quad (4.59)$$

which is defined for all Y and can deal with positive and negative skewness. John and Draper (1980) proposed an alterative transform to allow for values across the real line

$$h(Y; \lambda) = \begin{cases} \dfrac{\text{sign}(Y)(|Y| + 1)^{\lambda} - 1}{\lambda} & \text{if } \lambda \neq 0 \\ \text{sign}(Y)\text{Ln}(|Y| + 1) & \text{if } \lambda = 0 \end{cases}. \quad (4.60)$$

Equation (4.60) reduces to Eq. (4.58) where $\lambda_2 = 1$ when Y is positive. Manley (2002) proposed another transform for negative values that is supposedly better at transforming highly skewed distributions into nearly symmetric normal-like distributions and is of the form

$$h(Y; \lambda) = \begin{cases} \dfrac{\exp(\lambda Y) - 1}{\lambda} & \text{if } \lambda \neq 0 \\ Y & \text{if } \lambda = 0 \end{cases}. \quad (4.61)$$

Yeo and Johnson (2000) proposed a new family of power transformations that can be used across the real line of Y having many of the same properties of the Box–Cox transforms. These transforms are

$$h(Y; \lambda) = \begin{cases} \dfrac{(Y + 1)^{\lambda} - 1}{\lambda} & \text{if } \lambda \neq 0 \text{ and } Y \geq 0 \\ \text{Ln}(Y + 1) & \text{if } \lambda = 0 \text{ and } Y \geq 0 \\ \dfrac{-[(-Y + 1)^{2-\lambda} - 1]}{2 - \lambda} & \text{if } \lambda \neq 2 \text{ and } Y < 0 \\ -\text{Ln}(-Y + 1) & \text{if } \lambda = 2 \text{ and } Y < 0. \end{cases} \quad (4.62)$$

If Y is strictly positive then the Yeo–Johnson transform reduces to the Box–Cox transform of $Y + 1$. If Y is strictly negative, then the Yeo–Johnson transform reduces to the Box–Cox transform of $-Y + 1$ but with power $2 - \lambda$. For a mixture of positive and negative values, the Yeo–Johnson is a mixture of different transforms. For positive values near zero, Box–Cox transforms provide a much larger change in small values than Yeo–Johnson transforms.

Despite the long history of the data transformations, their use must be handled with extreme caution. Not only do they often destroy the error structure of the data but also interpretation of the model parameters is almost impossible. After data transformation, the regression parameters are on the transformed scale, often a scale that is not of interest to the researcher. Also, despite their claims, most of these transforms fail to produce exact normality, at best they produce near normality (Sakia, 1992). As will be later shown, however, when combined with model transformations, data transformations have a new found utility.

Transform-Both-Sides Approach

Carroll and Ruppert (1988) suggest that one should not transform either the model or the data, but one should transform the model AND the data. This leads to the model

$$h(Y; \lambda) = h(f(x; \theta); \lambda) + \varepsilon. \quad (4.63)$$

Equation (4.63) is called the transform-both-sides (TBS) approach. The transformation of Y is used to remove both skewness in the distribution of the data and to remove any dependence the variance may show on the mean response. The transformation of $f(x; \theta)$ maintains the nature of the relationship between x and Y in the transformed domain allowing the parameter estimates to have the same meaning they would have in the original domain.

Early applications of the transform-both-sides approach generally were done to transform a nonlinear problem into a linear one. One of the most common examples is found in enzyme kinetics. Given the Michaelis–Menten model of enzyme kinetics

$$v = \dfrac{V_{\text{max}} S}{K_m + S} \quad (4.64)$$

which is a one-site enzyme model where v is velocity of the reaction, V_{max} the maximal velocity, K_m the concentration that produces 50% of the maximal velocity, and S the initial substrate concentration, inversion leads to

$$\frac{1}{v} = \left(\frac{K_m}{V_{max}}\right)\frac{1}{S} + \frac{1}{V_{max}} \qquad (4.65)$$

which is a linear model with $1/S$ as the independent variable and $1/v$ as the dependent variable. V_{max} and K_m can then be solved directly using standard linear regression techniques. This transformation is called the Lineweaver–Burke transformation and its use is illustrated in just about every single graduate level biochemistry textbook known to man. Consider however that Eq. (4.64) is actually

$$v = \frac{V_{max}S}{K_m + S} + \varepsilon \qquad (4.66)$$

where ε is the random deviation from the true velocity which is normally distributed with mean 0 and variance σ_2. After inverse transformation ε is no longer normally distributed. This is illustrated in Fig. 4.8. In this plot, data were simulated from a Michaelis–Menten model having a V_{max} of 100 and a K_m of 20. Stochastic variability was added from a normal distribution with a standard deviation of 3. The data were then transformed using the Lineweaver–Burke transform. After the Lineweaver–Burke transformation, the variability around the model predicted values is no longer a constant, but varies as a function of the substrate concentration. Other linearizing transforms in enzyme kinetics, such as the Eadie–Hofstee transform, also have the same problem. It wasn't until the 1980's that researchers began to criticize these transforms and began advocating nonlinear regression techniques instead for estimation of enzyme kinetic parameters. Today, these transforms are used mostly for obtaining initial estimates or indicating how many binding sites may be present in the system.

One particularly useful transform, however, is the natural-log transform when the error model is the exponential

$$Y = f(x; \theta)\exp(\varepsilon). \qquad (4.67)$$

Ln-transformation of both sides of the equation leads to

$$Ln(Y) = Ln[f(x; \theta)] + \varepsilon \qquad (4.68)$$

which results in normality of the error term. The Ln-transformation is also useful for a proportional error or constant coefficient of variation model of the type

$$Y = f(\theta; x)(1 + \varepsilon). \qquad (4.69)$$

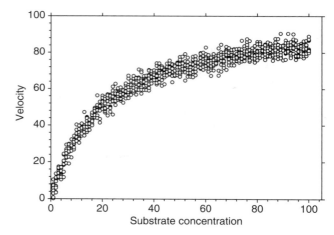

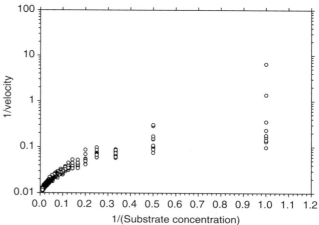

Figure 4.8 Scatter plot of simulated data from a Michaelis-Menten model with $V_{max} = 100$ and $K_m = 20$ (top) and Lineweaver–Burke transformation of data (bottom). Stochastic variability was added by assuming normally distributed constant variability with a standard deviation of 3.

In fact, the proportional error model and exponential error model are equal for small values of σ. To see this, the function $\exp(x)$ if first written as a MacLaurin series

$$e^x = 1 + \frac{1}{1!}x + \frac{1}{2!}x^2 \ldots + \frac{1}{n!}x^n. \qquad (4.70)$$

Looking at the first two terms on the right hand side of Eq. (4.70) and substituting into Eq. (4.67) gives

$$Y = f(x; \theta)(1 + \varepsilon), \qquad (4.71)$$

which is the proportional error model given in Eq. (4.69). Hence, the two models are equivalent for small σ and often, particularly in the population pharmacokinetic literature, one will see either Eq. (4.67) or Eq. (4.71) used to model proportional error. For large σ, the approximation breaks down because higher order terms in the series were not considered. Of course, this suggests that an alternative, possibly more accurate error structure, for the exponential distribution may be written as the second-order MacLaurin series

$$Y = f(x; \theta)(1 + \varepsilon + 0.5\varepsilon^2). \qquad (4.72)$$

Carroll and Ruppert (1988) were the first to present a general methodology for the TBS approach. Given the model in Eq. (4.63) any suitable transform can be used, either Box–Cox [Eq. (4.58)], John–Draper [Eq. (4.60)], Yeo–Johnson [Eq. (4.62)], or Manley [Eq. (4.61)]. Most often a Box–Cox transform is used. To estimate λ and θ one uses a modification of the method to estimate λ in a Box–Cox transformation. First create a dummy variable D that is zero for all observations. Then regress

$$k(x; \theta; \lambda) = \frac{[h(Y; \lambda) - h[f(x; \theta); \lambda]]}{\bar{Y}_{geo}^{\lambda}} \qquad (4.73)$$

against D where $\bar{Y}_{geo}$ is the geometric mean of Y [Eq. (4.57)]. For example, using a Box–Cox transform $k(x; \theta; \lambda)$ would be

$$k(x; \hat{\theta}; \lambda) = \frac{\left[\left(\frac{Y_i^{\lambda} - 1}{\lambda} \right) - \left(\frac{[f(x; \hat{\theta})]^{\lambda} - 1}{\lambda} \right) \right]}{\bar{Y}_{geo}^{\lambda}}. \qquad (4.74)$$

The residual from this fitting this model is the same as the residual from the transformed model and the least-squares estimates of θ and λ are the maximum likelihood estimates. The estimate of the mean square error can be calculated by

$$MSE = \hat{\sigma}^2 = \frac{\left[h(Y_i; \hat{\lambda}) - h(f(x; \hat{\theta}); \lambda) \right]^2}{n - p} \qquad (4.75)$$

where p is the number of estimated parameters in θ and λ. The difficulty with this method is the estimation of the standard errors of θ and λ. The standard error of the estimates obtained from nonlinear regression are consistent for θ asymptotically when σ approaches 0. However, the same is not true for λ—the standard error of the estimates are inconsistent. Often, however, one is not really interested in the value of λ. λ is more of a nuisance parameter than a parameter of interest. In most cases, the standard errors for θ may be used from the TBS approach. However, if one if truly interested in the

standard errors of both θ and λ, a bootstrap approach is recommended.

Transform-Both-Sides Approach with Accompanying Residual Variance Model

Carroll and Ruppert (1988) point out that even though a transformation may transform a distribution to normality, there is no guarantee that the transform will lead to homoscedasticity. Hence one may need to find a suitable transformation and a suitable residual variance model. This leads to the model

$$h(Y; \lambda) = h(f(x; \theta); \lambda) + g(\Phi; z; \theta; x)\varepsilon. \qquad (4.76)$$

Estimation of the model parameters in Eq. (4.76) can be done using the methods presented in previous sections. The only difficulty Carroll and Ruppert (1988) indicate with these methods is that θ and λ are often highly correlated and that the precision of the parameter estimates are not as great as when only either θ or λ are in the model. Ruppert et al. (1989) present the utility and application of this method to analyzing the E_{max} model with enzyme kinetic data.

Conclusions

At the two extremes of data analysis are hypothesis testing, where specific questions about the data are tested, and exploratory data analysis, where relationships between the variables are explored and any hypotheses that may be tested are based on after having seen the data (i.e., data driven or posthoc analyses). Under guidelines presented by the International Conference on Harmonization [ICH; (1998)], which were designed for the hypothesis testing mode, transformation of key variables should be specified before the analysis is conducted, during the design stage of the study, along with the rationale for the transformation, the idea being that often the data are insufficient to guide the analyst towards a suitable transformation. Buck (2002) showed using Monte Carlo simulation of normal and log-normal data in an analysis of variance setting for a 2-period crossover that with 32 subjects and a coefficient of variation of 20%, which is low variability for pharmacokinetic data, identifying the correct transformation occurred in only 70% of the cases. Often one has sufficient knowledge of the variable of the interest to know whether the suitable transformation is a priori. For example, the FDA requires pharmacokinetic data be log-transformed prior to analysis regardless of the observed distribution of the data because it is well known that the primary pharmacokinetic parameters, AUC and C_{max}, are log-normally distributed (United States Department of Health and Human Services et al., 2001) Another rationale for specifying the transform a priori is that by allowing the transform to be found posthoc, the results from the study then become study specific (Keene, 1995). An appropriate transformation identified in one study may not be the appropriate one in another.

In the past, exploratory data analysis was basically an "anything goes" approach to data analysis. The current regulatory environment is trying to move away from that philosophy to a more structured one. Current ICH guidelines also apply to studies that are exploratory in nature, but the a priori specification and data analysis plan can describe more general and descriptive in nature. As such, using the data to find a suitable transform is entirely valid and appropriate, although the problem of consistency across studies may remain. Later, confirmatory studies should then specify the transformation a priori and not be described in generalities.

EXAMPLE: EFFECT OF WEIGHTING ON THE PHARMACOKINETICS OF INTRAVENOUSLY ADMINISTERED DFMO

α-Dimethylornithine (DFMO) is a selective, irreversible inactivator of ornithine decarboxylase (ODC), the rate limiting enzyme in the biosynthesis of putrescine and the polyamines, spermidine and spermine. Haegle et al. (1981) administered DFMO to six healthy men in single doses of 5 and 10 mg/kg by intravenous administration given as a 5-min infusion. Serial blood samples were collected and assayed for DFMO. The mean data are presented in Table 4.4 and plotted in Fig. 4.9. It should be pointed out that compartmental modeling of this type of data (mean concentration—time data) is not statistically correct. Either individual subjects should be modeled one by one or the data should be pooled and a nonlinear mixed effects model approach taken to analyze the data. Nevertheless, it is common to see in the pharmacology and physiology literature modeling of mean data.

Plotting the mean data suggested the kinetics of DFMO to be at least biphasic. First, the intravenous data were fit using SAAM II to a 2-compartment model using the noncompartmental estimate for clearance (CL) as the initial value, 1.2 mL/(min/kg). The initial estimates for central volume (V1) and peripheral volume (V2) were divided equally between the noncompartmental estimate for volume of distribution at steady-state, 150 mL/kg. Intercompartmental clearance (Q2) was guessed to be about 1/10th systemic clearance based on trial and error. A power of the mean residual variance model was used for this data. The final parameter estimates are presented in Table 4.5. The fitted model showed a clear and obvious trend in the residuals with early time points underpredicted and later time-points overpredicted (data not shown).

Next a 3-compartment model was tried with the starting values set equal to the final values for the 2-compartment model and the new model parameters set to 1.6 mL/(min/kg) for Q3 (which was approximately equal to systemic clearance) and 150 mL/(min/kg) for V3 (which was approximately equal to the value of central volume). Final parameter estimates are in Table 4.6 with a

Table 4.4   Mean DFMO plasma concentration-time data in healthy male volunteers after intravenous administration.

Time (min)	Concentration (ng/mL)	
	5 mg/kg	10 mg/kg
5	No sample	90379.5
7	24448.6	87446.4
10	24539.6	67807.4
20	23337.3	49352.6
35	19019.6	37492.6
50	14556.2	31972.6
65	12661.5	26489.0
125	7852.0	15521.7
245	3516.1	6795.3
365	1603.2	3151.7
485	746.9	1639.6
785	182.2	491.9
1085	72.9	236.8
1445	36.4	Missing

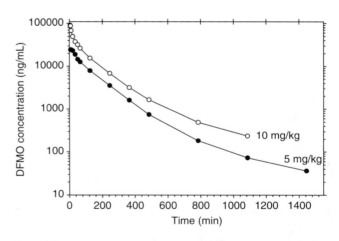

Figure 4.9   Mean concentration–time profile for DFMO administered as a 5-min intravenous infusion of 5 and 10 mg/kg. Data are presented in Table 4.4. The shape of the curve indicates that a multicompartment model is needed.

Table 4.5 Final parameter estimates for the data in Table 4.4 under a 2-compartment model expressed in terms of clearance and volume.

Parameter	Model term	Units	Value	Standard error	CV (%)
Clearance	CL	mL/(min/kg)	1.57	0.0434	2.7
Central volume	V1	mL/kg	204	7.90	3.9
Intercompartmental clearance	Q2	mL/(min/kg)	0.11	0.0019	17.3
Compartment 2 volume	V2	mL/kg	45	4.10	9.18

Akaike Information Criterion: 8.515

Table 4.6 Final parameter estimates for the data in Table 4.4 under a 3-compartment model expressed in terms of clearance and volume.

Parameter	Model term	Units	Value	Standard error	CV (%)
Clearance	CL	mL/(min/kg)	1.48	0.0475	3.2
Central volume	V1	mL/kg	83.3	4.12	4.9
Intercompartmental clearance	Q2	mL/(min/kg)	9.33	1.88	20.3
Compartment 2 volume	V2	mL/kg	77.8	5.32	6.8
Intercompartmental clearance	Q3	mL/(min/kg)	0.278	0.0573	20.7
Compartment 3 volume	V3	mL/kg	68.7	8.12	11.8

Akaike Information Criterion: 8.361

goodness of fit plot shown in Fig. 4.10. The 3-compartment model was a significant improvement over the 2-compartment model, but there was still a trend in residuals early after dosing. Prior to 20 min the model underpredicted and then between 20 and 100 min overpredicted concentrations. Later time points did not show a trend in residuals.

Next a 4-compartment model was examined. Initial estimates were the final estimates under the 3-compartment model. The initial estimate for Q_4 was 1 mL/min/kg, while V_4 was set equal to 70 mL/kg. Final parameter estimates are shown in Table 4.7 and a goodness of fit plot is shown in Fig. 4.11. The 4-compartment model was a significant improvement over the 3-compartment model. The over- and underpredictions seen within the first 100 min of dosing were not present. A residual plot showed no trend in the residuals (Fig. 4.11). Additional compartments to the model showed no further improvement to the model fit.

The effect of different residual variance models on the parameter estimates and goodness of fit of the 4-compartment model was then examined. Weights of 1 (OLS), $1/Y$, $1/Y^2$, $1/\hat{Y}$, $1/\hat{Y}^2$, and $\left[A + B\hat{Y}^C\right]$ were examined. The results are presented in Table 4.8 and the goodness of fit plots of shown in Fig. 4.12.

For the OLS model, a 4-compartment model could not even be estimated. The parameter estimate for Q_4 kept reaching its lower bound and eventually became zero. Hence for this residual variance model, a 3-compartment model was fit. The goodness of fit plot showed that at later time points the model began to significantly underpredict concentrations. When inverse observed or

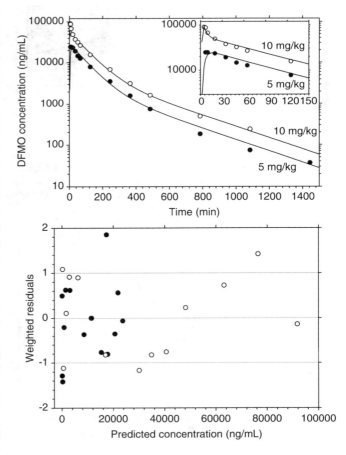

Figure 4.10 Mean concentration–time profile (top) and residual plot (bottom) for DFMO administered as a 5-min intravenous infusion of 5 and 10 mg/kg when a 3-compartment model was fit to the data. Parameter estimates are given in Table 4.6. Data are presented in Table 4.4.

Table 4.7 Final parameter estimates for the data in Table 4.4 under a 4-compartment model expressed in terms of clearance and volume.

Parameter	Model term	Units	Value	Standard error	CV (%)
Clearance	CL	mL/(min/kg)	1.50	0.027	1.9
Central volume	V1	mL/kg	69.1	3.84	5.6
Intercompartmental clearance	Q2	mL/(min/kg)	9.77	1.45	14.5
Compartment 2 volume	V2	mL/kg	58.8	4.05	6.9
Intercompartmental clearance	Q3	mL/(min/kg)	0.142	2.34E-2	16.7
Compartment 3 volume	V3	mL/kg	56.8	3.82	6.7
Intercompartmental clearance	Q4	mL/(min/kg)	1.62	0.365	22.5
Compartment 4 volume	V4	mL/kg	79.1	17.7	22.5

Akaike Information Criterion: 7.826

inverse predicted concentrations were used as the weights, there was little difference in the corresponding parameter estimates and goodness of fit plot. But a dramatic difference between the two sets of estimates and goodness of fit plots was observed when the data were weighted by observed squared concentrations or predicted squared concentrations. The model fit using squared predicted concentrations was dismal in predicting DFMO concentrations. For both models, the standard error of the parameter estimates became so large that the 95% confidence interval for these parameters included zero. This did not occur when the weights were inverse observed or inverse predicted concentrations. That the standard errors changed as a function of the weights was not unexpected [see Eq. (4.17)]. What was unexpected was how much a composite parameter like V_{ss} would change with the different estimates. V_{ss} ranged from 227 mL/kg using OLS to 394 mL/kg with WLS and inverse predicted squared concentrations as the weights. Noncompartmental estimates place V_{ss} at around 300 mL/kg. Clearly, the choice of weights can have a dramatic impact on the parameter estimates obtained with a compartmental model and whether a parameter can be considered to be statistically significant.

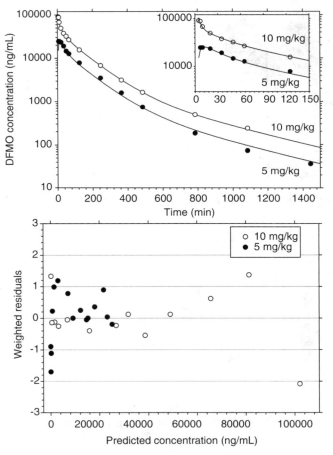

Figure 4.11 Mean concentration–time profile (top) and residual plot (bottom) for DFMO administered as a 5-min intravenous infusion of 5 and 10 mg/kg when a 4-compartment model was fit to the data. Parameter estimates are given in Table 4.7. Data are presented in Table 4.4.

Table 4.8 Effect of weighting on the parameter estimates for the data in Table 4.4 under a 4-compartment model.

Weights parameter	1 (OLS)	1/Y	1/Y²	1/Ŷ	1/Ŷ²	1/(A+ BŶ^C)
CL	1.52	1.49	1.47	1.48	2.36	1.46
V1	74.5	71.0	69.2	70.1	109*	69.5
Q2	10.0	10.9	11.0*	10.6	16.8*	11.6
V2	63.5	61.7	59.5*	61.1	92.7*	60.0
Q3	0.872	0.0895	0.104*	0.0923	0.187*	1.54
V3	89.5	56.8	45.5*	62.4	76.5*	66.0
Q4	NA	1.26	1.64*	1.27	2.88*	0.122*
V4	NA	75.6	76.1*	72.8	115.9*	139*
Vss	227	265	250	266	394	334

Legend: NA, for the OLS residual variance model, the parameters associated with the 4th compartment (Q4, V4) could not be estimated. At most three compartments could be identified. The symbol* denotes that 95% confidence interval contains zero; NA, could not be estimated (see text for details).

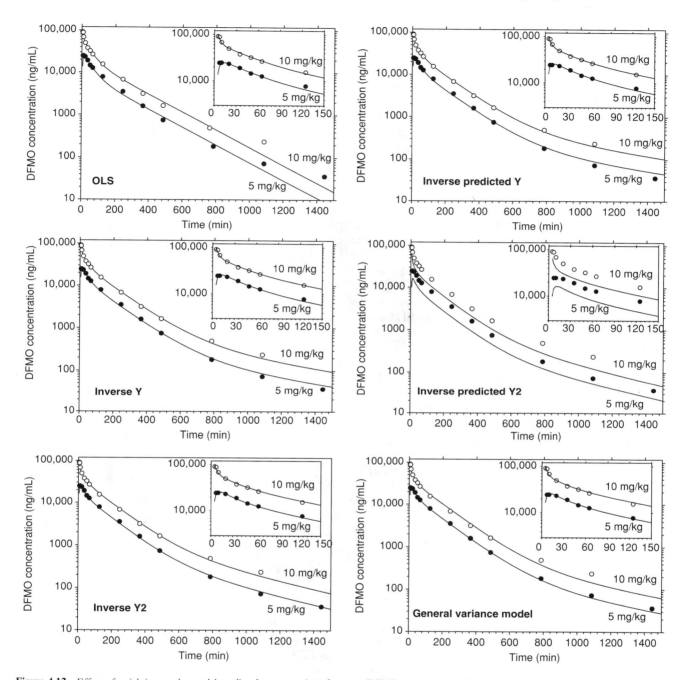

Figure 4.12   Effect of weighting on the model predicted concentrations for mean DFMO concentration data. Mean concentration-time profile for DFMO administered as a 5-min intravenous infusion of 5 and 10 mg/kg when fit to a 4-compartmentl model. Left top plot is OLS model predictions (weights equal 1). Left middle plot has 1/Y as the weights. Left bottom plot has 1 Y^2 as the weights. Right top plot has 1/$\hat{Y}$ as the weights. Right middle plot has 1/$\hat{Y}^2$ has the weights. Right bottom plot has 1 (A + B$\hat{Y}^2$) as the weights. Parameter estimates are given in Table 4.8. Data are presented in Table 4.4.

EXAMPLE: APPLICATION OF THE TRANSFORM-BOTH-SIDES APPROACH TO A PHARMACODYNAMIC MODEL

XomaZyme-791 (XZ-791) is a monoclonal antibody coupled to an immunotoxin, Ricin toxin A, developed to recognize an antigen present on ovarian, colorectal, and osteogenic sarcoma tissues. In a Phase I study, 17 patients having a least one measurable lesion with no prior monoclonal antibody therapy were dosed with XZ-791 for 1 h daily for 5 days with doses ranging from 0.02 to 2 mg (kg/day) (Byers et al., 1989). Patients were monitored daily through Day 6 and then at Day 15, 28, and 60. Blood chemistries were assessed on each study day and at predose. Investigators noted a drop in albumin concentration that reached a maximal change after around 10 days of dosing. The data are presented in Table 4.9. An E_{max} model was used to assess the relationship between dose and percent change in albumin in an attempt to determine the dose that decreased the albumin concentration by less than 20%. OLS was used to determine the model parameter estimates. The maximal change in albumin concentration (E_{max}) was estimated at $-38.0\% \pm 5.5\%$, whereas the dose that produced a 50% decrease in albumin (D_{50}) was estimated at 6.2 ± 3.9 mg. The mean square error was 75.6. The resulting goodness of fit plot and residual plot for the model are shown in Fig. 4.13. The model appeared to be an adequate fit to the data and no heteroscedasticity appeared to be present, so the choice of OLS appeared to be a good one. However, a test for normality of the residuals showed that the residuals were slightly skewed and were not normally distributed (p = 0.0186). Hence, the assumption of normally distributed residuals was violated.

To account for the skewness, the transform-both-sides methodology was used with a Box–Cox transformation. The geometric mean to the data was -27.1%. The SAS code to do the analysis is shown in Chapter Appendix 2. E_{max} was estimated at $-43.1 \pm 6.3\%$, whereas D_{50} was estimated at 11.3 ± 2.9 mg. λ was estimated at -1.39. The resulting goodness of fit plot is shown in Fig. 4.14. The fit appeared to be very similar to the untransformed E_{max} model, but this time the p-value testing the

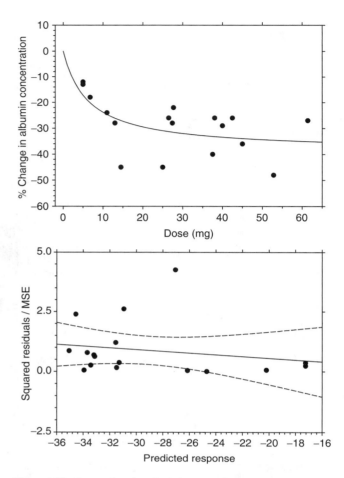

Figure 4.13   Scatter plot of maximal change in albumin concentration (top) in patients dosed with XomaZyme-791 and model predicted fit (solid line). Data were fit to a E_{max} model using ordinary least-squares. Bottom plot is residual plot of squared residuals divided by MSE against predicted values. Solid line is least-squares regression line and dashed lines are 95% confidence interval.

hypothesis of normality of the residual was 0.565. Hence, with the transform-both-sides methodology, the assumption of normality of the residuals was not violated and the fit was less biased than the OLS approach. At this point examination of the HAT matrix may be useful to determine if there are any influential observations, which there were not. The SAS code to compute the HAT matrix and transform-both-sides methodology with residual variance model is given in the chapter appendix. Going back to the problem at hand, the dose that produced a 20% decrease in albumin (f) can be estimated by

$$D_{80} = \frac{f}{1-f} D_{50} \qquad (4.77)$$

so setting f = 0.2 with D_{50} equal to 11.3 mg, then the estimated dose is 2.8 ± 0.7 mg.

Table 4.9   Maximal percent change in albumin concentration in patients treated with XomaZyme-791 as reported by Byers et al. (1989).

Subject	Dose (mg)	Maximal percent change (%)
1	5.0	−12
2	5.0	−13
3	13.0	−28
4	11.0	−24
5	14.5	−45
6	6.8	−18
7	42.5	−26
8	37.5	−40
9	25.0	−45
10	38.0	−26
11	40.0	−29
12	26.5	−26
13	27.7	−22
14	27.4	−28
15	45.0	−36
16	61.4	−27
16	52.8	−48

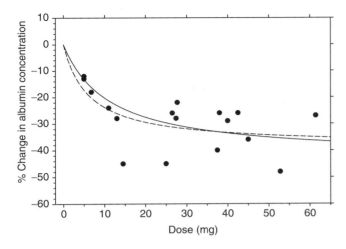

Figure 4.14 Scatter plot of maximal change in albumin concentration in patients dosed with XomaZyme-791 and model predicted fit. Data were fit to a E_{max} model using ordinary least-squares (dashed line) and using the transform-both-sides methodology with a Box–Cox transformation (solid line).

SUMMARY

In summary, residual variance models offer greater flexibility to regression models by relaxing the assumption of constant variance and provide greater insight into the data generating mechanism by explaining the variability in the data. The choice of residual variance model should be based on the data and theoretical considerations of the data and what is known about the data generating mechanism. In addition to the constant variance assumption in OLS, one other assumption regarding the model is that the residuals are normally distributed. Sometimes, even a valid structural model, violates this assumption, in which case a suitable transformation is needed. Much of the statistical literature regarding transformations revolves around transforming the response variable. However this make interpretation of the parameters problematic since the estimated parameters after transformation are not on the original scale of the data. Hence, the transform-both-sides approach is advocated, wherein both the response variable and the model is transformed using the same transformation. Sometimes a transform-both-sides approach with residual variance model is needed. Suitable use of these techniques allows for more efficient and unbiased parameter estimation.

Recommended Reading

Carroll, R.J. Ruppert, D. Transformation and weighting in regression. New York: Chapman and Hall, 1988.

Davidian, M. and Carroll, R.J. Variance function estimation. *Journal of the American Statistical Association* 1987; 82:1079–1091.

Davidian, M. and Giltinan, D.M. Nonlinear models for repeated measures data. New York: Chapman and Hall, 1995.

Davidian, M. and Haaland, P.D. Regression and calibration with nonconstant error variance. *Chemometrics and Intelligent Laboratory Systems* 1990; 9:231–248.

Sakia, R.M. Box–Cox transformation: A review. *The Statistician* 1992; 41: 169–178.

APPENDIX 1: CORRECTED APPENDIX TO GILTINAN AND RUPPERT (1989)

There are two errors in the SAS code presented by Giltinan and Ruppert (1989). These can be fixed using the following corrections, which are highlighted in bold.

```
Find the procedure:
  proc nlin;
    parms gamma=1;
    bounds gamma > −1.5, gamma < 1.5;
    g=(resid)*( (taudot/pred)**gamma);
    model = g;
    output out=seven parms=gamma;
```

```
And change it to:
  proc nlin;
    parms gamma=1;
    bounds gamma > −1.5, gamma < 1.5;
    model dummy =
      resid*(taudot/pred)**
      (0.5*gamma);
    output out=seven parms=gamma;
```

```
Find the data step:
  data eight;
    merge six seven;
    v = pred**(2*gamma);
    wt = 1/v;
```

```
And change it to:
  data eight;
    merge six seven;
    v = pred**gamma;
    wt = 1/v;
```

APPENDIX 2: SAS CODE USED TO COMPUTE THE TRANSFORM-BOTH-SIDES PARAMETER ESTIMATES IN THE XOMAZYME-791 EXAMPLE

```
dm 'clear log';
dm 'clear list';
options ls=90;
proc datasets kill; run; quit;
data z791;
  input dose alb;
  zero = 0;
```

```
   logalb = log(alb);
cards;
5.0000     12.0000
5.0000     13.0000
13.0000    28.0000
11.0000    24.0000
14.5000    45.0000
6.8000     18.0000
42.5000    26.0000
37.5000    40.0000
25.0000    45.0000
38.0000    26.0000
40.0000    29.0000
26.5000    26.0000
27.7000    22.0000
27.4000    28.0000
45.0000    36.0000
61.4000    27.0000
52.8000    48.0000

proc means data=z791 noprint;
  var logalb;
  output out=meaneff mean=mean;
run; quit;
data meaneff;
  set meaneff;
  zero = 0;
  gm = exp(mean);
  keep zero gm;
proc sort data=meaneff; by zero; run
proc sort data=z791; by zero; run;

data z791;
  merge z791 meaneff;
  by zero;
run; quit;
proc nlin;
  title1 'Standard OLS Model';
  parms emax=50, ed50 = 20;
  model alb = -emax*dose/(dose +
  ed50);
  output out=emax1 residual=residual
  predicted=pred;
run; quit;
proc univariate normal data=emax1;
  var residual;
run; quit;
proc nlin;
  title2 'Transform-both-sides';
```

```
  parms emax=50 ed50=20, lambda1=1;
  yhat = emax*dose/(ed50 + dose);
  a = (alb**lambda1 - 1)/lambda1;
  b = (yhat**lambda1 - 1)/lambda1;
  model zero = (a - b)/gm**lambda1;
  output out=tbs residual=residual
  predicted=predicted;
run; quit;
proc univariate normal data=tbs;
  var residual;
run; quit;


/*************************************************
This next block computes the HAT matrix
*************************************************/

data parms;
  set parms;
  zero = 0;
  if _type_ = 'FINAL' then output;
  keep emax ed50 zero;
proc sort data=parms; by zero; run;
proc sort data=tbs; by zero; run;
data tbs;
  merge tbs parms;
  by zero;
run; quit;

proc iml;
  use tbs var {dose ed50 emax zero alb gm};
  read all;
  d_emax = -dose/(ed50 + dose);
  d_ed50 = emax#dose/(ed50 + dose)##2;
  x = d_emax||d_ed50;
  q = x * inv(x` * x) * x`;
  n = nrow(dose);
  hat = j(n, 1, .);
  do i = 1 to n;
    hat[i] = q[i,i];
  end;
  invhat = 1/hat;
  create hat var {dose ed50 emax zero alb
  gm hat invhat};
  append var {dose ed50 emax zero alb gm
  hat invhat};
run; quit;

proc print data=hat; run; quit;
```

Handwritten margin notes:
$(y^{\lambda_1} - 1)/\lambda_1$
$(\hat{y}^{\lambda_1} - 1)/\lambda_1$

Chapter 5

Case Studies in Linear and Nonlinear Modeling

I may not have gone where I intended to go, but I think I have ended up where I intended to be.

—Douglas Adams (1952–2001), author of the Hitchhiker's Guide to the Galaxy

INTRODUCTION

Linear and nonlinear models are the backbone of pharmacokinetic and pharmacokinetic–pharmacodynamic models. A thorough understanding of linear and nonlinear modeling is needed before one can truly understand how to develop more complex or realistic models. In this chapter the application of these models to five real-life data sets will be examined. The first case study will be the application of allometric scaling to predict the pharmacokinetics of a protein in humans based on animal data. The second case study will be the analysis of dose proportionality for a new chemical entity. The third case study will be the development of a limited sampling model to predict area under the curve given a few well-timed samples which can then be used in future clinical trials as a surrogate for exposure. The fourth case study will be the development of a pharmacokinetic model for cocaine following intravenous, inhalational, and intravenous administration. Lastly, a pharmacokinetic model will be developed for a new oncolytic drug. A pharmacodynamic model will be

then developed to predict the presence or absence of adverse events. These two models will then be combined to find an optimal dosing strategy for the drug.

LINEAR REGRESSION CASE STUDY: ALLOMETRIC SCALING

Allometric scaling is an empirical technique used to explore relationships between physiological variables (e.g., cardiac output, heart rate, and organ weights) and physical characteristics (e.g., total body weight, body surface area, or maximum lifespan potential). The interrelationship between physiologic and physical variables can be used to relate one relationship with any other, thereby implying that all mammals have in common some basic "physiological design" and can be compared as "physical systems." Allometry "*can be used to study the underlying similarities (and differences) in drug disposition between species, to predict drug disposition in an untested species, to define pharmacokinetic equivalence in various species, and to design dosage regimens for experimental animals*" (Mordenti, 1986).

Adolph (1949) proposed that anatomic and physiologic variables were related to total body weight by the power function

$$Y = \theta_1 x^{\theta_2} \exp(\varepsilon) \qquad (5.1)$$

where Y is the dependent variable, x is the independent variable, θ_1 and θ_2 are scaling parameters, and ε independent, normally distributed residuals with zero mean and variance σ^2. In allometry, the independent variable, x, is usually total body weight.

The premise behind allometric scaling of pharmacokinetic parameters is that since many physiological parameters are a function of the size of an animal, then similarly pharmacokinetic parameters such as clearance and volume of distribution should also be a function of the size of an animal (Ritschel et al., 1992). Allometric scaling has been used to retrospectively compare the pharmacokinetics of a drug across species and to prospectively extrapolate a drug's pharmacokinetics from animals to humans. In many published studies, allometric scaling appears to hold for a variety of drugs with widely diverse structures and pharmacokinetics (unless one assumes that only drugs in which allometric scaling has been successful are submitted for publication). For systemic clearance, θ_2 tends to lie between 0.6 and 0.8; for volume of distribution between 0.8 and 1.0. The reader is referred to Chappell and Mordenti (1990) for an excellent review of allometric scaling in pharmacokinetics.

Mordenti et al. (1991) compared the pharmacokinetics of relaxin, a protein proposed for use in pregnant women at or near term to increase cervical ripening, across species using allometric scaling. Figure 5.1 plots the systemic clearance for mouse, rat, rabbit, rhesus monkey, and humans. Taking the natural log of both sides of Eq. (5.1) leads to

$$\mathrm{Ln}(Y) = \theta_2 \mathrm{Ln}(x) + \mathrm{Ln}(\theta_1) + \varepsilon, \qquad (5.2)$$

which transforms a nonlinear problem into a linear one. Fitting Eq. (5.2), $\mathrm{Ln}(\theta_1)$ was found to be 1.795 ± 0.115 and θ_2 was 0.796 ± 0.0418 with a coefficient of determination (R^2) of 0.9918; overall, an excellent fit. The value of θ_2 was also very close to its theoretical value of 0.8. Thus, excellent agreement in the systemic clearance of relaxin across species was observed.

Now suppose data were available only in animal species and it was of interest to predict the pharmacokinetics of relaxin in humans. Fitting Eq. (5.2) to only the animal data gives, $\mathrm{Ln}(\theta_1) = 1.763 \pm 0.155$, $\theta_2 = 0.776 \pm 0.0680$, and coefficient of determination of 0.9849. Overall, the precision of the model was slightly less than the previous one. The predicted value for a 62.4 kg adult female is then

$$\mathrm{CL} = \exp(\theta_1)W^{\theta_2} = \exp(1.763)62.4^{0.776} \qquad (5.3)$$

or 144 mL/min. Compared to the observed value 175 mL/min, the relative difference was only 18%, which would suggest that allometric scaling of the pharmacokinetics in animals would have lead to a useful prediction of relaxin pharmacokinetics in humans.

Bonate and Howard (2000) have argued that prospective allometric scaling leads to an artificially high degree of confidence because the prediction interval for the predicted pharmacokinetic parameter is not taken into account. Based on the animal data, the prediction interval for the clearance in a 62.4 kg female human can be calculated. Given the following, $MSE = 0.08943$, $n = 4$, $t_{n-2, 0.05(2)} = 4.303$, $S_{xx} = 19.334$, $X_0 = 4.134$ ($= \mathrm{Ln}(62.4\,\mathrm{kg})$), and $\bar{x} = -0.591$ (average weight of all animal species in log-domain), then the standard error of prediction is

$$\mathrm{SE}\left[\hat{Y}(x_0)\right] = \sqrt{0.08943\left[\frac{1}{m} + \frac{1}{4} + \frac{(4.134 + 0.591)^2}{19.334}\right]}. \qquad (5.4)$$

Assuming the best case scenario and letting the number of replicate measurements (m) equal ∞, then the standard error of $\hat{Y}(x_0) = 0.354$. The 95% prediction interval will be given by

$$[1.763 + 0.776\mathrm{Ln}(62.4)] \pm 4.303 \times 0.354$$
$$4.970 \pm 1.523. \qquad (5.5)$$
$$\{3.447, 6.493\}$$

The corresponding prediction interval for a 62.4 kg adult female after back transformation to the original domain was 31–661 mL/min. The 95% prediction interval across all species is presented in Fig. 5.2. Notice that in the log-domain, the confidence intervals were symmetric, but were asymmetric when transformed back to the original domain. It is this exponentiation that leads to very large prediction intervals, which should not be surprising because the model from animals weighing less than 5.5 kg was extrapolated to a 62.4 kg human. Common sense would indicate the prediction should have

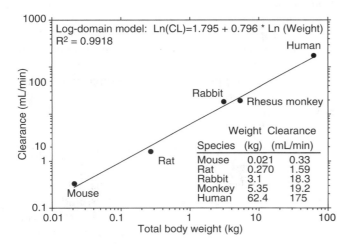

Figure 5.1 Allometric scaling of relaxin clearance. Data presented by Mordenti et al. (1991). Solid line is linear least squares fit to Ln–Ln transformed data.

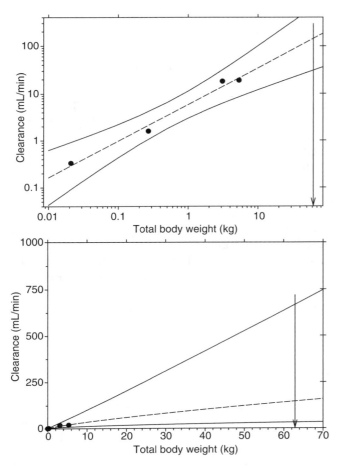

Figure 5.2 Prospective allometric scaling of relaxin clearance using only animal data. Data presented by Mordenti et al. (1991). Top plot is Ln–Ln scale. Bottom plot is linear scale. Solid line is 95% prediction interval. Prediction intervals are symmetric in the Ln-domain but become asymmetric when exponentiated back to the original domain. Arrow indicates where an adult human female (62.4 kg) falls on the line.

poor precision. Despite the problems with it, prospective allometric scaling is used by many to predict starting doses in humans for first time in man studies (Boxenbaum and Dilea, 1995). For more information on allometric scaling the reader is referred to Mahmood (2004, 1996, 1999).

LINEAR REGRESSION CASE STUDY: DOSE PROPORTIONALITY

For a linear pharmacokinetic system, measures of exposure, such as maximal concentration (C_{max}) or area under the curve from 0 to infinity (AUC), are proportional to dose

$$Y \propto \text{Dose}, \tag{5.6}$$

which can be expressed mathematically as

$$Y = c(\text{Dose}) \tag{5.7}$$

where c is a proportionality constant greater than zero. If Y is AUC then 1/c is the clearance of the drug. Under such a linear system, all concentration–time profiles when normalized to dose are superimposable. Technically, there is no intercept in Eq. (5.7) which means at zero dose the dependent variable is zero. Table 5.1 presents a summary of pharmacokinetic parameters and their relationship with dose assuming dose proportionality. If linear pharmacokinetics does not hold, then nonlinear pharmacokinetics is occurring, which means that measures of exposure increase in a disproportionate manner with increasing dose. It is important to remember that essentially all physiologic processes are nonlinear, but that there may be a range of concentrations in which the processes are essentially linear. In drug development, it is essential to determine whether the pharmacokinetics of a new drug candidate for a given dose range are linear or nonlinear.

One experimental design that is used to assess linearity, called an ascending single dose tolerance design, is to administer the drug of interest to a group of volunteers and observe them for adverse events, while at the same time collecting blood samples for assaying plasma or serum drug concentrations at the completion of the study. Once it has been determined that the dose produced no serious or limiting adverse events, a larger dose is given to the next set of volunteers. This process is repeated until a dose is given that has adverse events of such nature that it would be unethical to give the same dose or greater doses to other subjects. This last dose is called the minimal intolerable dose, whereas the dose given prior to the last dose is called the maximum tolerated dose.

Yin and Chen (2001) have studied different experimental designs for dose proportionality and have concluded that alternate panel designs wherein the same

Table 5.1 Pharmacokinetic parameters and their relationship to dose assuming dose proportionality.

Proportional	Independent
Maximal concentration	Time to maximal concentration
AUC(0 − τ)	Half life
AUC	Rate constants
Minimal concentration	Clearance
Concentration at steady state	Bioavailability
Amount excreted in urine	Fraction excreted unchanged in urine
	Volume of distribution

Reprinted from Gough et al. (1995) with permission from the Drug Information Association. Copyright, 1995.

subject is studied in alternate panels is superior in terms of parameter estimation than sequential panel designs wherein the same subject is studied in sequential panels, and that both alternate and sequential designs are superior to single panel designs wherein each subject is dosed once. For example, suppose there are six doses to be studied. In a sequential design, subjects may take doses 1, 2, and 3 or 4, 5, and 6, whereas subjects in an alternate design might take doses 1, 3, and 5 or 2, 4, and 6.

Once the study is completed and the plasma or serum samples are analyzed for drug concentrations and AUC and Cmax are determined for each subject. AUC and Cmax are treated as the dependent variables (Y) in the analysis. At this point, there are a number of ways to assess for dose proportionality. The Statisticians in the Pharmaceutical Industry/Pharmacokinetics UK Joint Working Party (SPI/PUK JWP) have reviewed the statistical methods used to assess dose proportionality and have published a summary of their findings (Gough et al., 1995). These methods will now be summarized. In the untransformed regression approach, the simple linear model is fit to the data

$$Y = \theta_0 + \theta_1(\text{Dose}) + \varepsilon \tag{5.8}$$

and θ_0 is tested for zero equality. If θ_0 equals zero, then Eq. (5.7) holds and the drug is dose proportional. If θ_0 does not equal zero then dose linearity (which is distinct from dose proportionality) is declared. A modification of the simple linear model is to fit a quadratic polynomial to the data

$$Y = \theta_0 + \theta_1(\text{Dose}) + \theta_2(\text{Dose})^2 + \varepsilon \tag{5.9}$$

and test for whether θ_0 and θ_2 both equal zero. Dose nonproportionality is declared if either parameter is significantly different than zero. Often since the variance of Y increases with increasing dose, a variance model other than constant variance needs to be used.

Alternatively, a common variant of Eq. (5.8) is to divide both sides by dose creating a dose-normalized summary measure. If the kinetics are linear, then a scatter plot of dose normalized Y versus dose would yield a flat line of zero slope. Hence, a test for dose proportionality would be to test whether $\theta_1 = 0$ in the linear model

$$\left(\frac{Y}{\text{Dose}}\right) = \theta_0 + \theta_1(\text{Dose}) + \varepsilon. \tag{5.10}$$

Lastly, another model referred to as the power model of dose proportionality is to expand Eq. (5.7) to

$$Y = \exp(\theta_1)(\text{Dose})^{\theta_2} \exp(\varepsilon) \tag{5.11}$$

where $\exp(\theta_1) = c$ and $\theta_2 = 1$. Taking the Ln-transformation yields

$$\text{Ln}(Y) = \theta_1 + \theta_2 \text{Ln}(\text{Dose}) + \varepsilon \tag{5.12}$$

where θ_2, the slope, measures the proportionality between Dose and Y. A test for dose proportionality is then to test whether $\theta_2 = 1$. The advantage of this method is that often the usual assumptions regarding homoscedasticity apply and alternative variance models are unnecessary.

Smith et al. (2000) argue that it is insufficient to simply hypothesis test for dose proportionality using regression methods because an imprecise study may lead to large confidence intervals around the model parameters that indicate dose proportionality but are in fact meaningless. If Y(h) and Y(l) denote the value of the dependent variable, like Cmax, at the highest (h) and lowest (l) dose tested, respectively, and the drug is dose proportional then

$$\frac{Y(h)}{Y(l)} = \frac{h}{l} = r \tag{5.13}$$

where r is a constant called the maximal dose ratio. Dose proportionality is declared if the ratio of geometric means Y(h)/Y(l) equals r. Smith et al. (2000) argue a more rigorous approach to determine dose proportionality would then be to use a bioequivalence-type approach to the problem and declare dose proportionality only if the appropriate confidence interval for r is entirely contained within some user-defined equivalence region $\{\Theta_l, \Theta_h\}$ that is based on the drug's safety, efficacy, or registration considerations.

For the power model, the predicted geometric mean at the high dose is given by $e^{\theta_0} h^{\theta_1}$ while for the geometric mean for the low dose is given by $e^{\theta_0} l^{\theta_1}$. Dose proportionality then implies that

$$\frac{e^{\theta_0} h^{\theta_1}}{e^{\theta_0} l^{\theta_1}} = \frac{h}{l} = r \tag{5.14}$$

which can be rewritten as

$$\left(\frac{h}{l}\right)^{\theta_1 - 1} = r^{\theta_1 - 1}. \tag{5.15}$$

Setting up a confidence interval for $r^{\theta_1 - 1}$ and taking the natural log gives

$$\text{Ln}(\Theta_l) < (\theta_1 - 1)\text{Ln}(r) < \text{Ln}(\Theta_h). \tag{5.16}$$

Solving for β_1 gives

$$1 + \frac{\text{Ln}(\Theta_l)}{\text{Ln}(r)} < \theta_1 < 1 + \frac{\text{Ln}(\Theta_h)}{\text{Ln}(r)}. \qquad (5.17)$$

Hence, if the $(1-\alpha)\%$ confidence interval for θ_1 is entirely contained within the equivalence region $\{1 + \text{Ln}(\Theta_l)/\text{Ln}(r), 1 + \text{Ln}(\Theta_h)/\text{Ln}(r)\}$ then dose proportionality is declared. If not, then dose nonproportionality is declared. No scientific guidelines exist for choice of α, Θ_l, or Θ_h, although Smith et al. (2000) suggest bioequivalence guidelines of 0.10, 0.80, and 1.25, respectively.

As an example, Table 5.2 presents the results from a first time in man study for a new chemical entity. This was a single dose ascending study where a cohort consisted of two to four subjects, except at the maximum tolerated dose $(27.3 \, \text{mg/m}^2)$ where nine subjects were dosed to gain better experience with the drug at that dose level. The simple linear model analysis [Eq. (5.8)] of the data, using actual dose received, gave an intercept of 4.54 with a standard error of 0.22. The p-value from the T-test was <0.001 indicating lack of dose proportionality. Although a test for normality on the residuals failed to indicate nonnormality, a residual plot showed a distinct trend in the fit of the model suggesting that the simple linear model was inadequate. When a power model was used to fit the data, the slope was estimated at 1.27 with a 90% confidence interval of $\{1.11, 1.43\}$. Using 19.4 (62.1 mg/3.2 mg), 0.10, 0.80, and 1.25 for r, α, Θ_l, and Θ_h, respectively, the critical region was $\{0.92, 1.08\}$. The 90% confidence interval for β_1 was not contained in the critical region. The residuals under this model were normally distributed and had no systematic deviations upon examination of the residual plot. Hence, the data were not dose proportional under the doses studied. For every doubling of dose there will be a 2.4-fold $(2^{1.27})$ increase in AUC, which will be 20% higher than expected (2.4/2.0). Similar results would have been obtained had the analysis been done using dose expressed

in mg/m^2. One might then conclude that in this case the deviation from proportionality was actually quite small and may even be clinically irrelevant.

The regression approach to dose proportionality answers the question "are the pharmacokinetics of the drug linear?" If the answer is no, then the question becomes "is there a range of doses over which the kinetics are linear?" This question may then require an analysis of variance approach with multiple comparisons between the dose groups. Which method to choose in determining dose proportionality is debatable. The SPI/PUK JWP analyzed a variety of different datasets and all the methods studied produced roughly equivalent results. They stress that all the assumptions of the regression analysis methods should be thoroughly examined before that statistical conclusions are accepted, a statement that really applies to all statistical analyses. Currently, however, opinion leaders in the field tend to favor the power model since it more closely approaches the theoretical foundation for dose proportionality.

LINEAR REGRESSION CASE STUDY: LIMITED SAMPLING STRATEGIES

Some drugs have narrow therapeutic windows such that small increases in concentration may lead to an increased risk in toxicity. For these narrow therapeutic window drugs, e.g., digoxin, phenytoin, lithium, and gentamicin, dose individualization is common. Under this strategy, plasma concentrations are monitored and if concentrations are "toxic" or "sub-therapeutic" the dose is adjusted to bring concentrations back into the window. Many oncolytic drugs also have narrow therapeutic windows and are not routinely monitored, but in cases where monitoring is done, concentrations are usually monitored to increase the chance of efficacy and not necessarily for safety concerns. Probably the most important pharmacokinetic parameter in oncology is AUC, the idea being that this parameter is a better

Table 5.2 AUC data after single dose administration of a new chemical entity.

				Dose (mg/m²)			
2.3	4.6	7.7	11.6	15.4	20.5	27.3	36.3
24.0 [3.2]	140.2 [8.7]	277.1 [20.4]	747.5 [27.3]	896.8 [31.3]	841.9 [31.0]	2162.9 [46.0]	1807.8 [61.0]
57.6 [5.0]	106.5 [7.8]	167.6 [15.7]	499.6 [24.4]	500.8 [31.7]	1313.4 [42.6]	1583.9 [57.3]	1512.0 [62.1]
137.0 [4.5]	57.8 [8.9]	485.9 [17.1]	257.6 [20.9]	1062.8 [25.6]	873.0 [52.0]	2238.4 [45.0]	
106.8 [4.9]				1079.0 [26.0]		1318.4 [37.1]	
						990.1 [57.0]	
						1274.8 [52.9]	
						1171.4 [60.6]	
						873.5 [52.4]	
						929.7 [52.4]	

Note: AUC values are in ng·h/mL. Values in brackets are the actual dose the patient received in mg.

measure of "exposure" and correlates better with efficacy than other parameters, such as maximal concentration or trough concentrations. To complicate matters, AUC can vary up to tenfold for some drugs in patients receiving the same dose. Hence, even at a safe dose for some individuals, others may experience adverse events, further highlighting the need for therapeutic drug monitoring.

In order to measure the AUC in an individual, many blood samples must be collected making its routine use prohibitive, timeconsuming, and costly. One approach used to avoid having to collect multiple blood samples is a so-called "limited sampling strategy" where one or two blood samples are drawn and these are used to predict the AUC for that individual. Under this approach, AUC is treated as the dependent variable and the observed concentrations are treated as the independent variables, the rationale being that AUC itself is a linear function of the weighted average concentration between two adjacent time points. For example, using the linear trapezoidal rule,

$$AUC(0 - last) = \sum_{i=2}^{n} 0.5(t_i - t_{i-1})(C_i + C_{i-1}) \quad (5.18)$$

where t is the time, C the concentration, and n the number of observations for that subject. The weights are simply the difference in time between two adjacent points. For model development, complete pharmacokinetic profiles are developed from a large number of representative patients. AUC is calculated for each subject and used as the model development data set. Linear regression techniques are then used to identify the subset of time points that have the greatest predictive capability. In general, the more time points included in the model, the greater the accuracy of the model, which comes at the expense of ease of use and cost.

It should also be noted that for most, if not all, of the models presented in the literature using this approach, the concentrations used to estimate AUC are the sole variable types used in model development. It is entirely possible that other patient characteristics, such as age or sex, may be useful predictor variables in the model, as well. Further, using drug concentration as an independent variable violates the assumption that the independent variables are known with certainty. Drug concentrations are not known with certainty—they are measurements subject to assay variability, operating error, etc. A more technically correct approach to the problem would be an error-in-variables approach to the problem, although this is never done in practice. Once the model is developed, an independent validation data set is used to characterize the model.

van Warmerdam et al. (1994) presents a review of the limited sampling approach in oncology, while van den Bongard et al. (2000) presents a very useful review of how AUC data may be used to guide dose administration in oncology. This approach has been used for many oncolytic agents, including carboplatin (Asai et al., 1998), doxorubicin (Ratain, Robert, and van der Vijgh, 1991), and 5-fluorouracil (Moore et al., 1993). It should be noted, however, that although this approach tends to focus on AUC as the dependent variable, it is not limited to AUC. Indeed, any pharmacokinetic parameter can be used as the dependent variable in the analysis.

An example will now be presented. In the development of a new drug, plasma concentration data were collected from 24 subjects at times 0, 0.5, 1, 1.5, 2, 3, 4, 6, 8, 12, 18, 24, 36, and 48 h postdose. From this data, the noncompartmental estimate of AUC was calculated. Of particular interest to the researchers was whether one or two samples early on in the timecourse of the kinetic profile of the drug could be used to predict AUC. Since it was problematic to expect patients to remain at the clinic longer than 4 h, the data set was limited to the first 4-h postdose.

The data are shown in Table 5.3. Note that all the concentration data were highly correlated with each other (Table 5.4), which may lead to collinearity problems if not recognized a priori. Since both the AUC and

Table 5.3 Listing of concentration-time data and corresponding AUC for a new drug.

Subject	Concentration (ng/mL)						AUC (ng/h)/mL
	0.5 h	1 h	1.5 h	2 h	3 h	4 h	
1	18.4	30.8	35.4	39.5	37.9	34.5	331.3
2	24.9	33.5	39.0	44.6	38.3	32.1	251.1
3	17.3	27.9	33.0	30.5	31.4	27.8	220.4
4	14.9	24.9	32.6	33.8	34.6	31.9	305.5
5	18.3	26.8	29.1	31.1	30.0	22.0	256.0
6	18.8	30.0	35.2	35.5	35.6	27.5	253.4
7	29.0	43.2	51.1	54.5	49.2	41.4	389.4
8	9.0	14.8	17.3	22.6	24.2	22.1	321.6
9	28.9	39.9	45.7	45.1	33.8	26.4	225.2
10	29.6	42.4	42.4	41.7	34.3	25.3	230.3
11	21.9	31.1	35.2	39.4	31.8	22.7	173.8
12	13.0	20.4	24.2	24.7	24.7	21.3	203.2
13	15.5	25.3	27.7	32.5	27.4	26.2	255.0
14	14.8	24.3	27.4	30.4	30.8	28.2	279.9
15	14.8	22.0	27.5	30.7	28.5	25.6	236.1
16	19.1	29.0	32.8	34.1	29.3	23.6	205.5
17	13.8	23.4	25.8	29.7	27.5	25.1	254.1
18	18.0	28.7	34.2	39.0	38.9	33.7	423.8
19	19.4	28.2	33.3	34.8	33.7	30.1	279.2
20	15.4	26.7	25.1	31.1	27.8	23.6	243.3
21	19.8	29.2	34.9	33.5	29.8	28.4	244.8
22	18.2	27.5	31.8	36.2	34.3	29.7	283.0
23	12.7	18.8	24.8	27.1	25.2	22.6	220.9
24	11.3	15.3	20.1	23.1	20.1	19.9	268.1

Table 5.4 Pearson's correlation coefficient between plasma concentration data presented in Table 5.3. *log transformed*

	0.5 h	1 h	1.5 h	2 h	3 h	4 h
0.5 h	1.0000	0.9701	0.9577	0.9256	0.7689	0.5172
1 h		1.0000	0.9597	0.9375	0.8319	0.5999
1.5 h			1.0000	0.9499	0.8677	0.6820
2 h				1.0000	0.9088	0.7348
3 h					1.0000	0.8864
4 h						1.0000

Note: All correlations were statistically significant at $p < 0.01$.

concentration data were skewed, the Ln-transformation on both AUC and concentration was used to stabilize the skewness. As a start, simple linear regression was used wherein each time point was used as the independent variable to see how each variable does individually (Table 5.5). Only the 3-h and 4-h time points were statistically significant at $p < 0.05$. The 3-h time point was significant at $p = 0.0286$, whereas the 4-h time point was significant at 0.0005. But notice what happened when the two variables were entered into the model jointly (Table 5.6). Not only did the p-value for both independent variables increase, the sign of the relationship between Ln-transformed AUC and Ln-transformed concentration at 3-h postdose changed from positive (see Table 5.5) to negative (see Table 5.6). These two changes (increase in p-value and sign changes) and the correlation between concentrations at 3-h and 4-h ($r = 0.89$) were indicative of a collinearity problem. Indeed, the condition number of the bivariate model was 9386, which was higher than the condition numbers of the simple linear models (1391 and 1444 for the 3-h and 4-h concentrations alone, respectively).

To help identify a final model, sequential variable selection using backwards elimination was done with SAS. A p-value of 0.05 was required to stay in the model. The final model is shown in Table 5.7. Although the final model identified the 4-h time point as a significant covariate, it did not identify the 3-h time point as

Table 5.5 Simple linear regression summary of Ln-transformed AUC against Ln-transformed concentration using data in Table 5.3.

Independent variable	Intercept Estimate	Intercept Std error	Slope Estimate	Slope Std error	Coefficient of determination
Ln (0.5 h)	**5.65**	0.42	−0.0392	0.146	0.0020
Ln (1 h)	**5.48**	0.53	0.0228	0.160	0.0009
Ln (1.5 h)	**5.33**	0.60	0.0673	0.173	0.0068
Ln (2 h)	**4.83**	0.70	0.207	0.199	0.0468
Ln (3 h)	**3.91**	0.70	**0.479**	0.205	0.1996
Ln (4 h)	**3.09**	0.61	**0.752**	0.184	0.4319

Note: Bold values were statistically significant at $p < 0.05$.

Table 5.6 Linear regression summary of Ln-transformed AUC using the 3- and 4-h times points as independent variables.

Parameter	Estimate	Standard error	p-Value
Intercept	3.314	0.582	<0.0001
Ln (3 h)	−0.680	0.352	0.0665
Ln(4 h)	1.394	0.374	0.0013

Note: The adjusted coefficient of determination was 0.4720.

Table 5.7 Final model produced using backwards stepwise linear regression of Ln-transformed AUC using the concentration data in Table 5.3.

Parameter	Estimate	Standard error	p-Value
Intercept	3.255	0.464	<0.0001
Ln (1.5 h)	−0.559	0.137	0.0006
Ln(4 h)	1.285	0.192	<0.0001

Note: The criteria to stay was a p-value of ≤ 0.05. The adjusted coefficient of determination was 0.6520

such. Instead the algorithm identified the 1.5-h time point as important. How could this be since the simple linear model did not even identify the 1.5-h as being statistically significant when tested alone? There are two answers. One is that sequential procedures do not necessarily lead to the same model as individual simple linear models. When all possible models were computed on the data set, using adjusted R^2 as the criteria, the best fit model was the 1.5-, 3-, and 4-h time points, which showed an adjusted R^2 of 0.6613, which was slightly better than the final model chosen using backwards elimination. Using another criterion, Mallow's C_p, the best model used the 1.5-h and 4-h time points and had an adjusted R^2 of 0.6520. The second answer is collinearity among the predictors may lead to an unstable model. The model that had all the independent variables included had a condition number of 82440, which was unstable, so that when different variables were included in the model, significant model parameters may have appeared not to be significant.

To further understand the impact of measurement error on the model parameters, the SIMEX algorithm was applied using a model containing only the 1.5-h and 4-h time points. The assay had a coefficient of variation of about 5% based on the bioanalytical validation of standards and controls in plasma having a known amount of drug added. The resulting SIMEX model was

$$Ln(AUC) = 2.95 - 0.686 \times Ln(C_{1.5h}) + 1.51 \times Ln(C_{4h})$$

$$(5.19)$$

with an adjusted coefficient of determination of 0.6288. The errors-in-variables parameter estimates were similar to the parameter estimates assuming no error in the independent variables, but were not identical. To see how the estimate of measurement error affected the SIMEX parameter estimates, a sensitivity analysis was conducted where the assay measurement error was varied from 0 to 20%. Figure 5.3 presents the results. The SIMEX parameter estimates were sensitive to the choice of measurement error. As measurement error increased the attenuation of the parameter estimates increased and pulled the parameter estimates toward zero. Still, the model parameter estimates were somewhat robust when the measurement error was less than 5%, which it was in this case, indicating that future use of parameter estimates assuming no error in the independent variables will be acceptable.

In summary, blindly using sequential variable selection procedures or all possible regressions can lead to misleading and conflicting models. It is better to use simple linear models initially and see what is important, then use these results to build more complicated models, keeping in mind the effect the correlation between the independent variables may have on the model development process. It may become necessary to use alternative regression techniques, such as ridge regression or principal component analysis, to stabilize the parameter estimates.

NONLINEAR REGRESSION CASE STUDY: PHARMACOKINETIC MODELING OF COCAINE AFTER INTRAVENOUS, SMOKING INHALATION ("CRACK COCAINE"), AND INTRANASAL ("SNORTING") ADMINISTRATION

Cocaine is a notorious drug of abuse that is administered via a number of routes of administration, including intranasal (snorting), intravenous, and inhalational ("crack cocaine"). Based on the rank order of addictive potential, inhalational > intravenous > intranasal. Bonate et al. (1996) developed a physiological based model of cocaine pharmacokinetics and showed that the rank order of addictive potency correlated with the maximal brain concentrations observed with each route of administration, i.e., maximal brain cocaine concentrations were as follows: inhalation > intravenous > intranasal ("snorting") after equimolar doses. Metabolically, cocaine is almost exclusively degraded to inactive metabolites, the primary ones being ecgonine methyl ester and benzoylecgonine.

Jeffcoat et al. (1989) administered cocaine to four to six human volunteers using three routes of administration: intravenous (20.5 mg), intranasal (94.3 mg), and inhalational (39.5 mg). Dosing via the inhalational route occurred as follows. Subjects were asked to inhale and hold for 30 s. This process was repeated 10 times over a 5 min period. For modeling purposes, the inhalational route was modeled as a series of 10 bolus doses of 3.95 mg every 30 s. For intranasal administration, two "lines" of cocaine were made and subjects were asked to snort the drug in both lines in a 30-s period. A typical "snort" lasts about 5 s, which for all practical purposes is a bolus dose. Hence, for modeling purposes, intranasal drug administration was treated as two bolus doses: a 47.15 mg bolus at time 0 and a second dose of 47.15 mg 15 s later. For intravenous administration, drug administration was modeled as a 1 min infusion of 20.5 mg into the central compartment. Serial blood samples were collected and plasma concentrations of cocaine and benzoylecgonine were determined by high performance liquid chromatography. For our purposes, however, only the cocaine data will be modeled since benzoylecgonine is an inactive metabolite. The data are plotted in Figure

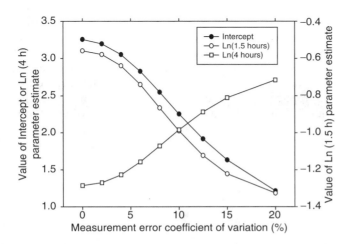

Figure 5.3 Scatter plot of SIMEX parameter estimates when the coefficient of variation in the measurement error was varied from 0 to 20% based on the data in Table 5.3.

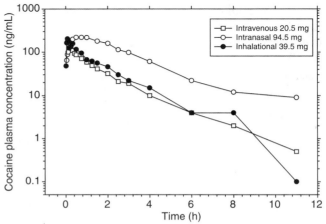

Figure 5.4 Scatter plots of observed plasma cocaine concentration after intravenous, inhalational, and intranasal administration. Data reported by Jeffcoat et al. (1989).

Table 5.8 Cocaine plasma concentrations (ng/mL) after intravenous, intranasal, and inhalational routes of administration as reported by Jeffcoat et al. (1989).

time (h)	Intravenous		Inhalational		Intranasal	
	Mean	Standard deviation	Mean	Standard deviation	Mean	Standard deviation
0.017					48.0	29.0
0.050			65.0	39.0	164.0	81.0
0.083	180.0	56.0	88.0	15.0	203.0	88.0
0.117			101.0	40.0	177.0	64.0
0.167	125.0	60.0	126.0	68.0	125.0	39.0
0.250	118.0	38.0	172.0	68.0	136.0	65.0
0.333	110.0	37.0	198.0	54.0	158.0	73.0
0.417	94.0	29.0				
0.500	87.0	23.0	220.0	39.0	116.0	49.0
0.750	71.0	22.0	220.0	50.0	95.0	52.0
1.000	59.0	12.0	217.0	51.0	67.0	43.0
1.250	49.0	14.0			62.0	37.0
1.500	41.0	9.0	180.0	58.0	56.0	27.0
2.000	32.0	6.6	159.0	50.0	46.0	25.0
2.500	21.0	7.0	114.0	36.0	30.0	17.0
3.000	19.0	5.0	98.0	35.0	22.0	9.0
4.000	10.0	0.0	61.0	17.0	15.0	7.0
6.000	4.0	2.8	22.0	12.0	4.0	2.5
8.000	2.0	0.0	12.0	5.0	4.0	2.5
11.000	0.5	1.0	9.0	1.0	0.1	1.6

5.4 and presented Table 5.8. On a log-scale the data appeared to exhibit a biexponential decline. Hence, a 2-compartment model was chosen as a base model. Rather than attempt to fit all the data simultaneously, the modeling process was done by order of their absorption complexity.

Hence, intravenous data were modeled first, followed by inhalational, then intranasal. Once the pharmacokinetics of each individual route of administration was established, all model parameters were then estimated simultaneously. Initial values for cocaine pharmacokinetics after intravenous administration were estimated using noncompartmental methods. Total systemic clearance was estimated at 100 L/h and volume of distribution at steady-state was estimated at 232 L. Central compartment clearance and intercompartmental clearance were set equal to one-half total systemic clearance (50 L/h), whereas central and peripheral compartment volumes were set equal to one-half volume of distribution (116 L). Data were weighed using a constant coefficient of variation error model based on model-predicted plasma concentrations. All models were fit using SAAM II (SAAM Institute, Seattle, WA). An Information-Theoretic approach was used for model selection, i.e., model selection was based on the AIC.

The first model examined was a 2-compartment model (Model 1) in Figure 5.5. A scatter plot of observed concentrations with model predicted overlay is shown in Fig. 5.6. The AIC of Model 1 was 2.560. Clearance, central volume, intercompartmental clear-

ance, and peripheral volume were estimated at 103 ± 2.3 L/h, 121 ± 8.2 L, 65.0 ± 16.3 L/h, and 62.2 ± 7.8 L, respectively. All parameter estimates were precisely estimated with coefficients of variation less than 25%. When a third compartment was added, the AIC decreased, but the standard errors of the parameter estimates were much larger. Also, the 95% confidence interval for central volume was so wide that its lower bound was less than zero. Hence, it was decided that the base model should be a 2-compartment model.

The parameter estimates were fixed from Model 1 and model development proceeded with the inhalational (si) route of administration. The initial model treated the inhaled dose as going directly into an absorption compartment with first-order transfer (k_a) into the central compartment (Model 2 in Fig. 5.5). To account for the fact that some of the inhaled cocaine was exhaled and that there may have been first-pass metabolism prior to reaching the sampling site, a bioavailability term was included in the model (F_{si}).

Initial parameter estimates for the first-order rate constant were arbitrarily set equal to 2/h and inhalational bioavailability was set equal to 0.9. After fitting the model, the estimate of k_a was 660 per hour. Hence, in essence, all the drug reached the systemic compartment almost immediately. The model was modified, removing the dosing compartment, and allowing the drug to be treated as an intravenous model with variable bioavailability (Model 3 in Fig. 5.5). Under this model the bioavailability of the inhaled dose was 62.6 ± 4.3%.

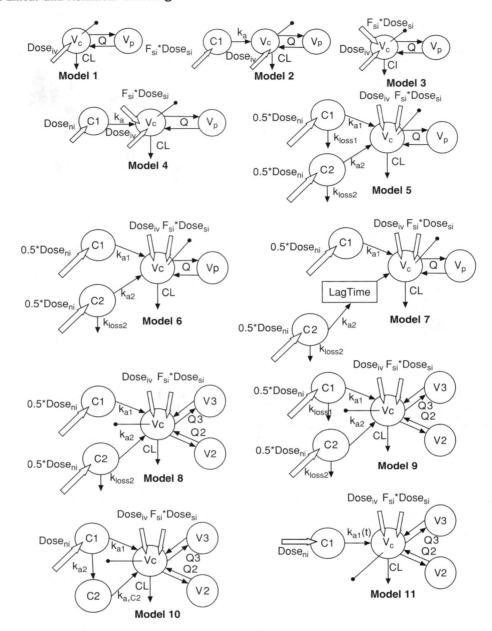

Figure 5.5   Models used in the development of the pharmacokinetics of cocaine.

A scatter plot of the observed data with model predicted overlay is shown in Fig. 5.7. The fit appeared to be adequate. The inhalational bioavailability term was then fixed and model development proceeded to intranasal administration.

Cocaine is known to have vasoconstrictive properties. It would be expected that following intranasal administration, the vasculature would constrict slowing the absorption of cocaine into the blood stream. Hence, the absorption kinetics would become time dependent. As an initial model, Model 4 in Fig. 5.5 was examined. In this model, intranasal (ni) absorption was treated as a

first-order process (k_a) using an initial value of 1 per hour. Normally, such a model would be unidentifiable but because data were available from other routes of administration, all model parameters were estimable. After fitting, k_a was 1.04 ± 0.14 per hour. The AIC for the model (which includes all other routes of administration) was 3.845. The fitted model is shown in Fig. 5.8. The model clearly overpredicted the maximal concentration and subsequent concentrations after intranasal administration.

A second absorption model was examined where the dose was split into components (Model 5 in

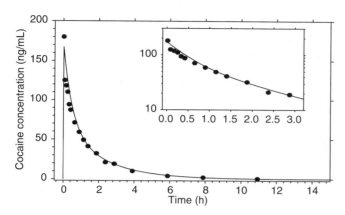

Figure 5.6 Scatter plot and model predicted overlay of cocaine plasma concentrations after intravenous administration. The final model was Model 1 in Fig. 5.5. Inset plot is 0–3 h postdose in the semi log domain.

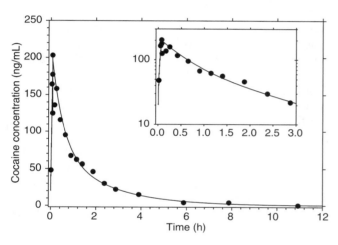

Figure 5.7 Scatter plot and model predicted overlay of cocaine plasma concentrations after inhalational administration. The final model was Model 3 in Fig. 5.5. Inset plot is 0–3 h post dose in the semilog domain.

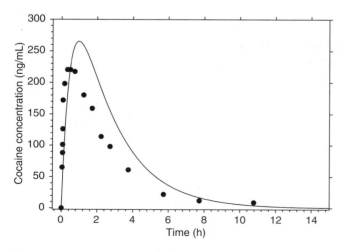

Figure 5.8 Scatter plot and model predicted overlay of cocaine plasma concentrations after intranasal administration. The final model was Model 4 in Fig. 5.5.

Fig. 5.5). This model was an attempt to model dose administration as two separate doses, one associated with each line of cocaine. The first model studied was a general model where one-half the total dose goes into an absorption compartment with absorption rate constant into the central compartment (k_{a1}) and first-order loss prior to reaching the central compartment (k_{loss1}). The second dosing compartment was treated the same as the first dosing compartment with terms (k_{a2} and k_{loss2}). Loss from the dosing compartment represented presystemic metabolism by pseudocholinesterases found in blood and tissues and nonenzymatic hydrolysis. Fitting this model resulted in k_{loss1} being equal to zero, so this rate constant was removed from the model. The resulting model (Model 6 in Fig. 5.5) resulted in an AIC of 3.574, an improvement over Model 5. The absorption rate constants, k_{a1} and k_{a2}, were estimated at 2.77 ± 0.26 per hour and 0.19 ± 0.045 per hour, respectively. That k_{a2} was smaller than k_{a1} was consistent with the hypothesis that vasoconstriction after the first dose will slow the absorption of later doses. The rate of loss from the second dosing compartment was 0.13 ± 0.023 per hour. The goodness of fit is shown in Fig. 5.9. The model appeared to be quite satisfactory in predicting intranasal administration.

At this point, all parameters were unfixed and treated as estimable. After fitting the AIC increased to 3.666, but this AIC has five more estimable parameters. Figure 5.10 presents the goodness of fit plots for all routes of administration. The second dosing compartment in Model 6 seemed to act like a slow release depot for cocaine. To see if further improvement in the absorption model could be obtained, a time-lag was added between C2 and the central compartment (Model 7 in Fig. 5.5). The AIC of this model was 3.691, which offered no

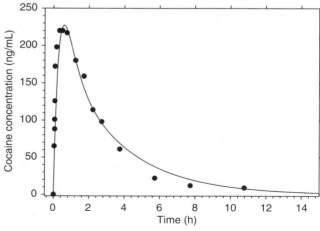

Figure 5.9 Scatter plot and model predicted overlay of cocaine plasma concentrations after intranasal administration. The final model was Model 6 in Fig. 5.5 with only the absorption parameters related to intranasal administration treated as estimable; all other model parameters were fixed.

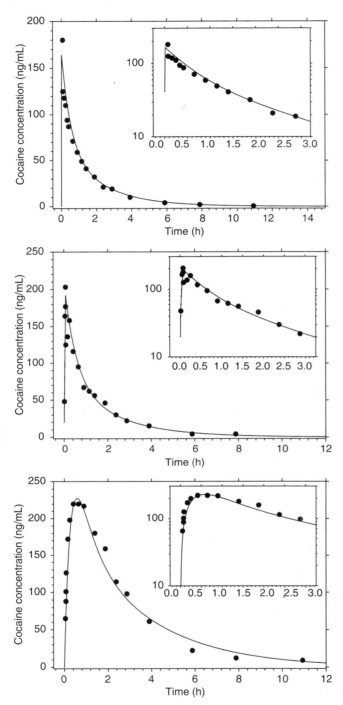

Figure 5.10 Scatter plot and model predicted overlay of cocaine plasma concentrations after intravenous (top), inhalation (middle), and intranasal (bottom) administration. The model used was Model 6 in Fig. 5.5 with all model parameters treated as estimable. Insets are in the semilog domain.

further improvement over Model 6. Further, the 95% confidence interval for the time-lag was { − 0.98, 1.33 h}, which contained zero. Therefore, Model 7 was discarded. Two alternative models were examined where in one model a lag-compartment between C1 and the

central compartment was examined with no lag compartment between C2 and the central compartment and a model with a two lag-compartments, one between C1 and the central compartment and another between C2 and the central compartment. In both alternative models, the estimated lag times were essentially zero, so these models were discarded.

Earlier in model development, a 3-compartment model was tested and its inclusion in the model was questionable. To see whether with the additional data a 3-compartment model should be used, the model estimates for the third compartment were set equal to 1/10 the intercompartmental clearance and peripheral volume values. Table 5.9 presents the model parameter estimates. The AIC of the Model 8 was 3.567, an improvement over Model 6. Visual examination of the goodness of fit plots, however, showed an improvement in fit with intravenous and inhalational administration, but now the intranasal route was not as well predicted (Fig. 5.11). That loss from the second dosing compartment occurred but not from the first dosing compartment, and it did not make much sense. Hence, first-order loss from C1 was added back into the model under two different conditions (Model 9 in Fig. 5.5). In the first condition, the rate of loss from C1 was treated as equal to the rate of loss from C2. With this model the AIC was 3.584, which was not an improvement over Model 8. Under the second condition, unique rate constants for each dosing compartment were examined. Like Model 5, the rate of loss from C1 kept hitting its lower bound of zero, indicating the k_{loss1} should be removed from the model. Both these models were then discarded.

At this point Model 8 should be considered the final model, but the goodness of fit of the intranasal model was not entirely satisfactory nor was the precision of the parameter estimates. So, after pondering how might cocaine be absorbed, two entirely different absorption models were considered. In the first model, intranasal cocaine was dosed into a single compartment at time 0 and then again 15 s later. Some fraction of the cocaine in the dosing compartment was rapidly absorbed directly into the central compartment with first-order rate constant k_{a1} while the remaining drug in the dosing compartment was absorbed into a lag compartment with first-order rate constant k_{a2}. From the lag-compartment, drug was absorbed into the central compartment with first-order rate constant $k_{a, C2}$. This model is shown as Model 10 in Fig. 5.5. Model parameter estimates are presented in Table 5.10. The AIC of Model 10 was 3.383, indicating that this model was better than Model 8. The goodness of fit plots are shown in Figure 5.12. This new intranasal absorption model seemed to have better predictive properties than Model 8.

Table 5.9 Parameter estimates for the cocaine data in Table 5.8 under a 3-compartment model expressed in terms of clearance and volume (Model 8).

Parameter	Model term	Units	Value	Standard error	CV (%)
Clearance	CL	L/h	101	1.6	1.6
Central volume	Vc	L	85.2	13.8	16.0
Intercompartmental clearance to compartment 2	Q2	L/h	28.7	8.5	29.5
Volume of compartment 2	V2	L	40.9	7.0	16.4
Intercompartmental clearance to compartment 3	Q3	L/h	342	156	45.7
Volume of compartment 3	V3	L	51.4	11.2	21.8
Inhalation bioavailability	F_{si}	%	60.7	5.1	8.5
Rate of loss from C2	k_{loss2}	per h	0.13	2.19E-2	16.6
Absorption rate constant from compartment C1	k_{a1}	per h	2.32	0.27	11.6
Absorption rate constant from compartment C2	k_{a2}	per h	0.17	4.08E-2	24.6

Akaike Information Criterion: 3.567

The second absorption model examined a time-dependent absorption rate constant. In this model, intranasal cocaine was dosed into a single compartment at time 0 and then again 15 s later. Absorption occurred directly from the dosing compartment into the central compartment via the rate constant k_{a1}, which was allowed to vary with time. A variety of time-dependent functions for k_{a1} could be examined, but a simple one was

$$k_{a1}(t) = A + B \exp(-kt) \qquad (5.20)$$

where $k_{a1}(t)$ equals $A + B$ at time 0 and A at infinite time. This model is Model 11 shown in Fig. 5.5. After fitting the model, the resulting AIC was 3.391, slightly worse than Model 10. The goodness of fit is shown in Fig. 5.13 while Table 5.11 presents the model parameter estimates. The resulting model was a good fit to all routes of administration. So which absorption model was the best model? From a strict AIC point of view the best absorption model was Model 10, which had the lowest AIC. Model 8 was substantially different from both Model 10 and Model 11 and can be discarded as a candidate model, but the difference in AIC between Model 10 and Model 11 was only 0.008.

While Model 10 had a slight edge over Model 11, interpreting Model 10 was problematic. What does Compartment C2 represent? A lag compartment? Is a model that does not have time-dependent parameters even reasonable for cocaine after intranasal administration? Model 11 can be more easily interpreted from a physiological perspective and was more consistent with theory. It is known that after cocaine is administered, absorption rapidly slows down leading to the nasal passages becoming almost a depot compartment for the

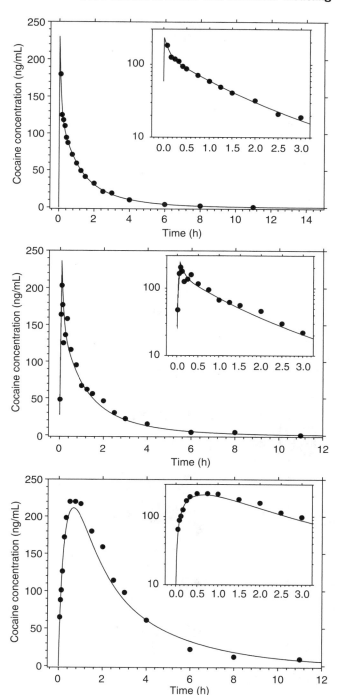

Figure 5.11 Scatter plot and model predicted overlay of cocaine plasma concentrations after intravenous (top), inhalation (middle), and intranasal (bottom) administration. The model used was Model 8 in Fig. 5.5. Insets are in the semilog domain.

drug. Model 11 was consistent with this observation. But Model 11 is not without its own problems in interpretation because k_{a1} in Model 11 never returns back to baseline, which does not happen. At some point in time, k_{a1} must return to baseline. So Model 11 would

Table 5.10   Parameter estimates for the cocaine data in Table 5.8 under a 3-compartment model expressed in terms of clearance and volume for all routes of administration (Model 10).

Parameter	Model term	Units	Value	Standard error	CV (%)
Clearance	CL	L/h	100.2	1.6	1.6
Central volume	V_c	L	65.6	10.5	16.0
Intercompartmental clearance to compartment 2	Q2	L/h	30.2	7.4	24.3
Volume of compartment 2	V2	L	42.0	5.6	13.3
Intercompartmental clearance to compartment 3	Q3	L/h	548	137	25.0
Volume of compartment 3	V3	L	66.8	8.6	12.8
Inhalation bioavailability	F_{si}	%	59.7	5.3	8.9
Absorption rate constant from compartment C1 to central compartment	k_{a1}	Per h	1.11	7.97E-2	7.2
Absorption rate constant from compartment C1 to compartment C2	k_{a2}	Per h	2.63E-2	3.85E-3	14.6
Absorption rate constant from compartment C2 to central compartment	$k_{a, C2}$	Per h	0.48	5.63E-2	11.7

Akaike Information Criterion: 3.383

probably fail with repeated dose administration over long periods of time (hours as opposed to seconds). But without repeated administration data, such a model where k_{a1} returns to baseline cannot not be developed. So despite having a slightly worse AIC than Model 10, Model 11 was considered the final model.

To see how well Model 11 predicted an independent data set, pharmacokinetic data reported by Cone (1995) was used. Cone administered 22.2 mg cocaine intravenously over 10 s, 42 mg by inhalational administration, and 28.4 mg by intranasal administration to six male subjects. Exact details of how each inhaled cocaine

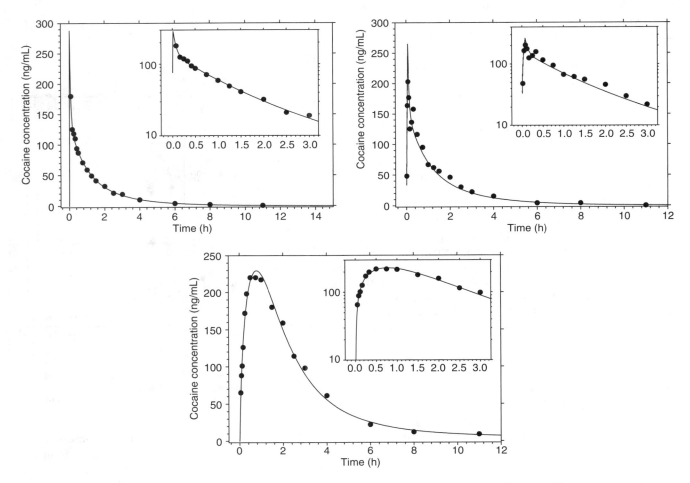

Figure 5.12   Scatter plot and model predicted overlay of cocaine plasma concentrations after intravenous (top), inhalation (middle), and intranasal (bottom) administration. The model used was Model 10 in Fig. 5.5. Insets are in the semilog domain.

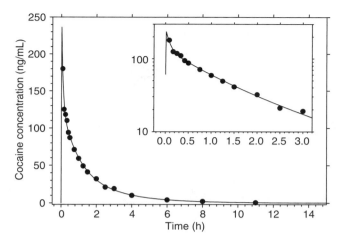

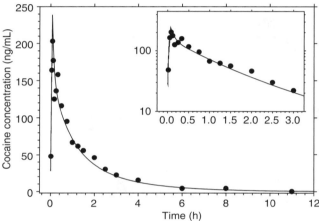

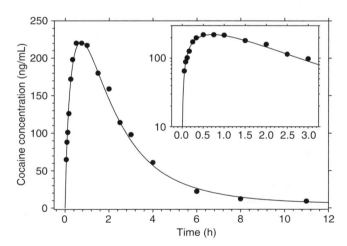

Figure 5.13 Scatter plot and model predicted overlay of cocaine plasma concentrations after intravenous (top), inhalation (middle), and intranasal (bottom) administration. The model used was Model 11 in Fig. 5.5. Insets are in the semilog domain.

dose administered was not reported, so it was assumed that cocaine administration was in 10-s interval intervals like in the model development data set. With intranasal administration, cocaine was snorted in two equal por-

Table 5.11 Parameter estimates for the cocaine data in Table 5.8 under a 3-compartment model expressed in terms of clearance and volume for all Routes of administration (Model 11) where the absorption rate constant (k_{A1}) was modeled as a function of time.

Parameter	Model term	Units	Value	Standard error	CV (%)
Clearance	CL	L/h	101	1.6	1.6
Central volume	V_c	L	81.9	11.6	14.2
Intercompartmental clearance to compartment 2	Q2	L/h	27.1	7.4	27.2
Volume of compartment 2	V2	L	39.7	5.9	15.0
Intercompartmental clearance to compartment 3	Q3	L/h	399	147	36.7
Volume of compartment 3	V3	L	55.4	9.6	17.3
Inhalation bioavailability	F_{si}	%	60.7	5.2	8.5
Absorption rate constant after intranasal administration					
$= k_{a1} = A + B \exp(-kt)$	A	Per h	2.54E-2	3.96E-3	15.6
	B	Per h	1.27	9.51E-2	7.6
	k	Per h	1.07	9.89E-2	9.2

Akaike Information Criterion: 3.391

tions, one line in each nostril, over a period of one min. One subject failed to self administer the inhalational cocaine dose and was not used in the modeling process. The mean concentration-time data, with standard deviations, are shown in Table 5.12.

The model predicted concentrations overlaid with the observed concentration-time data are shown in Fig. 5.14. Model 11 did a reasonable job of predicting concentrations early in the concentration–time profile but underpredicted concentrations later in the profile. Based on this comparison, Model 11 was not completely

Table 5.12 Mean cocaine plasma concentrations (ng/mL) after intravenous, intranasal, and inhalational routes of administration as reported by Cone (1995).

time (h)	Intravenous Mean	SD	Inhalational Mean	SD	Intranasal Mean	SD
0.00	3.2	7.8	5.0	8.1	6.0	8.7
0.02	217.8	95.6	7.5	8.7	192.4	69.3
0.05	194.0	78.3	17.3	13.7	194.6	65.4
0.08	174.4	67.7	27.2	20.4	179.8	80.7
0.17	160.2	56.7	42.8	22.7	141.6	43.4
0.25	141.8	44.0	53.2	24.3	144.4	54.4
0.33	125.5	41.2	55.0	21.3	107.0	33.1
0.50	99.3	30.3	59.8	21.1	95.8	28.0
0.75	76.7	19.0	60.8	20.0	77.2	22.9
1.00	61.2	13.9	61.7	15.3	63.4	17.5
1.50	46.8	11.3	51.3	19.4	49.4	9.3
2.00	37.5	13.2	45.5	20.8	42.2	11.3
3.00	22.8	11.1	40.0	9.6	28.4	5.3
4.00	16.8	11.5	28.8	10.6	21.2	5.4
6.00	8.7	11.1	20.8	11.9	17.0	4.6
12.00	6.0	9.6	10.5	8.7	11.2	7.2

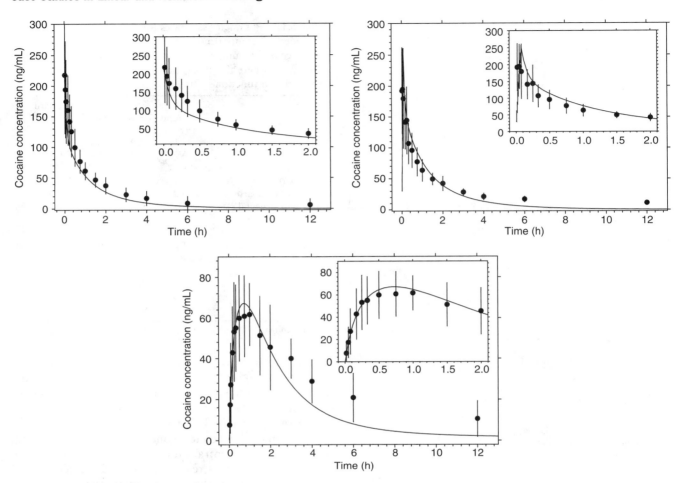

Figure 5.14 Scatter plot and model predicted overlay of cocaine plasma concentrations after intravenous (top), inhalation (middle), and intranasal (bottom) administration. The model used was Model 11 in Fig. 5.5. The observed data are the validation data set reported by Cone (1995) and presented in Table 5.12. Model parameters are shown in Table 5.11. Error bars are the standard deviation. Insets are in the semi-log domain.

adequate. But, examination of the Cone data showed that the disposition profiles were different from the Jeffcoat et al. data, even after taking into account differences in dosing. The concentration–time profiles were quite similar up to about 4 h after dosing but thereafter the Cone data began to diverge leading to a longer terminal elimination half-life than the Jeffcoat et al. data. Hence, these data sets were not directly comparable, possibly because of the different assays used to measure cocaine (high performance liquid chromatography with ultraviolet detection versus gas chromatography with mass spectral detection).

Data sets that are not directly comparable are a common problem in model validation because it is assumed that the validation data set is exchangeable with the model development data set, which may not be the case. In this instance, the two concentration–time profiles were not superimposable after correcting for differences in dose and hence must have different pharmacokinetic models. And if two data sets have different

time courses and models, the question then becomes "Is the model development set more representative of the pharmacokinetics of the drug or is the validation data set?" There is no way to answer this without additional data. But then again, there is no guarantee a third data set will be comparable to either of the previous data sets, which is why model validation is a Gestalt process. Focus cannot center on any particular aspect of the validation but instead must look at the process as a whole.

In summary, model development proceeded from the simplest route of administration (intravenous) to the most complex (intranasal). Model parameters were fixed whenever possible and the additional parameters were then estimated. Only when reasonable estimates for all model parameters were obtained were all parameters estimated simultaneously. Model comparisons were then made against a set of candidate models until a reasonable model was obtained that characterized all routes of administration. Was the final model a universal model applicable to all routes of administration and dosing regimens? Unlikely. Could a better model have been found? Probably. Was the model reasonable, consistent with theory, and interpretable? Yes, and because it was, the final model is useful and can be used as a starting point for pharmacokinetic-pharmacodynamic models.

NONLINEAR REGRESSION CASE STUDY: PHARMACOKINETIC MODELING OF A NEW CHEMICAL ENTITY

In the development of a new chemical entity for the treatment of solid tumors, called Drug X, the drug was given to volunteers as a 15 min intravenous infusion in doses of 10, 20, 33, 50, 70, 90, and 120 mg/m^2, at doses of 100 mg/m^2 for 1 h, and 160 mg/m^2 for 3 h. Serial blood samples were collected for 72 h. Plasma concentrations were averaged by dose (n = 2–6 subjects per group) and are presented in Fig. 5.15 and Table 5.13.

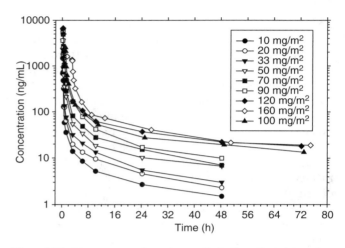

Figure 5.15 Mean concentration—time profile for Drug X administered as an intravenous infusion. Insets are in the semilog domain.

Table 5.13 Mean drug concentrations after intravenous infusion of Drug X.

Dose (mg/m^2)	10	20	33	50	70	90	120	160	100
Sample size	7	3	4	5	6	2	5	4	7
Infusion duration	15 min	15 min	15 min	15 min	15 min	15 min	15 min	3 h	1 h
Time (h)	Drug concentration (ng/mL)								
0	0	0	0	0	0	0	0	0	0
0.17	686	1463	2256	3559	5681	3605	6458		
0.25	725	1789	1471	3575	4919	5771	6686		
0.33	479	1435	895	2341	2690	2452	5009		
0.5	128	319	300	624	944	1935	2029		2390
0.75	58.1	125	134	351	482	812	1114		
1									2529
1.08									2099
1.25	35.6	63.6	76.2	212	283	490	495		962
1.5								1606	622
2									405
3								1358	
3.08								1296	
3.25	13.9	19.8	31.7	54.4	81.7	166	168	750	
3.5								485	
4								320	141
6								163	
6.25	8.5	13.3	20.7	33.9	48.5	78.6	106		
7									86
9								86.0	
10.25	5.2	9.5	13.3	18.4	27.8	42.0	62.1		
11									52.3
13								73.3	
24.25	2.7	4.6	5.5	10.2	15.3	17	37.1		
25									27.5
27								40.7	
48.25	1.5	2.3	3.0	6.7	7.0	9.9	22.2		
49									19.3
51								21.4	
72.25								18.1	
73									13.4
75								18.9	

The plasma concentrations appeared to decline in a biphasic or higher manner. The data were fit using SAAM II under a 2-compartment model with constant coefficient of variation error model. Starting values were estimated using a grid search. Central volume was set to $12 \, \text{L/m}^2$, peripheral volume was set equal to $300 \, \text{L/m}^2$, and both total systemic clearance and intercompartmental clearance were set to $20 (\text{L/h})/\text{m}^2$. A quick plot of the data indicated that the general shape of the model predicted concentrations were what was needed for the fitting, but the observed values were higher than predicted.

The parameter estimates for the 2-compartment model are presented in Table 5.14 with the observed and model fitted data plotted in Fig. 5.16. A plot of observed versus predicted concentrations showed that at higher concentrations there was less agreement between the observed and predicted concentrations. Although the parameter estimates were estimated with good precision, a clear trend in the residual plot was observed. The model predictions tended to overpredict the 24 and 48-h concentration data and there was a slight discrepancy at 72 h although these were only a few data points. The residual plot demonstrated the inadequacy of the 2-compartment model.

Hence, another compartment was added to the 2-compartment model creating a 3-compartment model. The starting value for the new intercompartmental clearance term was the intercompartmental clearance under the 2-compartment model, while the volume of the new compartment was set equal to 1/10, the volume of Compartment 2. The final parameter estimates are shown in Table 5.15 while Fig. 5.17 shows the model fit overlay plot.

The addition of a 3-compartment model dropped the Akaike Information Criterion (AIC) from 5.788 to 5.134. Although the model fit under the 3-compartment model was better than the 2-compartment model, a trend in the weighted residuals versus time plot was still apparent indicating that the model tended to underpredict (from 1 to 12 h), then overpredict (from 20 to

Table 5.14 Final parameter estimates for the data in Table 5.13 under a 2-compartment model expressed in terms of clearance and volume.

Parameter	Model term	Units	Value	Error	CV (%)
Clearance	CL	L/h/m^2	18.8	0.8	4.3
Central volume	V1	L/m^2	12.0	1.0	8.6
Intercompartmental clearance to C2	Q2	L/h/m^2	19.1	1.7	8.7
Compartment 2 (C2) volume	V2	L/m^2	281.9	2.5	9.0

Akaike Information Criterion: 5.788

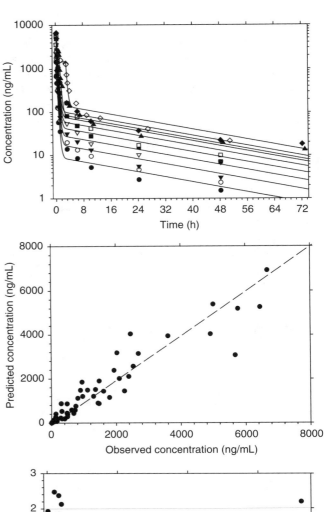

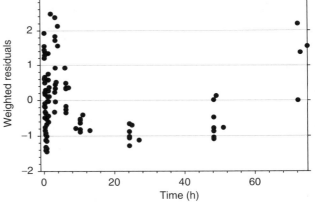

Figure 5.16 Top plot is mean concentration–time profile for Drug X administered as an intravenous infusion (Table 5.13). Solid lines are predicted values based on a 2-compartment model fit to the data. Model parameter estimates are shown in Table 5.14. Middle plot is scatter plot of observed versus predicted concentrations under the fitted model. Bottom plot is weighted residual plot versus time. Insets are in the semi-log domain. Symbols are defined in Fig. 5.15.

50 h), and finally underpredict again (greater than ~50 h). A plot of observed versus predicted concentrations also confirmed that there was some model deviation occurring even with the 3-compartment model.

Table 5.15 Final parameter estimates for the data in Table 5.13 under a 3-compartment model expressed in terms of clearance and volume.

Parameter	Model term	Units	Value	Error	CV (%)
Clearance	CL	$L/h/m^2$	18.4	0.5	2.7
Central volume	V1	L/m^2	6.5	0.5	7.3
Intercompartmental clearance to C2	Q2	$L/h/m^2$	11.8	0.7	5.7
Compartment 2 (C2) volume	V2	L/m^2	353.6	36.5	10.3
Intercompartmental clearance to C3	Q3	$L/h/m^2$	14.6	1.2	8.3
Compartment 3 (C3) volume	V3	L/m^2	20.4	2.0	9.8

Akaike Information Criterion: 5.134

The 3-compartment model was then expanded to a 4-compartment model. The parameter estimates are shown in Table 5.16 while Fig. 5.18 presents the model fit overlay plot. The addition of another compartment decreased the AIC from 5.134 to 4.979, a small change. There was little change in the observed versus predicted plot but the weighted residuals showed less trend over time. At this point, the analyst must make a decision. Was the 3-compartment model better than the 4-compartment model? The answer is not as clear-cut as the choice between the 2- and 3-compartment models. The precision of the parameter estimates under the 3-compartment model was better than the 4-compartment model, but there was less trend in the residual plot of the 4-compartment model. The AIC offered little guidance since the change from a 3-compartment model to a 4-compartment model was a decrease of only 0.155 units. Holistically, the 4-compartment model appeared to be the superior model.

Later, a second study was done wherein subjects were infused with Drug X for 3 h once daily for 5 days with doses of 2, 4, 6.6, 10, 18, and 24 mg/m². Serial plasma samples were collected on Days 1 and 5 with trough samples collected on Days 2–4. The data are presented in Table 5.17. The data from the first and second study were combined and the 4-compartment model was refit. The final parameter estimates are presented in Table 5.18 and plots of the observed data and corresponding model fits are shown in Fig. 5.19. The model predicted fit appeared adequate overall, although some observations were discordant from the model, as shown in the goodness of fit plots (Fig. 5.20). Closer examination of these outliers revealed that they arose predominantly from the 90 mg/m² group. The mean concentrations from this group were based on two subjects and may not have been of adequate sample size to obtain reliable estimates of the concentration—time profile for this dose cohort.

The 90 mg/m² dose group was then removed from the data set and the model was refit. The final parameter

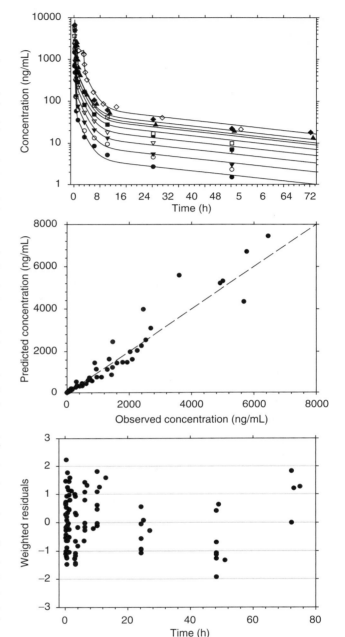

Figure 5.17 Top plot is mean concentration–time profile for Drug X administered as an intravenous infusion (Table 5.13). Solid lines are predicted values based on a 3-compartment model fit to the data. Model parameter estimates are shown in Table 5.15. Middle plot is scatter plot of observed versus predicted concentrations under the fitted model. Bottom plot is weighted residual plot versus time. Insets are in the semilog domain. Symbols are defined in Fig. 5.15.

estimates are presented in Table 5.19. Plots of the observed data and corresponding model predictions to the data are shown in Fig. 5.21. Removal of the 90 mg/m² dose group had little impact on the parameter estimates, although the goodness of fit plots shown in Fig. 5.22 appeared to be better behaved.

Table 5.16 Final parameter estimates for the data in Table 5.13 under a 4-compartment model expressed in terms of clearance and volume.

Parameter	Model term	Units	Value	Error	CV (%)
Clearance	CL	$L/h/m^2$	10.2	1.4	13.7
Central volume	V1	L/m^2	5.8	0.4	7.0
Intercompartmental clearance to C2	Q2	$L/h/m^2$	14.8	1.3	8.7
Compartment 2 (C2) volume	V2	L/m^2	2427.9	541.2	22.2
Intercompartmental clearance to C3	Q3	$L/h/m^2$	8.1	1.1	13.3
Compartment 3 (C3) volume	V3	L/m^2	69.1	20.7	30.0
Intercompartmental clearance to C4	Q4	$L/h/m^2$	12.9	1.2	9.0
Compartment 4 (C4) volume	V4	L/m^2	10.4	1.4	1.3

Akaike Information Criterion: 4.979

As a final test to see if the model might be over-parameterized, a 3-compartment model was fit to the data set without the $90 \, mg/m^2$ dose group. The para-meter estimates under the 3-compartment model are presented in Table 5.20. The model fits and goodness of fit plots will not be shown since they behaved similar to when a 3-compartment model was tested with the first data set. The parameter estimates were more precise, but there was still more trend in the residuals and the model failed to adequately capture the accumulation of Drug X seen with multiple dosing. Hence, it was decided the 4-compartment model would remain the final model with parameter estimates shown in Table 5.19.

To see how well the model performed using an independent data set, the model was used to simulate plasma concentrations of Drug X after 15 min infusions of 17, 25, 35, and $45 \, mg/m^2$ given once weekly for 3 weeks. The data were compared to actual data obtained from a third clinical study (Table 5.21). The observed concentrations and model predicted concentrations are shown in Fig. 5.23. Also, a plot of observed versus predicted concentrations is shown in Fig. 5.24. The average relative error between the observed and predicted

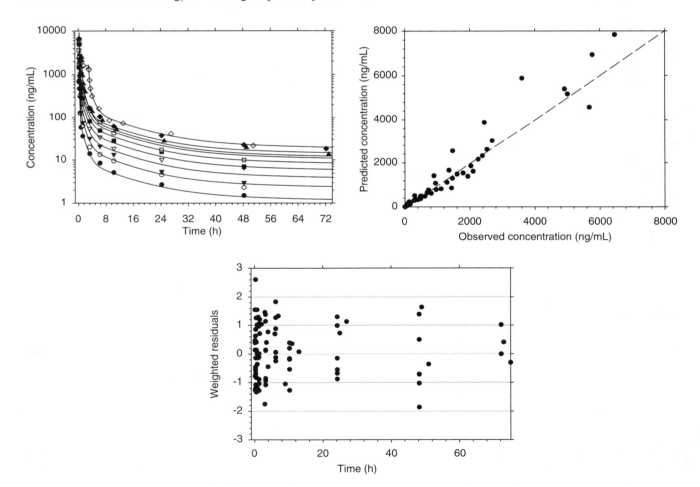

Figure 5.18 Top plot is mean concentration–time profile for Drug X administered as an intravenous infusion (Table 5.13). Solid lines are predicted values based on a 4-compartment model fit to the data. Model parameter estimates are shown in Table 5.16. Middle plot is scatter plot of observed versus predicted concentrations under the fitted model. Bottom plot is weighted residual plot versus time. Insets are in the semi-log domain. Symbols are defined in Fig. 5.15.

Table 5.17 Mean drug concentrations (ng/mL) after a once-weekly 3-h intravenous infusion of drug X.

Day	Time (h)	Relative time (h)	Sample size and dose					
			5 $2\,mg/m^2$	4 $4\,mg/m^2$	2 $6.6\,mg/m^2$	2 $10\,mg/m^2$	4 $18\,mg/m^2$	4 $24\,mg/m^2$
0	0	0	0	0	0	0	0	0
1	1.5	1.5	20.5	56.1	98.5	147.9	187.1	238
1	3	3	11.3	37.8	34.2	146.3	162.2	149.1
1	3.08	3.08	5.7	26.2	22.4	46.6	123.8	88
1	3.25	3.25	4.2	14.8	19.6	26.6	91.8	64.3
1	3.5	3.5	3.5	12.3	17.4	21.2	48.4	59
1	4	4	2.4	10.2	11.6	15.8	37.2	51.1
1	6	6	2	4.5	7.3	13.8	21.9	33.9
1	9	9	1.1	3.4	5.3	10.2	14.6	22.3
1	11	11	0.9		3.8			
2	0	24		1.5	2.3	2.3	6.8	7.3
3	0	48	2.8	2.2	3.7	3.3	8.9	9.3
4	0	72		2.2	4.4	4.2	11.9	12.1
5	0	96	1.9	2.8	4.0	5.7	22.0	69.4
5	1.5	97.5		47.8	105.5	177.1	179.5	294.4
5	3	99		29.8	32.8	110.9	174.6	194.1
5	3.08	99.08		28.8	25.5	53.8	143.3	137.5
5	3.25	99.25		17.8	21.2	36.9	94.0	103.1
5	3.5	99.5		15.1	20.2	33.8	66.5	100.1
5	4	100		14.1	16.8	26.4	51.6	77.4
5	6	102		10.6	12.6	16.9	33.7	56.1
5	9	105		6.7	10.0		24.5	36.1
5	11	107			7.8	13.2		
6	0	120		3.5	5.1	7.0	15.2	
7	0	144		2.0	3.9		13.2	
8	0	168	0.8	2.0	3.0	4.1	8.5	

Table 5.18 Final parameter estimates for the data in Table 5.13 and Table 5.17 under a 4-compartment model expressed in terms of clearance and volume.

Parameter	Model term	Units	Value	Standard error	CV (%)
Clearance	CL	$L/h/m^2$	14.3	1.4	9.5
Central volume	V1	L/m^2	5.6	0.4	6.4
Intercompartmental clearance to C2	Q2	$L/h/m^2$	10.9	0.9	9.6
Compartment 2 (C2) volume	V2	L/m^2	898.3	308.4	34.3
Intercompartmental clearance to C3	Q3	$L/h/m^2$	8.4	0.8	9.6
Compartment 3 (C3) volume	V3	L/m^2	63.7	13.2	20.9
Intercompartmental clearance to C4	Q4	$L/h/m^2$	11.8	1.0	8.5
Compartment 4 (C4) volume	V4	L/m^2	9.4	1.3	13.4

Akaike Information Criterion: 4.056

concentrations was −7.2% with a median of 0.05%. The range of relative errors was −142 to 75%, which was large. A plot of relative error versus predicted concentration (data not shown) indicated that the observations with the largest relative errors were the observations with the smallest concentrations. Overall, the model appeared to adequately characterize the independent data set, but the variability in the prediction was greater as the observed concentration increased and slightly underpredicted higher concentrations. This validation data set had a small number of patients and it may be that the mean concentrations reported were not entirely representative of the dosing groups that were studied.

In summary, this example further illustrated the model building process. Using data on-hand, representative models were examined and the best one was carried forward. With new data, the model was challenged and possibly changed. This process of comparing new models to old models continued throughout until a final candidate model was found. At the end, hopefully the analyst has a model that is useful and can be used to answer questions or test hypotheses about the drug.

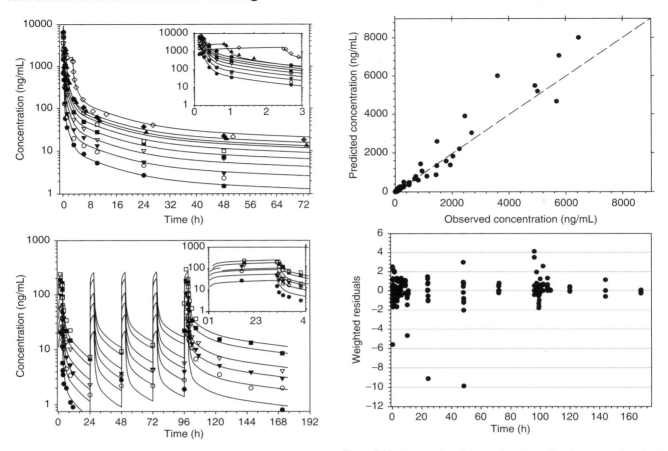

Figure 5.19 Top plot is mean concentration–time profile for Drug X administered as an intravenous infusion (Table 5.13). Bottom plot is mean concentration–time profile for Drug X administered as an intravenous infusion for 3 h. (Table 5.17). Model parameter estimates fitting both data sets simultaneously are shown in Table 5.18. Solid lines are predicted values based on a 4-compartment model fit to the data. Insets are in the semi-log domain. Goodness of fit plots and residual plots are shown in Fig. 5.20.

Figure 5.20 Scatter plot of observed versus predicted concentrations (top) and weighted residuals versus time (bottom) under a 4-compartment model fit to the data presented in Table 5.13 and Table 5.17. Model parameter estimates are shown in Table 5.18.

Table 5.19 Final parameter estimates for the data in Table 5.13 and Table 5.17 after removal the 90 mg/m^2 dose group in Table 5.13 under a 4-compartment model expressed in terms of clearance and volume.

Parameter	Model term	Units	Value	Standard error	CV (%)
Clearance	CL	L/h/m^2	14.4	1.3	9.2
Central volume	V1	L/m^2	5.5	0.4	6.4
Intercompartmental clearance to C2	Q2	L/h/m^2	10.8	0.9	8.4
Compartment 2 (C2) volume	V2	L/m^2	872.3	294.8	33.7
Intercompartmental clearance to C3	Q3	L/h/m^2	8.4	0.8	9.8
Compartment 3 (C3) volume	V3	L/m^2	64.0	13.7	21.4
Intercompartmental clearance to C4	Q4	L/h/m^2	11.6	1.0	8.6
Compartment 4 (C4) volume	V4	L/m^2	9.2	1.3	14.0

Akaike Information Criterion: 3.946

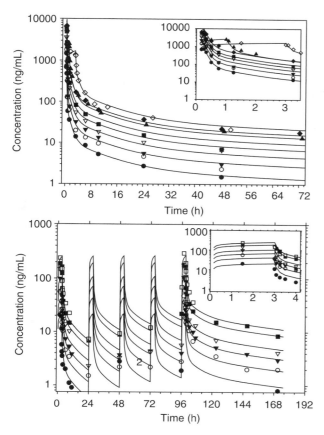

Figure 5.21 Top plot is mean concentration–time profile for Drug X administered as an intravenous infusion (Table 5.13). Bottom plot is mean concentration-time profile for Drug X administered as an intravenous infusion for 3-hours (Data presented in Table 5.17). Solid lines are predicted values based on a 4-compartment model fit to the data. Data from the 90 mg/m² dose group in Table 5.13 have been removed as an outlier dosing group. Model parameter estimates fitting both data sets simultaneously are shown in Table 5.19. Insets are in the semi-log domain. Goodness of fit plots and residual plots are shown in Fig. 5.22.

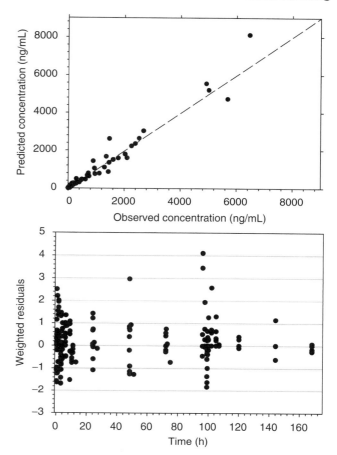

Figure 5.22 Scatter plot of observed versus predicted concentrations (top) and weighted residual plot (bottom) under a 4-compartment model fit to the data in Table 5.13 and Table 5.17 with the 90 mg/m² group removed as an outlier dosing group.

Table 5.20 Final parameter estimates for the data in Table 5.13 and Table 5.17 after removal the 90 mg/m² dose group in Table 5.13 under a 3-compartment model expressed in terms of clearance and volume.

Parameter	Model term	Units	Value	Standard error	CV (%)
Clearance	CL	L/h/m²	16.2	0.4	2.4
Central volume	V1	L/m²	6.5	0.4	6.7
Intercompartmental clearance	Q2	L/h/m²	13.2	0.6	4.7
Peripheral volume	V2	L/m²	481.5	41.2	8.7
Intercompartmental clearance	Q3	L/h/m²	13.3	0.6	7.4
Compartment 3 volume	V3	L/m²	23.1	2.0	8.8

Akaike Information Criterion: 4.017

NONLINEAR REGRESSION CASE STUDY: ASSESSING THE RELATIONSHIP BETWEEN DRUG CONCENTRATIONS AND ADVERSE EVENTS USING LOGISTIC REGRESSION

A common type of pharmacodynamic variable is where the response is not continuous, but qualitative. At its most simple extreme, the response either occurs or does not occur and the variable itself is said to be binary or dichotomous. In this case, the response can be coded using an indicator variable: '0' for the event does not occur or '1' for the event does occur. Many types of pharmacodynamic measures of this kind can be found, most notably with safety and efficacy variables. Theoretical and practical considerations indicate that when the pharmacodynamic measure is binary, the shape of the response function should be curvilinear.

That is, as the independent variable increases, the general shape of the response function is either monotonically increasing to a value of 1 or monotonically

Table 5.21   Mean drug concentrations after a 15 min intravenous infusion of Drug X.

Week	Day	Time	Relative time (h)	3 $17\,\mathrm{mg/m^2}$	3 $25\,\mathrm{mg/m^2}$	2 $35\,\mathrm{mg/m^2}$	2 $45\,\mathrm{mg/m^2}$
1	1	0.17	0.17	759	686	2477	3658
1	1	0.25	0.25	1555	2936	3588	3314
1	1	0.33	0.33	1185	958	3402	2613
1	1	0.5	0.5	587	576	701	994
1	1	0.75	0.75	197	276	287	450
1	1	1.25	1.25	95.7	139	178	258
1	1	3.25	3.25	36.0	31.0	50.1	63.1
1	1	6.25	6.25	18.5	15.7	38.7	32.2
1	1	10.25	10.25	12.7	8.8		19.5
1	1	24.25	24.25	4.7	4.1	15.8	13.0
1	1	48.25	48.25	2.5	2.0	8.1	9.7
3	1	0.00	336.00	1.6	17.6	5.1	5.1
3	1	0.17	336.17	1189	2540	3113	3289
3	1	0.25	336.25	1363	2010	3038	3049
3	1	0.33	336.33	616	987	3045	2324
3	1	0.50	336.50	242	271	1235	1958
3	1	0.75	336.75	150	195	490	539
3	1	1.25	337.25	87.7	95.3	216	274
3	1	3.25	339.25	35.6	33.5	65.5	78.7
3	1	6.25	342.25	20.7	15.5	40.0	39.3
3	1	10.25	346.25	9.8	12.7	30.2	38.6
3	1	24.25	360.25	7.1	8.0	17.1	19.7
3	1	48.25	384.25	4.9	4.8	13.4	14.0
3	1	72.25	408.25	3.7	4.6	10.9	10.9

decreasing to a value of 0 (Fig. 5.25). The response functions plotted in Fig. 5.25 are of the form

$$p(Y = 1) = \frac{\exp(\theta_0 + \theta_1 x)}{1 + \exp(\theta_0 + \theta_1 x)} \qquad (5.21)$$

where $p(Y = 1)$ is the probability of the response occurring. This particular function is called a simple logistic regression model (because there is only one independent variable) and is actually the cumulative distribution function for the logistic distribution. With such a model the response remains relatively constant until a point is reached after which the response changes monotonically to its asymptote. It should be pointed out that while most researchers use the logistic model, there are two competing models, the logit and probit models, that

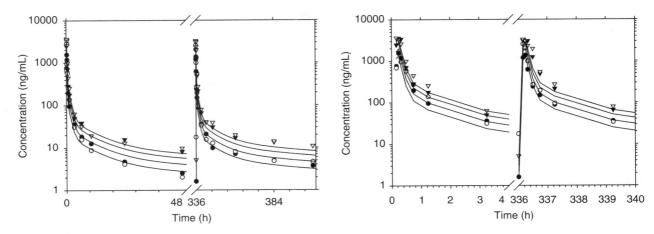

Figure 5.23   Mean concentration–time profile for Drug X administered as an intravenous infusion for 15 min compared to predicted concentrations simulated using a 4-compartment model with parameters found in Table 5.19. Data from Table 5.20. Bottom plot is first 4 h after dosing. A goodness of fit plot is shown in Fig. 5.24.

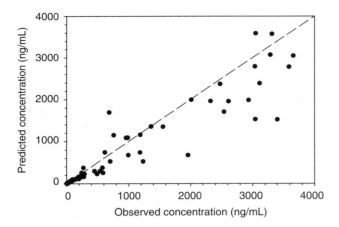

Figure 5.24 Scatter plot of observed versus simulated concentrations for Drug X. Observed concentrations were from an independent data set (Table 5.20). Model predicted concentrations were simulated using the final parameter estimates shown in Table 5.19.

produce almost identical results and for most data sets the three models cannot be distinguished. The reader is referred to Zelterman (1999) for details.

An interesting property of the logistic model is that it can be linearized by the following transformation. If $\pi(x)$ is the probability of the event occurring given x, then

$$g(x) = Ln\left[\frac{\pi(x)}{1 - \pi(x)}\right] = \theta_0 + \theta_1 x. \quad (5.22)$$

Equation (5.22) is referred to as the log-odds ratio or logit of the event occurring. The term in the brackets of Eq. (5.22) is referred to as the odds ratio. In the case of x itself being a binary variable, the log-odds ratio has a simple interpretation: it approximates how much more likely the event Y occurs in subjects with x = 1 than

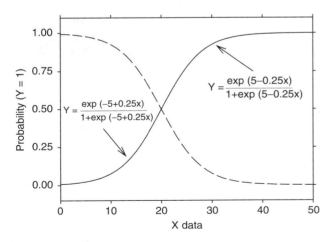

Figure 5.25 Examples of two logistic models. Both models have the same magnitude of parameters but with different signs leading to two different models: one which has decreasing probability with increasing x and the other with increasing probability with increasing x.

among those in which x = 0 on a logarithmic scale. The odds ratio is simply the exponent of the log odds ratio. When x is a continuous random variable, the interpretation of the log-odds ratio is more difficult because a reference point is needed. If x is the reference point, then the change in log odds ratio as x moves to x + c becomes $g(x + c) - g(x) = c\theta$ and the odds ratio then becomes $\exp(c\theta)$. For example, suppose the logit was $-2.73 + 0.2x$. The estimated odds ratio at x = 10 moving from x = 0 is $\exp(0.2 \times 10)$ or 7.4, which means that for every change in x of 10 units, the likelihood of the event occurring increases 7.4 times.

In order to estimate θ, maximum likelihood is often used. If the Y observations are independent then the joint probability or likelihood function is

$$L(\theta) = \prod_{i=1}^{n} \pi_i^{Y_i}(1 - \pi_i)^{1-Y_i}. \quad (5.23)$$

Since it is easier to maximize the log likelihood, Eq. (5.23) is transformed to

$$Ln[L(\theta)] = LL(\theta)$$
$$= \sum_{i=1}^{n} [Y_i Ln(\pi_i) + (1 - Y_i)Ln(1 - \pi_i)].$$
$$(5.24)$$

To find the value of θ that maximizes Eq. (5.24), $LL(\theta)$ is differentiated with respect to θ and the resulting expressions set equal to zero. These are, again, the set of normal equations to solve. Like the general nonlinear regression case, the normal equations for Eq. (5.24) cannot be solved directly, but must be solved iteratively using least squares or some variant thereof.

Also, like linear and nonlinear regression, the same inferences are of interest in logistic regression, e.g., $\theta_1 = 0$, and, also like nonlinear regression, the inferential procedures are based on asymptotic theory. Calculation of the variance–covariance matrix of the parameter estimates in logistic regression is done using methods presented in previous chapters. The standard error of the parameter estimates are then computed as the square root of the diagonal elements of the variance–covariance matrix. Once the standard error of the parameter estimate is obtained, confidence intervals and t-tests can be developed using standard methods. Some programs, such as SAS, do not present t-tests of the parameter estimates. Rather they present chi-squared statistics or Wald tests, which are test statistics that are squared. If $T = \theta/SE(\theta)$ then $\chi^2 = T^2$, which is distributed as a chi-squared random variate with 1 degree of freedom. SAS presents the χ^2 statistics and their corresponding p-values, which are identical to the p-values obtained from a t-test.

It is difficult to summarize a topic like logistic regression into a few paragraphs and an example because the issue is quite complex. Indeed, whole books have been devoted to the topic, one of the most referenced being Hosmer and Lemeshow (1989). Nevertheless, a few more points are worth mentioning. First, once an estimate of θ is obtained, the goodness of fit of the model must be examined and if the fit is adequate, the model should be examined for its predictability and inferential properties. Second, for the logistic regression model, the residuals are unique in that they may take on only the values of 0 or 1. The observation is either predicted or it is not. Hence the sum of squares will always be an integer. Also, the distribution of the residuals will not be normally distributed or centered at zero and any residual plots of predicted values versus residual will not be of value. However, a residual specific for logistic models, called deviance residuals has been developed, which is defined as

$$\text{dev}_i = \pm\sqrt{2[Y_i \text{Ln}(\pi_i) + (1 - Y_i)\text{Ln}(1 - \pi_i)]} \quad (5.25)$$

where the sign of dev is positive if $Y_i \geq \pi_i$ or negative if $Y_i < \pi_i$. Deviance residuals can be thought of as the contribution Y_i makes to the total likelihood. Deviance residuals, although they are not normally distributed, have a useful property in that the sum of squared deviance residuals equals the model deviance, which is akin to the residual sum of squares. A useful plot then is to plot the deviance residual versus index number, i, which may then be used to identify outlying observations. Lastly, influence measures, such as the HAT matrix and DFBETA, have been developed for logistic regression, but are beyond the scope of this section.

Often one does not have a binary variable, but rather a categorical variable with more than two levels. In this case, polychotomous logistic regression can be used. For example, the level of an adverse event may be classified into Grades I to IV. Begg and Gray (1984) have showed that an approximate method to polychotomous logistic regression is to do several binary logistic regressions. For example, with adverse events having Grades I to IV, one would fit the following models:

1. Grade I versus Grade II,
2. Grade I versus Grade III, and
3. Grade I versus Grade IV.

Begg and Gray (1984) showed that the individual parameter estimates are consistent and have relative efficiencies of greater than 90% compared to the model fit using all grade simultaneously. Loss of efficiency generally only occurs when the probability of the baseline category is low.

Now referring back to the previous example of a new oncolytic drug, safety data are collected as part of any clinical trial. In the first study of 42 patients the major adverse events in the study were Grade III or IV myalgia, phlebitis, asthenia, diarrhea, nausea, and vomiting using the National Cancer Institute Common Toxicity Criteria (1999). Of interest was whether the occurrence of any of these events was related to drug concentrations. Using noncompartmental methods, C_{max} and AUC were determined. One patient's AUC could not be calculated and was set equal to missing during the analysis. The data are presented in Table 5.22. Since the infusion rate and duration were quite different among patients, it would be difficult to develop dose-adverse event relationships between the variables. Hence, logistic regression was used to relate AUC and C_{max} to the presence or absence of these adverse events. Age, sex, and baseline performance status at entry in the study were included as covariates in the model. Model development proceeded in two stages. First, a full model was developed using all covariates and either AUC or C_{max}. Because AUC and C_{max} were correlated (Pearson's r: 0.4385, $p < 0.0001$), AUC and C_{max} were not included in the model at the same time to avoid collinearity issues. Covariates that were not significant in the full model at $p < 0.10$ were removed from the model and a reduced model was developed.

The results of the logistic regressions are shown in Table 5.23. Of the five adverse events, only two could be predicted based on pharmacokinetics: myalgia and nausea and vomiting. AUC was a significant predictor of myalgia with increasing AUC leading to increased probability of myalgia. Both AUC and C_{max} were predictive of nausea and vomiting with increasing AUC or C_{max} leading to an increase in the probability of nausea and vomiting. Sex was also predictive of nausea and vomiting with females having a greater baseline probability of nausea and vomiting than males, an observation seen with other drugs. Based on the $-2LL$, AUC gave slightly better predictions than C_{max} (45.756 for AUC versus 48.613 for C_{max}). Figure 5.26 presents the observed and predicted values for the nausea and vomiting data using AUC as the predictor for both males and females along with an index plot of the deviance residuals. None of the deviance residuals were unusual.

Given this information then it may be possible to devise a dosing regimen that minimizes the probability of adverse events. The goal is to find an AUC and C_{max} that minimizes the probability of both adverse events yet keeps AUC as large as possible since for many oncolytics AUC is the driving force for efficacy. Myalgia was a function of AUC, but nausea and vomiting were a function of both AUC and C_{max}. Figure 5.27 presents two plots. The top plot is the model predicted probability of

Table 5.22 Pharmacokinetics, patient characteristics, and adverse event data for a new oncolytic drug.

Subject	Pharmacokinetics		Patient characteristics			Adverse events				
	C_{max}	AUC	Age	Sex	PS	Myalgia	Phlebitis	Asthenia	Diarrhea	Nausea
1	654	442	61	0	0	0	0	0	0	0
2	369	269	52	1	1	0	0	0	1	0
3	800	545	49	0	1	0	0	1	0	0
4	1040	737	53	1	2	0	0	1	0	1
5	852	638	63	1	1	0	0	0	0	1
6	1783	963	60	0	0	0	0	0	0	0
7	1045	656	57	0	0	0	0	0	1	0
8	730	387	43	0	2	0	0	0	0	0
9	767	592	39	0	1	0	0	0	1	0
10	3052	1580	48	0	1	0	0	0	0	0
11	2637	1201	60	1	0	0	0	0	0	0
12	3002	1449	58	0	2	0	0	1	1	0
13	1882	871	44	1	2	0	0	0	0	0
14	1833	1226	67	1	2	0	0	0	0	1
15	3582	2588	55	1	0	0	0	1	1	0
16	3573	1698	60	1	1	0	1	1	1	1
17	7495	4364	74	1	1	0	0	0	1	0
18	5807	3186	60	0	0	0	1	1	0	0
20	1335	2208	57	0	1	0	0	1	0	0
21	3771	2135	40	1	1	0	0	0	0	0
22	6863	4339	55	0	0	0	1	1	0	1
23	6433	3607	68	1	0	0	0	1	0	1
24	8273	5129	66	0	1	0	0	0	0	1
25	3288	2558	61	0	2	0	0	0	1	0
26	3421	1992	50	1	0	0	1	1	0	0
27	5771	5259	53	0	2	0	0	0	1	0
28	2943	3622	73	1	1	1	0	1	1	1
30	5392	6946	37	0	1	0	1	0	0	0
31	5861	6882	56	0	1	1	1	1	0	0
32	7643	Missing	60	0	0	0	0	0	0	1
33	9718	7141	57	1	0	1	0	1	1	1
35	6740	7105	63	0	1	0	0	1	0	1
36	2078	8489	62	0	1	0	0	1	0	1
37	1213	4953	62	1	1	0	0	1	0	0
38	1829	8278	77	1	2	0	1	0	0	0
39	1761	8351	51	1	1	1	0	0	1	1
40	3211	6414	64	0	0	0	0	1	0	0
43	2190	4940	47	1	1	0	0	1	0	1
45	2267	6040	39	1	1	0	0	0	1	1
46	2994	6770	71	0	2	1	1	1	1	1
47	2643	5948	36	0	1	0	0	1	0	0
48	2867	6575	49	0	1	0	1	0	0	0
49	2464	6365	55	0	1	0	0	1	0	0

Legend: C_{max}, maximal drug concentration (ng/mL); AUC, area under the curve from time 0 to infinity (ng*h/mL); age in years; sex: males = 0, females = 1; PS, performance status; myalgia, presence (1) or absence (0) of Grade III or IV myalgia at any time during the trial; phlebitis, presence (1) or absence (0) of Grade III or IV phlebitis at any time during the trial; asthenia, presence (1) or absence (0) of Grade III or IV asthenia at any time during the trial; diarrhea, presence (1) or absence (0) of Grade III or IV diarrhea at any time during the trial; nausea, presence (1) or absence (0) of Grade III or IV nausea and vomiting at any time during the trial.

myalgia and nausea and vomiting in males and females as a function of AUC, and the bottom plot is the probability of nausea and vomiting in males and females as a function of C_{max}. Of the two adverse events, myalgia is a more serious adverse event since nausea and vomiting can be controlled with anti-emetics. To make the exercise more quantitative, what dosing regimen would have a probability of myalgia less than 10% and the probability of nausea and vomiting less than 50%?

The logistic regression model predicted that the probability of myalgia remained essentially constant to about 4000 (ng*h)/mL and then began to increase. A 10% chance of myalgia based on AUC occurred at about 5000 (ng*h)/mL. Because the probability of nausea and vomiting was different between the sexes, different dosing regimens were designed for males and females. The baseline probability of nausea and vomiting in males was about 7 and a 30% probability in nausea and vomit-

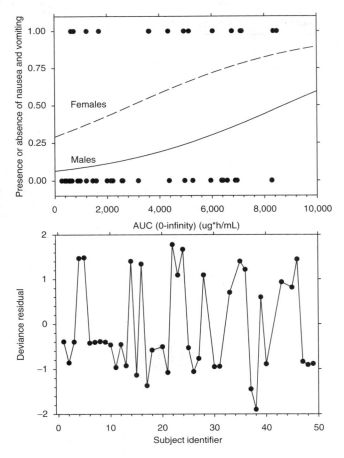

Figure 5.26 Top plot is observed data and fitted models for the nausea and vomiting data in Table 5.22 using AUC as the predictor for both males and females. Bottom plot is an index plot of deviance residuals.

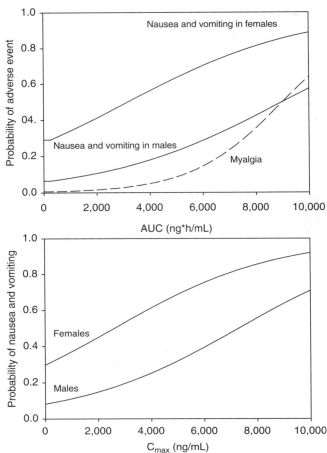

Figure 5.27 Top plot is model predicted probabilities of myalgia (dashed line) and nausea and vomiting (solid line) in males and females as a function of AUC. Bottom plot is model predicted probabilities of nausea and vomiting in males and females as a function of C_{max}.

ing based on AUC occurred at about 6000 ng*h/mL. Since the 5000 ng*h/mL needed for a 10% chance of myalgia was smaller than a 30% chance of nausea and vomiting, the AUC in males after dosing must be no larger than this value. But, nausea and vomiting was also a function of C_{max}. A 30% chance of nausea and vomiting in males based on C_{max} was about 5000 ng/mL. Hence, the desired dosing regimen in males must produce an AUC no larger than 5000 ng*h/mL and a C_{max} no larger than 5000 ng/mL. Using simulation and given the model parameters listed in Table 5.23, that dose was 80 mg/m² administered over 30 min. The model predicted AUC for this regimen was 4747 ng*h/mL with a maximal concentration at the end of infusion of 3744 ng/mL.

The baseline probability of nausea and vomiting in females was about 30% with a 50% chance occurring at about 3000 ng*h/mL. Females had higher baseline probability of nausea and vomiting and reached the maximal accepted percent of subjects experiencing the adverse event with smaller doses than males. Since 3000 ng*h/mL was smaller than the AUC needed for a 10% probability of myalgia, the AUC after dosing must be no larger than this value. A 50% chance of nausea and vomiting based on C_{max} was about 3000 ng/mL. Hence, the desired dosing regimen in females must produce an AUC no larger than 3000 ng*h/mL and a C_{max} no larger than 3000 ng/mL. Using simulation and given the model parameters listed in Table 5.23, that dose was 50 mg/m² administered over 30 min. The model predicted AUC was 2966 ng*h/mL with a maximal concentration at the end of infusion of 2340 ng/mL. Hence, the dosing regimen in males could be increased by 60% because of their greater tolerance for nausea and

Table 5.23 Model parameters from logistic regression analysis of data in Table 5.22.

Dependent variable	Model type	Intercept	C_{max}	AUC	Age	Sex	PS
Myalgia	Full	−6.5172	2.79E-4		0.0425	0.8097	0.5275
	Full	**−8.4067**		**6.38E-4**	0.0492	1.0741	−0.2836
	Reduced	**−5.0233**		**5.90E-4**			
Phlebitis	Full	−2.3339	1.96E-4		7.12E-3	−0.5243	0.1019
	Full	−2.5962		2.78E-4	0.0111	−0.5683	−0.3111
	Reduced	−2.4899		2.80E-4			
Asthenia	Full	−1.4178	6.9E-5		0.0283	−0.1361	−0.4216
	Full	−1.6014		1.86E-4	0.0295	−0.2041	−0.6910
Diarrhea	Full	−2.3341	1.00E-4		5.94E-3	0.8311	0.5541
	Full	−2.1271		−2.27E-6	0.0128	0.7030	0.3943
	Reduced						
Nausea	Full	−5.2820	3.36E-4		0.0445	1.5191	0.3655
	Full	−5.6029		2.90E-4	0.0495	1.7303	0.2205
	Reduced	**−2.4034**	**3.29E-4**			**1.5442**	
	Reduced	**−2.6635**		**3.04E-4**		**1.7722**	

Note: Bolded model parameters are statistically significant at $p < 0.05$.

vomiting compared to females. It should be kept in mind that efficacy was not considered here. It may be that the AUC needed for efficacy was larger than the maximal AUC that could be given to minimize the drug's side effects, in which case the drug may not be able to achieve efficacy without an unacceptable percent of subjects showing adverse events.

SUMMARY

This chapter presented many case studies in the application of linear and nonlinear modeling to real-life data sets. Some of the examples were relatively simple, whereas some were quite complex As might be apparent, there is no right approach to any problem and that the more complex the problem, the more approaches there are to solving a problem, none of them being the correct one. Hopefully the reader will begin to appreciate the power of modeling in being able to answer questions, "explain" data, and answer "what-if" questions.

Recommended Reading

Begg, C.B. and Gray, R. Calculation of polychotomous logistic and regression parameters using individualized regressions. *Biometrika* 1984; 71: 11–18.

Chappell, W.R. and Mordenti, J. Extrapolation of toxicological and pharmacological data from animals to humans. In: Testa, B. ed. *Advances in drug research*. New York: Academic, 1990: 1–116.

Gough, K., Hutcheson, M., Keene, O., Byrom, B., Ellis, S., and Lacey L. et al. Assessment of dose proportionality: Report from the statisticians in the pharmaceutical industry/pharmacokinetics UK Joint Working Party. *Drug Information Journal* 1995; 29: 1039–1048.

Hosmer, D.W. and Lemeshow, S. *Applied logistic regression*. New York: Wiley, 1989.

Smith, B.P., Vandenhende, F.R., DeSante, K.A., Farid, N.A., Welch, P.A., and Callaghan, J.T. et al. Confidence interval criteria for assessment of dose proportionality. *Pharmaceutical Research* 2000; 20: 1278–1283.

Chapter 6

Linear Mixed Effects Models

Truth is a thing of beauty. A beautiful model is not truth.

—the author with acknowledgements to Timothy Ferris (1944–), Popular science writer

INTRODUCTION

Linear mixed effects models are not commonly seen in analysis of pharmacokinetic data, but are more commonly seen in the analysis of pharmacodynamic data. Still, a good understanding of linear mixed effects models will lead to a better grasp of the nonlinear case, under which most population pharmacokinetic models are developed. The purpose of this chapter will be to introduce fixed and random effects, how they relate to linear mixed effects models, and to illustrate the use of these models in practice. For further details on linear mixed effects models, the reader is referred to the following texts. Verbeke and Molenberghs (1997, 2000) present excellent overviews on linear mixed models applied to longitudinal data, as does Fitzmaurice, Laird, and Ware (2004). Davidian and Gallant (1995) present these models as part of a comprehensive coverage of nonlinear models for repeated measures data. Longford presents a comprehensive overview of random coefficients models (1993). Another excellent book, one for the S-Plus system, is Pinheiro and Bates (2000).

In the chapters on Linear and Nonlinear Regression, it was assumed that the responses were independent, even within the same subject. With mixed effects models, the data are often longitudinal in nature, in the sense that multiple measurements are made on the same subject[1] over time. Responses may be unequally spaced, with an unequal number of observations per subject, and within a subject are often correlated. Also in the previous chapters it was assumed that any covariates, e.g., age, creatinine clearance, etc., were constant over time. With mixed effects models, this assumption is relaxed to allow the covariates to become time varying. For example, weight may be measured only at the beginning of a study, whereas hepatic enzymes may be measured throughout the study. In this case, weight is treated as a constant for a patient across time, but hepatic enzyme values may change as the study progresses. Hence, mixed effects models allow greater control over the sources of variability in a study, as well as incorporating patient-specific characteristics into the model making them far more flexible than the fixed effect models used in previous chapters.

FIXED EFFECTS, RANDOM EFFECTS, AND MIXED EFFECTS

In a designed experiment, whether a variable is a fixed or random effect depends on whether a researcher has control over that variable. A *fixed effect* is one where the researcher can choose the level(s) of the variable to represent the precise contrast of interest. For example, the doses of drug used in a study or the time points that

---

[1] The word "subject" will be used generically referring to an experimental unit, not necessarily to "subject" in the human sense.

blood samples are measured represent fixed effects. Fixed effect variables are also those whose levels in a study represent an exhaustive set of all possible levels. For example, using both males and females exhausts the possible levels of this variable, thus making sex a fixed effect.

Random effects are variables whose levels do not exhaust the set of possible levels and each level is equally representative of other levels. Random effects often represent nuisance variables whose precise value are not usually of interest, but are arbitrary samples from a larger pool of other equally possible samples. In other words, if it makes no difference to the researcher which specific levels of a factor are used in an experiment, it is best to treat that variable as a random effect. The most commonly seen random effect in clinical research are the subjects used in an experiment since in most cases researchers are not specifically interested in the particular set of subjects that were used in a study, but are more interested in generalizing the results from a study to the population at large.

To further delineate a random effect from a fixed effect, suppose a researcher studied the effect of a drug on blood pressure in a group of patients. Ignoring for a moment the specifics of how one measures blood pressure or quantifies the drug effect, if the researcher was interested in only those patients used in the study, then those patients would be considered a fixed effect. If, however, the researcher wanted to make generalizations to the patient population, and the patients that were used in the experiment were a random sample from the patient population, then patients would be considered a random effect. With that distinction now made, any linear model that contains both fixed and random effects is a linear mixed effects model.

SOURCES OF VARIABILITY

Most pharmacokinetic and pharmacodynamic data are longitudinal in nature, i.e., subjects are repeatedly measured on some variable over time, e.g., drug concentrations, blood pressure, etc. What follows will be based on this experimental design, although most of the materials can be applied to linear mixed effects models in general. Consider the following situation. A researcher weighs three subjects (in lbs.) on three occasions, one min apart. The data are presented in Table 6.1. Obviously, there is variability both within a subject and between subjects. Since the measurements were made only one min apart, it seems unlikely that a person's weight could fluctuate by 3 lbs (Subjects 2 and 3) in that time interval. Hence, the deviations within a subject must be

due to random, measurement error. A model for such a situation would be

$$Y_{ij} = \mu + S_i + \varepsilon_{ij} \tag{6.1}$$

where Y_{ij} is the jth measurement on the ith subject, $j = 1, 2, 3$ and $i = 1, 2, 3$; μ is the population mean, S_i the deviation of the ith subject from the population mean, and ε_{ij} the random deviation of the jth measurement from $\mu + S_i$. Because both S_i and ε_{ij} vary among individuals (and within individuals in the case of e_{ij}), they are random. A natural estimator for μ would be the grand mean of all observations

$$\hat{\mu} = \frac{\sum_{i=1}^{3} \sum_{j=1}^{3} Y_{ij}}{9} \tag{6.2}$$

and a natural estimator for S_i would be the average deviation a subject shows from the grand mean,

$$S_i = \bar{Y}_{i.} - \hat{\mu} \tag{6.3}$$

where $\bar{Y}_i$ is the average of all the measurements within a subject. The random error, ε_{ij}, would then be estimated by the deviation of an observed value from the expected value for that subject

$$\varepsilon_{ij} = Y_{ij} - \hat{\mu} - \bar{S}_i. \tag{6.4}$$

This is illustrated in Table 6.1. Note that the expected value, which is a measure of central tendency or population mean, of a linear model is the sum of the expectations, so that for Eq. (6.1)

$$E(Y) = E(\mu) + E(S_i) + E(\varepsilon_{ij}). \tag{6.5}$$

Assuming the S_i's across subjects sum to zero and ε_{ij}'s within a subject sum to zero, then

$$E(Y) = \mu \tag{6.6}$$

and

$$E(Y_i|S_i) = \mu + S_i. \tag{6.7}$$

Notice the difference between E(Y), the expected value for an individual randomly sampled from Y, and $E(Y_i|S_i)$, the expected value for a particular individual. If the expected value of individuals in their most general sense is of interest, then E(Y) is of interest. But as soon as the discussion moves to particular subjects, then $E(Y_i|S_i)$ becomes of interest.

Table 6.1 Example of between- and within-subject variability for individual weight measurements.

Subject (i)	Measurement (Y_{ij})			Mean (Y_i)	Deviation from the mean (S_i)
	Weight (1)	Weight (2)	Weight (3)		
1	190	191	189	190	17
2	154	154	157	155	−18
3	176	173	173	174	1
			Grand mean:	173	
Random errors (e_{ij}):					
	0	1	−1		
	−1	−1	2		
	2	−1	−1		

The generic equation for the variance of a linear combination of random variables is

$$\text{Var}\left(\sum_{i=1}^{k} a_i Y_i\right) =$$
$$\sum_{i=1}^{k} a_i^2 \text{Var}(Y_i) + 2\sum\sum_{i<j} a_i a_j \text{Cov}(Y_i, Y_j) \tag{6.8}$$

where $\text{Cov}(Y_i, Y_j)$ denotes the covariance between Y_i and Y_j. Assuming that the subject specific random effects are independent of the measurement errors, then

$$\text{Var}(Y) = \text{Var}(\mu) + \text{Var}(S) + \text{Var}(\varepsilon). \tag{6.9}$$

Since the variance of μ is zero, i.e., the population mean is a constant, then the variability of Y is

$$\text{Var}(Y) = \text{Var}(S) + \text{Var}(\varepsilon) = \sigma_s^2 + \sigma_\varepsilon^2 \tag{6.10}$$

or the total variability is equal to the variability between-subjects plus the variability within-subjects. Also, the variability within a subject is

$$\text{Var}(Y_i | S_i) = \sigma_\varepsilon^2. \tag{6.11}$$

Hence, Y has mean μ and variance $\sigma_s^2 + \sigma_\varepsilon^2$, or in mathematical notation, $Y \sim (\mu, \sigma_s^2 + \sigma_\varepsilon^2)$ and $Y_i \sim (\mu + S_i, \sigma_\varepsilon^2)$. Notice that at this point no assumptions regarding the distribution of Y have been made (normality or any such thing). σ_s^2 is often referred to as between-subject variability and reflects the variability in subject specific scores around μ. σ_ε^2 is sometimes called either intrasubject, within-subject or residual variability, because it represents variability that cannot be explained by some predictor variable and is a reflection of the variability of scores around a subject's true score, $\mu + S_i$. The reason residual variability cannot be explained is that it is im-

possible to determine if the deviation of Y_{ij} from $\mu + S_i$ is really measurement error or due to true random variability within a subject.

Now suppose that subjects are randomized into two treatment groups, a placebo group and a treatment group given a drug that causes weight loss. Equation (6.1) would be modified to include an effect due to the drug or placebo

$$Y_{ij} = \mu + S_i + \tau_k + \varepsilon_{ij} \tag{6.12}$$

where τ_k, k = 1 or 2, represents the treatment effect. In this case, the treatment effect is a fixed constant among subjects assigned to that group. Thus, Eq. (6.12) has both fixed effects (treatment effect) and random effects (subjects) and is referred to as linear mixed effect model.

A TWO-STAGE ANALYSIS

Since pharmacokinetic analyses are longitudinal in nature, the linear mixed effect model will be developed using a repeated measures approach, although the more general results apply to mixed effects models not involving repeated measures. The notation that will be used will be consistent with the statistical software package SAS, which is the leading software program used in the analysis of linear mixed effects models. In the first stage of the analysis, let Y_i be the $n_i \times 1$ vector of all the repeated measures data for the ith subject, i = 1, 2, ... k. Then the first stage is to model the Y_i for each subject as

$$Y_i = z_i \beta_i + \varepsilon_i \tag{6.13}$$

where z_i is an $n_i \times q$ matrix of known, fixed effect covariates modeling how the subject response changes over time (time-varying covariates), β_i is a vector of size q of subject-specific regression parameters, and ε_i is $n_i \times 1$ vector of subject specific residual errors, usually assumed to be normally distributed, independent, identically distributed, having mean zero and variance R_i, i.e., $\varepsilon_i \sim N(0, R_i)$. In the second stage, the β_i is modeled using multivariate regression

$$\beta_i = k_i\beta + U_i \qquad (6.14)$$

where k_i is an $n \times p$ matrix of known, fixed effect covariates for the ith subject, β is a vector of size p of unknown population regression parameters (note: $\beta \neq \beta_i$), and U_i is the vector of residual errors assumed to be normally distributed, independent and identically distributed with mean zero and general covariance matrix G_i, i.e., $U_i \sim N(0, G_i)$. U_i is the deviations of the ith subject from the population mean β.

Thus, the two-stage approach is to first summarize each subject individually and then use regression methods to summarize the so-called summary statistics for each subject using relevant covariates. However, the two-stage approach is not entirely satisfactory nor is it entirely valid (Verbeke and Molenberghs, 2000). First, it is not entirely satisfactory because information is lost when summarizing Y_i into β_i. Second, if the parameters of interest are in Eq. (6.14), then additional variability is added by the estimation of β_i, which is not taken into account during the regression analysis of Eq. (6.14). Also, the covariance matrix of $\hat{\beta}_i$ depends on the number of measurements in Y_i, as well as the time points at which the measurements were collected—an effect that is not taken into account in the second stage. Hence a more general approach to the model needs to be developed.

THE GENERAL LINEAR MIXED EFFECTS MODEL

The problems inherent in the two-stage approach can be avoided by combining Eqs. (6.13) and (6.14) to yield

$$\begin{aligned} Y_i &= z_i\beta_i + \varepsilon_i \\ &= z_i(k_i\beta + U_i) + \varepsilon_i \\ &= z_ik_i\beta + z_iU_i + \varepsilon_i \\ &= x_i\beta + z_iU_i + \varepsilon_i \end{aligned} \qquad (6.15)$$

where $x_i = z_ik_i$ is an $n_i \times p$ matrix of known fixed effect covariates specific to the ith individual. Equation (6.15) can be thought of as the sum of the population mean, deviation from the population mean, and deviation from the subject mean

$$Y_i = \underbrace{x_i\beta}_{\substack{\text{Population} \\ \text{Mean}}} + \underbrace{z_iU_i}_{\substack{\text{Subject} \\ \text{specific} \\ \text{deviation} \\ \text{from} \\ \text{population} \\ \text{mean}}} + \underbrace{\varepsilon_i}_{\substack{\text{Random} \\ \text{deviation} \\ \text{from} \\ \text{subject} \\ \text{mean}}} \qquad (6.16)$$

Figure 6.1 illustrates this relationship graphically for a 1-compartment open model plotted on a semi-log scale for two different subjects. Equation (6.15) has fixed effects β and random effects U_i. Note that if $z = 0$, then Eq. (6.15) simplifies to a general linear model. If there are no fixed effects in the model and all model parameters are allowed to vary across subjects, then Eq. (6.16) is referred to as a random coefficients model. It is assumed that U is normally distributed with mean 0 and variance G (which assesses between-subject variability), ε is normally distributed with mean 0 and variance R (which assesses residual variability), and that the random effects and residuals are independent. Sometimes R is referred to as within-subject or intrasubject variability but this is not technically correct because within-subject variability is but one component of residual variability. There may be other sources of variability in R, sometimes many others, like model misspecification or measurement variability. However, in this book within-subject variability and residual variability will be used interchangeably. Notice that the model assumes that each subject follows a linear regression model where some parameters are population-specific and others are subject-specific. Also note that the residual errors are "within-subject" errors.

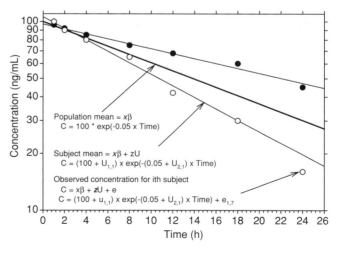

Figure 6.1 Plot demonstrating the relationship between the population mean, subject mean, and deviation from the subject mean for two different subjects using a 1-compartment open model plotted on a semilog scale.

By stacking all the Y_i's, x_i's, and z_i's, the complete model across all individuals can be written as

$$Y = x\beta + zU + \varepsilon, \qquad (6.17)$$

where Y is an $n \times 1$ vector of observations for the k subjects, x an $n \times p$ matrix of fixed effects, β a p-size vector of parameter estimates associated with the fixed effects, z an $n \times q$ matrix of random effects, U a q-size vector of parameter estimates associated with the random effects, ε an $n \times 1$ vector of residual for the k subjects, and n the total number of observations for all k subjects. It is assumed that $\beta \sim N(0, G)$, $\varepsilon \sim N(0, R)$, and $u_1, u_2, \ldots u_n$ is independent of $\varepsilon_1, \varepsilon_2, \ldots \varepsilon_n$. The matrices G and R are collectively referred to as the *variance components* of the model.

It follows that conditional on the random effects, the expected value for the ith subject is

$$E(Y_i | U_i) = x_i \beta + z_i U_i \qquad (6.18)$$

which is normally distributed with variance

$$Var(Y_i | U_i) = R_i. \qquad (6.19)$$

Equations (6.18) and (6.19) is referred to as the conditional model and implies that $Y \sim N(x\beta + zU, R)$. However, inference is not done on the conditional model but instead on the marginal distribution, which is obtained by integrating out the random effects. Under the marginal distribution, the expected value for the ith subject is

$$E(Y_i) = x_i \beta \qquad (6.20)$$

which is normally distributed with variance

$$Var(Y_i) = R_i + z_i G z_i^T = V_i. \qquad (6.21)$$

Hence, the marginal model implies that $Y \sim N(x\beta, zGz^T + R)$. Inference is based on this marginal model unless the data are analyzed within a Bayesian framework. The major difference between the conditional model and marginal model is that the conditional model is conditioned on the random effects, whereas the marginal model does not depend on the random effects. So, the expected value for a subject is the population mean in the absence of further information (the random effects), and the variance for that subject is the total variance, not just the within-subject variance, without any further knowledge on that subject.

As an example, consider a study where four subjects are dosed with an intravenous bolus solution of a drug that follows 1-compartment kinetics and plasma samples are collected at 1-, 2-, and 5-h post-dose. If the natural-log transformed drug concentrations are analyzed, the log-transformed plasma concentration–time profiles for each subject should follow a simple linear regression model

$$Ln(C) = \beta_0 + \beta_1 t + \varepsilon \qquad (6.22)$$

where C is the concentration, t the time, ε the residual error,

$$\beta_0 = Ln\left(\frac{Dose}{V_d}\right), \qquad (6.23)$$

V_d is the volume of distribution, and the negative of β_1 is the elimination rate constant. A linear mixed effect model is appropriate for this dataset. In this case, Y_i is a 3×1 vector of responses for each subject stacked on top of each other creating a Y vector with 12 rows. The other matrices are

$$x_i = \begin{bmatrix} 1 & 1 \\ 1 & 2 \\ 1 & 5 \end{bmatrix}, \beta = \begin{bmatrix} \beta_0 \\ \beta_1 \end{bmatrix}, \qquad (6.24)$$

z_i is a 3×4 matrix. x and z are all the x_i and z_i matrices, respectively, stacked on top of each other. Thus,

$$x = \begin{bmatrix} 1 & 1 \\ 1 & 2 \\ 1 & 5 \\ 1 & 1 \\ 1 & 2 \\ 1 & 5 \\ 1 & 1 \\ 1 & 2 \\ 1 & 5 \\ 1 & 1 \\ 1 & 2 \\ 1 & 5 \end{bmatrix}, z = \begin{bmatrix} 1 & 0 & 0 & 0 \\ 1 & 0 & 0 & 0 \\ 1 & 0 & 0 & 0 \\ 1 & 1 & 0 & 0 \\ 1 & 1 & 0 & 0 \\ 1 & 1 & 0 & 0 \\ 1 & 0 & 1 & 0 \\ 1 & 0 & 1 & 0 \\ 1 & 0 & 1 & 0 \\ 1 & 0 & 0 & 1 \\ 1 & 0 & 0 & 1 \\ 1 & 0 & 0 & 1 \end{bmatrix} U = \begin{bmatrix} U_1 \\ U_2 \\ U_3 \\ U_4 \end{bmatrix}, \varepsilon = \begin{bmatrix} \varepsilon_{11} \\ \varepsilon_{12} \\ \varepsilon_{13} \\ \varepsilon_{21} \\ \varepsilon_{22} \\ \varepsilon_{23} \\ \varepsilon_{31} \\ \varepsilon_{32} \\ \varepsilon_{33} \\ \varepsilon_{41} \\ \varepsilon_{42} \\ \varepsilon_{43} \end{bmatrix}.$$

$$(6.25)$$

The G matrix is then a diagonal matrix of size 4, i.e., the number of subjects,

$$G = \begin{bmatrix} G_1 & 0 & 0 & 0 \\ & G_2 & 0 & 0 \\ & & G_3 & 0 \\ & & & G_4 \end{bmatrix} = \begin{bmatrix} \sigma_1^2 & 0 & 0 & 0 \\ & \sigma_1^2 & 0 & 0 \\ & & \sigma_1^2 & 0 \\ & & & \sigma_1^2 \end{bmatrix}. \qquad (6.26)$$

The residual matrix for each individual, R_i, is a diagonal matrix of size 3, the number of observations,

$$R_i = \sigma^2 \begin{bmatrix} 1 & 0 & 0 \\ 0 & 1 & 0 \\ 0 & 0 & 1 \end{bmatrix}. \quad (6.27)$$

R then becomes a 12×12 matrix of R_i matrices

$$R = \sigma^2 \begin{bmatrix} 1 & 0 & 0 & & & & & & \\ 0 & 1 & 0 & & & & & & \\ 0 & 0 & 1 & & & & & & \\ & & & 1 & 0 & 0 & & & \\ & & & 0 & 1 & 0 & & & \\ & & & 0 & 0 & 1 & & & \\ & & & & & & 1 & 0 & 0 \\ & & & & & & 0 & 1 & 0 \\ & & & & & & 0 & 0 & 1 \\ & & & & & & & & & 1 & 0 & 0 \\ & & & & & & & & & 0 & 1 & 0 \\ & & & & & & & & & 0 & 0 & 1 \end{bmatrix}. \quad (6.28)$$

Not shown in Eq. (6.28) are all the remaining off-diagonal zero elements. Notice in Eq. (6.26) that the off-diagonal elements of G are zero, an indication that subjects are independent. Hence, diagonal elements of V, which is a 12×12 matrix, are

$$V_{ii} = \sigma^2 + \sigma_1^2 \quad (6.29)$$

with zero off-diagonal elements. In simplified terms, the total variance for Y is

$$\text{Var}(Y) = \sigma_1^2 + \sigma^2, \quad (6.30)$$

which is the sum of the between-subject and within-subject variability.

In the model presented above, the R matrix elements, or matrix of within-subject errors, are uncorrelated and of constant variance across all subjects. When this is the case, Eq. (6.15) is sometimes called the conditional independence model since it assumes that responses for the ith subject are independent of and conditional on the U_i's and β. At times, however, this may be an unrealistic assumption since it seems more likely that observations within a subject are correlated. For example, if the model were misspecified, then parts of the data over time would be more correlated than other parts (Karlsson, Beal, and Sheiner, 1995). Hence, it is more realistic to allow the within-subject errors to be correlated.

A variety of within-subject covariance matrices have been proposed (Table 6.2). The most common are the simple, unstructured, compound symmetry, first-order autoregressive [referred to as AR(1)], and Toeplitz covariance. The simple covariance assumes that observations within a subject are uncorrelated and have constant variance, like in Eq. (6.28). Unstructured assumes

Table 6.2 Structures of common within-subject covariance structures assuming three measurements per subject.

Structure	Example
Simple	$\begin{bmatrix} \sigma^2 & 0 & 0 \\ & \sigma^2 & 0 \\ & & \sigma^2 \end{bmatrix}$
Unstructured	$\begin{bmatrix} \sigma_{11}^2 & \sigma_{12}^2 & \sigma_{13}^2 \\ & \sigma_{21}^2 & \sigma_{23}^2 \\ & & \sigma_{33}^2 \end{bmatrix}$
Compound symmetry	$\begin{bmatrix} \sigma_1^2 + \sigma^2 & \sigma_1^2 & \sigma_1^2 \\ & \sigma_1^2 + \sigma^2 & \sigma_1^2 \\ & & \sigma_1^2 + \sigma^2 \end{bmatrix}$
First-order autoregressive	$\begin{bmatrix} \sigma^2 & \rho\sigma^2 & \rho^2\sigma^2 \\ & \sigma^2 & \rho\sigma^2 \\ & & \sigma^2 \end{bmatrix}$
Toeplitz	$\begin{bmatrix} \sigma^2 & \sigma_{12}^2 & \sigma_{13}^2 \\ & \sigma^2 & \sigma_{23}^2 \\ & & \sigma^2 \end{bmatrix}$

Note: σ refers to variances and covariances and ρ refers to correlations. More structures are available. See Wolfinger (1993) for details and additional structures.

no structure to the covariance that all variances and covariances are uncommon and unique to each subject. The problem with unstructured covariance matrices is that their use may sometimes lead to negative diagonal variance components, which cannot occur in reality. Compound symmetry assumes that the correlation between measurements is a constant. AR(1) assumes that measurements within a subject have a constant variance but are correlated with the correlation decreasing in proportion to the square of the correlation as time between measurements increases. For example, AR(1) assumes that the correlation between Measurement 1 and Measurement 2 is equal to ρ, that the correlation between measurement 1 and measurement 3 is ρ^2, etc. AR(1) is useful when the time interval between measurements is equal. For instance, in the prior example, there was 1 h between the measurement of the 1- and 2-h samples, and 3 h between the measurement of the 2- and 5-h samples. Hence, an AR(1) covariance may be inappropriate since the correlation between the first and second measurement may be greater than the correlation between the second and third measurement. A Toeplitz covariance assumes equal variance across measurements but unequal covariances. The difference between an unstructured and Toeplitz covariance is that the former assumes the variance between and among measurements is different, whereas the Toeplitz assumes the between measurement variances are the same but the covariances may be different.

There is another class of functions that assumes that ε_i can be decomposed into two components, one ($\varepsilon_{(1)i}$)

Table 6.3 Structures of common spatial covariance structures assuming three measurements per subject.

Structure	Example
Spatial power	$\sigma^2 \begin{bmatrix} 1 & \rho^{d_{12}} & \rho^{d_{13}} \\ & 1 & \rho^{d_{23}} \\ & & 1 \end{bmatrix}$
Spatial exponential	$\sigma^2 \begin{bmatrix} 1 & \exp\left(-\frac{d_{12}}{\rho}\right) & \exp\left(-\frac{d_{13}}{\rho}\right) \\ & 1 & \exp\left(-\frac{d_{23}}{\rho}\right) \\ & & 1 \end{bmatrix}$
Spatial Gaussian	$\sigma^2 \begin{bmatrix} 1 & \exp\left(-\frac{d_{12}^2}{\rho^2}\right) & \exp\left(-\frac{d_{13}^2}{\rho^2}\right) \\ & 1 & \exp\left(-\frac{d_{23}^2}{\rho^2}\right) \\ & & 1 \end{bmatrix}$

Note: σ refers to variances and covariances and ρ refers to correlations. d_{ij} is the Euclidean distance between the ith and jth measurement. More structures are available. See Wolfinger (1993) for details and additional structures.

has constant variance and the other is a component of serial correlation ($\varepsilon_{(2)i}$), such that $\varepsilon_i = \varepsilon_{(1)i} + \varepsilon_{(2)i}$ with $\varepsilon_{(1)i}$ and $\varepsilon_{(2)i}$ being independent. The covariance matrices generated from this decomposition are referred to as spatial covariances. Three examples are the Gaussian, exponential, and power functions (Table 6.3 and presented graphically in Fig. 6.2). These functions all have decreasing correlation between measurements with increasing time separating measurements, have a correlation of 1 when the time distance is 0, and a correlation of zero when the time interval between measurements is infinite. The advantage of these functions is that if subjects are sampled at unequal time intervals or if the subjects are measured at the same time and are unequally spaced, then the correlation structure between measurements can still be estimated.

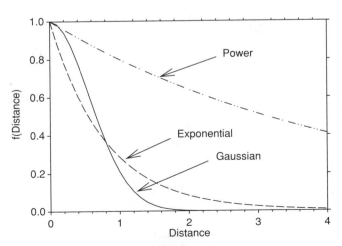

Figure 6.2 Plot of exponential, Gaussian, and power serial correlation functions as a function of distance between measurements. The underlying correlation between measurements was 0.8.

ESTIMATION OF THE MIXED EFFECT MODEL PARAMETERS

In the case of the mixed effects model, not only does β get estimated, but so do U and V which requires an estimate of G and R. Thus, estimation using least squares is no longer appropriate, whereas generalized least squares, which minimizes

$$(Y - x\beta)^T V^{-1}(Y - x\beta), \qquad (6.31)$$

is more appropriate. In order to minimize this function a reasonable estimate of V, and hence G and R, must be made. G and R are usually best estimated by likelihood based methods, either maximum likelihood (ML) or restricted maximum likelihood (REML), which take advantage of the assumption that the random effects and residuals are normally distributed. ML maximizes the log-likelihood objective function

$$LL(G, R) = -\frac{1}{2}Ln|V| - \frac{1}{2}q^T V^{-1}q - \frac{n}{2}\left[1 + Ln\left(\frac{2\pi}{n}\right)\right] \qquad (6.32)$$

while REML maximizes

$$LL(G, R) = -\frac{1}{2}Ln|V| - \frac{1}{2}Ln|x^T V^{-1}x| - \frac{n-p}{2}q^T V^{-1}q - \frac{n-p}{2}\left[1 + Ln\left(\frac{2\pi}{n-p}\right)\right] \qquad (6.33)$$

where $q = Y - x(x^T V^{-1}x)^{-1}x^T V^{-1}Y$, $|.|$ is the determinant function, and p is the rank of x, e.g., the number of estimated fixed effects. Rather than maximize the log-likelihood function directly, most software programs minimize -2 times the log-likelihood function ($-2LL$) for greater numerical stability and that it is easier to find the minimum of a function rather than its maximum. Notice that Eq. (6.33) requires the inverse of $x^T V^{-1}x$ for its solution, which may lead to unstable inverse matrices or may not exist at all. The reader is referred to Searle (1997), Verbeke and Molenberghs (1997), and Littell et al. (1996) for further details. The solution to the linear mixed effect model also assumes that the parameters of G, the covariance matrix of the random effects, are positive semidefinite and that R is positive definite.[2]

Most programs actually minimize $-2LL$ of these functions using a Newton–Raphson method. Littell et al. (1996) indicate that the advantage of using a

---

[2] A symmetric matrix is positive semidefinite if all its eigenvalues are nonnegative. A positive definite matrix is one where all its eigenvalues are strictly positive and nonzero.

Newton–Raphson approach, as opposed to other methods, such as an expectation–maximization approach, is that the matrix of second derivatives of the objective function, evaluated at the optima, is immediately available. By denoting this matrix, H, $2H^{-1}$, is an asymptotic variance–covariance matrix of the estimated parameters G and R. Another method to estimate G and R is the noniterative MIVQUE0 method. Using Monte Carlo simulation, Swallow and Monahan (1984) have shown that REML and ML are better estimators than MIVQUE0, although MIVQUE0 is better when REML and ML methods fail to converge.

Once an estimate of G and R are obtained, denoted $\hat{G}$ and $\hat{R}$, respectively, β and U are usually estimated by simultaneously solving the mixed model equations

$$\begin{bmatrix} x^T\hat{R}^{-1}x & x^T\hat{R}^{-1}z \\ z^T\hat{R}^{-1}x & z^T\hat{R}^{-1}z + \hat{G}^{-1} \end{bmatrix} \begin{bmatrix} \hat{\beta} \\ \hat{u} \end{bmatrix} = \begin{bmatrix} x^T\hat{R}^{-1}Y \\ z^T\hat{R}^{-1}Y \end{bmatrix} \quad (6.34)$$

(Henderson, 1985). The solutions to Eq. (6.34) are

$$\hat{\beta} = \left(x^T\hat{V}^{-1}x\right)^{-1}x^T\hat{V}^{-1}Y \quad (6.35)$$

$$\hat{u} = \hat{G}z^T\hat{V}^{-1}\left(Y - x\hat{\beta}\right). \quad (6.36)$$

Note that these equations are simple extensions to least squares equations presented in previous chapters. Modifications to these equations are needed if G is near singular; see Henderson (1985) for details. The covariance of the parameter estimates $(\hat{\beta}, \hat{u})$ is estimated by

$$\text{Cov}\begin{pmatrix} \hat{\beta} \\ \hat{u} \end{pmatrix} = \hat{C} = \begin{bmatrix} x^T\hat{R}^{-1}x & x^T\hat{R}^{-1}z \\ z^T\hat{R}^{-1}x & z^T\hat{R}^{-1}z + \hat{G}^{-1} \end{bmatrix}^{-} \quad (6.37)$$

where the superscript "-" denotes the generalized inverse. Notice that element C_{11} in C is similar to the formula for the covariance matrix for β under weighted least squares.

There are a number of advantages to using ML or REML. First, the parameter estimates are consistent, i.e., as the sample size increases, the estimates themselves converge towards the true population values, while at the same time, their standard errors decrease. Second, the estimates are also asymptotically normally distributed. Third, the variance of the ML or REML estimators is smaller than estimators using any other method. Hence, if G and R are known, then $\hat{\beta}$ is the best linear unbiased estimate (BLUE) of β, and $\hat{U}$ is the best linear unbiased predictor (BLUP) of U (Henderson, 1985). The word "best" is in terms of minimum mean square error. If G and R are unknown and are estimated using ML or REML, then these estimates are the empirical BLUEs and BLUPs for β and U, respectively.

Harville (1977) summarizes the literature on the properties of ML and REML methods. Both ML and REML have similar merits. When the between-subject variability is larger relative to the residual variance, then ML generates a variance estimate of between-subject variability that is smaller than the true value. However, when between-subject variability is smaller relative to residual error, then the ML estimator is the preferred estimator for between-subject variability. ML or REML produce unbiased estimators of residual variance and either can be used for its estimation. When the number of estimable parameters is small, ML and REML produce similar results. As the number of estimable model parameters increases, ML and REML estimates will start to diverge. Also, ML estimates of variance components tend to be smaller than their true values because REML takes into account the loss of degrees of freedom associated with estimation of the fixed effects. To understand why this is important, think about the simple variance estimator for a univariate distribution with n observations

$$\hat{\sigma}^2 = \frac{\sum_{i=1}^{n}(x_i - \bar{x})}{n}. \quad (6.38)$$

Equation (6.38) is known to be biased because it fails to take into account the estimation of $\bar{x}$. However, if the denominator in Equation (6.38) is changed to $(n-1)$, where the loss of a single degree of freedom occurs because of the estimation of $\bar{x}$, then the result is an unbiased estimator for the variance. The same analogy is made for ML and REML estimation with mixed effects models.

Because ML and REML require iterative methods, there will be instances wherein convergence cannot be achieved. One method to solve this problem is to provide better starting parameters or use some other optimization algorithm. The default optimization method in the MIXED procedure in SAS is Newton–Raphson optimization. Verbeke and Molenberghs (2000) provide an example where Newton–Raphson optimization failed, but Gauss–Newton optimization did not. They also point out that convergence problems with ML or REML arise from estimation of the variance components, not from the fixed effects, because estimation of G and R requires optimization [Eqs. (6.32) or (6.33)], but estimation of β and U can be solved directly [Eqs. (6.35) and (6.36)]. Convergence difficulties in this instance may be overcome by using different starting values for the variance components. Another situation that may lead to convergence problems is when a variance component is small, which may result in a nonpositive definite G matrix. One solution to this problem is recoding the variable to a different scale, thereby artificially enlarging the variance. Another problem sometimes observed is when an infinite likelihood error occurs with any of the spatial covariance matrices. The immediate solution is to examine for duplicate observations within a subject taken at the same time. This results in an attempt to raise zero to a power, which is an undefined function. If duplicate observations are observed, then the mean at that time point can be substituted.

INFERENCE FOR THE FIXED EFFECT PARAMETER ESTIMATES

For inferences regarding the fixed effect parameters in the model, one common method to assess the significance of the estimates is to use a Z-test in which the parameter estimate $(\hat{\beta})$ is divided by its asymptotic standard error $[\text{SE}(\hat{\beta})]$ and compared to a Z-distribution

$$Z = \frac{\hat{\beta} - \beta}{\text{SE}(\hat{\beta})} \sim N(0, 1). \qquad (6.39)$$

Z-tests are valid for large sample sizes, but are typically biased upwards, resulting in inflated Z-scores and Type I error rate, because of their underestimation in the variability of $\hat{\beta}$. Note that the covariance matrix $\hat{C}$ [Eq. (6.37)] uses an estimate of G and R in its calculation and that no correction in Z is made for the uncertainty in $\hat{G}$ and $\hat{R}$. Rather than adjust for the inflation, most software packages account for the bias by comparing Z to a t-distribution, which has wider tails than a Z-distribution, and adjust the degrees of freedom accordingly.

A variety of different methods exist that estimate the degrees of freedom, all of which are conditioned on the variance–covariance structure of the model. Only for balanced data is the default degrees of freedom in SAS (the containment method), which is based on the degrees of freedom containing the effect of interest, valid. If the data are unbalanced, the appropriate degrees of freedom should be calculated from the data. The most common, but by no means the only, method used is Satterthwaite's correction, a method that is computationally intensive and will not be derived herein. The reader is referred to Verbeke and Molenberghs (1997) for details. It has been concluded that all of the different degrees of freedom approximations may lead to different results, but that for longitudinal data, the differences between the methods will be minimal (Verbeke and Molenberghs, 2000). Only for very small samples and for cases outside the context of longitudinal data may the methods lead to severe differences.

An alternative method to determining the significance of a model parameter is the likelihood ratio test (LRT) comparing a fitted model with the parameter of interest having p_1 estimable parameters and a fitted model without the parameter of interest having p_2 estimable parameters. Note that p_1 and p_2 include all fixed and estimable random effects in the model. If the difference in the $-2LL$ functions is larger than the critical value from a chi-squared distribution with p_1-p_2 degrees of freedom, the full model will be considered the superior model and the parameter of interest should be retained in the model. Verbeke and Molenberghs (2000) point out that the LRT is not valid if the models were fit using REML because although the ML function is invariant to one-to-one reparameterization of the fixed effects while REML is not. Also, REML deals with linear combinations of the observed variables whose expectations are zero, resulting in error contrasts that are free of any fixed effects in the model. Hence, linear mixed effects models dealing with different fixed effect structures cannot be compared on the basis of the REML functions. Verbeke and Molenberghs (2000) present an example where the difference in likelihood functions (reduced–full) was negative under REML, something that cannot occur. They conclude that the LRT should only be done using ML estimates. In summary, caution needs to be expressed in inference for the fixed effects because the results are conditional on the random effects. Also, inference for the fixed effects using the LRT or information criterion should be based on ML estimates, not REML estimates, whereas Z-type tests can be used using either REML or ML estimates.

INFERENCE FOR THE VARIANCE COMPONENTS

In most cases, the fixed effect parameters are the parameters of interest. However, adequate modeling of the variance–covariance structure is critical for assessment of the fixed effects and is useful in explaining the variability of the data. Indeed, sometimes the fixed effects are of little interest and the variance components are of primary importance. Covariance structures that are overparameterized may lead to poor estimation of the standard errors for estimates of the fixed effects (Altham, 1984). However, covariance matrices that are too restrictive may lead to invalid inferences about the fixed effects because the assumed covariance structure does not exist and is not valid. For this reason, methods need to be available for testing the significance of the variance components in a model.

One method might be to use a Z-test, similar to the one developed for fixed effects. SAS, as well as many of other programs, present such estimates of the variance components and their standard errors. One might then naively calculate a Z-score for a variance and conclude that the variance is statistically significant from zero. This method is not advised since variance components are often skewed and are not normally distributed, which Z-scores are assumed to be, at least asymptotically (McLean and Sanders, 1988). Hence, another measure should be used.

An alternative test would be to use the LRT comparing two models with the same mean structure, but with nested covariance structures since only newly added variance components are being added. Whatever the method used, testing for the significance of variance components is problematic since the null hypothesis that the estimate equals zero lies on the boundary of the parameter space for the alternative hypothesis. In other words, consider the hypothesis test $H_o: \sigma^2 = 0$ versus. $H_a: \sigma^2 > 0$. Notice that the alternative hypothesis is lower bounded by the null hypothesis. The LRT is not valid under these conditions because the test statistic is no longer distributed as a single chi-squared random variable, but becomes a mixture of chi-squared random variables (Stram and Lee, 1994).

Naïve use of the chi-squared distribution leads to p-values that are greater than they should be, resulting in accepting the null hypothesis (that the additional variance component is not needed) too often. Stram and Lee (1994) showed that in the simplest case, where one new random effect is being added or removed from a model, the distribution of the LRT is a 50:50 mixture of chi-squared random variables with p_1 and $p_1 + 1$ degrees of freedom. Table 6.4 presents critical values from a 50:50 mixture of chi-squared distributions with p_1 and $p_1 + 1$ degrees of freedom. In the case of 1 degree of freedom, the bias is small. However, the bias could be substantial

for testing many new variance components simultaneously. Interestingly, however, is the case where the variance term being tested is a covariance term. For example, suppose the variance–covariance matrix was defined as

$$\Omega = \begin{bmatrix} \omega_1^2 & \omega_{12} \\ \omega_{12} & \omega_2^2 \end{bmatrix} \qquad (6.40)$$

where ω_1^2 and ω_2^2 are nonzero diagonal variances and the hypothesis test was defined as $H_o: \omega_{12} = 0$ versus $H_a: \omega_{12} \neq 0$. In this case, the boundary issue does not apply because an off-diagonal covariance term can take positive, zero, or negative values. Hence, the usual LRT is valid (D. Stram, personal communication). But if the hypothesis test was defined as $H_o: \omega_{12} = 0$ versus. $H_a: \omega_{12} > 0$ then the boundary issue would apply and the usual LRT would not be valid.

One method to adjust for boundary problems is to use simulation. First, replace the unknown parameters by their parameter estimates under the null model. Second, simulate data under the null model ignoring the variability in treating the unknown parameters as fixed. Third, the data is then fit to both the null and alternative model and the LRT statistic is calculated. This process is repeated many times and the empirical distribution of the test statistic under the null distribution is determined. This empirical distribution can then be compared to mixtures of chi-squared distributions to see which chi-squared distribution is appropriate.

Pinheiro and Bates (2000) illustrate this technique using the S-Plus programming language. They point out that in their example, the 50:50 mixture of chi-squared distributions is not always successful; that in their example, a 65:35 mixture was a better approximation, although it has been suggested that the reason Pinheiro and Bates observed a 65:35 mixture, instead of the theoretical 50:50 mixture predicted by Stram and Lee, was because Pinheiro and Bates ignored the variability in the parameter estimates used to simulate data under the null model (Verbeke, personal communication). They conclude that there really are no good rules of thumb for approximating the distribution of the LRT for nested models and that one should simply use the p-values obtained using the naïve chi-squared distribution, keeping in mind that these values will be conservative. Alternatively, one might use a smaller p-value for declaring significance, such that if one were interested in keeping model terms where $p < 0.05$, then a critical value of 0.01 might be used instead. Lastly, one could simply ignore this issue, which is probably the most common solution to the problem.

Table 6.4 Critical values from a 50:50 mixture of chi-squared distributions with p_1 and $p_1 + 1$ degrees of freedom.

p_1	Significance Level						
	0.1	0.05	0.025	0.01	0.005	0.0025	0.001
1	3.81	5.14	6.48	8.27	9.63	11.00	12.81
2	5.53	7.05	8.54	10.50	11.97	13.43	15/36
3	7.09	8.76	10.38	12.48	14.04	15.59	17.61
4	8.57	10.37	12.10	14.32	15.97	17.59	19.69
5	10.00	11.91	13.74	16.07	17.79	19.47	21.66
6	11.38	13.40	15.32	17.76	19.54	21.29	23.55
7	12.74	14.85	16.86	19.38	21.23	23.04	25.37
8	14.07	16.27	18.35	20.97	22.88	24.74	27/13
9	15.38	17.67	19.82	22.52	24.49	26.40	28.86
10	16.67	19.04	21.27	24.05	26.07	28.02	30.54

Reprinted with permission from Table C.1 in Fitzmaurice, G.M., Laird, N.M., and Ware, J.H. *Applied longitudinal analysis*, Wiley, 2004. Copyright 2004.

ESTIMATION OF THE RANDOM EFFECTS AND EMPIRICAL BAYES ESTIMATES (EBEs)

Traditional frequentist interpretations of statistics make no room for prior or previous knowledge about an estimate for some parameter. For instance, suppose hemoglobin A_1c concentration was assayed in 15 people after receiving diabetic therapy for 3 months and a mean decrease from baseline of 16% was observed. However, also suppose the same experiment was performed 6 months later in another set of 15 people having the same age, weight, and sex and the decrease was found to be 3%. What was the population mean change on diabetic therapy? Frequentist data interpretation looks at one set of data at a time. Frequentist evaluation of the most recent experiment does not take into account the results from the previous experiment. Bayesians argue that prior knowledge should be included in an estimate of the true population value. It is beyond the scope of this chapter to detail Bayesian estimation methods or to compare and contrast the frequentist versus Bayesian argument. The reader is referred to Carlin and Louis (1996) or Lee (1997) for further details.

The basic tool that Bayesians use derives from Bayes theorem, from which it is known that the

$$p(\theta|x) \propto p(\theta)p(x|\theta) \qquad (6.41)$$

where p(.) is the probability, $p(\theta|x)$ is the probability of θ given x, θ is the parameter to be estimated, and x is the data used to estimate θ. Basically, Eq. (6.41) states that the probability of observing θ given x is proportional to the probability of θ occurring times the probability of observing x given θ. In its easier to remember form, the

posterior $\propto$ prior $\times$ likelihood.

In the case of normal prior and likelihood, the posterior distribution is a normal distribution with a weighted mean of the prior value mean and observed data mean with weights proportional to the inverse of their respective variances. The posterior variance is a weighted average of the individual variances.

As an example, based on data in the literature, the mean and standard deviation of some parameter in the population was estimated at 275 with a standard deviation of 12. An experiment was conducted and the sample mean and standard deviation was estimated at 300 and 10, respectively. Using the historic data as the prior distribution, the posterior distribution mean was estimated at 290 with a standard deviation of 7.7. This is illustrated in Figure 6.3. Notice that the mean was a compromise between the observed data and the historic

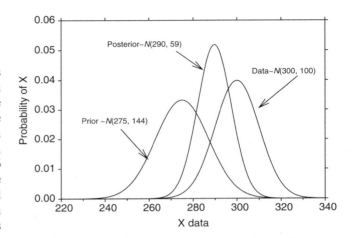

Figure 6.3 Plot illustrating the posterior distribution as a function of the prior distribution and likelihood distribution.

data. Hence, Bayes estimates attempt to make a compromise between what is observed and what was theorized. This compromise is sometimes called *shrinkage* because the posterior data distribution is shrunk towards the prior. Shrinkage has the effect of pulling extreme observations toward the population mean, even if the distribution is heavy tailed.

In the linear mixed model it is assumed that the marginal model for the ith subject is given by

$$Y_i = x_i\beta + z_iU_i + \varepsilon_i. \qquad (6.42)$$

Another assumption is that ε_i is normally distributed with mean 0 and variance R_i and that U_i is normally distributed with mean 0 and variance G. The latter assumption is the prior distribution of the parameters U_i. Once data are collected, the posterior distribution of U_i can be generated conditional on Y_i. Estimation of U_i is given by the average of the values for the ith subject and the population mean. If the subject mean is higher than the population mean then this would suggest that U_i is positive. Given the assumptions for the model, the expected value of U_i given the subject mean is

$$E(U_i|Y_i) = \hat{U}_i = \hat{G}z_i^T\hat{V}^{-1}(Y_i - x_i\hat{\beta}). \qquad (6.43)$$

From this then, the expected value for $\hat{Y}_i$ is

$$\begin{aligned} \hat{Y}_i &= x_i\hat{\beta} + z_i\hat{U}_i \\ &= x_i\hat{\beta} + z_i\hat{G}z_i^T\hat{V}^{-1}(Y_i - x_i\hat{\beta}) \\ &= \left(I_{n_i} - z_i\hat{G}z_i^T\hat{V}^{-1}\right)x_i\hat{\beta} + z_i\hat{G}z_i^T\hat{V}^{-1}Y_i \end{aligned} \qquad (6.44)$$

Making the substitution $zGz^T = V - R$, then

$$\hat{Y}_i = \left(I_{n_i} - \left(\hat{V}_i - \hat{R}_i\right)\hat{V}_i^{-1}\right)x_i\hat{\beta} + \left(\hat{V}_i - \hat{R}_i\right)\hat{V}_i^{-1}Y_i$$
$$= \hat{R}_i\hat{V}_i^{-1}x_i\hat{\beta} + \left(I_{n_i} - \hat{R}_i\hat{V}_i^{-1}\right)Y_i$$

(6.45)

Since these equations use either the ML or REML estimates of all the model parameters, e.g., $\hat{V}$ and $\hat{G}$, instead of the true parameters, the resulting estimates are called empirical Bayes estimates (EBEs) or sometimes James–Stein estimators (James and Stein, 1960). EBEs of random effects in a linear mixed model can be interpreted as a weighted average of the population average ($x\beta$) and the observed data Y_i with weights $\hat{R}_i\hat{V}_i^{-1}$ and $I_{n_i} - \hat{R}_i\hat{V}_i^{-1}$, respectively. If the between-subject variability is large relative to the within-subject variability then $\hat{R}_i\hat{V}_i^{-1}$ will be small. Conversely, if within-subject variability is large then $\hat{R}_i\hat{V}_i^{-1}$ will be large as well. Thus, greater weight will be given to the population average if the within-subject variance is large compared to the between-subject variance and conversely, more weight will be given to the subject profile if the within-subject variance is small compared to the between-subject variability. The net effect is shrinkage of the estimates toward the prior. One practical consequence of shrinkage is that an empirical estimate of the variance of a random effect based on the EBEs will always lead to a smaller estimate of the true variability.

On a last note, because all the model parameters in Eq. (6.43) are estimated, the true variability in U is underestimated. The estimate $\hat{U}_i$ does not take into account the variability introduced by replacing an unknown parameter with its estimate. Also, as will be seen, EBEs are extremely sensitive to the prior distribution assumption. When the prior is not valid, the EBEs themselves become highly suspect.

MODEL SELECTION

Selecting a mixed effects model means identifying a structural or mean model, the components of variance, and the covariance matrix for the residuals. The basic rationale for model selection will be parsimony in parameters, i.e., to obtain the most efficient estimation of fixed effects, one selects the covariance model that has the most parsimonious structure that fits the data (Wolfinger, 1996). Estimation of the fixed effects is dependent on the covariance matrix and statistical significance may change if a different covariance structure is used. The general strategy to be used follows the ideas presented in

Diggle (1988). The basic strategy is as follows and is illustrated in Fig. 6.4:

1. Include the random effects to be included in the model.
2. Choose an initial variance–covariance model.
3. Use statistical and graphical methods to compare various variance–covariance structures and select one of them.
4. Using the selected variance–covariance structure, reduce the model as necessary.

Model selection can be done using the LRT or information criteria. This general approach has been advocated by Wolfinger (1993; 1996) and Verbeke and Molenberghs (2000) as being useful in identifying an appropriate model. Each of these steps will now be elaborated. It should be stressed that there is overlap in these steps and that there may be several iterations of the process.

In the first step, an overparameterized model is chosen because underparameterized models tend to introduce spurious autocorrelations among the residuals. If the experiment is designed in the sense that all subjects are measured at the same time points with the same treatments and all variables are categorical, a saturated model with all categorical variables and their interactions are suggested. If time is treated as a continuous variable, which may be the case if not all subjects are measured at the same time, as may be the case in a Phase III study, the concept of a saturated model breaks down. Verbeke and Molenberghs (2000) suggest using smoothed average trends or individual profiles to choose how best to model time. For example, a smoothed plot may show that the response changes curvilinearly over

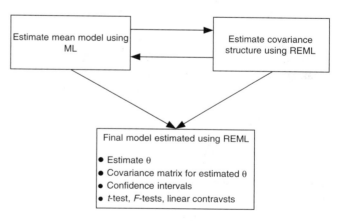

Figure 6.4 Schematic of how the mean structure affects the covariance matrix and vice versa and how they both influence the final model. Redrawn from Fig. 3.7 in Verbeke, G. and Molenberghs, G. *Linear mixed models in practice: A SAS-oriented approach.* Springer, New York, 2000, p. 120. Copyright *Springer 1997.*

time and that a treating time as a quadratic polynomial model may be appropriate.

In the second step, the random effects (which comprise the G matrix) to be included in the model are identified. The random effects to be included are typically a subset of the mean effects in the model, although this is not a requirement. For example, time and time squared might be treated as fixed effects such that the population response changes in a quadratic manner over time, but that time alone (and not time squared) is treated as a random effect, thereby implying that there is between-subject variability in the linear rate of change across subjects, but no between-subject variability in the quadratic rate of change. If the time effect or any other continuous covariate is treated as a polynomial, do not include the polynomial term as a random effect if the inferior terms are not significant (Morrell, Pearson, and Brant, 1997). The same applies to interaction terms. Do not include interaction terms if either of the component terms are not significant (Diggle, 1988).

On the other hand, there may be cases where a random effect is included in the model but not in the mean model. One case would be in a designed experiment where subjects were first randomized into blocks to control variability before assignments to treatments. The blocks the subjects were assigned to are not necessarily of interest—they are nuisance variables. In this case, blocks could be treated as a random effect and not be included in the mean model. When the subject level covariates are categorical (class) variables, such as race, treating random effects beyond random intercepts, which allows each subject to have their own unique baseline, is not usually done.

At this stage, time-varying random effects should be examined by plotting the residuals obtained using a simple OLS estimate of β, ignoring any serial correlation or random effects in the model, against time. If this plot shows no trends and is of constant variance across time, no other random effects need to be included in the model, save perhaps a random intercept term. If, however, a systematic trend still exists in the plot then further random effects need to be included in the model to account for the trend.

In the third step, the residual covariance structure (the R matrix) is chosen, conditional on the set of random effects chosen for the model. In helping to choose a covariance model, one guideline provided by Verbeke and Molenberghs (2000) is that for highly unbalanced data with many measurements made on each subject, it can be assumed that the random effects predominate and can account for most of the variability in the data. In this case, one usually chooses a simple residual error model, usually the simple covariance matrix. Indeed, the first model examined should be one where the residual

variance is treated as simple, i.e., all the observations are independent within a subject. However, sometimes a more complex residual error structure is necessary in which the residual error term is decomposed into a term for measurement error and a serial correlation term. The most frequently used serial correlation models are the exponential, Gaussian, and power models. All three models may be examined and the information criteria then used to see which model is superior. If the covariance model is overparameterized, starting values for the covariances may need to be specified or the Fisher scoring method, used during the early iterations of the optimization process. One model combination that should be avoided is an unstructured random effect covariance matrix and unstructured residual variance matrix because the resulting model is overparameterized and singular.

The last step is model reduction. Fixed and random effects that appear to be nonsignificant can now be removed, keeping in mind the boundary issue with the LRT. Once the final model is identified, it is refit using REML to obtain the unbiased estimates of the variance parameters.

SENSITIVITY TO THE MODEL ASSUMPTIONS

The linear mixed effect model assumes that the random effects are normally distributed and that the residuals are normally distributed. Butler and Louis (1992) showed that estimation of the fixed effects and covariance parameters, as well as residual variance terms, were very robust to deviations from normality. However, the standard errors of the estimates can be affected by deviations from normality, as much as five times too large or three times too small (Verbeke and Lesaffre, 1997). In contrast to the estimation of the mean model, the estimation of the random effects (and hence, variance components) are very sensitive to the normality assumption. Verbeke and Lesaffre (1996) studied the effects of deviation from normality on the empirical Bayes estimates of the random effects. Using computer simulation they simulated 1000 subjects with five measurements per subject, where each subject had a random intercept coming from a 50:50 mixture of normal distributions, which may arise if two subpopulations were examined each having equal variability and size. By assuming a unimodal normal distribution of the random effects, a histogram of the empirical Bayes estimates revealed a unimodal distribution, not a bimodal distribution as would be expected. They showed that the correct distributional shape of the random effects may not be observed if the error variability is large compared to the between-subject variability.

If one is interested only in the estimates of the fixed effects and variance components, then it is unnecessary to test the assumption of normality of the random effects. However, if inferences are to be drawn from the empirical Bayes estimates, then it is suggested to test the normality assumption. Pinheiro and Bates (2000) suggest using QQ-plots. Verbeke and Lesaffre (1996; 1997) argue that the only valid method to check for random effects normality is by comparing the model of interest to a model where the distributional assumptions of the random effects have been relaxed. They suggest that the comparator model contain random effects having a mixture of normal distributions, what they call the heterogeneity model. They suggest fitting models with differing numbers of underlying components, leading to a series of nested models that can then be tested using the LRT. The reader is referred to Verbeke and Molenberghs (2000) for more details.

RESIDUAL ANALYSIS AND GOODNESS OF FIT

Residual analysis, when used to assess goodness of fit in a linear mixed effects model, is usually done with the same methods as in linear or nonlinear models. However, two type of residuals arise with a mixed effects model. If interest centers on a particular individual then conditional residuals (ε_{ci}) are of interest

$$\varepsilon_{ci} = Y_i - \left(x_i\hat{\beta} + z_iU_i\right). \qquad (6.46)$$

If however, interest centers on a individual averaged across all possible random effects, then the marginal residuals (ε_{mi}) are of interest

$$\varepsilon_{mi} = Y_i - x_i\hat{\beta} \qquad (6.47)$$

If there are no random effects in the model, then the two residuals are equal. Residual analysis can be done on either the raw conditional or marginal residuals. However, as with the linear model, residual analysis in this manner is complicated by the fact that the variance of the residuals is unknown. A data point with a small residual may be of more importance because it has a smaller standard error than an observation with a larger residual but correspondingly larger standard error.

Hence, raw residuals are often standardized by some quantity, usually its standard deviation, to account for the unequal variance of the residuals. If the estimate of the standard deviation is based on the observation in question the method is called internal studentization, but if the observation is not included in the estimate of the standard deviation, then the method is called external studentization. Studentized residuals can be estimated

by both methods. Another type of residual is Pearson residuals, which standardize the residuals by the standard deviation of the observation (not the residual) in the marginal case and by the standard deviation of the conditional observation in the conditional case. Lastly, another class of residuals are scaled residuals, which are useful for detecting improper covariance structures. If C is the Cholesky decomposition of $\hat{V}$ such that

$$CC^T = Var\,(\hat{Y}) = \hat{V} \qquad (6.48)$$

then the scaled residuals are calculated using the marginal residuals

$$r_c = C^{-1}\varepsilon_m. \qquad (6.49)$$

Scaled residuals have zero mean and are approximately uncorrelated. Once the residuals are scaled or standardized then it is appropriate to compare residuals directly for influence and outliers.

A common metric for goodness of fit (although in actuality it is more a measure of predictability) in a linear model is the coefficient of determination (R^2), which measures the proportion of variance explained by the model to the total variance in the observations. In the case of a mixed effects model, R^2 is not a proper statistic because it fails to account for between-subject variability. Consider the effect-time data shown in the top plot in Fig. 6.5. Herein data were simulated from 50 subjects having a mean baseline of 100 with a standard deviation of 60. The effect over time increased by 1 unit per unit time. No random error was added to the observations. Looking at the naïve pooled analysis of the data using a simple linear regression model, the slope was estimated at 1.0, which is an unbiased estimate of the slope, but the standard error was so large the 95% confidence interval (CI) contained zero, {−1.0, 3.0}. So, the conclusion would be reached that time is not a significant predictor for effect. The coefficient of determination for this model was 0.02.

But, look at the bottom plot of Fig. 6.5. In this plot, effect is plotted by individual. Clearly, there is a time effect. The effect of between-subject variability is obscuring this relationship, however. A linear mixed effects model analysis of this data showed time to be highly significant (p < 0.0001) with a point estimate of the slope being 1.00. The standard error of the slope was <1E-6 so the 95% CI could not be determined. The coefficient of determination for this model should be 1.0 after accounting for between-subject variability.

One way to calculate the coefficient of determination in a mixed effects model is to fit a null model and compute the residual sum of squares (SS_{null}). The

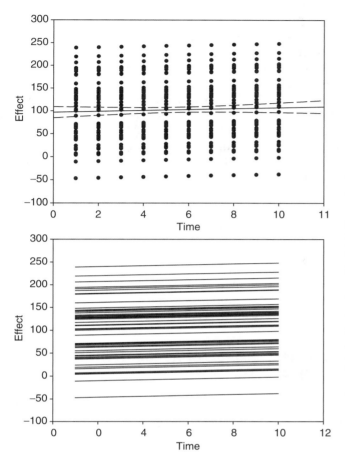

Figure 6.5 Simulated time–effect data where the intercept was normally distributed with a mean of 100 and a standard deviation of 60. The effect was linear over time within an individual with a slope of 1.0. No random error was added to the model—the only predictor in the model is time and it is an exact predictor. The top plot shows the data pooled across 50 subjects. Solid line is the predicted values under the simple linear model pooled across observations. Dashed line is the 95% confidence interval. The coefficient of determination for this model was 0.02. The 95% confidence interval for the slope was {−1.0, 3.0} with a point estimate of 1.00. The bottom plot shows how the data in the top plot extended to an individual. The bottom plot shows perfect correspondence between effect and time within an individual. The mixed effects coefficient of determination for this data set was 1.0, as it should be. This example was meant to illustrate how the coefficient of determination using the usual linear regression formula is invalid in the mixed effects model case because it fails to account for between-subject variability and use of such a measure results in a significant underestimation of the predictive power of a covariate.

coefficient of determination, which will be denoted as Ω^2 to indicate a mixed effects model, can then be estimated as

$$\hat{\Omega}^2 = 1 - \frac{SS_{full}}{SS_{null}} \qquad (6.50)$$

where SS_{full} is the residual sum of squares from the full mixed model (Xu, 2003). In this example, the null model was a linear mixed model without time as a fixed effect. SS_{null} was 9.1667, whereas SS_{full} was 1.02E-11. Hence, $\hat{\Omega}^2 \cong 1$, as would be expected. The trick in finding Ω^2 is

determining the appropriate null model, although in many cases it is simply the model without any fixed effects. There is not any substantial difference in using ML or REML to estimate Ω^2 (Xu, 2003).

INFLUENCE ANALYSIS

The basic experimental unit in a linear or nonlinear model is the observation itself—each observation is independent of the others. With a mixed model, the basic experimental unit is the subject that is being repeatedly sampled. For example, a patient's CD4-count may be measured monthly in an AIDS clinical trial. While a particular observation may be influential, of more interest is whether a particular subject is influential. Hence, influence analysis in a mixed effects model tends to focus on a set of observations within a subject, rather than at the observation level. That is not to say that particular observations are not of interest. Once an individual is identified as being influential, the next step then is to determine whether that subject's influence is due to a particular observation.

In a linear model, influence in the x direction is assessed using the HAT matrix

$$HAT = x(x^Tx)^{-1}x^T. \qquad (6.51)$$

A similar statistic can be developed in linear mixed effects models

$$HAT_1 = x(x^T\hat{V}^{-1}x)^{-1}x^T\hat{V}^{-1} \qquad (6.52)$$

where $\hat{V}$ is the total variance of the model given by $z\hat{G}z^T + \hat{R}$ and HAT_1 denotes that this is only one type of HAT matrix that can be developed. Another type of HAT matrix can be developed using the Cholesky decomposition of $\hat{V}$, $CC^T = \hat{V}$, namely

$$HAT_2 = C^{-1}x(x^T\hat{V}^{-1}x)^{-1}x^T(C^T)^{-1}. \qquad (6.53)$$

Both $tr(HAT_1)$ and $tr(HAT_2)$ equal rank(x). With HAT_2, however, it is possible to have negative diagonal elements, which may appear unusual. However, it may be that the surrounding observations have such profound influence that the negative HAT_2 observation has a negative weight (screening effect) (Schabenberger, 2003).

In a linear or nonlinear model, influence can be assessed by removing each observation one by one. In mixed effects models, each subject can be removed one by one, as a starting point. A number of metrics can then be developed using these case deletion data sets. One is an overall measure of influence called the likelihood distance (LD_{-i}). Let LL be the log-likelihood of the complete case data set and $LL_{(-i)}$ be the log-likelihood for the full data set based on the parameter estimates using the data set with the case deleted fitted using the same algorithm as the complete case model, ML or REML. Then

$$LD_{-i} = 2\{LL - LL_{(-i)}\}. \qquad (6.54)$$

Note that $LL_{(-i)}$ is not the log-likelihood with the ith case deleted. The log-likelihood of the complete case is based on, say n observations. The log-likelihood of the reduced data set will be based on $< n$ observations so that comparing LL to $LL_{(-i)}$ is not valid. Hence the need to determine the log-likelihood of the complete case data set using the parameter estimates of the reduced data set.

Similar to the linear regression case, influence diagnostics for linear mixed models can be developed using case deletion. These extensions include Cook's distance, DFFITs, COVRATIO, and PRESS residuals. For example, a linear mixed effects extension to DFFITS is

$$\text{DFFITs}_{(-i)} = \left(\hat{\beta} - \hat{\beta}_{(-i)}\right)^{T} \text{Var}\left(\hat{\beta}_{(-i)}\right)\left(\hat{\beta} - \hat{\beta}_{(-i)}\right)/\text{rank}(x)$$

$$(6.55)$$

where $\hat{\beta}_{(-i)}$ is the estimate of the fixed effect parameters with the ith case removed. The reader is referred to Schabenberger (2003) and Demidenko and Stukel (2005) for details on other influence diagnostics and how they are calculated.

HANDLING MISSING AND CENSORED DATA

Missing and censored data in the context of linear mixed models is more problematic than in linear models because of the repeated nature of the dependent variable. In general, however, when the dependent variable is missing at random or missing completely at random, then imputation techniques are not needed to "fill in" missing values and are not a serious problem unless there are very large differences in the drop-out pattern between treatment groups. If the covariates are missing, then indeed some imputation method may be needed. However, all imputation techniques discussed with linear models when applied to longitudinal data fail to take into account the correlated nature of observations within the same individual. This topic is discussed in much further detail in the chapter on practical issues related to nonlinear mixed effects models and the reader is referred there for details.

SOFTWARE

Linear mixed effect software can be found in most statistical packages. Within SAS (SAS Institute, Cary, NC) is the MIXED procedure, which is used for all the linear mixed effect analyses done in this chapter. Three excellent books on using the MIXED procedure are Littell et al. (1996) and Verbeke and Molenberghs (1997; 2000). Within S-Plus (Insightful Corp., Seattle, WA) is the LME function, of which Pinheiro and Bates (2000) is a useful resource. WinNonlin Professional (Pharsight Corp., Mountain View, CA) also has a linear mixed effect model module. The choice between the three depends on the level of programming savvy of the analyst and the degree of comfort an analyst has at using each program. There are, however, subtle differences between the packages primarily in the number of options each offers and it should be recognized that because of these differences the results from each package may vary.

EXAMPLE: ANALYSIS OF A FOOD EFFECT PHASE I CLINICAL TRIAL

Besides repeated measures data, linear mixed effects models are more commonly used to analyze traditional experimental designs with fixed treatment regimens and sample collection schedules. In these studies, subjects are treated as random effects. As an example, an analysis of variance will be done using linear mixed models in a food-effect study. Testing for whether food has an effect on a drug's pharmacokinetics is a common clinical study in the development of new drugs since food can either increase or decrease the absorption of orally administered drugs (Singh, 1999). The most common study design for immediate release formulations is the one recommended by the Food and Drug Administration (2002): a single dose, two-period, two-treatment, two-sequence crossover study. That guidance suggests that the two treatments consist of drug administration in the fasting state and drug administration within 30 min of consuming a high fat meal. If the geometric mean ratio for the fed to fasted treatments falls entirely within the interval 80 to 125% for both area under the curve from time 0 to infinity [$AUC(0-\infty)$] and maximal drug concentration (C_{max}) then food has no effect on the drug's pharmacokinetics.

To assess whether food impacted the pharmacokinetics of a new drug, such a study was conducted in 12 healthy, male subjects. Plasma samples were collected and analyzed for drug concentrations. $AUC(0-\infty)$ was calculated using the linear trapezoidal rule and C_{max} was determined from direct observation of the data.

AUC$(0-\infty)$ and C_{max} are presented in Table 6.5. Two subjects did not return to the clinic and did not complete the study. Hence, these subjects had only data from Period 1. Natural-log transformed AUC$(0-\infty)$ and C_{max} were used as the dependent variables. The analysis of variance consisted of sequence, treatment, and period as fixed effects. Subjects nested within sequence were treated as a random effect using a random intercept model. The model was fit using REML. Table 6.6 presents the results. The 90% CI for the ratio of treatment means for both AUC$(0-\infty)$ and C_{max} were entirely contained within the interval 80–125%. Hence, it was concluded that food had no effect on the pharmacokinetics of the drug.

EXAMPLE: MODELING TUMOR GROWTH

In the development of a new oncolytic, an experiment was conducted wherein mice subcutaneously implanted with A549 human lung tumors were randomized to four treatment groups:

1. Saline once daily by intraperitoneal (IP) administration (control group)
2. Drug X 10 mg/kg once daily by oral (PO) administration for 28 days
3. Drug X 100 mg/kg once daily by PO administration for 28 days, and
4. Drug X 100 mg/kg once daily by IP administration for 28 days.

On days 1, 5, 8, 12, 15, 20, 22, 26, 29, and 33 the mouse weight, tumor length, and tumor width were measured. Length and width were converted to tumor volume which was used as a surrogate for tumor growth. Seven (7) mice were randomized into each treatment group. Of interest to the researchers were the following questions:

Table 6.5 AUC and C_{max} estimates from a 2-period crossover food-effect study.

Subject	Sequence	Period 1 AUC$(0-\infty)$	Period 2 AUC$(0-\infty)$	Period 1 C_{max}	Period 2 C_{max}
1	AB	9074.83	8366.08	726	842
2	AB	7183.59	8962.48	603	735
3	BA	6625.54	11412.18	811	784
4	AB	5136.37	12383.78	550	670
5	BA	11387.68	9838.2	588	887
6	BA	11190.42	10026.18	767	597
7	BA	10883.88	Missing	641	Missing
8	AB	8723.98	10359.55	598	669
9	BA	8456.65	9574.34	859	624
10	AB	10056.91	10234.52	672	782
11	AB	7893.45	7934.59	570	773
12	BA	8797.77	Missing	699	Missing

Note: Treatment A is fasting; treatment B is fed.

Table 6.6 Results of analysis of variance of data in Table 6.5 after Ln-transformation using REML.

Analysis of variance summary				
	AUC		C_{max}	
Fixed effects	F-value	p-Value	F-value	p-Value
Sequence	2.09	0.1651	1.05	0.3183
treatment	0.53	0.4777	3.01	0.0999
period	2.94	0.1036	2.38	0.1405
Least squares means	Estimate (90% CI)		Estimate (90% CI)	
Fast	8937 (8028, 9948)		663 (617, 714)	
Fed	9490 (8622, 10446)		731 (685, 781)	
Ratio of means : Fed to fast (90% CI)				
	AUC	1.06 (1.05, 1.07)		
	C_{max}	1.10 (1.09, 1.11)		

1. Did Drug X have a differential effect on mean tumor volume overall compared to controls at the end of study?
2. Was there a difference in mean tumor volume between the Drug X 100 mg/kg dose groups after PO and IP administration at the end of study?
3. Did Drug X slow the rate of tumor growth compared to controls?

The raw data are presented in Appendix 1 at the end of the chapter.

This study design is a traditional repeated measures design. Figure 6.6 presents a scatter plot of mean tumor volume and standard deviation for each treatment group over time. Tumor volume appeared to increase in a curvilinear manner for each treatment group. Looking at the mean values one might easily conclude that at the 100 mg/kg IP dose level, tumor volume was significantly smaller than controls and that there might be a difference between 100 mg/kg PO versus IP. Additionally, tumor volume variability did not remain constant over time, but increased as time increased. Increasing variance over time will violate the assumption of homoscedasticity of the residuals if one were to fit tumor volume to a general linear model. Thus, a variance model will be needed or some transformation needs to be found such that tumor volume variance remains essentially constant over time.

Many researchers have shown that tumor growth tends to grow exponentially. Hence, a log-transformation might be useful here. Figure 6.7 presents the mean tumor volume and standard deviation on a log scale. Ln-transformed tumor volume appeared to grow more linearly, although there was some small curvature to the growth curve. More importantly, tumor volume

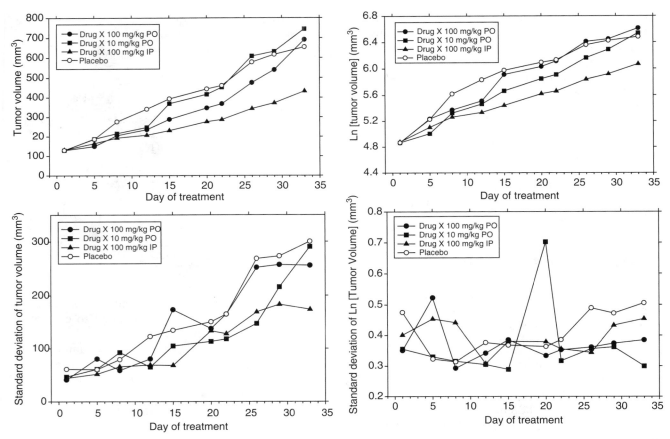

Figure 6.6 Mean (top) and standard deviation (bottom) of tumor volume in mice with A549 human lung carcinoma. Mice were dosed with saline, Drug X 10 mg/kg PO, Drug X 100 mg/kg PO, or Drug X 100 mg/kg IP once daily for 28 days.

Figure 6.7 Mean (top) and standard deviation (bottom) of tumor volume in log-scale in mice with A549 human lung carcinoma. Mice were dosed with saline, Drug X 10 mg/kg PO, Drug X 100 mg/kg PO, or Drug X 100 mg/kg IP once daily for 28 days.

variability remained relatively constant, which is what was desired. Hence, the difference between groups was examined using models with Ln-transformed tumor volume as the dependent variable using ML estimation. In a repeated measures analysis, time can be treated as a either a categorical or continuous variable. Time will first be treated as a categorical variable. In a traditional repeated measures analysis, treatment group, subject nested within group, day, and group by day interaction are all treated as fixed, categorical effects, while animal weight can be treated as a continuous covariate. The test for treatment group is not made using the residual variance, but instead calculated using the variance term for subject within treatment group. This model implicitly assumes that the correlation between observations is one of compound symmetry, which models all the covariances and correlations among observations as equal. Under this model, day ($p < 0.0001$) and group by day interaction ($p = 0.0131$) were both highly significant.

Interpreting main effects (day) in the presence of interactions can be difficult and controversial. Most books do not recommend interpreting main effects in the presence of an interaction arguing that such main effects are meaningless and instead recommend analyzing the main effects at each level of the interaction factor. In this case, this would involve testing for differences in treatment groups on each study day. When an analysis of variance was performed on Day 33 (data at the end of study), the p-value for treatment groups was 0.1040, indicating that Drug X had no differential effect on tumor growth nor was there a difference in route of administration.

Sometimes a suitable transformation, such as an inverse transform, can be found to remove the interaction, but in this case, the presence of an interaction is of specific interest because a significant interaction indicates that the treatments have a differential effect on the rate of tumor growth. So attempting to remove the interaction is not an option here.

Using a general linear model (GLM) approach to repeated measures data with time treated as a categorical variable is limited in two respects. First, such a model assumes a compound symmetry covariance matrix which defines the correlations between observations to be constant. In the case of unequally spaced data, such as with this example, such a covariance structure may be inappropriate. Second, when the dependent variable is missing at random, a GLM approach to the analysis may delete entire subjects (not just observations) leading to low power at detecting treatment effects when the data are treated as a multivariate repeated measures problem. In this case no missing data were present, so the latter problem is not an issue.

To explore the effect of the within-subject covariance structure on the analysis conclusions, many different within-subject covariance structures were explored within PROC MIXED in SAS, including simple, compound symmetry, Toeplitz, spatial power, spatial exponential, and spatial Gaussian. Treatment group, subject nested within group, day, and group by day interaction were all treated as fixed, categorical effects, while animal weight was treated as a continuous covariate. Numerator degrees of freedom were estimated using Satterthwaite's correction. Model parameters were estimated with ML. The results are presented in Table 6.7.

What should be immediately apparent is that the choice of the within-subject covariance can have a tremendous impact on the p-value for the fixed effects. In this example, the p-value for treatment group ranged from highly significant ($p < 0.0001$ assuming a simple covariance matrix) to nonsignificant ($p = 0.2381$ assuming a spatial power or Gaussian covariance). What should then be apparent is that the AIC selected a Toeplitz covariance as the best model, whereas the AICc and BIC both selected either the spatial power or spatial Gaussian covariance. With the Toeplitz covariance matrix, 10 covariance terms must be estimated, whereas with the spatial power or spatial Gaussian only two covariance parameters must be estimated. Both the AICc and BIC impose a heavier penalty for the number of estimable parameters in a model than the AIC, and so these

former two measures tend to select models with fewer estimable parameters than the AIC. It should be noted that the results obtained with PROC MIXED using a compound symmetry covariance were slightly different than those obtained with PROC GLM, the reason being that the mixed effects models were fit using ML. Had the mixed effects models been fit using REML, the mixed effects model under compound symmetry would have been identical to the GLM model. In this case, using a traditional repeated measures analysis, a significant treatment by time interaction was discovered. Using a different covariance structure ameliorated the significance of the interaction and resulted in a model whose only significant factor was day of administration. Hence, under this approach, Drug X was no different from controls and did not slow the rate of tumor growth. Nor was the difference between IP and oral routes of administration significant.

An alternative method to treating time as a categorical variable is to treat time as a continuous variable and to model time using a low-order polynomial, thereby reducing the number of estimable parameters in the model. In this case, rather than modeling the within-subject covariance the between-subject covariance is manipulated. Subjects are treated as random effects, as are the model parameters associated with time. The within-subject covariance matrix was treated as a simple covariance structure. In this example, time was modeled as a quadratic polynomial. Also, included in the model were the interactions associated with the quadratic term for time.

The results are presented in Table 6.8. Again, different between-subject covariance structured resulted in different results. The AIC and AICc selected the unstructured covariance (which has seven estimable covariance parameters) as the best model, whereas the BIC selected the simple covariance (which has four estimable covariance parameters) as the best model.

At this stage, different within-subject covariance structures, along with between-subject covariances, can

Table 6.7 Summary of linear mixed effect model analysis to tumor growth data using a repeated measures analysis of covariance treating time as a categorical variable.

	Simple	Compound symmetry	Toeplitz	Power	Exponential	Gaussian
		R-matrix covariance structure				
−2LL	385.8	216.6	−129.0	−108.3	81.8	−108.3
AIC	469.8	302.6	−27.0	−22.3	167.8	−22.3
AICc	485.1	318.7	−3.8	−6.3	183.9	−6.3
BIC	525.8	359.9	40.9	35.0	225.1	35.0
		p-Values for fixed effects				
Group	<0.0001	0.0700	0.2211	0.2381	<0.0001	0.2381
Day	<0.0001	<0.0001	<0.0001	<0.0001	<0.0001	<0.0001
Weight	0.0064	0.0929	0.8622	0.4493	0.1276	0.4493
Group × Day	0.5505	0.0016	0.1415	0.0327	0.5891	0.0327

Table 6.8 Summary of linear mixed effect model analysis to tumor growth data using a repeated measures analysis of covariance treating time as a continuous variable.

	G-matrix covariance structure		
	Simple	Compound symmetry	Unstructured
−2LL	−57.3	145.5	−66.2
AIC	−23.3	175.5	−26.2
AICc	−21.0	177.3	−23.0
BIC	−0.7	195.5	0.4
	p-Values for fixed effects		
Group	0.9304	0.7874	0.9444
Day	<0.0001	<0.0001	<0.0001
Group × Day	0.0035	0.0134	0.0119
Day2	<0.0001	0.0015	<0.0001
Group × Day2	0.0131	0.2587	0.0182
Weight	0.7064	0.4544	0.7153

Note: Day2 corresponds to day of treatment squared (day^2).

be examined. In this analysis, Toeplitz, spatial power, spatial exponential, and spatial Gaussian were examined against an unstructured G-matrix. Table 6.9 presents the results. Changing the within-subject covariance structured resulted in little change in the p-values for the fixed effects, but did improve the overall goodness of fit. The AIC selected the Toeplitz as the best model, whereas the AICc and BIC selected either the spatial power or spatial exponential model. At this point, heterogeneous covariance structures could be examined, such as allowing unique between-subject variability across treatment groups. When such a model was fit (which has 26 estimable covariance terms) the resulting AIC, AICc, and BIC were −57.6, −47.3, and −11.0, respectively, indicating that the additional covariance terms did not really improve the model. Further, regardless of the discrimination criteria used, all three showed

that weight was not statistically significant and could be removed from the model.

Model development has proceeded at finding an overparameterized model. A suitable covariance structure (unstructured G-matrix, spatial power R-matrix) has been found and so the next step then was model reduction. Weight was not statistically significant and was removed from the model. The resulting model had an AIC of −58.7 and a BIC of −33.4, indicating that removal of weight from the model was a wise choice as its inclusion did not improve the model fit. Removal of the treatment group variable, despite being not significant, should remain in the model since the day by group interaction was significant. Models with interaction effects that do not include the main effect may sometimes lead to confounding and inestimable model parameters. Hence, the fixed effects remained as is and the focus shifted to the covariance parameters.

Examination of the covariance parameters indicated that the variance component associated with day by group interaction was near zero. Removal of the variance component associated with day by treatment interaction resulted in a model with an AIC, AICc, and BIC of −58.1, −55.8, −35.5, respectively. The final model resulted in goodness of fit measures that were better than any other model considered so far. Recall that with ML estimation the variance components tend to be underestimated. The final model was then fit using REML. The results, and its comparison to ML, are presented in Table 6.10. Notice that the goodness of fit measures were different between ML and REML. That is because these metrics are not comparable between the estimation methods. Also notice that that variance components for REML were indeed larger than for ML. Figure 6.8 presents a scatter plot of observed versus predicted tumor volumes after back-transformation to

Table 6.9 Summary of linear mixed effect model analysis to tumor growth data using a repeated measures analysis of covariance treating time as a categorical variable using an unstructured G-matrix.

	R-matrix covariance structure					
	Simple	Compound symmetry	Toeplitz	Power	Exponential	Gaussian
−2LL	−66.2	−66.2	−109.5	−96.8	−96.8	−86.2
AIC	−26.2	−24.2	−57.5	−56.8	−56.8	−44.2
AICc	−23.0	−20.7	−52.0	−53.6	−53.6	−40.6
BIC	0.4	3.7	−22.9	−30.2	−30.2	−16.2
	p-Values for fixed effects					
Group	0.9444	0.9444	0.9310	0.9652	0.9652	0.9571
Day	<0.0001	<0.0001	<0.0001	<0.0001	<0.0001	<0.0001
Group × Day	0.0119	0.0119	0.0033	0.0052	0.0052	0.0059
Day2	<0.0001	<0.0001	<0.0001	<0.0001	<0.0001	<0.0001
Group × Day2	0.0182	0.0182	0.0028	0.0128	0.0128	0.0139
Weight	0.7153	0.7153	0.8696	0.6977	0.6977	0.7729

Note: Day2 corresponds to day of treatment squared (day^2).

Table 6.10 Comparison of ML and REML goodness of fit metrics and p-values for significance of fixed effects for tumor growth example under the final model (unstructured G-matrix, spatial power R-matrix).

Discrimination criteria	ML	REML
−2LL	−92.1	4.7
AIC	−58.1	14.7
AICc	−55.8	14.9
BIC	−35.5	21.3
Fixed effects	p-value	p-value
Group	0.9645	0.9712
Day	<0.0001	<0.0001
Group × Day	0.0221	0.0340
Day2	<0.0001	<0.0001
Day2 × Group	0.0120	0.0172
Variance Components	Estimate	Estimate
Between-subject	0.1065	0.1236
Day	5.50×10^{-4}	6.36×10^{-4}
Covariance (Day, between-subject)	-3.62×10^{-3}	-4.14×10^{-3}
Residual	0.0389	0.0435

Note: Day2 corresponds to day of treatment squared (day^2).

the original domain. There was good concordance between observed and model predicted volumes. Examination of the residual plots and distribution of the residuals (Fig. 6.9) did not indicate any significant bias or trend in the model predictions. Figure 6.10 presents scatter plots of observed data for the first mouse in each treatment group and the model predicted volumes. Overall, the model appeared to be an adequate fit to the data.

However, a test for normality on the residuals indicated that the residuals were not normally distributed (p < 0.01). Of what impact was this violation on the model inferences? Probably little. First, it is well known

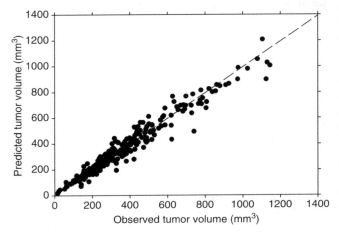

Figure 6.8 Scatter plot of observed versus predicted tumor volume. Dashed line is the line of unity.

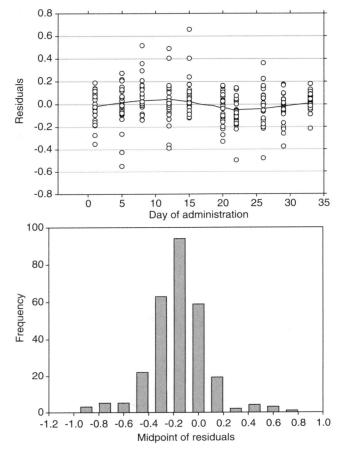

Figure 6.9 Scatter plot of residuals versus day of drug administration (top) and histogram of residuals (bottom). Solid line in top plot is the LOESS fit to the data.

that an F-test in an ANOVA is relatively robust to departures from normality. Second, the nonnormality in this case was not due to heavy tails, which would tend to inflate the residual variance estimate and decrease the power to detect significant fixed effects. Third, the skewness and kurtosis of the residuals was 0.19 and 2.95, respectively. Theoretically, for a normal distribution the skewness should be 0 with a kurtosis of 3. The nonnormality of the residuals appeared to be due to a slight skewness in the residuals, not due to a kurtosis violation. Kurtosis deviations tend to have more impact than skewness deviations. Hence, the nonnormality violation was ignored.

Now, returning to the questions posed by the researchers. When analysis of variance was done on Day 33 data only, the p-value for treatment group was 0.1587. Thus, there was no apparent difference in mean tumor volumes among treatments nor was there a difference between IP and PO administration of Drug X. Basically, Drug X could not be distinguished from placebo at the doses given despite the apparent difference in

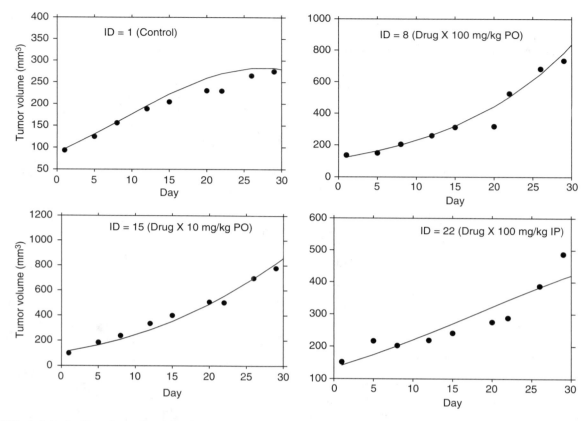

Figure 6.10   Individual subject plots and model predicted values for the first subject in each treatment group.

the mean plots. The inability to distinguish between placebo and Drug X may have been due to a combination of moderate between-subject variability with small sample size leading to low statistical power.

SUMMARY

Linear mixed effects models are primarily used in pharmacodynamic analysis or in the statistical analysis of pharmacokinetic parameters. Linear mixed effects models could also be used to analyze concentration-time data from a 1-compartment model with bolus administration after Ln-transformation. The advantages to using mixed effects in an analysis are that observations within a subject may be correlated and that in addition to estimation of the model parameters, between- and within-subject variability may be estimated. Also, the structural model is based on the population, not on data from any one particular subject, thus allowing for sparse sampling. Most statistical packages now include linear mixed effects models as part of their analysis options, as do some pharmacokinetic software (Win-Nonlin). While linear mixed effects models are not cov-

ered in most pharmacokinetic texts, their application is increasing and since they form a special case of nonlinear mixed effect modeling, the analysis method used to perform population pharmacokinetic analysis, a working understanding of this class of models is useful for the pharmacokineticist.

Recommended Reading

Cnaan, A., Laird, N.M., and Slasor, P. Using the general linear mixed model to analyse unbalanced repeated measures and longitudinal data. *Statistics in Medicine* 1997; 16: 2349–2380.

Littell, R.C., Milliken, G.A., Stroup, W.W., and Wolfinger, R.D. *SAS system for mixed models.* Cary, NC: SAS Institute, Inc., 1996.

Verbeke, G. and Molenberghs, G. *Linear mixed models in practice: A SAS-oriented approach.* New York: Springer 1997.

Wolfinger, R.D. Heterogeneous variance–covariance structures for repeated measures. *Journal of Agricultural, Biological, and Environmental Statistics* 1996; 1: 205–230.

Wolfinger, R.D. An example of using mixed models and PROC MIXED for longitudinal data. *Journal of Biopharmaceutical Statistics* 1997; 7: 481–500.

APPENDIX 1: TUMOR VOLUME DATA

		Control group							
		Weight	Volume	Weight	Volume	Weight	Volume	Weight	Volume
Group	Day	Mouse 1	Mouse 1	Mouse 2	Mouse 2	Mouse 3	Mouse 3	Mouse 4	Mouse 4
1	1	25.7	93.3	28.4	107.9	25.5	160.1	23.6	226.5
1	5	25.8	124.5	29.6	193.6	28.6	209.1	23.7	287.6
1	8	24.2	155.6	28.6	220.3	28.7	358.4	23.8	364.1
1	12	24.6	188.1	29.0	277.2	29.5	491.8	24.2	479.2
1	15	26.7	204.2	28.3	366.5	28.5	552.5	24.4	566.8
1	20	25.6	230.0	20.0	435.2	29.2	670.3	24.3	585.8
1	22	25.4	229.1	29.2	442.8	29.7	698.3	24.8	635.1
1	26	26.8	264.7	30.7	579.5	30.1	973.2	25.9	855.4
1	29	26.5	274.6	30.1	691.6	29.9	1026.4	25.3	878.4
1	33	26.4	273.8	29.1	765.1	30.6	1078.7	25.9	925.9

		Weight	Volume	Weight	Volume	Weight	Volume
Group	Day	Mouse 5	Mouse 5	Mouse 6	Mouse 6	Mouse 7	Mouse 7
1	1	25.5	73.9	24.6	183.8	29.0	64.8
1	5	25.2	123.9	25.5	222.9	28.6	141.5
1	8	25.0	222.0	25.1	282.9	28.6	327.7
1	12	25.5	226.6	25.0	302.7	29.6	421.6
1	15	25.0	271.8	25.5	366.1	29.1	426.3
1	20	26.4	310.3	26.4	418.2	28.8	454.7
1	22	26.1	313.3	26.0	435.9	29.1	469.2
1	26	27.3	337.7	27.2	382.9	29.4	650.1
1	29	27.0	404.6	26.8	409.1	30.0	627.3
1	33	26.1	463.4	26.7	415.9	29.8	862.0

		Drug X (100 mg/kg) PO							
		Weight	Volume	Weight	Volume	Weight	Volume	Weight	Volume
Group	Day	Mouse 8	Mouse 8	Mouse 9	Mouse 9	Mouse 10	Mouse 10	Mouse 11	Mouse 11
2	1	28.3	135.8	27.0	127.1	24.9	61.4	23.9	84.6
2	5	30.1	149.5	26.0	116.5	25.3	62.2	25.5	106.4
2	8	30.4	204.2	26.1	167.9	25.0	116.5	25.8	105.3
2	12	30.1	258.5	26.3	237.7	25.5	155.7	25.8	141.0
2	15	29.4	311.9	25.9	302.7	24.8	176.4	25.3	154.8
2	20	30.0	317.7	26.2	404.0	25.3	303.1	25.9	154.8
2	22	30.2	525.3	26.3	422.3	25.2	291.2	26.0	184.3
2	26	31.4	682.3	27.2	455.5	26.4	622.4	27.0	240.1
2	29	31.2	734.8	27.8	804.8	26.0	489.8	25.1	266.5
2	33	30.4	1145.2	27.0	909.4	26.0	685.4	25.9	306.1

		Weight	Volume	Weight	Volume	Weight	Volume
Group	Day	Mouse 12	Mouse 12	Mouse 13	Mouse 13	Mouse 14	Mouse 14
2	1	28.7	201.1	27.0	136.4	25.2	162.7
2	5	27.1	244.5	28.0	167.4	24.3	199.1
2	8	27.2	380.9	27.8	222.2	23.7	240.3
2	12	27.4	320.6	28.5	259.6	23.8	278.7
2	15	27.1	472.4	28.4	282.3	23.5	318.2
2	20	26.1	530.0	28.3	343.7	22.6	369.8
2	22	26.8	484.4	29.4	320.6	22.8	349.3
2	26	28.3	499.5	29.4	444.3	24.1	383.3
2	29	27.9	726.7	29.9	426.9	24.7	323.8
2	33	27.5	820.2	29.9	517.6	25.0	450.6

Note: Weight in grams; volume in mm^3.

Drug X (10 mg/kg) PO

		Weight	Volume	Weight	Volume	Weight	Volume	Weight	Volume
Group	Day	Mouse 15	Mouse 15	Mouse 16	Mouse 16	Mouse 17	Mouse 17	Mouse 18	Mouse 18
3	1	27.1	99.1	25.6	129.0	28.5	162.7	27.6	117.0
3	5	23.4	183.8	25.1	142.2	29.2	184.0	28.3	202.3
3	8	20.1	237.1	26.0	165.3	29.6	240.3	24.3	210.7
3	12	24.0	334.1	26.2	173.2	30.1	153.8	28.4	255.9
3	15	23.9	399.4	25.9	304.2	29.7	230.0	27.9	290.5
3	20	25.1	506.9	27.0	305.3	30.1	236.3	28.4	366.9
3	22	25.1	500.9	26.4	398.7	19.4	241.9	18.4	373.2
3	26	25.9	696.6	27.6	620.0	30.0	379.5	29.0	516.9
3	29	25.4	777.7	27.4	621.0	30.0	373.5	28.4	516.9
3	33	25.0	975.8	26.7	807.9	30.1	352.0	27.8	619.0

		Weight	Volume	Weight	Volume	Weight	Volume
Group	Day	Mouse 19	Mouse 19	Mouse 20	Mouse 20	Mouse 21	Mouse 21
3	1	27.1	65.7	28.8	142.9	25.4	190.4
3	5	27.1	60.1	29.8	213.2	25.2	328.1
3	8	27.3	124.5	29.9	223.0	25.7	308.4
3	12	27.2	172.1	28.5	304.2	25.6	337.9
3	15	26.6	262.8	29.0	354.3	25.3	740.9
3	20	27.5	404.6	30.0	435.7	24.0	656.7
3	22	17.6	393.8	29.5	482.4	24.4	773.3
3	26	29.1	438.9	30.1	479.2	26.9	1125.0
3	29	29.1	573.9	29.7	423.4	26.9	1130.1
3	33	29.3	786.5	29.7	562.2	27.4	1105.4

Drug X (100 mg/kg) IP

		Weight	Volume	Weight	Volume	Weight	Volume	Weight	Volume
Group	Day	Mouse 22	Mouse 22	Mouse 23	Mouse 23	Mouse 24	Mouse 24	Mouse 25	Mouse 25
4	1	26.5	151.6	30.1	129.5	24.1	84.1	26.8	164.8
4	5	25.6	216.6	28.5	139.2	27.2	102.8	27.8	206.7
4	8	26.3	202.2	28.7	157.6	26.7	125.4	27.2	222.9
4	12	26.7	218.5	29.5	184.5	27.3	174.6	27.8	239.7
4	15	25.4	240.9	28.3	234.5	26.6	189.8	26.8	239.8
4	20	27.2	275.2	28.7	289.9	28.2	249.9	28.0	276.8
4	22	27.6	288.0	29.8	265.9	29.1	245.1	28.9	277.7
4	26	29.1	387.2	31.0	317.6	29.8	296.5	28.9	269.8
4	29	29.1	487.4	30.2	358.7	28.7	315.0	28.6	338.7
4	33	28.3	488.4	29.4	516.6	28.2	386.9	28.5	379.3

		Weight	Volume	Weight	Volume	Weight	Volume
Group	Day	Mouse 26	Mouse 26	Mouse 27	Mouse 27	Mouse 28	Mouse 28
4	1	28.6	117.0	26.6	198.5	26.7	74.5
4	5	26.4	155.6	27.5	225.5	26.0	106.7
4	8	25.9	181.3	27.7	321.0	26.3	141.0
4	12	26.2	140.9	28.2	342.2	27.7	150.7
4	15	25.8	139.3	28.5	362.4	26.9	210.7
4	20	26.9	52.9	29.2	512.8	27.7	275.7
4	22	26.9	27.6	30.0	586.6	28.0	319.4
4	26	27.9	21.0	30.8	729.0	28.7	380.9
4	29	27.8	18.5	30.1	780.5	28.7	305.3
4	33	27.3	15.8	29.5	838.2	28.3	403.1

Note: Weight in grams; volume in mm^3.

Chapter 7

Nonlinear Mixed Effects Models: Theory

Tortured data will confess to anything.

—Fredric M. Menger (1937–), Candler Professor
of Chemistry, Emory University

INTRODUCTION

Nonlinear mixed effects models are similar to linear mixed effects models with the difference being that the function under consideration f(x, θ) is nonlinear in the model parameters θ. Population pharmacokinetics (PopPK) is the study of pharmacokinetics in the population of interest and instead of modeling data from each individual separately, data from all individuals are modeled simultaneously. To account for the different levels of variability (between-subject, within-subject, interoccasion, residual, etc.), nonlinear mixed effects models are used. For the remainder of the chapter, the term PopPK will be used synonymously with nonlinear mixed effects models, even though the latter covers a richer class of models and data types. Along with PopPK is population pharmacodynamics (PopPD), which is the study of a drug's effect in the population of interest. Often PopPK and PopPD are combined into a singular PopPK-PD analysis.

The primary goal of PopPK is to obtain a model relating concentration to dose and individual covariates. A PopPD model then relates drug concentrations to effect. A secondary goal is to obtain estimates of the mean pharmacokinetic parameters and the sources of variability in the population. The advantage of nonlinear mixed effects models is that the data need not be "rich," or dense, as in a nonlinear regression analysis of single-subject data. The data do not have to follow any particular structured sampling time schedule and may have irregular sampling times. Further, the data may be "sparse" with as little as one observation per subject, "rich" with many observations per subject, or a combination of both with some subjects having many samples collected in a dosing interval while others have only a few. Table 7.1 lists some of the strengths and weaknesses of the population approach. A major hindrance to implementing population methods in drug development is that it is mathematically and statistically complex, and compared to the number of pharmacokineticists in general there are few modelers who specialize in the methodology.

PopPK has created a paradigm shift in the role and influence of pharmacokinetics in drug development. In the time since the early 1980s when Sheiner, Beal, and colleagues (1980; 1981; 1977) introduced population methods to the pharmacokinetic community, PopPK has reinvigorated the use of compartmental and mechanistic models to a field that was being increasingly drawn toward noncompartmental, summary statistic-like approaches to data analysis. Today, PopPK is an integral component in regulatory applications for drug marketing approval as it summarizes pharmacokinetic data obtained across many phases of drug development. PopPK was even granted its own Guidance for Industry, issued by the Food and Drug Administration (FDA) in 1999, something that noncompartmental methods have not been able to achieve (United States Department of Health and Human Services et al., 1999). Also, the Common Technical Document, which is set to become

Table 7.1 Strengths and weaknesses of the population pharmacokinetic-pharmacodynamic approach.

Strengths

- Data generated from population of interest
- Use is made of more data than is possible with traditional pharmacokinetic and pharmacodynamic study designs, particularly with unbalanced data
- Population methods can analyze sparse data and integrate data from different sources
- Population subgroups can be identified, which otherwise might not have been found
- Important covariates which explain subject variability can be identified
- A model based approach that facilitates inclusion of prior knowledge, thus enhancing understanding and statistical power
- Can overcome ethical barriers that prohibit traditional Phase 1 studies from being performed, e.g., children
- Information obtained may be used for individualized prediction of dose
- Model may be used to develop what if scenarios
- Facilitates inclusion of prior knowledge, thus increasing understanding

Weaknesses

- Perceived as complicated and difficult to implement
- Few "experts" available for consultation and education
- Often misunderstood as a quick fix for poorly designed studies
- Methods are difficult to understand
- Less power than Phase 1 studies
- Very expensive
- Time consuming
- Difficult to review
- Different analysts may develop different models
- Database issue and data management issues that must be resolved

Reprinted and modified with permission from Tett, S., Holford, N.H., and McLachlan, A.J. Population pharmacokinetics and pharmacodynamics: An underutilized resource. *Drug Information Journal* (1998); 32: 693–710. Copyright © 1998, Drug Information Association.

the standard format for new marketing applications in regions that subscribe to the International Conference on Harmonization, has an entire subsection dedicated to the results of population analyses. Despite these advances, population methods are not routinely taught at the graduate level and pharmaceutical companies still have difficulty recruiting individuals with PopPK experience.

APPLICATION OF POPPK IN DRUG DEVELOPMENT

Perhaps the area where PopPK has made the largest impact is in drug development. Prior to the introduction of NONMEM as a commercial software package, there was little one could do with pharmacokinetic data collected from Phase 3 clinical studies beyond, perhaps, summary statistics and correlations between some summary measure of the pharmacokinetic data, like the mean or median concentration in a subject, and subject

covariates. Today, depending on the company and the drug under consideration, PopPK can have no impact in how the drug is developed or can be a major driver in how the drug is developed. In most cases, the role of PopPK in drug development is probably somewhere in between.

It is in the product label, which is the major source of information for clinicians on the safe and effective use of a drug (Marroum and Gobburu, 2002), where PopPK analysis has had major impact. Olson et al. (2000) examined all the NDAs submitted to the FDA by Parke–Davis, prior to its merger with Pfizer, from the 10 years between 1990 and 2000 and found a PopPK analysis was included in the submission for 12 drugs. Sixty-five (65) project team members who worked on these drugs were surveyed on their perception of how PopPK analysis impacted the development of the drug. A total of 79% felt that the results of the PopPK analysis were reflected in the product label. Seven of 12 drugs had information from the PopPK analysis included in the product label. It was also noteworthy that 74% of the respondents felt that PopPK analysis led to more assurance about decisions made during the development of the drug, while only 47% felt that PopPK analysis facilitated approval of the drug.

An example of how PopPK analyses are reported in the product label can be found in the product label for Xeloda (capecitabine), which is manufactured by Hoffman-La Roche:

> *"A population analysis of pooled data from two large controlled studies in patients with colorectal cancer (n = 505) who were administered XELODA at 1250 mg/m² twice a day indicated that gender (202 males and 303 females) and race (455 white/Caucasian patients, 22 black patients, and 28 patients of other race) have no influence on the pharmacokinetics of 5'-DFUR [5'-deoxy-5-fluorouridine], 5-FU [5-fluorouracil], and FBAL [α-fluoro -β-alanine]. Age has no significant influence on the pharmacokinetics 5'-FDUR and 5-FU over the age range 27–86 years. A 20% increase in age results in a 15% increase in AUC of FBAL."*

The label clearly states that what follows are from the results of a PopPK analysis, what was the sample size, and what were the results from the analysis—that race and sex have no impact on the pharmacokinetics of Xeloda®.

PopPK may also be used to shorten development times of new drugs. Since the year 1997 a slowdown in the number of new drug applications submitted to the FDA has occurred almost every year. Along with that is the almost exponential growth in research and development spending by pharmaceutical companies. Hence, companies are producing fewer drugs having spent more money in the process. In an effort to increase the productivity of pharmaceutical companies, the FDA (2004) has issued their "critical path initiative" which aims to decrease clinical development times. One of the processes by which the FDA believes pharmaceutical companies can increase efficiency is through model-based drug development, a view that has been expressed by others (Lesko et al., 2000). The question then becomes where in drug development can such model-based analyses improve the process. Peck, Rubin, and Sheiner (2003) have suggested that with the Food and Drug Administration Modernization Act (FDAMA) of 1997, which changed the standard of drug approval from safety and efficacy from at least two controlled trials to safety and efficacy from a single controlled trial plus confirmatory evidence, that mechanistic modeling and simulation could, in certain situations, such as when the pharmacology of the drug is well understood, be used as the confirmatory evidence for drug approval.

In summary, PopPK has had a major influence how pharmacokinetic data are reported and analyzed. Its role in drug development will only increase as computers become faster, as more pharmacokineticists become familiar with it, and project managers and clinicians become more comfortable with its use. Indeed, there is a trend in job advertisements for pharmacokineticists to have experience in population-based methods as a requirement for hiring. Surprisingly, however, few universities actually teach population-based methods, which may be a reflection on the newness of the technology or the difficulty in obtaining grants to research this approach. Regardless, the small number of centers where population methods are taught combined with the paucity of pharmacokineticists with experience in population-based methods has resulted in a high industrial demand. One of the purposes of this book is to provide pharmacokineticists with the statistical and modeling background necessary to perform PopPK analyses.

THE NONLINEAR MIXED EFFECTS MODEL

Nonlinear mixed effects models consist of two components: the structural model (which may or may not contain covariates) and the statistical or variance model. The structural model describes the mean response for the population. Similar to a linear mixed effects model, nonlinear mixed effects models can be developed using a hierarchical approach. Data consist of an independent sample of n-subjects with the ith subject having n_i-observations measured at time points $t_{i,1}, t_{i,2}, \ldots t_{i,ni}$. Let Y be the vector of observations, $Y = \{Y_{1,1}, Y_{1,2}, \ldots Y_{n,1}, Y_{n,2}, \ldots Y_{n,ni})^T$ and let ε

be the same size vector of random intraindividual errors. In Stage 1 (intraindividual variation level), the model describing how the mean response profile changes over time is

$$Y = f(x; t; \beta) + \varepsilon \quad (7.1)$$

where x is a matrix of fixed effect covariates specific to the subject and β is a vector of estimable regression parameters. For simplicity, x will include t from this point. The regression function f depends on β in a nonlinear manner. At Stage 2 (interindividual variation level), the possibility that some of the β (denoted β_i, $\beta_i \in \beta$) can vary across individuals (with mean $\mu_{\beta i}$ and variance $\omega^2_{\beta_i}$) is allowed, i.e., $\beta_i \sim (\mu_{\beta i}, \omega^2_{\beta_i})$, and can be "explained" by a set of subject-specific covariates z. In other words, β_i is not fixed across individuals, but allowed to vary, and that variability may be explained by subject-specific covariates. This stage is referred to as a covariate submodel and relates how subject-specific covariates (z) predict the subject-specific regression parameters (β_i), i.e.,

$$\beta_i \sim \left(h(z; \theta), \omega^2_{\beta_i} \right) \quad (7.2)$$

where θ is a vector of estimable regression parameters. Collectively the set of all $\omega^2_{\beta_i}$ is referred to as the variance–covariance matrix, denoted Ω. Those βs that do not vary across individuals are referred to as fixed effects, whereas those β_is that do vary across individuals are referred to as random effects. The structural model across all individuals is then

$$Y = f(\beta; \theta; x; z). \quad (7.3)$$

For simplicity, the set of estimable regression parameters $\{\beta, \theta\}$ shall be denoted as θ.

As a pharmacokinetic example, for the 1-compartment model after single dose intravenous administration, Y would be drug concentration, x would consist of dose (D) and sample time (t), and β would consist of clearance (CL) and volume of distribution (V)

$$\beta = \begin{bmatrix} \mu_{CL} \\ \mu_{V} \end{bmatrix}. \quad (7.4)$$

If clearance and volume of distribution were treated as correlated random effects, then ω^2_{CL} and ω^2_V denote the between-subject variability for clearance and volume of distribution, respectively, and

$$\Omega = \begin{bmatrix} \omega^2_{CL} & \omega_{CL, V} \\ & \omega^2_{V} \end{bmatrix} \quad (7.5)$$

where $\omega_{CL,\,V}$ is the covariance between clearance and volume of distribution. Now further suppose that an individual's age was linearly related to clearance. Then clearance could be modeled as

$$CL_i = \theta_1 + \theta_2 Age_i + \eta_i \qquad (7.6)$$

where CL_i is the average clearance for an individual with Age_i, θ_1 and θ_2 are the intercept and slope, respectively, Age_i is the age of the ith subject, and η_i is the deviation of the ith individual from mean clearance of the population having Age_i. The ηs are assumed to be independent, have mean zero, and constant variance ω^2. In Eq. (7.3), age would comprise the set z. The hierarchical nonlinear mixed effects model can then be written as

$$\begin{bmatrix} CL \\ V \end{bmatrix} \sim \left(\begin{array}{c} \theta_1 + \theta_2 Age, \\ \mu_V \end{array} \quad \begin{bmatrix} \omega_{CL}^2 & \omega_{CL,\,V} \\ & \omega_V^2 \end{bmatrix} \right) \qquad (7.7)$$

$$Y = f(D; t; CL; V; Age)$$
$$= \frac{D}{V} \exp\left(-\frac{\theta_1 + \theta_2 Age}{V} t \right). \qquad (7.8)$$

At this point no assumptions have been made regarding the distribution of the random effects other than their scale.

Residual variance models were described in detail in the chapter on variance models and weighting. What was detailed in that chapter readily extends to nonlinear mixed effects models. As might be expected, residual variance models model the random, unexplained variability in the regression function f. Hence, the structural model is extended to

$$Y = f(\theta; \Phi; x; z; \varepsilon) \qquad (7.9)$$

where ε is the residual term and Φ are residual variance model parameters. All other variables are the same as before. Common variance functions are:

- Additive error

$$Y = f(\theta; x) + \varepsilon \qquad (7.10)$$

- Constant coefficient of variation (CV) or proportional error

$$Y = f(\theta; x)(1 + \varepsilon) \qquad (7.11)$$

- Exponential error

$$Y = f(\theta; x) \exp(\varepsilon) \qquad (7.12)$$

- Combined additive and proportional

$$Y = f(\theta; x)(1 + \varepsilon_1) + \varepsilon_2. \qquad (7.13)$$

Under all these models, the generic residuals are assumed to be independent, have zero mean, and constant variance σ^2. Collectively the set of all residual variance components, σ^2, is referred to as the residual variance matrix (Σ), the elements of which are not necessarily independent, i.e., the residual variance components can be correlated, which is referred to as *autocorrelation*. It is generally assumed that ε and η are independent, but this condition may be relaxed for residual error models with proportional terms (referred to as an $\eta - \varepsilon$ interaction, which will be discussed later).

Returning to the previous structural model, a complete nonlinear mixed effects model may be written as

$$Y_{ij} = \left(\frac{D_i}{V_i} \exp\left[\frac{-(\theta_{1i} + \theta_{2i} Age_i + \eta_i) t_{ij}}{V_i} \right] \right) \exp(\varepsilon_{ij}) \qquad (7.14)$$

where D_i is the dose administered to the ith subject, V_i the volume of distribution for the ith subject, clearance is modeled as a random effect that is a linear function of age, η_i the deviation for the ith subject from the population mean clearance such that η has mean 0 and variance ω^2, t_{ij} the time, and ε has mean 0 and variance σ^2. Collectively Ω is equal to Eq. (7.5) and Σ is a scalar equal to σ^2, since there is only one residual error term.

THE STRUCTURAL OR BASE MODEL

The first step in the development of a PopPK model is to identify the base or structural model, which is the model that best describes the data in the absence of covariates. It may be, however, that a covariate has such a profound influence on a particular model parameter, one may choose to include that covariate into the base model right from the start. For instance if a drug is eliminated from the body exclusively by the kidney, such as topotecan or the aminoglycosides, then creatinine clearance (CrCL) may be very highly correlated with systemic clearance and so CrCL may be built into the model from the beginning stages. If previous studies have identified a structural model one typically proceeds from there. In the absence of a known base model, one plan of attack is to try a variety of base models, 1-, 2-, and 3-compartment models with different absorption models (if the drug is given by extravascular administration) and choose the best model using a combination of likelihood ratio test (LRT), Akaike information criterion (AIC), and graphical examination using residual plots, etc. Once the base model is identified, covariate submodels are then developed.

For Phase 3 data, it is not uncommon to find that there are large "gaps" in the concentration–time profile. For example, in an out-patient study where drug is dosed once a day in the morning, one often sees no data collected from 10 to 22 h after drug administration since this would place sample collection in the evening when most physician's offices are not open for business. For a 1-compartment model this might not be a problem, but for a drug exhibiting multiphasic pharmacokinetics this is problematic since it might not be possible to differentiate when one phase of the concentration–time profile ends and another phase begins. One strategy then is to augment the dataset with data from Phase 1 studies where concentration data are available during the missing interval and "fill-in" the gap in the concentration–time profile. If the Phase 1 data were collected in healthy normal volunteers and the Phase 3 data collected in subjects, a binary covariate (0 = healthy, 1 = subject) can be included into the covariate submodel to account for differences in pharmacokinetics between healthy subjects and subjects with the disease.

MODELING RANDOM EFFECTS

Although one is usually more often interested in estimates of the population mean for a parameter, sometimes one is just as interested in the variability of the parameter among subjects in a population. Indeed, in order to do any type of Monte Carlo simulation of a model, one needs both an estimate of the mean and variance of the parameter. Keep in mind, it is not the variance or standard error of the *estimate* of a parameter being discussed, but how much the value of that parameter varies from individual to individual. Such variability makes the parameter a random effect, as opposed to a fixed effect that has no variability associated with it.

On the other hand, it is sometimes seen in the literature that the estimation of the random effects are not of interest, but are treated more as nuisance variables in an analysis. In this case, the analyst is more interested in the fixed effects and their estimation. This view of random effects characterization is rather narrow because in order to precisely estimate the fixed effects in a model, the random effects have to be properly accounted for. Too few random effects in a model leads to biased estimates of the fixed effects, whereas too many random effects lead to overly large standard errors (Altham, 1984).

Random effects are useful, not only for quantifying the variability in a population, but also for being able to

determine an individual's empirical Bayes estimate (EBE) for some parameter, e.g., an individual's clearance. Also, if an EBE of a parameter is available, one can use the estimate to examine for groups of subpopulations that may be of interest or one can look for correlations between subject-specific characteristics, like age or weight, and the parameter of interest. When a covariate is introduced into a model, then the variability associated with that parameter should be decreased since the change in parameter values is predictable based on the covariate.

In a population analysis, there are usually two sources of variability: between-subject variability (BSV), sometimes called intersubject variability, and residual variability. Between-subject variability refers to the variance of a parameter across different individuals in the population. In this text, intersubject variability will be used interchangeably with between-subject variability. Residual variability refers to the unexplained variability in the observed data after controlling for other sources of variability. There are other sources of variability that are sometimes encountered in the pharmacokinetic literature: interoccasion variability (IOV) and interstudy variability. Each of these sources of variability and how to model them will now be discussed.

Modeling Between Subject Variability (BSV)

One would not expect that a parameter in a model will be a constant across all individuals. For example, one would not expect clearance or volume of distribution to be a constant value for all individuals, i.e., not every subject would be expected to have a volume of distribution of 125 L for example. One could begin by assuming that all model parameters are random and that there will be some variability in their values across individuals. However, assuming that all parameters are random is not realistic either because it may be that the right type of data has not been collected or not enough data has been collected to estimate the variability of a particular parameter in a population and so the model will need to be simplified by treating that parameter as a fixed effect. For example, suppose a drug exhibits biexponential kinetics, it is not uncommon to see with Phase 3 data that the BSV in intercompartmental clearance and/or peripheral volume of distribution cannot be estimated. Another common situation is the inability to estimate the BSV of the absorption rate constant for an orally administered drug with sparse pharmacokinetic data. In both cases, the parameters may be treated as a fixed effect across individuals. Hence, a model may consist some parameters that are fixed across all individuals and some parameters that are allowed to vary across individuals.

For cases where the variability across individuals can be estimated, the choice of how to model the variability is often based on the type of data. Pharmacokinetic data is often modeled on an exponential scale since pharmacokinetic model parameters must be constrained to be greater than zero and are often right skewed. Hence, the model parameter for the ith subject (θ_i) is written as

$$\theta_i = \theta_\mu \exp(\eta_i) \qquad (7.15)$$

where θ_μ is the population mean and η_i is the deviation from the mean for the ith subject with zero mean and variance ω^2. Under this model, the variance estimate ω^2 is the variance in the log-domain, which will not have the same magnitude as θ_μ. For example, the population mean clearance may be 100 L/h with a between-subject log-standard deviation of 0.5 L/h. One can use the equation

$$CV(\%) = \sqrt{\exp(\omega^2) - 1} \times 100\% \qquad (7.16)$$

to convert the variance on a log-scale to a coefficient of variation (CV) in the original scale. Hence, in the example, the coefficient of variability for clearance would be 53% in the population. It is often reported in the literature that a useful approximation to CV(%) is simply the square root of $\omega^2 \times 100\%$ (see Fig. 7.1). There are a number of reasons for why this approximation is valid and useful. First, for first-order approximation estimation methods (which will be discussed later in the chapter), Eq. (7.15) is equivalent to

$$\theta_i = \theta_\mu(1 + \eta_i). \qquad (7.17)$$

The expected value of Eq. (7.17) is θ_μ with variance $\theta_\mu^2 \omega^2$. Using the standard equation for CV(%)

$$
\begin{aligned}
CV(\%) &= \frac{\sqrt{\text{variance}}}{\text{mean}} \times 100\% \\
&= \frac{\sqrt{\theta_\mu^2 \omega^2}}{\theta_\mu} \times 100\% \\
&= \sqrt{\omega^2} \times 100\%
\end{aligned} \qquad (7.18)
$$

Hence, Eq. (7.18) is exactly equal to the CV(%) under first-order approximation. The problem lies with conditional estimation methods because then Eq. (7.15) is not expressed as Eq. (7.17). However, the approximation is still valid because as $\omega^2 \to 0$, then $\exp(\omega^2) \to 1$, and $\exp(\omega^2) - 1 \to 0$. Hence, $\exp(\omega^2) - 1 \to \omega^2$ as $\omega^2 \to 0$. In other words, because the limit of exponentiation approaches 1.0 as ω^2 approaches zero, then $\exp(\omega^2) - 1$

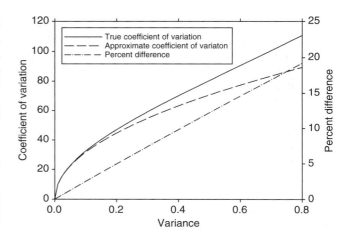

Figure 7.1 Line plot of the coefficient of variation of a log-normal distribution as a function of the population variance using the true equation $\left(\sqrt{\exp(\omega^2) - 1} \times 100\%\right)$ and the approximate equation $\left(\sqrt{\omega^2} \times 100\%\right)$. The approximation's accuracy increases as $\omega^2 \to 0$ since then $\exp(\omega^2) \to 1$ and begins to show significant percent error when the variance is greater than ~ 0.4.

approaches zero, as does its square root. This is the same as taking the square root of ω^2 in the first place. Although, it has been argued that even for large ω^2 the approximation is still valid because of the large uncertainty in estimating ω^2. The "added accuracy" of Eq. (7.16) may not really represent added accuracy but could just as well be added garbage (Beal, 1997). Beal suggests that rather than reporting CV%, one should report "apparent CV%" using Eq. (7.18), a value that is on the CV scale and is mildly related to an actual but unknown CV. In a review of the literature it seems that which formula one uses is a matter of personal preference with no equation seen as superior to the other.

In the simplest case, all the random effects are uncorrelated, in which case the variance–covariance matrix can be expressed as a diagonal or simple matrix. For example, if ω_{CL}^2 is the variance for clearance and ω_v^2 is the variance for volume of distribution, then the variance–covariance matrix (which will be referred to synonymously with the term "covariance matrix") can be expressed as

$$\Omega = \begin{bmatrix} \omega_{CL}^2 & 0 \\ 0 & \omega_v^2 \end{bmatrix}. \qquad (7.19)$$

More often than not, the random effects are not uncorrelated but are correlated with each other and so a covariance term ($\omega_{CL, v}$) is added to the variance–covariance matrix

$$\Omega = \begin{bmatrix} \omega_{CL}^2 & \\ \omega_{CL, v} & \omega_v^2 \end{bmatrix}. \qquad (7.20)$$

Such a matrix with nonzero off-diagonal elements is sometimes referred to as an unstructured or block matrix. It should be noted that the elements on the diagonal of Ω are referred to as the variance terms, while the off-diagonal elements are the covariance terms. Collectively, both Ω and all residual variance terms are referred to as the *variance components* of the model. The correlation between the random effects can be calculated using the standard formula

$$\rho = \frac{\omega_{CL, V}}{\sqrt{\omega_{CL}^2 \omega_V^2}}. \qquad (7.21)$$

Holford, Gobburu, and Mould (2003) have shown that not including a covariance term when one is needed results in more bias in the resulting parameter estimates than an overparameterized model having an unnecessary covariance term. Their results are consistent with linear mixed effects models where an overparameterized covariance structures lead to poor estimation of the standard errors but an underparameterized covariance results in biased inference about the fixed effects (Altham, 1984).

Sometimes the situation is encountered where two random effect parameters are so highly correlated that convergence cannot be achieved. In this case, one parameter can be treated as being perfectly correlated with the other parameter and the random effect model for both parameters can be written as a function of only one parameter. For example, suppose CL and V have variance–covariance matrix given in Eq. (7.20) with a very large condition number, i.e., CL and V are very highly correlated. The random effects model may be rewritten as

$$CL_i = \theta_{\mu, CL} \exp\left(\eta_{i, CL}\right) \qquad (7.22)$$

$$V_i = \theta_{\mu, V} \exp\left(\theta_3 \eta_{i, CL}\right) \qquad (7.23)$$

without loss of information, where now Ω is a scalar equal to the variance of CL and θ_3 is the ratio of the standard deviations

$$\theta_3 = \frac{\omega_V}{\omega_{CL}}. \qquad (7.24)$$

The variance of V is then

$$\text{Var}(V) = \theta_3^2 \text{Var}(CL). \qquad (7.25)$$

Keep in mind, though, that as other random effects or covariates enter the model, the correlation between the correlated parameters may decrease and this trick is no longer necessary.

To illustrate this technique, a simulation was conducted. Concentration–time data from 125 individuals with intense serial sampling after single dose administration was simulated using a 1-compartment model with first-order absorption. Clearance, volume of distribution, and k_a had typical values of 3.7 L/h, 227 L, and 0.7 per hour, respectively. All parameters were modeled as log-normal. Ω was 3×3 with values

$$\Omega = \begin{bmatrix} CL & V & k_a \\ 0.1 & & \\ 0.16 & 0.3 & \\ 0 & 0 & 0.1 \end{bmatrix}. \qquad (7.26)$$

Thus the correlation (defined as r) between CL and V, calculated as

$$r = \frac{0.16}{\sqrt{0.1}\sqrt{0.3}} = 0.92 \qquad (7.27)$$

was 0.92. Residual variability was proportional having a variability of 0.003 (5.5%). The model was then fit using first-order conditional estimation with interaction (which is discussed in later sections) having the true values as initial estimates. The model minimized with no errors and had an OFV of 13409. The final structural model parameter estimates (standard errors) was 3.65 (0.104) L/h, 220 (11.0) L, and 0.698 (0.0215) per hour for CL, V, and k_a, respectively. Ω was estimated at

$$\Omega = \begin{bmatrix} CL & V & k_a \\ 0.0893 & & \\ 0.142 & 0.264 & \\ 0 & 0 & 0.101 \end{bmatrix}. \qquad (7.28)$$

with a residual variance of 0.00422 (6.5%). The model fitted correlation between CL and V was 0.92. But an examination of the largest (3.18) and smallest eigenvalue (0.00417) showed a condition number of 762. Hence, the model was moderately unstable, as expected of having so high a correlation between CL and V.

The model was then refit with V redefined using Eq. (7.23). The refit model minimized successfully with no errors and had an OFV of 14005, an increase of 596! The new structural model parameter estimates (standard error in parentheses) were 4.32 (0.186) L/h, 295 (22.8) L, and 0.636 (0.0223) per hour for CL, V, and k_a, respectively. ω_{CL} was estimated at 0.33 L/h for CL and 0.33 per hour for ω_{k_a} with a residual variance of 0.0123 (11.1%). θ_3 was estimated at 1.72 (0.146). The true ratio of the standard deviations was 1.73. Reparameterization resulted in a better estimate of the variance of both CL and V, with essentially no change in k_a. But, although θ_3 was accurately estimated, CL, V, and k_a had slightly greater bias and slightly larger standard errors under the new model. However, this model was more stable having a condition number of 102. In summary, a trade-off resulted between accuracy and numerical precision. Normally there is a balance between bias versus variance (accuracy versus precision) in the estimation of model parameters. The shared variance term shifts that balance toward a model that had slightly more bias in the parameter estimates but was more stable than the original model.

In contrast to pharmacokinetic model parameters which are often modeled assuming an exponential scale, model parameters from a pharmacodynamic model are sometimes modeled on an arithmetic scale

$$\theta_i = \theta_\mu + \eta_i \qquad (7.29)$$

where θ_μ is the population mean and η_i is the deviation from the mean for the ith subject with zero mean and variance ω^2. The standard deviation in the population is simply the square root of ω^2 and the CV in the population is

$$CV(\%) = \frac{\omega}{\theta_\mu} \times 100\%. \qquad (7.30)$$

Whether to model a pharmacodynamic model parameter using an arithmetic or exponential scale is largely up to the analyst. Ideally, theory would help guide the choice, but there are certainly cases when an arithmetic scale is more appropriate than an exponential scale, such as when the baseline pharmacodynamic parameter has no constraint on individual values. However, more often than not the choice is left to the analyst and is somewhat arbitrarily made. In a data rich situation where each subject could be fit individually, one could examine the distribution of the fitted parameter estimates and see whether a histogram of the model parameter follows an approximate normal or log-normal distribution. If the distribution is approximately normal then an arithmetic scale seems more appropriate, whereas if the distribution is approximately log-normal then an exponential scale seems more appropriate. In the sparse data situation, one may fit both an arithmetic and exponential scale model and examine the objective function values. The model with the smallest objective function value is the scale that is used.

One last note is that BSV can vary among groups. For example, in modeling Phase 2 data from subjects having a particular disease and Phase 1 data from healthy normal volunteers, which tend to be more homogeneous than subjects, it may be necessary to allow separate variance components for each group. For example, clearance may be written as

$$CL = \theta_{\mu,\,CL} \exp{(D\eta_1 + (1 - D)\eta_2)} \qquad (7.31)$$

where D is an indicator variable that takes values of either '0' (if the subject is healthy) or '1' (if the subject has disease), η_1 has zero mean and variance ω_1^2, η_2 has zero mean and variance ω_2^2, ω_1^2 is the variance of subjects with disease, and ω_2^2 is the variance of healthy volunteers. In this manner, each group has their own degree of variability that is smaller than had BSV been estimated without regard to the disease state.

Modeling Interoccasion Variability (IOV)

It is well known that the pharmacokinetics of an individual can change over time due to many factors. Pharmacokinetics may change over large spans of time due to aging or fluctuations in weight, for example, or they may change over shorter periods of time, even within a day, due to diet or presence of concomitant medications, among others. However, these changes are regular and predictable and may therefore be described by time-dependent covariate functions. However, often the reason for a change in pharmacokinetics within an individual is unknown. But, whatever the reason, it may not be physiologically realistic to assume that a single model with subject-specific model parameters applies for that subject forever. Such changes in variability are said to reflect intraindividual variability and when the pharmacokinetics for a subject are characterized on different occasions, the variability introduced on each occasion is random and said to be interoccasion variability (IOV). Failure to include IOV in a model may result in biased parameter estimates (Karlsson and Sheiner, 1993).

A quick test for IOV is to modify the data set treating each subject measured on each occasion as a separate and unique subject. The difference in residual variance between the original data set and the modified data set reflects the degree of IOV (Hossain et al., 1997). This works only if there is sufficient data collected on each occasion. For example, there may be only one observation during a series of occasions in which case IOV cannot be identified using this approach. When IOV is not included in a model, that variability is included in the residual variability term. Hence, residual variability is inflated when IOV is not included in the model.

Using Monte Carlo simulation, Karlsson and Sheiner (1993) estimated the impact of IOV on structural model parameter estimates and variance components. Not including IOV in the model can lead to appreciable bias in the structural model parameter estimates, but which parameter is affected and to what extent depends on many different variables with no clear pattern emerging. Ignoring IOV always inflates the residual variance estimate. However, when BSV is large relative to IOV, the bias in the estimate of BSV is negligible. On the other hand, when IOV is large relative to BSV, then biases in the estimates of BSV were large.

Karlsson and Sheiner (1993) presented an easy method to estimate IOV. In order to estimate IOV serial pharmacokinetic data must be collected on each subject on each occasion. If only a single sample is available on each occasion an estimate of IOV cannot be calculated. Begin by assuming that each subject has pharmacokinetic data collected on O occasions, j = 1, 2, ... O, and that the model parameter for the ith subject (θ_i) is written as

$$\theta_i = \theta_\mu \exp(\eta_i). \tag{7.32}$$

Assuming that IOV only affects the variability in the data, the model parameter can be written as

$$\theta_i = \theta_\mu \exp(\eta_i + \eta_1 OCC_1 + \eta_2 OCC_2 + \ldots \eta_o OCC_o) \tag{7.33}$$

where η_1 is the deviation from the population mean due to variability from Occasion 1, η_2 is the deviation from the population mean due to variability from Occasion 2, etc. OCC_j is coded as 1 if the sample was collected on the jth occasion and 0 otherwise. Hence, the IOV model is equivalent to

$$\theta_i = \begin{cases} \theta_\mu \exp(\eta_i + \eta_1 OCC_1) & \text{If Occasion 1} \\ \theta_\mu \exp(\eta_i + \eta_2 OCC_2) & \text{If Occasion 2} \\ \quad \ldots \\ \theta_\mu \exp(\eta_i + \eta_o OCC_o) & \text{If Occasion O} \end{cases} \tag{7.34}$$

It is assumed that each η_j has zero mean and variance ω_j^2.

As an example, suppose subjects are dosed once daily for 5 days and that serial plasma samples are collected on Days 1 and 5. An IOV model for a model parameter may be written as

$$\theta_i = \theta_\mu \exp(\eta_i + \eta_1 DAY_1 + \eta_2 DAY_5) \tag{7.35}$$

where DAY_1 equals '1' if the sample was collected on Day 1 and '0' otherwise and DAY 5 equals '1' if the sample was collected on Day 5 and '0' otherwise.

There may be many different occasions within a study and hence many levels of IOV. For example, suppose subjects were randomized to receive once daily

dosing for 5 days in two different periods, now there are two levels of IOV: day and period. One could change the IOV model to assume that the data in Period 2 simply reflect two more days of sampling, in which case the IOV model could be changed to

$$\theta_i = \theta_\mu \exp(\eta_i + \eta_1 DP_{11} + \eta_2 DP_{15} + \eta_3 DP_{21} + \eta_4 DP_{25}) \tag{7.36}$$

where DP_{11} equals 1 if the sample was collected on Day 1 in Period 1 and 0 otherwise, etc. In this manner one obtains a variance estimate for IOV across days. But a more parsimonious model would be to treat days and period as two different levels of IOV and to write the IOV model as

$$\theta_i = \theta_\mu \exp(\eta_i + \eta_1 DAY_1 + \eta_2 DAY_5 + \eta_3 PRD_1 + \eta_4 PRD_2) \tag{7.37}$$

where PRD_1 equals 1 if the sample was collected in Period 1 and 0 otherwise, and PRD_2 equals 1 if the sample was collected in Period 2 and 0 otherwise. In this manner one obtains a variance across days and a variance estimate across periods.

The problem with this approach is that if one models IOV exactly as above and then attempts to estimate the EBE for the parameter, what one obtains is an estimate of the parameter on each occasion. But that may not be wanted. What is really wanted is an estimate of the parameter for that subject across all occasions, i.e., Eq. (7.32). To obtain this estimate, IOV in Eq. (7.35) is decomposed to

$$\theta_i = \theta_\mu \exp(\eta_i) \exp(\eta_1 DAY_1 + \eta_2 DAY_5). \tag{7.38}$$

$\theta_\mu \exp(\eta_i)$ then estimates the parameter across occasions controlled for IOV.

In practice, at first one may wish to try to obtain a separate estimate of the variance on each occasion, i.e., obtain estimates of ω_1^2, ω_2^2, etc. If the variance terms are approximately equal (in general if the ratio of the largest to smallest variance component is less than four, the variances are treated as equivalent) then one can assume that $\omega_1^2 = \omega_2^2 = \ldots \omega_j^2$, or that there is a common variance between occasions, and reestimate the model. If, however, there is a trend in the variances over time then one may wish to treat η_j as a function of time. Alternatively, one may wish to examine whether IOV can be explained by any covariates in the data set. For most data sets, such complex IOV models cannot be supported by the data and these complications will not be explored any further.

Modeling Interstudy Variability (ISV)

Sometimes one has to perform a single PopPK analysis from data pooled across many different studies, a so-called "meta-analysis." An example of this is the PopPK analysis of docetaxel reported by Bruno et al. (1996) wherein data from 547 subjects enrolled in two Phase 1 studies and 22 Phase 2 studies were analyzed. The advantage of such an analysis is that the analysis is now integrated across studies with greater power at detecting possible covariate relationships than an analysis of any single study. Also, performing multiple PopPK analyses on a drug can lead to the situation where one analysis might identify an important covariate, but another analysis does not owing to restrictions in the study entrance criteria or randomly associated with accrual. Is the covariate important or not? By having a single analysis, this problem is less likely to occur. However, a pooled PopPK analysis has another problem. By combining data sets another source of variability is introduced into the data. It may be that some proportion of the total variability in the data is due to interstudy variability (ISV). ISV, which will be denoted as κ, becomes merged with BSV when the former is not controlled in the analysis. Laporte-Simitsidis et al. (2000), using Monte Carlo simulation, showed that failure to include ISV does not introduce any bias into the estimation of the fixed effects or the residual variance terms, but does inflate the estimate of BSV.

Controlling for ISV depends on how the analyst believes ISV affects the parameter of interest. In general, ISV can affect the model parameters in three different ways. Begin by assuming that there are S number of studies being pooled and that the model parameter for the ith subject (θ_i) be written as

$$\theta_i = \theta_\mu \exp(\eta_i). \qquad (7.39)$$

In Case 1, ISV does not add any variability into the model parameter, but does add a shift in location to the population mean. Then the model parameter can be written as

$$\theta_i = (\theta_\mu + \theta_1 Study_1 + \theta_2 Study_2 + \ldots \theta_s Study_s) \exp(\eta_i) \qquad (7.40)$$

where $Study_j = 1$ when the ith subject is in $Study_j$ and $Study_j = 0$ otherwise. In Case 2, ISV does not shift the location, but does affect the variability. In this case the model parameter can be written as

$$\theta_i = \theta_\mu \exp(\eta_i + \eta_1 Study_1 + \eta_2 Study_2 + \ldots \eta_s Study_s) \qquad (7.41)$$

such that η_j has zero mean and variance ω_j^2. Typically one assumes that $\omega_1^2 = \omega_2^2 = \ldots \omega_s^2$ or that there is a common variance between studies. In Case 3, interstudy variability affects both a shift in location and the total variability of the data, such that the model parameter can now be written

$$\theta_i = (\theta_\mu + \theta_1 Study_1 + \theta_2 Study_2 + \ldots \theta_s Study_s) \\ \exp(\eta_i + \eta_1 Study_1 + \eta_2 Study_2 + \ldots \eta_s Study_s) \qquad (7.42)$$

with the same assumptions as in Case 1 and 2. Laporte-Simitsidis et al. (2000) showed that if the number of studies being pooled is less than 20 then it is probably not worth estimating ISV and, indeed, one cannot reliably estimate it for small sample sizes. This is not a surprising conclusion since one often needs large sample sizes to reliably estimate a variance. It should be noted that if this approach is taken, then adding IOV to a model can become very complex.

ISV could also affect the residual variability and this approach is often taken by analysts. For example, if the residual variability can be written as

$$Y = f(\theta; x)(1 + \varepsilon) \qquad (7.43)$$

then ISV can be written like in Case 1

$$Y = f(\theta; x)(1 + \varepsilon + \varepsilon_1 Study_1 + \varepsilon_2 Study_2 + \ldots \varepsilon_s Study_s) \qquad (7.44)$$

such that ε_j are independent with zero mean and variance σ_j^2. In this manner one can decompose the residual variance into a "pure" residual variance term and variance term due to study.

Modeling Residual Variability

Whatever variability remains unexplained due to intraindividual variability, model misspecification, assay error, dosing history errors, etc., is lumped into residual variability. Sometimes this variability is referred to as intrasubject variability, which is technically incorrect. For our purposes, this variability will be called residual variability and the model that accounts for such variability is called the residual variance model. The larger and more heterogeneous the residual variance, the greater the necessity to account for it in the overall model. Common variance models for pharmacokinetic data are given in Eqs. (7.11)–(7.13) with the most common being a proportional error model. For pharmacodynamic models, more often an additive model is used. In choosing a residual variance model, often the LRT and goodness of fit plots are used, although the latter may be insensitive to detect small improvements in fit. One strategy that is often employed is to use an additive and proportional error model throughout model development and then see if the residual model can be simplified, particularly if one of the residual variance components is near zero. A particularly useful residual variance model is

$$Y = f(x; \theta) + \left(\sqrt{1 - \theta_k + \theta_k \, f(x; \theta)^2} \right) \varepsilon \qquad (7.45)$$

where θ_k is allowed to vary between 0 and 1. If θ_k equals zero then the equation reduces to an additive error model and if θ_k equals 1, then the equation becomes a proportional error model. Such a model if useful is neither the additive nor proportional error model is acceptable.

Like other random effects, the residual error can be dependent on subject-specific covariates and as such, covariates can be included in the residual variance model. The classic example is when some blood samples were assayed with one analytical assay, while others were assayed with another type of assay. If an indicator variable, ASY, is defined such that every sample is assigned either a 0 or 1, depending on the reference assay, the residual error could then be modeled as

$$Y = f(\theta; x)[1 + ASY\varepsilon_1 + (1 - ASY)\varepsilon_2] \qquad (7.46)$$

subject to ε_1 being independent with zero mean and variance ω_1^2 and ε_2 being independent with zero mean and variance ω_2^2. Hence, the residual error model simplifies to the following cases

$$Y = \begin{cases} f(\theta; x)(1 + \varepsilon_1) & \text{if } ASY = 1 \\ f(\theta; x)(1 + \varepsilon_2) & \text{if } ASY = 0 \end{cases} . \qquad (7.47)$$

Analytical differences are often a key factor in interstudy variability, particularly because assay and assay variability can change over time.

Another example of distinct residual error models is when data from two different populations are studied. For example, data from healthy volunteers and subjects may be analyzed together. For whatever reason, possibly due to better control over dosing and sampling in healthy volunteers or because of inherent homogeneity in healthy volunteers, data from healthy volunteers have smaller residual variability than subjects. Hence, a residual error of the type

$$Y = f(\theta; x)[1 + H\varepsilon_1 + (1 - H)\varepsilon_2] \qquad (7.48)$$

may be more appropriate, where H is an indicator variable where H = 0 if the subject has the disease of interest

and H = 1 if the subject is healthy and ε_1 and ε_2 are defined as before. One modification of this residual variance model is where all the subjects in the data set have the illness, but some have an additional complicating factor, such as hepatic and/or renal failure. Another modification is where, for whatever reasons, subjects at one clinical site are more heterogeneous than subjects at another clinical site. Such a model was used in characterizing the pharmacokinetics of topotecan in subjects with solid tumors (Mould et al., 2002) and in characterizing the pharmacokinetics of oral busulfan in children (Schiltmeyer et al., 2003). One last example would be if the data consisted of a mixture of sparse data with few observations per subject and rich data with many observations per subject. In such a case then separate residual variance terms for dense and sparse data may be appropriate.

A further modification of this model is one presented by Kerbusch, Milligan, and Karlsson (2003) in an population pharmacodynamic analysis of saliva flow rate after administration of the M_3-muscarinic antagonist, darifenacin. Data were pooled from Phase 1 studies from healthy volunteers and a Phase 2 study from subjects with overactive bladder disease. Also, different formulations were used in many of the studies. Hence, the data set was quite heterogeneous and it was anticipated that the residual error might not be consistent across individuals. Residual error was modeled as

$$Y = f(\theta; x) + [f(\theta; x)\varepsilon_1 + \varepsilon_2] \exp(\eta_i) \qquad (7.49)$$

where now a variance component for BSV was added to the traditional additive plus proportional error model. Such a residual error model will minimize the influence of a few individuals who have poor fits on the overall fit of the model to the data. In this instance, FOCE with interaction was required to estimate BSV. Compared to the model having only an additive plus proportional error model, the additional variance component resulted in a significant decrease in the objective function value (-497) and the residual error decreased 4.4%.

Additionally, many sources of variability, such as model misspecification, or dosing and sampling history, may lead to residual errors that are time dependent. For example, the residual variance may be larger in the absorption phase than in the elimination phase of a drug. Hence, it may be necessary to include time in the residual variance model. One can use a more general residual variance model where time is explicitly taken into account or one can use a threshold model where one residual variance model accounts for the residual variability up to time t, but another model applies thereafter. Such models have been shown to result in significant model improvements (Karlsson, Beal, and Sheiner, 1995).

One assumption of the residuals is that they are uncorrelated. It may be that in a misspecified pharmacokinetic model where frequent sampling is done, regions of the concentration–time curve will show consistent deviations between the observed and predicted concentrations. In such a case, the assumption of independence can be called into question. In the chapter on linear mixed effects models, covariance models, such as the AR(1), spatial power, spatial exponential, and spatial Gaussian were introduced to account for such autocorrelation. The same models can be applied to nonlinear mixed effects models when there are many samples per subject, but with sparse data sampling, there is often insufficient data to use these covariance models. Karlsson, Sheiner, and Beal (1995) compared an AR(1) model to a standard, independent error model and showed how using such a model resulted in a significant improvement in the goodness of fit for an unidentified antihypertensive drug. Using Monte Carlo simulation, they also showed that population estimates were not as accurate when autocorrelated errors were not accounted for. In practice, spatial covariance models tend to increase run-times many orders of magnitude and should be saved for the last step in model building, such as when the final covariate model is identified.

In most PopPK analyses, the residual error model is given little attention. One almost universally sees a proportional or combined additive and proportional error model in published PopPK studies and rarely, if ever, does one see a more complex error model involving covariates. One reason might be that with an adequate model, other sources of variability usually are an order or magnitude or more than the residual variance, so little is gained in getting a more precise estimate of that parameter. More often, however, it is probably that residual error is neglected during the model development process, which is an unfortunate oversight.

Incorporating Fixed and Random Effects into the Structural Model

One of the most basic questions in any mixed effects model analysis is which parameters should be treated as fixed and which are random. As repeatedly mentioned in the chapter on Linear Mixed Effects Models, an overparameterized random effects matrix can lead to inefficient estimation and poor estimates of the standard errors of the fixed effects, whereas too restrictive a random effects matrix may lead to invalid and biased estimation of the mean response profile (Altham, 1984). In a data rich situation where there are enough observations per subject to obtain individual parameter estimates, i.e., each subject can be fit individually using

nonlinear regression, one could examine the distribution of the individual parameter estimates and see which parameters exhibit sufficient variability such that they warrant being treated as a random effect. While this may be a practical approach for Phase 1 data, wherein subjects are repeatedly sampled and it is not unusual to have 10 or more samples collected during a dosing interval, for most Phase 3 studies, the data are more often sparse and not amenable to individual analysis.

The analyst is then faced with the decision of what to do. One strategy is to treat all parameters as random effects. The Ω matrix is built as an unstructured matrix with variance and covariance terms for all model parameters. After optimization, the Ω matrix is examined for elements that are near zero. Those variances or covariances that are near zero are treated as fixed effects (i.e., set equal to zero) and correlations that are zero may also be set to zero, such as in a banded matrix. Pinheiro and Bates (1994) suggest examining the eigenvalues of Ω and see if any are near zero. Near zero eigenvalues and corresponding high condition number are suggestive of either an overparameterized Ω matrix or the relative magnitude of the model parameters are quite different. While this may be a useful approach, in practice it is difficult to implement, except for models with few random effects, because of convergence difficulties during optimization.

Another approach then is to first identify the fixed effects and then build the random effects matrix. However, there is an interaction between the random effects matrix and fixed effects such that the exclusion of a random effect may fail to identify a significant fixed effect. So what is an analyst to do? A common strategy is to first treat all structural parameters in the model as independent random effects, i.e., to use a diagonal covariance matrix. Random effects with near zero variance are treated as fixed effects. Second, whenever possible, use an unstructured covariance matrix between those random effects identified in the first step as being important. If the unstructured covariance model does not minimize successfully, then treat the covariance as a simple matrix (no covariances between diagonal elements). Lastly, once the final model is selected, obtain the EBE (which are discussed later in the chapter) for the random effects and generate a scatter plot correlation matrix. EBEs that appear correlated should then have a covariance term included in the covariance, otherwise the covariance is set equal to zero. Keep in mind, however, that this approach is sequential in that $A \rightarrow B \rightarrow C$, but model building is not necessarily sequential. The process may be iterative such that the process may need to be modified based on the data and model.

Some suggest that the inclusion of a random effect (i.e., variance term) should be reflected by a significant decrease in the objective function, such that the LRT is statistically significant at some α-level (Verbeke and Molenberghs, 1997). However, Wahlby, Jonsson, and Karlsson (2001) have shown that the LRT should not be used with confidence since the Type I error rate is sensitive to variance model misspecification, the assumption of residual normality, and the amount of information each subject contributes to the model. Furthermore, the LRT does not apply to the inclusion of a variance term (although this is no longer true for covariance terms) because the distribution is no longer chi-squared with a single degree of freedom (Stram and Lee, 1994). Others suggest that if a scatter plot of the EBEs indicates correlation between two random effects, then this is sufficient to include a covariance term between them. Unfortunately there is no single strategy that can identify which model parameters should be treated as fixed and which should be random. It is up to the analyst to chose a strategy that best reflects the data on hand. More often, as model development proceeds for a complex model, random effects are added and removed from the model and at the end (hopefully) are the random effects that best account for the variability in the data.

MODELING COVARIATE RELATIONSHIPS (THE COVARIATE SUBMODEL)

A key term in PopPK is 'covariate,' which has been used throughout the book and will now be more formally defined. A covariate is any variable that is specific to an individual and may influence the pharmacokinetics or pharmacodynamics of a drug. Covariates are classified as intrinsic factors (inherited, genetically determined), such as age, weight, height, and race, or extrinsic factors (subject to outside environmental influences), such as dose, degree of compliance, smoking status, and presence of concomitant medications (International Conference on Harmonization of Technical Requirements for Registration of Pharmaceuticals for Human Use, 1998a). In general, intrinsic covariates do not change over short spans of time or at all, whereas extrinsic covariates can change many times during a study. A notable exception to this rule is phenotypic expression of metabolism status, an intrinsic covariate, where a subject can covert from a normal or rapid metabolizer to a poor metabolizer due to the presence of some external inhibitor. Covariates can also be classified as either continuous (such as age), dichotomous (such as sex), or polychotomous/categorical (such as race). Table 7.2 presents a nonexhaustive listing of covariates that have been used in PopPK-PD analyses.

Table 7.2 Covariates that have been used in population pharmacokinetic-pharmacodynamic analyses.

- Weight and its surrogates, e.g., body surface area, lean body weight, etc.
- Age
- Race
- Sex
- Concomitant medications
- Clinical chemistry values, e.g., bilirubin, SGOT, etc.
- Hematologic values, e.g., white blood cell count
- Protein binding
- Dose
- Fast or slow absorption
- Formulation
- Diurnal variation
- Liver disease
- Renal disease
- Presence or absence of HIV or hepatitis
- Renal function markers
- Disease stage

One of the biggest reasons for using a population approach to modeling is that subject-specific characteristics can be built into the model through their associations with model parameters. For example, if volume of distribution is dependent on weight then weight can be built into the model, thereby reducing both between-subject variability in volume of distribution and unexplained, residual variability. When covariates are identified and the between-subject variability is sufficiently reduced, individualized dosage regimens become possible.

An excellent overview of this topic was presented by Philips (1999) and much of what will follow in this section will be based on that presentation. The question of whether a covariate is useful in explaining the random effects variability will be ignored in this section; it will be assumed that it does. Also, clearance will be used as the dependent variable and age as the independent variable (unless otherwise noted) but the relationships that will be discussed can be applied to any arbitrary covariate and model parameter.

In general, how the covariate is built into the model is dependent on the type of variable the covariate is. For continuous covariates, covariate submodels are generally of three different functions: linear, exponential, or power. Choosing which function broadly depends on the modeling approach taken. One such approach is covariate screening, in which given a PopPK model the EBE for a pharmacokinetic parameter is estimated for each individual. The EBEs are then plotted against subject-specific covariates and examined for a relationship between the two. If examination of the scatter plot shows a straight line, a linear model is usually used. However, if the plot shows curvature then exponential or power models are often used. More formally a regression line or generalized additive model (GAM) can be used to statistically test for curvature, nonlinearity, or break points. A judgment call is then made by the modeler as to the nature of the relationship between covariate and EBE and this relationship is taken forward into the covariate submodel.

A second approach is, postulate a series of competing models and then use a more rigorous statistical criteria to choose which function best describes the data. For example, one could build different covariate submodels, one for each function to be tested, with the model having the smallest AIC taken forward for further development. More will be discussed on these approaches later in the chapter and elsewhere in the book. It should be noted that rarely do published PopPK models justify the choice of covariate submodel used.

The linear covariate model should be obvious from previous chapters. For example, if clearance is linearly dependent on age then a model of the form

$$CL = \theta_1 + \theta_2 Age \qquad (7.50)$$

might be useful. For simplicity the subscripts 'i,' denoting individual subjects, and η, denoting deviations from the population mean having Age_i, are suppressed. Under this model, θ_1 represents clearance when age equals zero and θ_2 represents the change in clearance for unit change in age. Early studies using population approaches almost exclusively used linear covariate submodels.

When the dependent variable and the covariate show curvilinearity then power or exponential models may be useful. Exponential covariate models take the form

$$CL = \theta_1 \exp(\theta_2 Age). \qquad (7.51)$$

The shape of the relationship can be monotonically increasing or decreasing depending on whether θ_2 is positive or negative, respectively. θ_1 represents clearance when age equals zero, whereas θ_2 represents the change in Ln(CL) per unit change in age. Exponential models are linear on a Ln-scale and after Ln-transformation become

$$Ln(CL) = Ln(\theta_1) + \theta_2 Age. \qquad (7.52)$$

Representative line plots of the exponential model and its Ln-transformed form are illustrated in Fig. 7.2. The problem with the exponential model is if θ_2 is positive and large, then the model can very rapidly "blow-up" and lead to overflow errors. A more useful model for a curvilinear relationship is the power covariate model

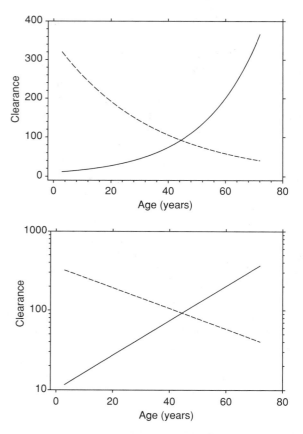

Figure 7.2 Line plot of an exponential model $CL = \theta_1 \exp(\theta_2 Age)$ in original (top) and Ln-transformed scale (bottom). Solid line has $\theta_2 > 0$, whereas dashed line has $\theta_2 < 0$.

$$CL = \theta_1(Age)^{\theta_2}. \qquad (7.53)$$

In this case, θ_1 represents clearance when age equals one and θ_2 represents the change in Ln(CL) per unit change in Ln(Age). If $\theta_2 > 0$ then clearance equals zero when age equals zero, which is physiologically appealing. If $\theta_2 \leq 0$ then clearance is undefined when age equals zero.

Power models are linear on a Ln–Ln scale. After Ln-transformation the power model becomes

$$Ln(CL) = Ln(\theta_1) + \theta_2 Ln(Age). \qquad (7.54)$$

Representative line plots for the power model and after Ln–Ln transformation are shown in Fig. 7.3. Power models are often used because of the allometric relationship between many physiological parameters and body weight. Adolph (1949) proposed that anatomic and physiologic variables were related to body weight by power functions. For example, brain weight is related to total body weight by the model

$$Brain\ Weight = 10\,(Weight)^{0.7} \qquad (7.55)$$

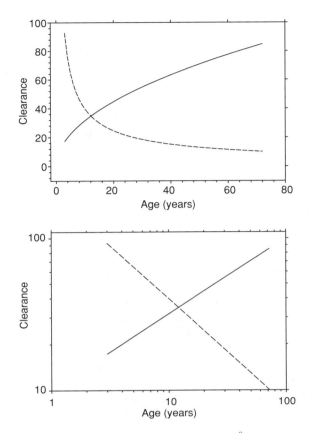

Figure 7.3 Line plot of a power model $CL = \theta_1(Age)^{\theta_2}$ in original (top) and Ln–Ln transformed scale (bottom). Solid line has $\theta_2 > 0$, whereas dashed line has $\theta_2 < 0$.

whereas cardiac output is related to total body weight by

$$\text{Cardiac Output (mL/min)} = 166(\text{Weight})^{0.79} \quad (7.56)$$

where weight is in kg (Davidian and Carroll, 1987). Because many physiological parameters are related to body weight then similarly pharmacokinetic parameters should also be a function of size (Ritschel et al., 1992). When weight or some other measure of size is the covariate, then there is a physiologic rationale for choosing a power model. When size is not the covariate, justification of the power model is often made empirically. Use of power models is more commonly seen in the literature than exponential models and are used almost as commonly as linear models.

Two continuous covariates can be modeled as either an additive effect or a multiplicative effect. For an additive effect model using age and weight as an example

$$CL = \theta_1 + \theta_2 \text{Age} + \theta_3 \text{Weight}. \quad (7.57)$$

This model assumes that age and weight act independent on clearance with intercept θ_1. The difference between any two ages, $\text{Age}_1 - \text{Age}_2$, is given by

$$\Delta = \theta_2(\text{Age}_2 - \text{Age}_1). \quad (7.58)$$

Hence, the difference between any two ages will be a constant for fixed weight. To include interaction between age and weight one could model clearance as

$$CL = \theta_1 + \theta_2 \text{Age} + \theta_3 \text{Weight} + \theta_4 (\text{Age})(\text{Weight}). \quad (7.59)$$

In this case, the difference between any two ages is given by

$$\Delta = \theta_2(\text{Age}_1 - \text{Age}_2) + \theta_4(\text{Age}_1 - \text{Age}_2)\text{Weight} \quad (7.60)$$

which is a function of weight and the difference in ages. Hence, the lines for clearance will not be parallel for any two ages (Fig. 7.4). If age and weight followed a power model then the model for independent multiplicative effects would be

$$CL = \theta_1(\text{Age})^{\theta_2} (\text{Weight})^{\theta_3} \quad (7.61)$$

whereas a model including interaction would be

$$CL = \theta_1(\text{Age})^{\theta_2} (\text{Weight})^{\theta_3} (\text{Age} \times \text{Weight})^{\theta_4}. \quad (7.62)$$

However, the use of interaction in covariate models is not common. (It is easy to see how these models could be expanded to three or more covariate or mixed and matched depending on the covariates). For example if age had a linear relationship with clearance, but weight followed a power model then one such covariate submodel might be

$$CL = (\theta_1 + \theta_2 \text{Age})(\text{Weight})^{\theta_3}. \quad (7.63)$$

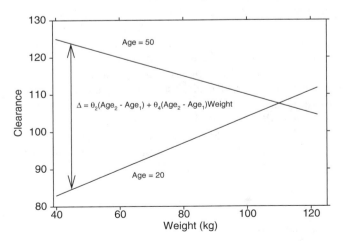

Figure 7.4 Line plot of a linear model including interaction for clearance as a function of age and weight. Clearance was modeled as CL = 25 + 2.2 (Age) + 0.75 (Weight) -0.02 (Age) (Weight). The difference between any two ages is not a constant but a function of the difference in age and weight.

For continuous covariates, there are more possibilities than linear models. Indeed, there are a wide, possibly infinite, number of models that can be developed between continuous covariates. What is important is that at the completion of the analysis, the relationship and parameters must be interpretable and defendable.

In practice, rarely are models of the exact form given by Eq. (7.57) or (7.61) used. The reason is that the scale, or range, and magnitude of the many covariates that may be in a model may be so different that the gradient, which is evaluated during the optimization process, may be unstable. To avoid this instability, covariates are often centered or standardized in the case of linear models or scaled in the case of power or exponential models. For example, if age had a mean of 40 years and a standard deviation of 8 and weight had a mean of 80 kg and standard deviation of 12, then Eq. (7.57) may be standardized using

$$CL = \theta_1 + \theta_2 \left(\frac{Age - 40}{8} \right) + \theta_3 \left(\frac{Weight - 80}{12} \right) \quad (7.64)$$

or scaled using

$$CL = \theta_1 + \theta_2 \left(\frac{Age}{40} \right) + \theta_3 \left(\frac{Weight}{80} \right) \quad (7.65)$$

or centered using

$$CL = \theta_1 + \theta_2(Age - 40) + \theta_3(Weight - 80). \quad (7.66)$$

It is not necessary to scale to the exact mean or median value of the data set. For example, many modelers will scale to a common covariate such as 65 years old for age or 70 kg for weight. The parameter estimates associated with covariates remain the same, but the intercept will change after centering. The parameter estimate associated with the covariates change, but the intercept remains the same after scaling. And all the parameter estimates will change after standardizing. The units of a regression parameter may also change after standardizing or scaling, but not after centering. An additional benefit of standardization, scaling, or centering is that the parameter estimates for a typical or reference subject can be easily defined. For example, returning back to Eqs. (7.64)–(7.66), drug clearance in a typical 40-year-old subject weighing 80 kg is equal to θ_1 if the data were standardized or centered or

$$CL = \theta_1 + \theta_2 + \theta_3 \quad (7.67)$$

if the data were scaled.

It should be noted that scaling in the original domain is the same as centering in the log–log trans-formed domain. In the chapters on linear and nonlinear regression, the importance of centering and standardization was extensively discussed and will not be further discussed here, except to say that these transformations are actually a reparameterization of the model that does not improve the fit of the model nor does it change the data. What these transformations do are by improving the stability of the optimization process as well as potentially providing parameter estimates that are more reflective of the average subject.

There is one caution in building covariate submodels and that is related to collinearity. In the chapters on linear regression, and nonlinear regression, it was shown how two or more covariates that are correlated can destabilize the inversion of the gradient matrix making the parameter estimates unstable. The same applies to PopPK analyses including two correlated covariates in the model, even if they are on different parameters, can lead to unstable parameter estimates. In the simple case where two correlated covariates, such as height and weight or weight and body surface area, are included in the linear model for a model parameter, Bonate (1999) showed that if the correlation between covariates was greater than 0.5, then the resulting population parameter estimates begin to show increasing bias and standard error. Also if one parameter was correlated with another, the bias and increase in standard errors is propagated to the other parameter as well. It was recommended that the eigenvalues be examined for values near zero, which are indicative of collinearity.

Another recommendation was to examine the correlation matrix of the covariates prior to the analysis and determine whether any two covariates were correlated. If any two correlated covariates were found to be important predictor variables, one could possibly transform the variables into a composite variable, such as the transformation of height and weight into body surface area or body mass index, or to use only the covariate with the greatest predictive value in the model and not to include the other covariate. An untested approach would be to use principal component analysis and then use one or more of the principal components as the covariate in a model.

When the covariate is categorical and dichotomous, three possible models are typically used: additive, fractional change, and exponential. To illustrate these models, it will be assumed that clearance is dependent on age in a linear manner and that clearance is also dependent on the sex of the subject. In an additive model, the effect of the dichotomous covariate is modeled as

$$CL = \theta_1 + \theta_2 Age + \theta_3 Sex \quad (7.68)$$

where Sex is coded as either 0 (male) or 1 (female). Hence, clearance can take on the following forms

$$CL = \begin{cases} \theta_1 + \theta_2 Age + \theta_3 & \text{if female} \\ \theta_1 + \theta_2 Age & \text{if male} \end{cases}. \quad (7.69)$$

θ_3 then represents the constant difference between males and females (Fig. 7.5). A more commonly used model is the fractional change model

$$CL = (\theta_1 + \theta_2 Age)(1 + \theta_3 Sex). \quad (7.70)$$

Hence, clearance can take the following forms

$$CL = \begin{cases} (\theta_1 + \theta_2 Age)(1 + \theta_3) & \text{if female} \\ \theta_1 + \theta_2 Age & \text{if male} \end{cases}. \quad (7.71)$$

The difference between females and males, Δ, is

$$\begin{aligned} \Delta &= (\theta_1 + \theta_2 Age)\theta_3 \\ &= \theta_1\theta_3 + \theta_2\theta_3\, Age \qquad (7.72) \\ &= \theta_1^* + \theta_2^* Age \end{aligned}$$

which shows that the difference between females and males is a linear function of age (hence the name proportional change model, see Fig. 7.6). One problem with the fractional change model is that it is possible for θ_3 to be greater than -1, which would cause clearance to be less than zero and be physiologically impossible. A method to constrain clearance which will always be greater than zero would be to use an exponential model

$$CL = (\theta_1 + \theta_2 Age) \exp(\theta_3 Sex) \quad (7.73)$$

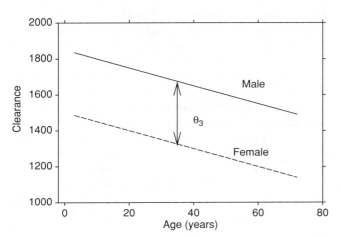

Figure 7.5 Line plot of a linear model for clearance as a function of age and sex, where sex is treated as an additive effect (no interaction).

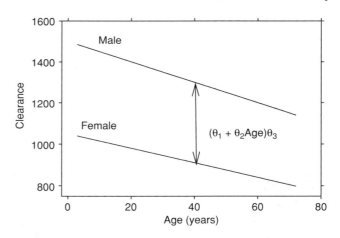

Figure 7.6 Line plot of a linear model for clearance as a function of age and sex, where sex is treated as an fractional change effect, which allows for interaction between sex and age.

and allow θ_3 to be unconstrained on the interval $\{-\infty, +\infty\}$. Hence, for males and females clearance can take on values

$$CL = \begin{cases} (\theta_1 + \theta_2 Age)\exp(\theta_3) & \text{if female} \\ \theta_1 + \theta_2 Age & \text{if male} \end{cases}. \quad (7.74)$$

The difference between females and males is

$$\begin{aligned} \Delta &= (\theta_1 + \theta_2 Age)(\exp(\theta_3) - 1) \\ &= \theta_1 \exp(\theta_3) - \theta_1 + \theta_2 \exp(\theta_3)Age - \theta_2 Age \\ &= \theta_1 \exp(\theta_3) - \theta_1 + (\theta_2 \exp(\theta_3) - \theta_2)Age \\ &= \theta_1^* + \theta_2^* Age \end{aligned} \quad (7.75)$$

where

$$\theta_1^* = \theta_1 \exp(\theta_3) - \theta_1 \quad (7.76)$$

and

$$\theta_2^* = \theta_2 \exp(\theta_3) - \theta_2 \quad (7.77)$$

which means that the exponential model also models the difference between females and males as a linear function of age (Fig. 7.7).

When the covariate is of two or more categories, pharmacokineticists often first try to convert the variable to a dichotomous variable, such as converting race into Caucasian versus others, and then use standard dichotomous modeling techniques to build the model. This practice is not entirely appropriate because categorization results in loss of information.

However, it may be a necessity because the number of subjects in some categories may be too small to make meaningful conclusions about them impossible. To truly

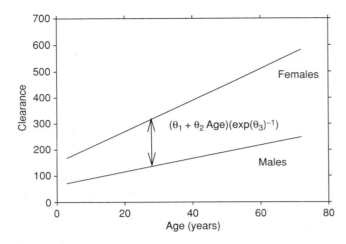

Figure 7.7 Line plot of a linear model between clearance and the covariates age and sex, where sex is treated as an exponential fractional change effect which allows for interaction between sex and age.

model categorical variables, one needs to convert the k-level categorical variable into a k-1 level dummy variable. For example, with race having levels Caucasian, Black, and Asian, the following dummy variables (X_1 and X_2) could be created:

Race	Variable 1 (X_1)	Variable 2 (X_2)
Caucasian	0	0
Black	1	0
Asian	0	1

Then any of the dichotomous models could be expanded to include the additional dummy variable. For example, using a fractional change model clearance could be modeled as

$$CL = (\theta_1 + \theta_2 Age)(1 + \theta_3 X_1 + \theta_4 X_2). \qquad (7.78)$$

Hence, clearance would take on the following values

$$CL = \begin{cases} \theta_1 + \theta_2 Age & \text{if race = Caucasian} \\ (\theta_1 + \theta_2 Age)(1 + \theta_3 X_1) & \text{if race = Black} \\ (\theta_1 + \theta_2 Age)(1 + \theta_4 X_2) & \text{if race = Asian} \end{cases}$$

$$(7.79)$$

Sometimes a continuous variable is categorized and then the categorical variable is included in the model. For example, if age were the covariate and there is a question about the clearance of a drug in the elderly, then age could be transformed to a dichotomous covariate (Age group) where subjects younger than 65 years take on a value of '0' and those older than or equal to 65 years a value of '1.' Clearance could then be modeled as

$$CL = \theta_1[1 + \theta_2(Age\ Group)]. \qquad (7.80)$$

If θ_2 were significantly different from zero then this provides evidence that a difference in clearance exists between the elderly and the young. In general, categorization of a continuous covariate results in loss of information with dichotomization resulting in maximal loss of information. Most statisticians dichotomize at the median but it has been recommended that three groups be used, instead of two, so that trends can be examined (Altman, 1991). There is also evidence to suggest that slightly greater power is achieved when subjects are categorized into equal numbers per group as opposed to equal bin width. In other words, suppose age ranged from 20 to 70 years old. For two groups with equal bin width, one bin might range from 20 to 45 years old with 30 observations, while the other bin ranges from 46 to 70 years old with the remaining 20 observations. On the other hand, for equal sample size per group, half the observations might be in the bin 20–37 years old with the other half in the bin 38–70 years old. For equal size groups, the width of the bins are most likely of unequal length. While it should not be a common practice to categorize continuous variables, there is a use for categorization in modeling practice.

In summary, covariate submodels are limited by the imagination of the modeler and indeed, reviewing the literature one can find many strange covariate submodels. The covariate submodels described here are the most common and many problems can be handled using them. Regardless of the covariate submodel used, good practices dictate that the reason for choosing the model be indicated.

MIXTURE MODELS

Mixture models represent an important tool in the population pharmacokineticist's arsenal in that discrete subpopulations contained within the distribution of a random effect which can be isolated and identified. For example, suppose clearance was significantly higher and more variable in males than females, naïvely generating a histogram may show a bimodal or multimodal distribution. Hence, clearance would appear to consist of a mixture of two distributions, one for males and one for females, each with their own unique mean and variance. Figure 7.8 presents a situation where clearance is a mixture of two normally distributed populations with a mixing proportion of 75% (i.e., 75% of the individuals are in Group 1 and the other 25% are in Group 2), where Group 2 is more variable and has a population mean twice that of Group 1. The histogram clearly identifies two subgroups. An analyst may then identify which group a subject is classified into and see whether any covariates are predictive of group classification. Using a

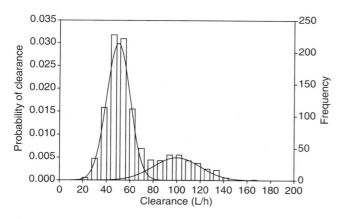

Figure 7.8 Histogram and line plot of a mixture two normal distributions. Group 1 is normally distributed with a mean of 50 and a standard deviation of 10. Group 2 is normally distributed with a mean of 100 and a standard deviation of 20. The proportion of subjects in Group 1 is 75%. The solid line is the probability distribution function for the population.

mixture model usually also decreases the variance associated with a random effect. In Fig. 7.8 the standard deviation of the total distribution is 0.61 L/h on a log-scale, which translates to a CV of 67%. But the standard deviation of the subpopulations is considerably smaller, 0.22 L/h for Group 1 and 0.27 L/h for Group 2, which translates to a CV of 22% and 27% for Group 1 and Group 2, respectively. Hence, the variance components become smaller using a mixture model because the total variance is decomposed into its components.

Mixture models must be defined by specifying the population characteristics of each subgroup, e.g., mean and variance, and the mixing proportion for each group, i.e., the probability that a subject will be classified into a particular subgroup. Rarely will the mixing proportion be known a priori, so often it is treated as an estimable parameter. For example, if clearance consists of two subpopulations, both of which are log-normal in distribution having different variances, the mixing model may be written as

$$CL_i = \begin{cases} \theta_1 \exp(\eta_{1i}) & \text{if Subject i is in Group 1} \\ \theta_1\theta_2 \exp(\eta_{2i}) & \text{if Subject i is in Group 2} \end{cases}$$
(7.81)

with mixing proportion θ_3, θ_1 is the mean of Group 1, and θ_2 is a multiplier such that $\theta_1\theta_2$ equals the population mean of Group 2. The bounds for the mixing proportion are [0, 1]. To ensure that boundary problems are not encountered, one trick is to model the mixing proportion as

$$\text{mixing proportion} = \frac{1}{1 + \exp(\theta_3)}$$
(7.82)

where θ_3 is allowed to be unconstrained. Thus, the mixing proportion approaches 1 as $\theta_3 \rightarrow -\infty$ while the mixing proportion approaches 0 when $\theta_3 \rightarrow \infty$. It is not uncommon to assume that the variance of both populations is the same and that the only difference between the subgroups is the shift factor, θ_2. In this case the mixture model simplifies to

$$CL_i = \begin{cases} \theta_1 \exp(\eta_{1i}) & \text{if Subject i is in Group 1} \\ \theta_1\theta_2 \exp(\eta_{1i}) & \text{if Subject i is in Group 2} \end{cases}$$
(7.83)

Although not constrained to only two subpopulations, mixture models can be expanded to many subgroups. Identification of a mixture should result in a decrease in the objective function value.

The classic example of use of a mixture model in nonlinear mixed effects modeling is when the drug is believed to be polymorphically metabolized, e.g., drugs metabolized by CYP 2D6, such that some proportion of subjects are "normal" or "extensive" metabolizers and the remainder are "poor" metabolizers. For example, Hussein et al. (2001) characterized the population pharmacokinetics of perhexiline, a drug used to treat angina, and found that clearance was bimodal with a mean of 21.8 L/h in Group 1 (88% of subjects) and 2.1 L/h in Group 2 (12% of subjects). There was little difference in between-subject variability, 69% in Group 1 and 86% in Group 2. They attributed the subjects in Group 2 to having CYP 2D6 deficiency in the metabolism of the drug. In practice, it is not uncommon to see that if clearance is bimodal it is necessary to treat volume of distribution as a bimodal distribution as well. It should also be noted that mixing proportions can be based on a selected covariate. In the current example, it is well known that extensive metabolizers and poor metabolizers in a group are to some extent dependent on the racial characteristics of that group. Therefore, one might assign mixing proportions to be dependent on race.

Another use of mixture models is seen with orally administered drugs that exhibit a lag-time. It is not uncommon to observe that some subjects do not exhibit a lag-time, while other subjects do. Treating lag-time as a random effect often results in bimodal distributions with some observations near zero and others greater than zero. Hence, one modeling trick is to treat the absorption model as a mixture model, such that

$$\left. \begin{aligned} k_a &= \theta_1 \exp(\eta_1) \\ ALAG1 &= \theta_2 \end{aligned} \right\} \text{If Group 1}$$

$$\left. \begin{aligned} k_a &= \theta_3 \exp(\eta_1) \\ ALAG1 &= 0 \end{aligned} \right\} \text{If Group 2}$$
(7.84)

where ALAG1 is the lag-time fixed to zero. In this manner, those subjects that do not show a lag-time are accounted for. However, in this case, a separate residual error model based on the identifying covariate may be more appropriate.

Mixture models can also be used in modeling residual variability. It may be that there is a group of subjects that do not really fit the model and so their presence increases the residual variability in the model. A mixture model of the form may be useful

$$Y = \begin{cases} f(\theta; x)(1 + \varepsilon_1) & \text{if Group 1} \\ f(\theta; x)(1 + \varepsilon_2) & \text{if Group 2} \end{cases} \quad (7.85)$$

where subjects are classified into two groups; one group having different variability than the other group.

The use of mixture models is not limited to identification of important subpopulations. A common assumption in modeling pharmacokinetic parameters is that the distribution of a random effect is log-normal, or approximately normal on a log-scale. Sometimes, the distribution of a random effect is heavy tailed and when examined on a log-scale, is skewed and not exactly normal. A mixture distribution can be used to account for the large skewness in the distribution. However, the mixture used in this way does not in any way imply the distribution consists of two populations, but acts solely to account for heavy tails in the distribution of the parameter.

When examining a distribution of parameter values, one question that is asked is whether the distribution consists of a mixture. Answering this question may not be readily apparent with pharmacokinetic parameters that are often log-normal in distribution. It may be easier to detect a mixture after Ln-transformation of a skewed distribution. The next question in any model using mixtures is how many subpopulations are there? One usually sees only two subpopulations used in PopPK analyses, but this choice is often rooted in convention and not statistically based. Using two groups is not a bad choice since rarely are mixtures in biology composed of more than two groups.

The first step towards inclusion of a mixture model in a PopPK analysis is often graphical examination of the histograms of the EBEs of the model parameters that are treated as random effects assuming no mixture is present in the distribution of the random effects (i.e., the model does not include a mixture distribution), with clear multimodality used as strong evidence that a mixture distribution should be included in the model. This approach is not ideal since in order to visually detect a bimodal distribution of two normally distributed random variates, the subpopulation means must be separated by at least two standard deviations (Schilling,

Watkins, and Watkins, 2002). Also, poor choice of the number of histogram bins can obscure a mixture. Wand (1997) showed how using the default S-Plus bin width can obscure the bimodality seen with British incomes. On the other extreme, too many bins can lead to a jagged histogram that really explains nothing about the data. Schilling, Watkins, and Watkins (2002) conclude that using a histogram to detect multimodality is *"unreliable unless the sample size is very large"* with false positives and false negatives frequently occurring.

A more statistically grounded approach may be to consider a QQ plot or a Fowlkes' plot (1979) of a random variable. If Y is the EBE of some parameter, like clearance, a Fowlkes' plot plots $(Y_{[i]} - \bar{Y})/s$ against $\Phi[(Y_{[i]} - \bar{Y})/s] - (i - 0.5)/n$, where $Y_{[i]}$ is the n-ordered sample values, $Y_1, Y_2, \ldots Y_n$ of the variable with mean $\bar{Y}$ and standard deviation s and $\Phi[.]$ is the standard normal density function. Observations from a single probability density will show a straight line with zero slope and intercept. Observations from two or more mixture densities will show cyclical patterns around zero. For a mixture of log-normal distributions, $Ln(Y)$ should be used, not untransformed Y, since the plot was devised for a mixture of normal distributions. However, Everitt (1996) suggests that these plots are only slightly more sensitive to detecting mixtures than simple histogram examination.

A common approach to determine whether mixture model inclusion improves goodness of fit is to use the LRT. The problem with this approach is that the LRT statistic is not distributed as a chi-squared random variable with q degrees of freedom anymore, where q is the difference in the number of estimable parameters between the full (with mixture) and reduced (without mixture) models. Wolfe (1971) showed that the distribution of the LRT statistic comparing m + 1 mixtures to a model with m mixtures is chi-squared distributed with $2v - 2$ degrees of freedom, where v is the number of extra parameters in the mixture model with m + 1 components. Later simulation studies have shown that Wolfe's results are a good rule of thumb but do not apply universally. Frame, Miller, and Lalonde (2003) showed that adding a mixture model to simulated data from a unimodal distribution resulted in a false-positive rate of about 8%, which is not much higher than the nominal Type I error rate of 5%. To guard against such false positives, they recommended that the 90% confidence interval for the mixing proportion not contain either 0 or 1 and that the confidence interval be entirely contained within the interval [0.047, 0.95].

Their results also showed that if the LRT was used to determine whether a mixture should be included in the model, the LRT did not follow a chi-squared distribution. Under a chi-squared distribution, a LRT of 5.99

would be needed for 0.05 level significance on two degrees of freedom. Their simulations showed that a value of 5.43 is needed for 0.05 level significance on two degrees of freedom. It has been the author's experience that if a mixture is present then adding an appropriate mixture model to a parameter in a pharmacokinetic model results in a highly significant LRT, not a LRT that is in the gray zone. In other words, when a mixture model works, it really works. Still, if one must be absolutely certain of the significance of the mixture to the model, more computer-intensive methods, such as the bootstrap, can be applied (McLachlan, 1987). Finally, again, physiology can also be applied in the decision to use a mixture model. If the analyst knows that subpopulations are likely, such as in the case of CYP 2D6 polymorphisms, then it is often reasonable to evaluate a mixture model without statistical justification.

ESTIMATION METHODS

Suppose $Y = f(x, \theta, \eta) + g(z, \varepsilon)$ where $\eta \sim (0, \Omega)$, $\varepsilon \sim (0, \Sigma)$, x is the set of subject-specific covariates $\{x, z\}$, Ω is the variance–covariance matrix for the random effects in the model (η), and Σ is the residual variance matrix. NONMEM (version 5 and higher) offers two general approaches towards parameter estimation with nonlinear mixed effects models: first-order approximation (FO) and first-order conditional estimation (FOCE), with FOCE being more accurate and computationally difficult than FO. First-order (FO) approximation, which was the first algorithm derived to estimate parameters in a nonlinear mixed effects models, was originally developed by Sheiner and Beal (1980; 1981; 1983). FO-approximation expands the nonlinear mixed effects model as a first-order Taylor series approximation about $\eta = 0$ and then estimates the model parameters based on the linear approximation to the nonlinear model. Consider the model

$$C_{ij} = \frac{D}{V + \eta_{i,v}} \left(\frac{k_a + \eta_{i,k_a}}{(k_a + \eta_{i,k_a}) - (k_{10} + \eta_{i,k_{10}})} \right)$$

$$\left\{ \exp\left[-(k_{10} + \eta_{i,k_{10}})t \right] - \exp\left[-(k_a + \eta_{i,k_a})t \right] \right\} + \varepsilon_{ij}$$

$$(7.86)$$

which is a 1-compartment model with first-order absorption, where C is concentration, the subscripts denote the jth sample for the ith subject, $i = 1, 2, \ldots n$, D is the dose, V population volume of distribution, k_a the population absorption rate constant, k_{10} the population elimination rate constant, η_i the deviation from the population mean for the ith subject, and ε the random

error. There are two random effects in this model, η and ε. All ηs in the model are assumed to be multivariate normally distributed with mean 0 and variance ω^2. Collectively, the vector of all model parameters is $\theta = \{k_a, k_{10}, V\}$ and the matrix of all ω^2s is the Ω matrix

$$\Omega = \begin{bmatrix} \omega_{k_a}^2 & 0 & 0 \\ 0 & \omega_{k_{10}}^2 & 0 \\ 0 & 0 & \omega_v^2 \end{bmatrix} \qquad (7.87)$$

In this example the off-diagonal elements of Ω are assumed to be 0, but they do not have to be independent and are often not. ε is assumed to be normally distributed with mean 0 and variance σ^2. In this example, ε is one term, but it does not have to be. If ε consists of more than one term, then collectively the set of residuals is the Σ matrix.

The expected value of Eq. (7.86) is

$$E(C_{ij}) = f(t; \theta; D)$$
$$= \frac{D}{V} \left(\frac{k_a}{k_a - k_{10}} \right) [\exp(-k_{10}t_{ij}) - \exp(-k_a t_{ij})]$$
$$(7.88)$$

which is the model given that the ηs equal 0 or in other words, the population mean. This makes sense, because the expected value for any individual, in the absence of further knowledge, would be the population mean. Now, if the variance of C_{ij} were known then weighted least squares or some modification thereof could be used to estimate the population parameters. Given that there are two random effects that enter into the model nonlinearly, the variance of C_{ij} cannot be estimated analytically, but must be estimated numerically or by some type of approximation.

Sheiner and Beal (1980; 1981; 1983) proposed taking a first-order Taylor series approximation around the set of ηs evaluated at $\eta = 0$ to find the variance. Recall that Taylor series approximations, which are linear polynomials, take a function and create an approximation to the model around some neighborhood. The derivatives of Eq. (7.86) to the model are

$$\left. \frac{\partial f(t_{ij}; \theta; D)}{\partial \eta_V} \right|_{\eta_v = 0} = -\frac{f(t_{ij}; \theta; D)}{V} \qquad (7.89)$$

$$\left. \frac{\partial f(t_{ij}; \theta; D)}{\partial \eta_{k_a}} \right|_{\eta_{k_a} = 0} = \frac{f(t_{ij}; \theta; D)}{k_a} - \frac{f(t_{ij}; \theta; D)}{(k_a - k_{10})} -$$
$$\frac{Dt_{ij}}{V} \left(\frac{k_a}{k_a - k_{10}} \right) \exp(-k_a t_{ij}) \qquad (7.90)$$

$$\frac{\partial f(t_{ij}; \theta; D)}{\partial \eta_{k_{10}}}\bigg|_{\eta_{k_{10}}=0} = \frac{f(t_{ij}; \theta; D)}{k_a - k_{10}} -$$

$$\frac{Dt_{ij}}{V}\left(\frac{k_a}{k_a - k_{10}}\right)\exp(-k_{10}t_{ij})$$

(7.91)

where $f(t_{ij}, \theta; D)$ is defined in Eq. (7.88). Recall that the first-order Taylor series approximation to a function $f(x, y)$ evaluated at x_0 and y_0 is

$$f(x, y) = f(x_0, y_0) + \frac{\partial f}{\partial x}(x - x_0) + \frac{\partial f}{\partial y}(y - y_0). \quad (7.92)$$

Hence, the first-order Taylor series approximation to Eq. (7.86) evaluated at $\eta = 0$ is

$$C_{ij} = f(t_{ij}; \theta; D) + \frac{\partial f(t_{ij}; \theta; D)}{\partial \eta_V}\eta_{i, v}$$

$$+ \frac{\partial f(t_{ij}; \theta; D)}{\partial \eta_{k_a}}\eta_{i, k_a} + \frac{\partial f(t_{ij}; \theta; D)}{\partial \eta_{k_{10}}}\eta_{i, k_{10}} + \varepsilon_{ij}^*.$$

(7.93)

Notice that the approximation is exact, but that $\varepsilon \neq \varepsilon^*$. The reason is that the residual in Eq. (7.93) includes the truncation error for the approximation plus the residual error term, ε. Equation (7.93) can be thought of as a linear model

$$\underbrace{C_{ij}}_{Y} \cong \underbrace{f(t_{ij}; \theta; D)}_{\beta_0} + \underbrace{\frac{\partial f(t_{ij}; \theta; D)}{\partial \eta_V}\eta_{i, v}}_{x_1\beta_1} +$$

$$\underbrace{\frac{\partial f(t_{ij}; \theta; D)}{\partial \eta_{k_a}}\eta_{i, k_a}}_{x_2\beta_2} + \underbrace{\frac{\partial f(t_{ij}; \theta; D)}{\partial \eta_{k_{10}}}\eta_{i, k_{10}}}_{x_3\beta_3} + \underbrace{\varepsilon_{ij}^*}_{\varepsilon_{ij}},$$

(7.94)

where x is the partial derivative and β represents η. In matrix form, Eq. (7.93) can be written as

$$C_{ij} \cong f(t_{ij}; \theta; D) +$$

$$\begin{bmatrix} \frac{\partial f(t_1; \theta; D)}{\partial \eta_V} & \frac{\partial f(t_1; \theta; D)}{\partial \eta_{k_a}} & \frac{\partial f(t_1; \theta; D)}{\partial \eta_{k_{10}}} \\ \frac{\partial f(t_2; \theta; D)}{\partial \eta_V} & \frac{\partial f(t_1; \theta; D)}{\partial \eta_{k_a}} & \frac{\partial f(t_1; \theta; D)}{\partial \eta_{k_{10}}} \\ \cdots & \cdots & \cdots \\ \frac{\partial f(t_{n_i}; \theta; D)}{\partial \eta_V} & \frac{\partial f(t_{n_i}; \theta; D)}{\partial \eta_{k_a}} & \frac{\partial f(t_{n_i}; \theta; D)}{\partial \eta_{k_{10}}} \end{bmatrix}\begin{bmatrix} \eta_{i, v} \\ \eta_{i, k_a} \\ \eta_{i, k_{10}} \end{bmatrix} + \begin{bmatrix} \varepsilon_1 \\ \varepsilon_2 \\ \cdots \\ \varepsilon_{n_i} \end{bmatrix}$$

$$= f(t_{ij}; \theta; D) + R_i\eta + \varepsilon_i,$$

(7.95)

where n_i is the number of observations for the ith subject,

$$R_i = \begin{bmatrix} \frac{\partial f(t_1; \theta; D)}{\partial \eta_V} & \frac{\partial f(t_1; \theta; D)}{\partial \eta_{k_a}} & \frac{\partial f(t_1; \theta; D)}{\partial \eta_{k_{10}}} \\ \frac{\partial f(t_2; \theta; D)}{\partial \eta_V} & \frac{\partial f(t_2; \theta; D)}{\partial \eta_{k_a}} & \frac{\partial f(t_2; \theta; D)}{\partial \eta_{k_{10}}} \\ \cdots & \cdots & \cdots \\ \frac{\partial f(t_{n_i}; \theta; D)}{\partial \eta_V} & \frac{\partial f(t_{n_i}; \theta; D)}{\partial \eta_{k_a}} & \frac{\partial f(t_{n_i}; \theta; D)}{\partial \eta_{k_{10}}} \end{bmatrix}$$

(7.96)

$$\eta = \begin{bmatrix} \eta_{i, v} \\ \eta_{i, k_a} \\ \eta_{i, k_{10}} \end{bmatrix}$$

(7.97)

and

$$\varepsilon_i = \begin{bmatrix} \varepsilon_1 \\ \varepsilon_2 \\ \cdots \\ \varepsilon_{n_i} \end{bmatrix}.$$

(7.98)

The variance of Eq. (7.93) is the variance of a linear combination of random variables

$$Var(C_i) \cong R\Omega R^T + \sigma^2 I, \quad (7.99)$$

where I is the identity matrix of size $n_i \times 3$. Given the variance of C_{ij}, weighted least-squares or some modification thereof can then be minimized to obtain estimates of θ, σ^2, and Ω. NONMEM uses extended least-squares as its objective function. Hence, NONMEM minimizes the following function

$$S(\theta; \Omega; \sigma^2) =$$

$$\sum_{i=1}^{n}\sum_{j=1}^{n_i}\left\{\frac{[C_{ij} - f(t_{ij}; \theta; D)]^2}{Var(C_{ij})} + Ln\left[|Var(C_{ij})|\right]\right\}$$

(7.100)

where $|.|$ denotes the determinant of the variance matrix, $f(t_{ij}; \theta; D)$.

This original FO-approximation algorithm to provide population estimates has proven surprisingly adequate for many pharmacokinetic–pharmacodynamic problems and was also important in the past when computer processor speed was slower than it is today. However, more recent algorithms are developed around the marginal likelihood. The joint probability distribution for Y_i and η_i can be written as

$$p(Y_i, \eta_i | \theta, \Omega, \Sigma) = L_i(\theta, \Omega, \Sigma | Y_i, \eta_i)$$

$$= p(Y_i | \theta, \Sigma, \eta_i)p(\eta_i | \Omega) \quad (7.101)$$

$$= l_i h$$

where $L_i(\cdot)$ is the likelihood for the ith individual given Y_i and η_i, $p(Y_i | \theta, \Sigma, \eta_i)$ is the conditional probability density of the observed data, and $p(\eta_i|\Omega)$ is the conditional density of η_i. Since η_i is not observable, the marginal distribution of Y_i can be written as

$$p(Y_i|\theta, \Omega, \Sigma) = \int p(Y_i|\theta, \Sigma, \eta_i) p(\eta_i|\Omega) d\eta. \quad (7.102)$$

The likelihood function can then be expressed as

$$L(\theta, \Omega, \Sigma) = \prod_i p(Y_i|\theta, \Omega, \Sigma). \quad (7.103)$$

Assuming that $\eta \sim N(0, \Omega)$ and $\varepsilon \sim N(0, \Sigma)$ then

$$p(Y_i|\theta, \Sigma, \eta_i) = (2\pi)^{-n_i/2}|\Sigma|^{-1/2}$$
$$\exp\left(-\frac{1}{2}(Y_i - f(x_i, \theta, \eta_i))^T\Sigma^{-1}(Y_i - f(x_i, \theta, \eta_i))\right) \quad (7.104)$$

and

$$p(\eta_i|\Omega) = (2\pi)^{-q/2}|\Omega|^{-1/2}\exp\left(-\frac{1}{2}\eta_i^T\Omega^{-1}\eta_i\right). \quad (7.105)$$

Hence, the marginal distribution can be written as

$$p(Y_i|\theta, \Omega, \Sigma) =$$
$$\int (2\pi)^{-(n_i+q)/2}|\Sigma|^{-1/2}|\Omega|^{-1/2}\exp\left(-\frac{1}{2}\Psi(\eta_i)\right)d\eta \quad (7.106)$$

where

$$\Psi(\eta_i) =$$
$$(Y_i - f(x_i, \theta, \eta_i))^T\Sigma^{-1}(Y_i - f(x_i, \theta, \eta_i)) + \eta_i^T\Omega^{-1}\eta_i \quad (7.107)$$

For a linear mixed effects models, both ε and η are normally distributed random variables and the marginal distribution is itself a normal distribution (see book appendix for details) provided η and ε are independent. After some matrix manipulation, the integral in Eq. (7.102) can be analytically expressed and the likelihood function can be explicitly written. For a nonlinear mixed effects model, the integral in Eq. (7.102) cannot be analytically expressed (although there are specific cases where this is true) and the integration must be done by numeric approximation. The reason why the integral is intractable is that ε and η are no longer independent because the residual variance matrix depends on the estimation of the between-subject variance matrix, i.e., the estimate of ε depends on the estimate of η. $f(x, \theta, \Omega)$ being a nonlinear function adds a further complication

to evaluating the integral. What differentiates the various software packages and their estimation routines is how the marginal distribution is approximated.

One type of approximation is the Laplacian approximation.[1] Given a complex integral, $\int f(x)dx, f(x)$ is reexpressed as $\exp[Ln(f(x)] = \exp[g(x)]$. $g(x)$ can then be approximated using a second-order Taylor series approximation about the point x_0

$$g(x) \approx g(x_0) + (x - x_0)g'(x_0) + \frac{(x - x_0)^2}{2!}g''(x_0). \quad (7.108)$$

The integral then becomes

$$\int f(x)dx = \int \exp[g(x)]dx$$
$$\approx \int \exp\left[g(x_0) + (x - x_0)g'(x_0) + \frac{(x - x_0)^2}{2!}g'(x_0)\right]dx. \quad (7.109)$$

Notice that Eq. (7.109) is being integrated with respect to x. Therefore $g(x_0)$ can be pulled outside the integral and the equation rewritten as

$$\int f(x)dx \approx$$
$$\exp[g(x_0)]\int \exp\left[(x - x_0)g'(x_0) + \frac{(x - x_0)^2}{2!}g''(x_0)\right]dx. \quad (7.110)$$

At this point a brief diversion is needed. The moment generating function for a random variable X that is normally distributed with mean μ and variance σ^2 is

$$M_x(t) = \int \frac{1}{\sqrt{2\pi\sigma^2}}\exp(Xt)\exp\left(-\frac{(X - \mu)^2}{2\sigma^2}\right)dx$$
$$= \int \frac{1}{\sqrt{2\pi\sigma^2}}\exp\left(Xt - \frac{(X - \mu)^2}{2\sigma^2}\right)dx$$
$$= \exp\left(\mu t + \frac{t^2\sigma^2}{2}\right). \quad (7.111)$$

---

[1] I am indebted to Yaning Wang, PhD, for deriving these equations and allowing me to reprint them.

Notice that the integrand in Eq. (7.110) is similar in form to the middle line in Eq. (7.111) where $X = (x - x_0)$, $\mu = 0$, $t = g'(x_0)$, and $\sigma^2 = -g''(x_0)^{-1}$. Hence,

$$
\int f(x)dx \approx \exp[g(x_0)]\sqrt{2\pi\sigma^2}\exp\left(\frac{\sigma^2 t^2}{2}\right)
$$
$$
= \exp[g(x_0)]\sqrt{\frac{2\pi}{g''(x_0)}}\exp\left(\frac{-g'(x_0)^2}{2g''(x_0)}\right). \tag{7.112}
$$

Here now is the second diversion. First, let -2 times the log-likelihood ($-2LL_i$) be defined as $-2Ln[l_i(\eta_i, \theta, \Sigma)] = \Phi(\eta_i, \theta, \Sigma)$. Using the chain rule for derivatives,

$$
\frac{dy}{dx} = \frac{dy}{du}\frac{du}{dx}, \tag{7.113}
$$

it can be shown that the gradient (the matrix of first-order derivatives with respect to η) of $-2LL$ for the ith subject is

$$
\nabla_i(\eta) = \frac{d[-2LL_i,]}{d\eta} = -2\frac{l_i'}{l_i} \tag{7.114}
$$

and by rearrangement

$$
\frac{l_i'}{l_i} = \frac{\nabla_i(\eta)}{-2}. \tag{7.115}
$$

Then, the Hessian (the matrix of second-order derivatives with respect to η) of $-2LL$ for the ith subject is equal to

$$
\nabla_i^2(\eta) = \frac{d\nabla_i(\eta)}{d\eta} = -2\left(\frac{l_i'}{l_i}\right)' \tag{7.116}
$$

and by rearrangement

$$
\left(\frac{l_i'}{l_i}\right)' = \frac{\nabla_i^2(\eta)}{-2}. \tag{7.117}
$$

Since the between-subject random effects, η, are multivariate normal then

$$
h = \frac{1}{\sqrt{2\pi}|\Omega|^{1/2}}\exp\left(-\frac{1}{2}\eta'\Omega^{-1}\eta\right) \tag{7.118}
$$

with first derivative

$$
h' = \frac{1}{\sqrt{2\pi}|\Omega|^{1/2}}\exp\left(-\frac{1}{2}\eta'\Omega^{-1}\eta\right)(-\Omega^{-1}\eta). \tag{7.119}
$$

Therefore,

$$
\frac{h'}{h} = -\Omega^{-1}\eta \tag{7.120}
$$

and

$$
\left(\frac{h'}{h}\right)' = -\Omega^{-1}. \tag{7.121}
$$

Since the integrand is

$$
f(\eta) = l_i(\eta, \theta, \Sigma)h(\eta, \Omega), \tag{7.122}
$$

then

$$
g(\eta) = Ln[l_i(\eta, \theta, \Sigma)] + Ln[h(\eta, \Omega)] \tag{7.123}
$$

with first and second derivatives

$$
g'(\eta) = \frac{l_i'}{l_i} + \frac{h^i}{h_i} = -\frac{\nabla_i(\eta)}{2} - \Omega^{-1}\eta \tag{7.124}
$$

$$
g''(\eta) = \left(\frac{l_i'}{l_i}\right)' + \left(\frac{h^i}{h_i}\right)' = -\frac{\nabla_i^2(\eta)}{2} - \Omega^{-1}. \tag{7.125}
$$

Hence,

$$
\begin{aligned}
&-2Ln[L_i(\theta, \Sigma, \Omega|Y_i, \eta_i)] \\
&= -2Ln\int l_i(\eta, \Sigma, \theta)h(\eta, \Omega)d\eta \\
&\approx -2Ln\left\{l_i(\hat{\eta}, \Sigma, \theta)h(\hat{\eta}, \Omega)\sqrt{\frac{2\pi}{|g''(\hat{\eta})|}}\right. \\
&\quad\left. \exp\left(-\frac{1}{2}g'(\hat{\eta})^T g''(\hat{\eta})^{-1}g'(\hat{\eta})\right)\right\} \\
&\approx -2Ln[l_i(\hat{\eta}, \Sigma, \theta)] - 2Ln[h(\hat{\eta}, \Omega)] \\
&\quad -2Ln\left[\sqrt{\frac{2\pi}{|g''(\hat{\eta})|}}\right] \\
&\quad -2Ln\left[\exp\left(-\frac{1}{2}g'(\hat{\eta})^T g''(\hat{\eta})^{-1}g'(\hat{\eta})\right)\right] \\
&\approx \Phi(\hat{\eta}) - 2Ln\left[\frac{1}{\sqrt{2\pi}|\Omega|^{1/2}}\right] \\
&\quad -2Ln\left[-\frac{1}{2}\hat{\eta}\Omega^{-1}\hat{\eta}\right] - Ln\left[\frac{2\pi}{|g''(\hat{\eta})|}\right] \\
&\quad + g'(\hat{\eta})^T g''(\hat{\eta})^{-1}g'(\hat{\eta}) \\
&\propto \Phi(\hat{\eta}) + Ln|\Omega| + \hat{\eta}\Omega^{-1}\hat{\eta} + Ln|g''(\hat{\eta})| \\
&\quad + g'(\hat{\eta})^T g''(\hat{\eta})^{-1}g'(\hat{\eta}).
\end{aligned} \tag{7.126}
$$

After making the appropriate substitutions defined previously

$$-2\text{Ln}[L_i(\theta, \Sigma, \Omega|Y_i, \eta_i)] \propto \Phi(\hat{\eta}) + \text{Ln}|\Omega| +$$

$$\hat{\eta}_i \Omega^{-1} \hat{\eta}_i + \text{Ln}\left|\Omega^{-1} + \frac{\nabla_i^2(\hat{\eta})}{2}\right| -$$

$$\left(\frac{\nabla_i(\hat{\eta})}{2} + \Omega^{-1}\hat{\eta}_i\right)^T \left(\Omega^{-1} + \frac{\nabla_i^2(\hat{\eta})}{2}\right)^{-1} \left(\frac{\nabla_i(\hat{\eta})}{2} + \Omega^{-1}\hat{\eta}_i\right)$$

$$(7.127)$$

If $\hat{\eta}$ is the mode of the conditional density of η then the last term in Eq. (7.127) is zero because the gradient is zero. This last equation is the function that is minimized by NONMEM using the Laplace option.

With first-order conditional estimation (FOCE) in NONMEM, the Hessian is approximated as

$$\nabla_i^2(\hat{\eta}) \approx \frac{1}{2}\nabla(\hat{\eta})'\nabla(\hat{\eta}), \qquad (7.128)$$

which is a type of first-order approximation. FOCE is sometimes described as a first-order Taylor series approximation of the nonlinear mixed effects model around the posterior mode of η. Because both FOCE and Laplace options depend on a conditional estimate of η (denoted $\hat{\eta}$), both FOCE and Laplace are referred to as conditional estimation algorithms.

Coincidentally, using both Eq. (7.128) and setting $\hat{\eta} = 0$ results in an equivalent parameterization to the likelihood function for FO-approximation. Hence, the FO-approximation can be developed using a Laplacian approach or through a Taylor series approximation to the nonlinear mixed effects model itself. This duality leads to two different conclusions regarding the distribution of the random effects. Under the Laplacian derivation, normality is assumed, but no such assumption is made using the Taylor series derivation. Hence, there is confusion in the literature in that some report that the FO-approximation depends on normality, but others state that FO-approximation does not depend on normality. The normality assumption depends on the basis for the approximation. Beal (2004, personal communication) has stated that normality is not needed for valid FO-approximation and that the assumption of normality is less important than the accuracy of the Taylor series. In practice, when the ηs themselves are examined, rarely are they exactly normally distributed, so that as long as they are approximately normal with good symmetry the FO-approximation will seem to be valid.

NONMEM also has a number of options available for estimation: interaction, centering, and hybrid. The derivation just described is predicated on η and ε being independent. However, consider the model

$$Y = f(x, \theta, \eta) + f(x, \theta, \eta)\varepsilon, \qquad (7.129)$$

which is a proportional random error model. ε is clearly not independent of η because the value of the former depends on the value of the latter. In this case, there is an interaction between η and ε. With the NONMEM estimation algorithm, FOCE with interaction (FOCE-I), such an interaction is accounted for in the estimation of the likelihood. FOCE-I is generally not useful when the residual variance is large or the amount of data per individual is small nor is it useful for simpler homoscedastic error models. Under the hybrid model, certain elements in the set of all η are constrained such that $\hat{\eta}$ is fixed to zero, while the remaining elements allow $\hat{\eta}$ to vary. Hence, some elements of η are fit using FO-approximation, while the remaining elements are fit using FOCE. It is assumed that η has mean zero and when the population model is a good fit to the observed data then the mean η (denoted $\bar{\eta}$) will be close to zero and such a fit is referred to as 'centered.' None of the estimation algorithms just presented guarantee a centered fit. With the centering option in NONMEM, the likelihood function is modified to result in a more 'centered' fit by forcing the interindividual error terms to be distributed about zero.

There is not a lot of experience in the literature about NONMEM's hybrid or centering options to suggest when they might be appropriate. One output feature in NONMEM is a t-test of the mean η against the null hypothesis that its value equal zero. The NONMEM manuals indicate that if the p-value for one of the mean ηs is small and the goodness of fit of the predicted model is poor, centering may be of value. Using centering tends to result in models that are no worse in fit than models that are uncentered and may significantly improve the goodness of fit. However, it is strongly encouraged not to routinely use centering as centering may mask a poor model. Centering can also be used with conditional estimation to reduce computing times of complex models. Examples of the use of centering in this instance can be found in Zuideveld et al. (2002a; 2002b). The NONMEM manuals also suggest that hybrid models may be useful when the model is a change-point model (e.g., includes a lag-time or some other discontinuity) and anecdotal evidence suggests that the hybrid method may be useful when lag-times are included as random effects in an extravascular administration model (in which case they are functioning as change points). An example of the use of the hybrid method can be found in Friberg et al. (2002) and Cox et al. (2004).

Within NONMEM, a generalized least-squares-like (GLS-like) estimation algorithm can be developed by iterating separate, sequential models. In the first step, the model is fit using one of the estimation algorithms (FO-approximation, FOCE, etc.). The individual predicted values are saved in a data set that is formatted the same as the input data set, i.e., the output data set contains the original data set plus one more variable: the individual predicted values. The second step then models the residual error based on the value of the individual predicted values given in the previous step. So, for example, suppose the residual error was modeled as a proportional error model

$$Y = F(1 + \varepsilon), \qquad (7.130)$$

where F is the predicted value. The second step would model the residual error as

$$Y = F_{\text{current step}} + F_{\text{previous step}}\varepsilon, \qquad (7.131)$$

where $F_{\text{previous step}}$ is the individual predicted value stored from the previous step. This process can be iterated until the parameter estimates converge to some set of stable values, although in most cases the algorithm is implemented as a two-step process. The reader is referred to Wahlby et al. (2001) for an application.

With SAS, version 8.0 and higher, a nonlinear mixed effects model procedure called NLMIXED is available. NLMIXED offers FO-approximation (called the FIRO method) and Laplace method, but does not offer a FOCE or FOCE-I option. Instead, SAS offers more exact integral approximations than does NON-MEM. In particular, adaptive and nonadaptive Gaussian quadrature may be used. Both methods are numerical techniques used to evaluate integrals, like Simpson's rule or the trapezoidal rule to evaluate area under the curve, but are much more accurate. SAS also offers importance sampling, which approximates an integral using Monte Carlo simulation. Pinheiro and Bates (1995) compared conditional estimation, Laplacian, adaptive and nonadaptive Gaussian quadrature, and importance sampling using simulation and two actual data sets (one of which was the infamous theophylline data set). Gaussian quadrature only seemed to give accurate results when the number of abscissas was greater than 100, which makes it very computationally inefficient. Importance sampling, while producing accurate and reliable results, was also computationally inefficient compared to Laplacian and adaptive Gaussian quadrature methods. Of the methods studied, the authors concluded that Laplacian and adaptive Gaussian quadrature gave the best mix of efficiency and accuracy of the methods studied. There is almost no experience in the

pharmacokinetic literature with these methods so it is difficult to make recommendations on their use. My own personal experience with NLMIXED is that it is much slower than NONMEM or NLME in S-Plus and since it is not designed for pharmacokinetic models is more difficult to use.

The NLME function in S-Plus offers three different estimation algorithms: a FOCE algorithm similar to NONMEM, adaptive Gaussian quadrature, and Laplacian approximation. The FOCE algorithm in S-Plus, similar to the one in NONMEM, was developed by Lindstrom and Bates (1990). The algorithm is predicated on normally distributed random effects and normally distributed random errors and makes a first-order Taylor series approximation of the nonlinear mixed effects model around both the current parameter estimates θ and the random effects η. The adaptive Gaussian quadrature and Laplacian options are similar to the options offered by SAS.

In general, the following order applies in terms of accuracy and computer time: importance sampling > adaptive Gaussian quadrature > Laplacian > FOCE > Lindstrom and Bates FOCE method > FO-approximation. The major difference in these algorithms is in variance component estimates. The structural model parameters usually compare pretty well from one algorithm to the next, but the variance components may be quite different. Also, FO-approximation tends to differ from the conditional estimates as the amount of data per individual decreases or as the degree of between-subject variability decreases. However, FO-approximation is often useful as a starting algorithm to obtain initiate parameter estimates for more accurate estimation methods.

To illustrate how these algorithms may differ in their estimates, a simple simulation was conducted. A total of 100 subjects were simulated under a Phase 2 clinical study design where $\sim 1/3$ of the subjects had two samples collected, 1/3 had four samples collected, and 1/3 had six samples collected. If subjects were assigned to have two samples collected, samples were collected randomly from the time intervals (0–6 h) and (6–24 h). If subjects were assigned to have four samples collected, samples were collected randomly from the time intervals (0–2 h), (2–4 h), (4–10 h), and (10–24 h). If subjects were assigned to have six samples collected, samples were collected randomly from the time intervals (0–2 h), (2–4 h), (4–6 h), (6–10 h), (10–16 h), and (16–24 h). The sample time windows were arbitrarily chosen to cover the entire concentration–time profile and to capture the absorption and elimination phases.

Concentration–time data were simulated following a once-daily 50 mg dose from a 1-compartment model with first-order absorption at steady-state where the absorption rate constant (k_a) was fixed to 0.7 per hour. Clearance was log-normal in distribution having a population mean of 8000 mL/h and a log-standard deviation of 0.32 mL/h, i.e., 32% CV. Volume of distribution was log-normal in distribution having a population mean of 200 L and a log-standard deviation of 0.32 L, i.e., 32% CV. Residual error was log-normal in distribution having a standard deviation of 0.145 ng/mL (15% CV). Simulated concentration–time data were fit in NONMEM using FO-approximation, FOCE, FOCE-I, and Laplacian estimation. The same data were also fit in SAS using FO-approximation, adaptive Gaussian quadrature with a quadrature tolerance of 0.001, importance sampling using a quadrature tolerance of 0.001, and Laplacian estimation. The starting values for clearance and volume of distribution were 8000 mL/h and 200 L, respectively. All starting values for variance components were set at 0.1. k_a was fixed at 0.7 per hour. The simulation was repeated 100 times using a 2.6 GHz Pentium® 4 personal computer.

Initial attempts to model the random effects in SAS resulted in poor estimates or estimates that failed to move beyond the initial values. Success was finally achieved when the random effects were modeled using the following form (using clearance as an example)

$$CL = \exp(\theta_1 + \eta_1), \qquad (7.132)$$

where θ is brought inside the exponent. The starting value for clearance and volume of distribution were the log-transformed population value. The population estimate for clearance after successful convergence is then $\exp(\theta_1)$.

Figure 7.9 presents box and whisker plots of the final parameter estimates for the simulation by estimation method. All estimation algorithms had equal variability across simulations, i.e., no estimation method appeared more precise than the others. The SAS algorithms were more accurate in regards to estimating clearance and, except for SAS's FO-approximation, were more accurate in estimating volume of distribution. Within NONMEM, the rank order of accuracy was FO-approximation < FOCE ≅ Laplacian < FOCE-I for clearance but was FO-approximation < FOCE ≅ FOCE-I < Laplacian for volume of distribution. Hence, the conditional estimation algorithms within NONMEM were more accurate than FO-approximation. Little difference was observed between the estimation algorithms in the estimates of the between-subject variance components. However, residual variance estimates were more precise using SAS algorithms than NONMEM algorithms in general. The most precise estimate of residual variance was NONMEM's FOCE-I

algorithm. Not shown was that SAS's algorithms were slightly slower than NONMEM's algorithm resulting in longer optimization times.

This simulation was then repeated only this time concentration–time data were simulated from a Phase 1 study where each subject had samples collected at 0, 0.5, 1, 1.5, 2, 3, 4, 5, 6, 8, 10, 12, 18, and 24 h after dosing. In the *previous simulation*, the number of observations per subject ranged from two to six, but in this simulation each subject had 14 observations collected during the dosing interval. All other conditions remained unchanged. The results are presented in Fig. 7.10. No difference was observed between the data rich and data sparse designs for any of the estimable parameters, except with the data rich design the BSV estimate for volume of distribution was more accurate and precise for all software packages as compared to the sparse sampling design. Increasing the number of observations per subject actually had very little impact on the parameter estimates. These simulations illustrate that under certain conditions one algorithm may be better than another, but there is little difference for many problems in the conditional estimation algorithms or between results of different software platforms. This is not to say that there will be no differences. Indeed, there will be differences sometimes between algorithms and software, but these differences will be problem specific and must be evaluated on a case by case basis. This example also illustrates that collecting more data per individual does not necessarily translate into better parameter estimates. More on the choice of estimation algorithms and sampling times will be presented in the next chapter.

MODEL BUILDING TECHNIQUES

One goal of population pharmacokinetic models is to relate subject-specific characteristics or covariates, e.g., age, weight, or race, to individual pharmacokinetic parameters, such as clearance. There are many different methods to determine whether such a relationship exists, some of which were discussed previously in the chapter, and they can be characterized as either manual or automated in nature. With manual methods, the user controls the model development process. In contrast, automated methods proceed based on an algorithm defined by the user a priori and a computer, not the user, controls the model development process. Consequently, the automated methods are generally considered somewhat less subjective than manual procedures. The advantage of the automated method is its supposed lack of bias and ability to rapidly test many different models. The advantage of the manual method is that the user

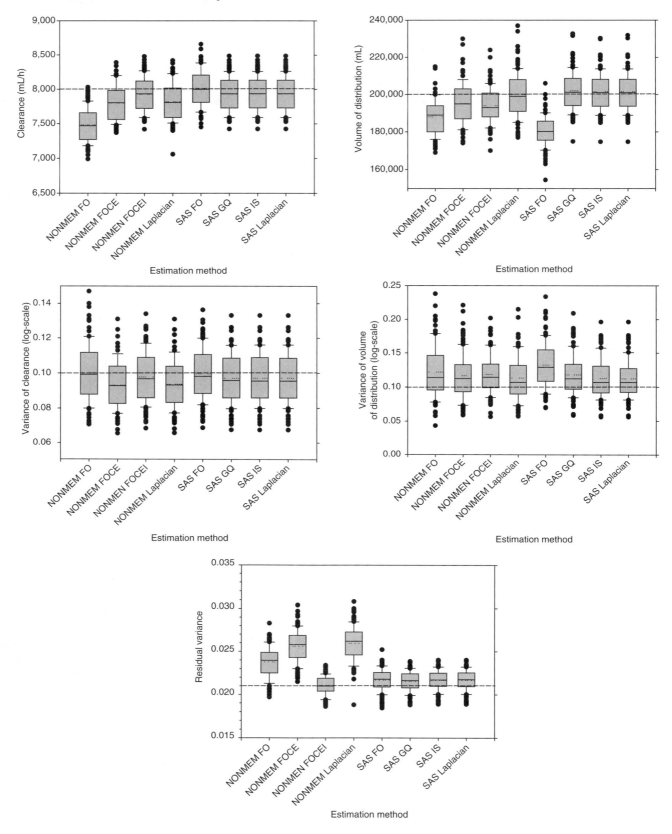

Figure 7.9 Box and whiskers plot comparing the parameter estimates under a sparse sampling design using various estimation algorithms.

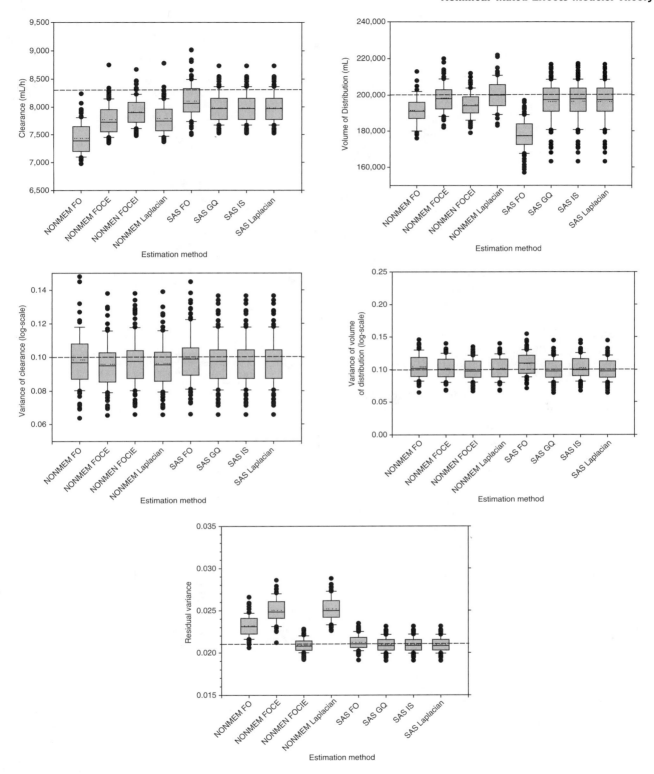

Figure 7.10 Box and whiskers plot comparing the parameter estimates under a rich sampling design using various estimation algorithms.

makes decisions and, hence, model development can be done "outside the box." In other words, with automated methods models are developed in a linear process A → B → C. With manual methods, models can be developed in a nonlinear process A → C (provided the analyst can think nonlinearly).

Most modelers still model using manual methods. One reason is that knowledge is obtained through the trial and error of model development. As model development proceeds, the user begins to understand the system and the data, even though an adequate model might not be found. Models that fail, tell the user something about the system. The same model development process that was done manually might be done automatically, but the level of knowledge gained by the user is not the same because with the manual process the user has to think where to go next and this usually leads to increased knowledge and understanding of the system. With automated methods, the process of deciding what model to try next is not passed onto the user and while some knowledge is gained upon review of the model development logs, the gain in knowledge is not as great as when done manually. Hence, this book will focus on manual model development.

Ette and Ludden (1995) elegantly describe the current state of building PopPK models, which were originally proposed by Maitre et al. (1991) and elaborated by Mandema et al. (1992). The stepwise process is as follows (Figure 11):

• Step 1: Determine the structural pharmacokinetic model.

The first step in the process is to develop a structural model, e.g., 2-compartment model open with lag-time, without covariates. At this point an over-parameterized model is preferred to an underparameterized model, especially with regards to the random effects.

• Step 2: Examine the distribution of the random effects.

The assumptions of the structural model regarding distribution of the random effects should be examined. Most population parameters are modeled assuming the random effects are log-normal. The random effects are assumed to be independent and have a normal distribution with mean 0 and variance ω^2. These assumptions should be tested. Other assumptions that should be tested include testing the residuals for homoscedasticity, normality, and lack of systematic deviations in the residuals over time. More about assumption testing will be presenting later in the chapter. If the assumptions are violated, remedial measures should be taken.

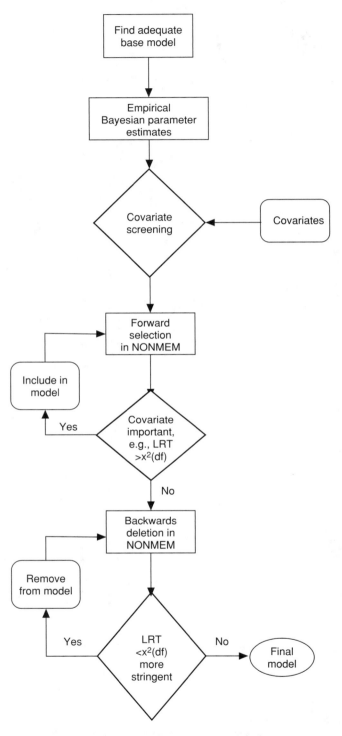

Figure 7.11 Flow chart of forward stepwise model building to a full covariate model followed by backwards deletion to a reduced, final covariate model.

● Step 3: Select the covariates for inclusion in the model.

It is this step that largely differentiates automated from manual methods, and modelers for that matter. The particular choice of how to test covariates in models is a matter of debate. One popular method is covariate screening, which treats the EBEs of the random effects as a random variable and then uses regression-based techniques to assess the relationship between the random effect and subject characteristics. For example, one might use linear regression of clearance against weight and determine if the T-test for the slope term associated with weight was statistically significant. Alternatives to linear regression include correlation analysis or use of generalized additive models. Some users evaluate the scatter plot of the data and then use "right between the eyes test," i.e., if a relationship is real and statistically significant, it should be visually noticeable and "hit you right between the eyes." The other method is to test the covariate directly in the nonlinear mixed effects model. These approaches will be discussed later in the chapter. Many modelers combine several of these approaches during covariate selection.

● Step 4: Build the model using covariates using stepwise model building strategies (usually forward selection followed by backwards deletion).

Step 4 may be redundant if the covariates were tested directly in the nonlinear mixed effects model. If the covariates were screened using some external method, e.g., regression models, then these covariates are included in the model in a forward stepwise manner. Improvement in the goodness of fit in the model is tested using either the LRT or T-test. In addition, reduction in parameter variability is expected as well. Further discussion of this topic will be made later in the chapter.

● Step 5: Evaluate the final parameter estimates
Like Step 2, the assumptions of the final model need to be tested before they can be accepted. Significant deviations from the assumptions of the model may lead to doubtful validity.

Most applications of PopPK methodology follow this general scheme but they are all flawed in the sense that they suffer from the same problems as are seen with stepwise regression, such as selection bias, overstated importance of retained covariates, and possibly invalid distributional assumptions (Wahlby, Jonsson, and Karlsson, 2002). However, it must be stressed that there is no universally accepted method for covariate selection in any regression-based model.

COVARIATE SCREENING METHODS

The first step in building a covariate model is to identify which covariates are to be examined. PopPK is largely an exercise in exploratory data analysis. However, more credibility is given to an analysis when the covariates to be chosen for inclusion in the model are selected prior to examining the data in accordance with ICH guidelines (1997). Further, the covariates selected should have some physiological rationale for their inclusion in the model and should result in some change (usually a change of ~20%) in the parameter across the range of covariates evaluated in the database. For example, if clearance correlated with age then the estimated clearance in the subject with the highest value of the covariate should be at least 20% different than the clearance in the subject with the lowest value of the covariate. It is important to remember that the Type I error rate increases as the number of covariates increases. In some cases, the level of significance associated with a selected covariate may be increased to help reduce the Type I error rate. The take-home message is that "covariates should be carefully chosen."

Covariate screening methods are used when there are a large number of covariates, such that evaluating every possible combination in a model is prohibitive. With this methodology, EBEs of the random effects are treated as "data" and then exploratory methods are used to assess the relationship between random effects and the covariate of interest. In other words, each individual's pharmacokinetic parameter, clearance for example, is estimated and treated as a being without measurement error. These Bayes estimates are then compared against subject-specific covariates for a "relationship" using either manual or automated methods.

Manual Covariate Screening Methods

Manual covariate screening methods come in one of two types. One is based on regression. The other is directly testing the covariate using the nonlinear mixed effects model software. Under a regression-based approach (EBE-method), the EBE of the parameter of interest is treated as the dependent variable and then using a linear or quadratic model, the dependent variable is regressed against the subject-specific covariate, e.g., clearance against weight. A drawback to this approach is that the effect of the covariate on the parameter is evaluated independently of the model. In other words, using this approach a trend between clearance and weight might be seen but due to correlations between say clearance and volume of distribution, when one actually adds weight to the model, little to no improvement is seen in the goodness of fit because the other correlated model parameters may change to accommodate the new covariate.

Alternatively, instead of using the EBE of the parameter of interest as the dependent variable, an estimate of the random effect (η) can be used as the dependent variable, similar to how partial residuals are used in stepwise linear regression. Early population pharmacokinetic methodology advocated multiple linear regression using either forward, backwards, or stepwise models. A modification of this is to use multiple simple linear models, one for each covariate. For categorical covariates, analysis of variance is used instead. If the p-value for the omnibus F-test or p-value for the T-test is less than some cut-off value, usually 0.05, the covariate is moved forward for further examination. Many reports in the literature use this approach.

It is not uncommon to see modifications to the EBE-method. For example, Verotta (1997) used regression trees for covariate identification. Frame et al. (2001) generated a primary database composed of the EBEs of the pharmacokinetic parameters along with demographic information. This dataset was sampled with replacement (bootstrapped) and a secondary dataset was generated with the same number of subjects as the primary dataset. This process was repeated 100 times creating 100 secondary datasets. Each secondary dataset was subjected to stepwise linear regression and the number of models that a particular covariate was identified (called the inclusion percentage) as being statistically significant was determined. Using an a priori defined cut-off criteria, those covariates that will be taken into the covariate submodel were then identified. Whether these modifications offer any improvement over "regular" EBE-based methods remains to be seen.

Linear models in general have been criticized as being too rigid in their structural form and might not detect a curvilinear relationship. For this reason, generalized additive models (GAMs) have been used instead and are more commonly seen in the literature than linear models (Mandema, Verotta, and Sheiner, 1992). Like linear regression models, the analyst can either develop a GAM for the EBE of the parameter itself, of the estimate of the random effect (η), or both. Using the EBE of the parameter itself as opposed to using the random effect as the dependent variable can sometimes lead to different covariate identification.

Because of the criticisms against linear models and GAMs there are those within the pharmacokinetic community who advocate a simple examination of the sca-

tter plot (or box and whisker plot in the case of a categorical variable) in choosing which covariates to move forward in model development. This approach, however, is too subjective and is likely to spot only the most obvious covariates. Covariates of marginal significance might not be detected nor might marginal covariates be consistently chosen across analyses. For these reasons, caution must be exercised if this approach is taken.

It should also be recognized that regression-based methods, whether they are linear models or GAMs, do not take into account whether a covariate is time dependent nor do they reflect the potentially correlated behavior of the parameters. These methods compare the value of a single dependent variable against the value of a single independent variable. If the independent variable varies with time then some summary of the independent variable must be used. For example, the baseline, the median value, or the value at the midpoint of the time interval on which the variable was collected are sometimes used.

A new type of covariate screening method is to use partially linear mixed effects models (Bonate, 2005). Briefly, the time component in a structural model is modeled using a penalized spline basis function with knots at usually equally spaced time intervals. Under this approach, the knots are treated as random effects and linear mixed effects models can be used to find the optimal smoothing parameter. Further, covariates can be introduced into the model to improve the goodness of fit. The LRT between a full and reduced model with and without the covariate of interest can be used to test for the inclusion of a covariate in a model. The advantage of this method is that the exact structural model (i.e., a 1-compartment or 2-compartment model with absorption) does not have to be determined and it is fast and efficient at covariate identification.

Direct Covariate Testing

Covariates can also be tested directly within the software program itself, although this is not technically a form of screening. For example, a model can be developed with and without the covariate of interest and the improvement in the goodness of fit with the covariate included in the model can be examined. If the goodness of fit is improved, then the covariate is kept in the model. Because it is difficult to detect meaningful improvements in goodness of fit graphically, albeit for only the most important covariates, most often model improvements are tested using the LRT. However, the LRT has some problems in its use (see the sections on Mixture Models and the next chapter for its limitations). Those concerns aside, covariate screening within the software package itself also has its own problems. First, the nature of the relationship between the covariate and pharmacokinetic parameter of interest must be determined. This is often done empirically by testing the covariate under a variety of different models, such as a linear and power model. Since a linear model and power model have the same number of estimable parameters, all other things being equal, the model having the lowest objective function value is deemed the superior model.

There is also the issue of Type I error rate, which is the rate at which a covariate is deemed statistically important when in fact it is not. Hypothesis testing a large number of models is referred to as *multiplicity* and results in an inflated Type I error rate. Because a large number of models are tested as some level of significance, usually $p < 0.05$, then $\sim 5\%$ of those models will be selected as being an improvement over the comparator model based on chance alone.

Ribbing and Jonsson (2004) performed a comprehensive set of simulations examining the Type I error rate, power, and selection bias (defined as the average parameter estimate minus the true parameter value) using direct covariate screening. They found that the power to detect a true covariate effect depended on a number of factors. First, power was influenced by the p-value used to declare significance under the LRT. A more stringent p-value decreases the power of the test. Second, power was also influenced by other covariates included in the model. This supports the simulation by Bonate (1999) who showed that as the correlation between covariates increased, even if they were not on the same pharmacokinetic parameter, such as age on clearance and weight on volume of distribution, larger standard errors of the parameter estimates resulted such that the T-test on the estimates were not different than zero when the correlation exceeded 0.5. Third, as the magnitude of the covariate effect increased so did power. Fourth, as the precision of the estimated covariate effect increased so did power. Lastly, power increased as the number of subjects increased.

In their study, Ribbing and Jonsson found that when only one covariate was in the model, 80% power was achieved with (i) 20 subjects having three samples per subject and high correlation ($\sim$0.85) between covariate and pharmacokinetic parameter, (ii) 100 subjects having three samples per subject and medium correlation ($\sim$0.50) between covariate and pharmacokinetic parameter, and (iii) 300 subjects having three samples per subject and low correlation ($\sim$0.15) between covariate and pharmacokinetic parameter. They also found that selection bias increased when the number of subjects decreased. In other words, the estimated value of the parameter relating the covariate to the pharmacokinetic parameter of interest was overestimated as the

number of subjects decreased. Hence, when the number of subjects in an analysis is small, low-powered covariates may appear to be statistically relevant when in fact they may not be. This outcome has implications for many fields where sparse data are available on a modest number of subjects, like in oncology or pediatrics. Ribbing and Jonsson suggest that forward stepwise covariate screening within the software program itself not be done on small to moderate sized datasets ($<$ 50–100 subjects) because of the high degree of selection bias. Further, if two covariates are correlated and there is no mechanistic basis for choosing one over the other, then the data should decide which covariate should be used, instead of discarding one at random.

Automated Covariate Screening Methods

A few automated covariate screening methods have been reported in the literature and almost universally these methods are purported to be better at identifying important, "real" covariates and have better goodness of fit than models developed using manual screening. These methods build the model directly using nonlinear mixed effects model software, an advantage of which is that the now time-varying covariates can be easily handled. Jonsson and Karlsson (1998) presented one such method (GAM42) wherein the covariate model is built in a stepwise manner in which both linear and nonlinear relationships between the covariates and model parameters are explored. The starting model is a structural model without covariates. In the second step, each covariate model is examined on each parameter individually. For each parameter-covariate combination, a linear model having a single slope between parameter and covariate is examined, as is a nonlinear function having two slopes with a break-point at the median of the covariate space. A shift from intercept model was used for categorical covariates. The model with the best improvement in goodness in fit and is statistically significant based on the LRT is then moved forward. This process is repeated until no further covariates are added. Backwards deletion is then done using a more stringent p-value to retain covariates in the model. Using simulation, this approach was shown to have good sensitivity at identifying important covariates that were continuous in nature, but was only adequate in identifying covariates that were categorical in nature. Further, the method was also shown to be prone to identifying nonreal covariates.

Another automated algorithm is the WAM (Wald's Approximation Method) algorithm developed by Kowalski and Hutmacher (2002). They showed that ranking Schwarz's Bayesian Criterion (larger is better)

$$SBC = LL - \frac{p - q}{2} Ln(n) \qquad (7.133)$$

for a series of models is equivalent to ranking

$$SBC = -\frac{LRT}{2} - \frac{p - q}{2} Ln(n), \qquad (7.134)$$

where LL is the log-likelihood, p the number of parameters in θ, Ω, and Σ for the full model, q the number of covariate parameters in θ restricted to zero (i.e., excluded from the full model to form a reduced model), and n the total number of observations. Using the full model, Kowalski and Hutmacher illustrated that the LRT comparing the full model to any reduced model can be approximated by

$$LRT^* = \theta^{(x)'} C^{-1} \theta^{(x)}, \qquad (7.135)$$

where $\theta^{(x)}$ is the set of parameter estimates related to the covariates and C is a partitioned variance-covariance matrix of parameter estimates related to the covariates. This calculation is similar to one for forming linear contrasts in an analysis of variance. Hence, under the WAM approach, rank all 2^k models (all possible combinations with and without the covariate of interest) using SBC* where LRT in Eq. (7.134) is replaced by LRT* in Eq. (7.135). Then fit the 10–15 models with the highest SBC* in NONMEM and select the model with the largest SBC as the final model. Because the WAM algorithm is an approximation, unlike the LRT, the distribution of LRT* is not necessarily chi-squared, so that using critical values based on the chi-squared distribution will not lead to nominal Type I error rates (e.g., a LRT* greater than 3.84 on one degree of freedom indicates that that model is significant at 0.05 is not correct).

Using actual data sets, Kowalski (2001) showed that five out of six case studies selected the same model as stepwise procedures but did not perform as well when the data were rich and FO-approximation was used. He concluded that WAM might actually perform better than FOCE at choosing a model. However, one potential drawback for this approach is that it requires successful estimation of the variance–covariance matrix, which can sometimes require special handling to develop (e.g., if the model is sensitive to initial estimates, the variance–covariance matrix may not be readily evaluated). Therefore, the WAM algorithm may not be suitable for automated searches if the model output does not always include the standard errors.

As an example, Phase 1 concentration–time data from 300 subjects (150 males and females; two to five observations per subject) were simulated using a 1-compartment model with first-order absorption of 20 mg Drug X with complete absorption. Clearance was linearly related to weight (in kg) and volume of distribution was 35% higher in females than males as follows

$$CL \, (mL/h) = 200(Weight)^{0.75}$$
$$V \, (mL) = 150000(1 + 0.35 \times Sex), \qquad (7.136)$$

where Sex was coded as '0' for males and '1' for females. The absorption rate constant (k_a) was fixed to 0.7 per hour. It was assumed that clearance and volume of distribution had 30% BSV, while k_a had 50% BSV. For simplicity, no random effects were correlated. The following covariate model was fit to the data

$$CL \, (mL/h) = \theta_1 \left(\frac{Weight}{75 \, kg}\right)^{\theta_4}$$
$$V \, (mL) = \theta_2(1 + \theta_5 Sex) \qquad (7.137)$$
$$k_a \, (per \, h) = \theta_3(1 + \theta_6 Sex)$$

using FOCE with interaction with the true model parameter values were used as initial estimates, except θ_6 for which a value of 0.25 was used as the initial value. Under the fitted model with all covariates

$$\hat{\theta} = \begin{bmatrix} 4940 \\ 152000 \\ 0.681 \\ 0.665 \\ 0.398 \\ 0.139 \end{bmatrix}, \hat{\theta}^{(x)} = \begin{bmatrix} 0.665 \\ 0.398 \\ 0.139 \end{bmatrix},$$

$$\hat{\Omega} = \begin{bmatrix} 0.107 & 0 & 0 \\ 0 & 0.0857 & 0 \\ 0 & 0 & 0.312 \end{bmatrix}$$

$$C = \begin{bmatrix} 0.188 & -0.00496 & -0.00726 \\ -0.00496 & 0.00316 & 0.00109 \\ -0.00726 & 0.00109 & 0.00736 \end{bmatrix}. \qquad (7.138)$$

For the model with and without sex as a covariate on volume of distribution, $\theta^{(x)T}$ was (0.665 0.139) and

$$LRT^* = \begin{pmatrix} 0.665 \\ 0.139 \end{pmatrix}^T \begin{pmatrix} 0.188 & -0.00726 \\ -0.00726 & 0.00736 \end{pmatrix}^{-1}$$
$$(0.665 \, 0.139) = 6.2, \qquad (7.139)$$

whereas the actual LRT value was 6.1. The results of the WAM analysis are presented in Table 7.3. Neither the

Table 7.3 Results from WAM analysis.

#	Covariate on pharmacokinetic parameter CL	V	k_a	OFV	NONMEM results Ref. model	LRT	SBC	SBC ranking	WAM results LRT*	p − q	SBC*	SBC* ranking
0	None	None	None	6201.4	—	71.7	−59.7	6	59.6	7	−53.6	6
1	Weight			6191.3	7	61.8	−58.0	5	50.1	8	−52.2	5
2		Sex		6135.7	7	6.1	−30.2	1	6.2	8	−30.3	1
3			Sex	6201.1	7	71.5	−62.9	8	59.4	8	−56.9	8
4	Weight	Sex		6132.6	7	3.0	−32.1	3	2.6	9	−31.9	3
5		Sex	Sex	6131.8	7	2.2	−31.7	2	2.3	9	−31.7	2
6	Weight		Sex	6191.3	7	61.7	−61.4	7	50.1	9	−55.6	7
7	Weight	Sex	Sex	6129.6	—	0.0	−34.0	4	0.0	10	−34.0	4

Legend: #, model number; OFV, NONMEM objective function value; LRT, likelihood ratio test; SBC, Schwarz's Bayesian criterion based on NONMEM OFV (larger is better); LRT*, likelihood ratio test based on Wald's approximation; SBC*, Schwarz's Bayesian criterion based on Wald's approximation (larger is better); p, total number of estimable parameter values plus all estimable covariance terms in reference model; q, number of estimable parameter values and estimable covariance terms in reduced model. SBC and SBC* ranking based on the largest value.

WAM or NONMEM analysis identified the data generating model (which was Model 4) as the "best" model based on SBC ranking. However, among the models examined, exact concordance among the rankings was observed. The exact model ranking was obtained using NONMEM screening compared to the WAM algorithm. Importantly, the WAM algorithm took about 30 s to complete, whereas the NONMEM runs took about 20 min. The biggest problem with the WAM algorithm is obtaining a model with many covariates, most of which may be spurious, that minimizes successfully without any covariance problems, such as R-matrix singularity. Beyond that, the algorithm is surprisingly easy to use and SAS and S-plus code to implement it can be obtained from the internet.

Sale (2001) proposed using a genetic algorithm (GA), which is a search-based algorithm to find some optimum, as a method for covariate screening. Using a "fitness" measure based on objective function plus number of estimable parameters and various penalty terms, the model with the smallest fitness measure was found using the GA. The GA model, which was identified in only 153 steps, was then compared to all possible 12,288 model combinations and found to be the best (lowest) in terms of fitness. Hence, the optimal model was identified after examining significantly fewer models than an all possible models approach.

Bies et al. (2003) compared the stepwise model building approach to the GA approach. Three different stepwise approaches were used: forward stepwise starting from a base model with no covariates, and a backwards elimination approach starting from a full model with all covariates, and then forward addition to a full model followed by backwards elimination to retain only the most important covariates. Bies et al. found that the GA approach identified a model a full 30 points lower based on objective function value than the other three methods and that the GA algorithm identified important covariates not identified by the other approaches. Further, the standard stepwise approaches all generated different models. This last result is disconcerting because it confirms that different modeling strategies can often lead to identification of different covariates. Unfortunately, although intriguing, GA optimization is not readily available to the average modeler and software to perform this method is not readily available. Once it becomes more readily available, GA model development may become the automated method of choice.

Comparison of the Covariate Selection Methods

There have only been a few studies comparing the different covariate selection methods with most using Monte Carlo comparisons where the true data generating model is known. It should be stressed at the outset that no method is universally superior to the others— they all sometimes choose the wrong covariates or miss important covariates. Most often the choice of selection method is a personal one dependent on the analysis and analyst.

Wu and Wu (2002) compared three different covariate screening methods: nonlinear least-squares based method (NL-based), EBE-based method, and direct covariate screening by inclusion in the model and LRT. In the NL-based method, the same model is fit to each individual using nonlinear regression and the parameter estimates for that subject are obtained. Correlation tests or regression-based models between the individual parameter estimates and individual covariates may then be used to determine whether a significant relationship exists between the variables. This method is difficult to implement in practice because it requires rich data for each subject. For Phase 3 studies where sparse pharmacokinetic data are often collected, this method is impractical since many subjects will have insufficient data to support even simple pharmacokinetic models. Hence, data from many subjects will be unavailable and often, even if parameter estimates could be obtained from individual subjects with sparse data, often these estimates are questionable.

In a study of a pharmacodynamic model of HIV viral load (HIV-1 RNA copies) over time with 31 covariates, the three different methods identified three different sets of important covariates. The NL-based method produced a set of covariates with the smallest number, whereas the LRT produced the largest set of important covariates. They concluded that EBE-based methods are the most reliable for covariate selection. They also found that nonparametric regression methods were more likely to select fewer important covariates than parametric regression methods. The authors then used Monte Carlo simulation to examine the power and Type I error rate of the methods.

They concluded that the Type I error rate for EBE-based methods were near the nominal level ($\alpha = 0.05$) under most cases. The Type I errors for the NL-based methods were near the nominal level in most cases, but were smaller under sparse data conditions and with small sample sizes. The LRT cases consistently inflated the Type I error rate and that, not surprisingly, the LRT was the most powerful of the methods examined. This latter result can be rationalized as thinking that the inflated Type I error rate acts as a constant to inflate statistical power at nonzero effect sizes. They concluded that the LRT was too liberal for sparse data, while the NL-based methods were too conservative, and that the EBE-based methods were the most reliable for covariate selection.

Wahlby, Jonsson, and Karlsson (2002) compared covariate identification by GAM screening to screening of covariates directly within NONMEM (NM–NM method). Within her analysis she examined two different GAM relationships: one between the EBE of the parameter itself and the covariate of interest (GAM(EBE)–NM method) and one between an estimate of the random effect (η) and the covariate of interest (GAM(η)–NM method). For simulated data sets, the GAM(η)–NM method and NM–NM method gave identical covariate models, although the GAM(EBE) method was not as sensitive at covariate detection as the GAM(η) method. When some parameters were fixed during fitting and not allowed to optimize within the NM–NM procedure, the sensitivity at covariate detection was diminished for that method.

In summary, the choice of covariate screening method is capricious. Modelers mostly use what they are comfortable with and may not even compare the results from different screening methods. The most reliable method would be screening covariates directly in NONMEM, but this method is also the slowest. Further,

while NM–NM screening appears to be the gold standard, it is not without its faults. Ribbing and Jonsson (2003) showed that with small datasets (50 subjects), weak covariate effects tend to get amplified (by as much as two-times its actual value) and show selection bias—an effect not due to the presence of competing covariates in the model. At this time, no recommendations can be made about which algorithm to use, although GAM(η), GAM(EBE), and NM–NM screening are the most often used methods.

TESTING THE MODEL ASSUMPTIONS

Karlsson et al. (1998) present a comprehensive list of assumptions made during a PopPK analysis and how to test them. The assumptions can be classified into the following groups:

- Estimation method used;
- Quality of the data;
- Structural model used;
- Covariate submodel(s) used;
- Variance model (between-subject, interoccasion, and residual variability) used; and
- General modeling aspects.

Each assumption will be dealt with specifically as follows and are presented are slightly different than Karlsson et al. (1998)

1. The model parameters are estimable and unique.

This assumption relates to whether the model is globally identifiable. Obviously if a model's parameters are not identifiable, there is no use attempting to fit such a model. This assumption is usually answered early on in model development since models that are not identifiable (at least a posteriori) are usually evident by their failure to converge successfully or produce nonsensical parameter estimates.

2. The model inputs are measured without error.

It is assumed that the inputs into our model, e.g., dosing history, sampling times, and covariates are error-free. This does not mean that variables are not random, simply that they are measured without error. Errors in the inputs can mask real relationships between the dependent and independent variables and as such, every effort should be made to use "clean" data in an analysis (Carroll, Ruppert, and Stefanski, 1995). A useful way to test the impact of errors in the analysis is to perform a sensitivity analysis and examine how the model parameters change. To do this, one randomly alters the inputs by some value and collect the output. Many different data sets are generated and the model parameters are summarized using descriptive statistics.

For example, to examine how sampling time errors might affect the results, the sampling times might be perturbed by 15 min from a uniform distribution. If dosing history was in question, one might randomly select 10% of the doses and double them or halve them or change the time of dose within a 30-min window. In this manner, one can gauge how stable the model is to input misspecification.

3. Missing data did not affect the analysis.

In any large clinical study, data are sometimes missing for a subject despite the best efforts of the sponsor conducting the study. This is problematic since missing data can represent a source of uncontrollable bias in the study analysis. Current ICH guidelines indicate that the results from an analysis containing missing data may still be valid provided the method to deal with the missing data is "sensible" and specified a priori in the data analysis plan (International Conference on Harmonization of Technical Requirements for Registration of Pharmaceuticals for Human Use, 1998b). There are no uniform guidelines for handling missing data, although some guidelines have been presented elsewhere in this book. Regardless of the method used, sensitivity analysis should be done to quantify the impact of the missing data on the modeling results.

4. Excluded data did not affect the analysis.

In analysis of population data, particularly with Phase 3 studies, observable data may be excluded from the analysis. Data may be excluded for a variety of reasons, but the most common reasons are that either data (either the dependent or independent variable) are missing or the data are suspect (for a variety of reasons) and are considered to be an outlier. One example is the case where the half-life of the drug is on the order of hours, but in one subject observable drug concentrations are present days or weeks after the last noted dosing event. Obviously something is wrong, either a wrong date of last dose administered, wrong date of sample collection, or bioanalytical error. Procedures for removal of data are usually specified in advance of the modeling effort in an attempt to develop objective procedures. In this case, it is common to exclude such observations. If the percentage of data excluded from the analysis is small (less than a 5%), the assumption that excluded observations will not affect the analysis is usually made. However, recent guidelines dictate that whenever data are excluded from an analysis, the precise reason for its removal should be documented and the impact of its exclusion quantified (International Conference on Harmonisation of Technical Requirements for Registration of Pharmaceuticals for Human Use, 1998b). If no method for dealing with data to be excluded is in the data analysis plan, then two analyses

should be done: one with the excluded data and one without the excluded data. The two datasets are then compared and differences between their results discussed.

5. The structural model was adequate.

At the heart of any analysis lies the question of whether the structural model was adequate. Notice that it was not said that the model was correct. No model is correct. The question is whether the model adequately characterizes the data (a descriptive model) and is useful for predictive purposes (a predictive model). Adequacy of the structural model for descriptive purposes is typically made through goodness of fit plots, particularly observed versus predicted plots, residual plots, histograms of the distribution of the random effects, and histograms of the distribution of the residuals. Adequacy of the model for predictive purposes is done using simulation and predictive checks.

6. The same structural model applies to all subjects at all occasions.

There is little reason to believe that the structural model may change over time or be different for different individuals, but the values of the model parameters themselves may change over time. If measurements within a subject can be grouped by occasions, e.g., different days or cycles, then by obtaining the EBEs for model parameters on each occasion, one can then determine if the values change over occasions by examining box and whisker plots or spaghetti plots of EBEs versus occasion. A large change or shift in mean is suggestive of time-varying model parameters.

7. An adequate covariate submodel building strategy was used.

Already discussed have been methods used to identify important covariates. At issue is whether the strategy used missed any important covariates or identified any false positives. There is no definitive method to answer this question.

8. The covariate submodel is appropriate.

Once a covariate is identified as having a significant relationship with a model parameter, the question is how best to model their relationship, e.g., linear, power, exponential, change point, etc. With covariate screening methods, by failing to detect a nonlinear relationship between covariate and model parameter, there is increased risk of failing to detect any relationship at all. Typically, one tests the relationship by studying other relationships and seeing whether the goodness of fit improves. For example, if a power model having the same number of model parameters as a comparator model has a smaller objective function value, the power model is considered the better model. Hence, covariate submodel adequacy is tested by exclusion, i.e., showing what it is not.

9. Any covariate parameter interactions are adequately modeled.

It is assumed that any interaction between covariates included in a model are accounted for. Residual plots obtained from a model without interaction can be used to assess for interaction between two covariates by plotting the residuals versus the product of the two covariates (du Toit, Steyn, and Stumpf, 1986). Lack of interaction should result in a distribution of residuals around zero. Interaction between covariates is indicated by any positive or negative trend in the plot.

10. The distribution of the random effects are adequately modeled.

In a population analysis, the between-subject random effects are assumed to be either log-normal or normal in distribution and are modeled accordingly. The distribution of the random effects can never truly be identified but an approximate estimate of its distribution can be made from the EBEs. For data rich in observations per subject, the EBEs are close approximations to the true estimates given the correct structural and variance model. For very sparse data, the EBEs are more dependent on the model assumptions than the data. Nevertheless, the distribution of the random effects should be examined for consistency with the modeled distribution. For example, if the distribution of random effects was modeled as a normal distribution, but the distribution of the EBEs showed right skewness, then a log-normal distribution may be more appropriate. Also, if a random effect was modeled as a normally distributed random variable or a log-normally distributed random variable, then it is assumed that in both cases $\eta \sim N(0, \omega^2)$. A histogram of the distribution of EBEs of η should show a mean of zero, have a sample variance less than the estimated population variance (ω^2), and be consistent with a normal distribution. If this is not the case, then the adequacy of the random effects model should be questioned. An alternative is to model the random effects nonparametrically, although this is beyond the scope of this book.

11. An appropriate correlation term is included between random effects.

It is assumed that any correlation between the random effects is accounted for in the final model. Adding a covariance term to a random effect is usually made on the basis of examination of the distribution of EBEs of the random effects, e.g., clearance versus volume of distribution, or the distribution of the random effects, e.g., η_{Cl} versus η_V. If the scatter plot indicates a trend or if a correlation analysis indicates a significant correl-

ation, a covariance term is usually added. Holford, Gobburu, and Mould (2003) have shown that including a nonreal covariance term is generally more forgiving than not including one when it should be present. Fortunately, no boundary issue exists with the LRT so its use is not problematic.

12. The residual variance model is adequate.

It is assumed that the residuals are independent, normally distributed, with mean zero and constant variance. These are standard assumptions for maximum likelihood estimation and can be tested using standard methods: examination of histograms, autocorrelation plots (ith residual versus lag-1 residual), univariate analysis with a test for normality, etc.

13. The estimation method is adequate for the analysis.

Since the likelihood integral is intractable for the nonlinear case, most software packages approximate it with the assumption being that the approximation is adequate. History has shown that these approximations perform well under most circumstances in pharmacokinetics and any bias introduced by the approximation is of acceptable magnitude. One test is to fit the final model with a more accurate estimation routine, i.e., fit the final model using Laplacian estimation if the model was developed with FOCE, and compare the two model fits. If the approximation is adequate, the parameters obtained from the two models will not be substantially different. Note that it is inappropriate to compare objective function values under the two estimation models.

14. The global minimum is found.

It is assumed that the final model parameter estimates are associated with the global minimum on the sum of squares response surface, i.e., are associated with the lowest objective function value. Usually this assumption is met since during the model development process many different starting values are tried and model development generally proceeds from simpler models to more complex models. The likelihood is that the final model will find the global minimum during model development. Still, as a final test, one might perturb the parameter estimates by some amount ($\sim 25\%$) and compare the perturbed model parameters with the unperturbed model parameters. Small changes in the model parameters tend to confirm a global minimum was found.

15. The computer software algorithms are correct and accurate.

This assumption is one that is rarely questioned. It is often assumed that the software is accurate and uses reliable algorithms. Surprisingly, this is not always the case. McCullough (1998, 1999, 1999) has shown that many popularly used statistical programs and spreadsheet programs fail to calculate accurately even the most simplest statistics, such as standard deviation. He concludes "caveat emptor," let the buyer beware, when it comes to the accuracy and reliability of statistical software. There have been no studies done examining the accuracy of nonlinear mixed effects model software. More on this topic will be discussed in the section on Consistency of Model Parameter Estimates in the next chapter.

16. The model can be used to simulate real-world data.

Given the final model and the same set of inputs (dosing history, subject characteristics, etc.) and experimental design (randomization scheme, sampling design, etc.) used to build the model, it is assumed that the final model can simulate data that are indistinguishable from the observed, real-world data. This assumption is easy enough to test. Data are simulated and plots of concentration–time data are generated. If the simulated concentration–time profile is indistinguishable from the real concentration–time data, the assumption is met. Alternatively, some summary measure of the data, such as AUC or C_{max}, can be simulated and compared to similar observed statistics obtained from other studies. The distribution of the simulated data to the observed data can then be compared and examined for substantive differences. Particular attention should be paid to the variance of the simulated data to the observations.

Obviously not all assumption tests can be applied at every stage of model development, although many should. At the least, many of these assumptions should be examined once a final covariate submodel or base model is developed. It should also be noted that many of these assumptions are tested by examination of the EBEs. As such, datasets that have few observations per subject will be of less value than datasets with many observations per subject since sparse data tend to produce EBEs that are more model dependent than data dependent. More will be said of the quality of the EBEs later in the chapter.

PRECISION OF THE PARAMETER ESTIMATES AND CONFIDENCE INTERVALS

The primary objective of a PopPK analysis is to estimate the population parameters and associated variance components. Along with those estimates is a desire to understand the precision of the model parameters obtained, i.e., standard errors, and to expect that these standard errors will be small since small standard errors are indicative of good parameter estimation. Estimation

of the standard errors of the model parameters is usually based on standard maximum likelihood theory assuming the number of individuals used in the estimation is large and the random effects and intraindividual errors are normally distributed, i.e., the standard errors are asymptotically normally distributed (Davidian and Giltinan, 1995).

In NONMEM, the default covariance matrix is a function of the Hessian (denoted as the R-matrix within NONMEM, which is not the same R-matrix within the MIXED procedure in SAS) and the cross-product gradient (denoted as the S-matrix within NONMEM) of the $-2LL$ function. The standard errors are computed as the square root of the diagonals of this matrix. An approximate asymptotic $(1 - \alpha)100\%$ confidence interval (CI) can then be generated using a Z-distribution (large sample) approximation

$$(1 - \alpha)100\%CI = \hat{\theta} \pm Z_{\alpha/2}SE_{\hat{\theta}}, \qquad (7.140)$$

where $\hat{\theta}$ is the final parameter estimate, $Z_{\alpha/2}$ is from a Z-distribution with $\alpha/2$ probability, e.g., 1.96 for 95% CI, and $SE_{\hat{\theta}}$ is the maximum likelihood standard error of $\hat{\theta}$. Alternatively, one could also estimate the standard errors based only on the gradient or on the Hessian.

A number of problems are noted with this approach. First, this approach assumes that the CI is symmetric and normally distributed, which for variance components may not be the case. Principally, for a given data set, BSV is harder to estimate such that asymptotic theory applies better to the estimates of the fixed effects than the variance components. Consequently, in most cases, the resulting estimate of the standard error of the variance components can only be used qualitatively. Second, the method assumes an infinite number of subjects in the data set, which is obviously wrong. Lastly, in practice, the covariance matrix may be inestimable because the Hessian is near singular, so-called R-matrix singularity, and cannot be reliably inverted. Sometimes the singularity can be resolved because the model is overparameterized and a simpler model removes the singularity. However, there are a number of alternative measures to assess the precision of the parameter estimates, even in the face of covariance matrix singularity, provided minimization is successful.

One method to estimate standard errors is the nonparametric bootstrap (see the book Appendix for further details and background). With this method, subjects are repeatedly sampled with replacement creating a new data set of the same size as the original dataset. For example, if the data set had 100 subjects with subjects numbered 1, 2, ..., 100. The first bootstrap data set may consist of subjects 10, 56, 75, 56, 9, 98, 10,.... 4. The model is fit to the bootstrap dataset and the parameter estimates are saved as $\theta_1^*, \Omega_1^*,$ and Σ_i^* where the * denotes they are bootstrap estimates for $\theta, \Omega,$ and Σ, respectively. This process is repeated many times and a matrix of bootstrap estimates is obtained. The standard error of the parameter estimates is calculated as the standard deviation of the distribution of bootstrap estimates. Usually to obtain reliable standard errors, only about 100 bootstrap data sets are needed. An approximate $(1 - \alpha)100\%$ CI can then be generated using Eq. (7.140) where $SE_{\hat{\theta}}$ is now the bootstrap estimate of the standard error. Alternatively, a more precise, possibly asymmetric, $(1 - \alpha)100\%$ CI can be obtained from the distribution of the bootstrap estimates, although at least 1000 bootstrap data sets are needed for this approach to be valid.

Yafune and Ishiguro (1999) first reported the bootstrap approach with population models. Using Monte Carlo simulation the authors concluded that usually, but not always, bootstrap distributions contain the true population mean parameter, whereas usually the CI does *not* contain the true population mean with the asymptotic method. For all of the parameters they studied, the asymptotic CIs were contained within the bootstrap CIs and that the asymptotic CIs tended to be smaller than the bootstrap CIs. This last result was confirmed using an actual data set.

Related to the bootstrap is the jackknife approach (see the book Appendix for further details and background) of which there are two major variants. The first approach, called the delete-1 approach, removes one subject at a time from the data set to create n-new jackknife data sets. The model is fit to each data set and the parameter pseudovalues are calculated as

$$P_i^* = n\hat{\theta} - (n - 1)\hat{\theta}_{(i)}, \qquad (7.141)$$

where n is the number of subjects, $\hat{\theta}$ is the estimate of the parameter under the original data set, and $\hat{\theta}_{(i)}$ denotes the jackknife estimate of the parameter with the ith-subject deleted from the dataset. The jackknife estimator of the parameter is the mean of the pseudovalues ($\bar{P}$), while the standard error of the parameter is calculated as

$$SE = \sqrt{\frac{\sum_{i=1}^{n} (P_i - \bar{P})^2}{n(n - 1)}} = \sqrt{\frac{n - 1}{n} \sum_{i=1}^{n} \left(\hat{\theta}_{(i)} - \bar{\hat{\theta}}_{(i)}\right)^2}.$$

$$(7.142)$$

For large data sets, the delete-1 jackknife may be impractical since it may require fitting hundreds of data sets. A modification of the delete-1 jackknife is the delete 10% jackknife, where 10 different jackknife data sets are created with each data set having a unique 10% of the data removed. Only 10 data sets are modeled using this jackknife modification. All other calculations are as before but n now becomes the number of data sets, not the number of subjects. The use of the jackknife has largely been supplanted by the bootstrap since the jackknife has been criticized as producing standard errors that have poor statistical behavior when the estimator is non-smooth, e.g., the median, which may not be a valid criticism for pharmacokinetic parameters. But whether one is better than the other at estimating standard errors of continuous functions is debatable and a matter of preference.

Another infrequently used method to generate a $(1 - \alpha)100\%$ CI is likelihood profiling, sometimes called objective function profiling or objective function mapping. The basic idea is to serially fix all the model parameters at their final parameter estimates (i.e., allow the parameters that are not being investigated to be estimated), then incrementally increase and decrease the value of the parameter of interest until the objective function value changes by a predetermined amount. These cut-off values are then deemed the confidence interval. For example, assuming a chi-squared distribution with a desired p-value of α on 1 degree of freedom, e.g., 3.84 for a 95% CI, the parameter values that change the objective function by ± 3.84 are deemed the 95% CI. In practice, this can be a tedious approach to do manually and is best when automated, although the method tends to be sensitive to its starting estimates and requires fine-tuning of the initial estimates (sometimes for each evaluation) by the user.

As an example of the different methods, the data set presented by Yafune and Ishiguro (1999) will be reexamined. The data set was from a Phase 1 dose-escalation study in 26 subjects. A single dose of Drug X was administered to three to five subjects per cohort as a 3-h intravenous infusion with doses ranging from 20 to 640 mg. Serial blood samples were collected for either 48 (in all cohorts) or 72-h (only in the last two cohorts) and the plasma drug concentration assayed. The data are presented in Table 7.4. Not detectable ("ND") data were treated as follows. Samples at time zero were set equal to missing. The first instance of "ND" was set equal to one-half the lower limit of quantification, i.e., samples were set equal to 12.5 ng/mL. All instances of "ND" after the first "ND" sample were treated as missing. A 4-compartment model using a simple diagonal

Table 7.4 Plasma drug concentrations (in ng/mL) in 26 healthy males as reported by Yafune and Ishiguro (1999).

#	0	0.5	1.5	3	3.25	3.5	4	4.5	5	6	7	9	12	24	48	72

Time after start of infusion (h)

#	0	0.5	1.5	3	3.25	3.5	4	4.5	5	6	7	9	12	24	48	72
					20 mg dose as a 3-h intravenous infusion											
1	ND	255	499	673	547	441	289	219	209	144	102	67	41	28	ND	
2	ND	258	501	576	422	323	248	208	158	105	72	55	33	ND	ND	
3	ND	277	483	584	440	346	285	178	134	91	66	42	27	ND	ND	
					40 mg dose as a 3-h intravenous infusion											
11	ND	630	957	1370	1040	904	680	510	390	260	182	114	59	ND	ND	
12	ND	528	946	1412	995	850	633	492	398	252	179	110	62	ND	ND	
13	ND	605	1052	1462	1070	866	650	574	390	289	198	104	51	ND	ND	
					80 mg dose as a 3-h intravenous infusion											
21	ND	971	1541	2092	1453	1293	911	722	541	374	258	153	88	29	ND	
22	ND	1196	1937	2404	1585	1132	970	690	536	350	223	154	90	41	ND	
23	ND	1268	2024	2487	1835	1504	1234	920	744	477	338	190	115	50	43	
24	ND	1292	2081	2719	2060	1761	1221	1051	794	502	347	181	136	62	ND	
25	ND	1101	1805	2613	2128	1725	1401	997	856	527	412	206	125	32	ND	
					160 mg dose as a 3-h intravenous infusion											
31	ND	2438	4438	5688	4525	4032	3050	2468	1966	1380	965	511	270	104	50	
32	ND	2114	3333	5033	4277	3973	2634	2125	1622	1195	806	489	237	98	48	
33	ND	1948	3710	5289	3894	3443	2679	2137	1648	1315	835	464	277	113	71	
34	ND	2051	3394	4994	3634	3424	2598	2101	1625	1169	755	463	268	85	52	
35	ND	1480	3326	3993	3384	2782	2330	1969	1645	1071	767	479	216	86	56	
					320 mg dose as a 3-h intravenous infusion											
41	ND	5791	10007	13622	9904	8848	6863	5554	4403	2772	2142	1124	664	192	48	33
42	ND	5277	9919	15114	9967	8705	7287	5470	4778	3537	2046	1268	664	221	61	36
43	ND	5470	9854	13401	10655	9113	7819	6231	4914	3604	2614	1327	788	204	80	59
44	ND	4340	7467	10548	9655	9031	6745	4913	3642	2194	1577	1126	517	166	68	32
45	ND	5633	8942	12570	9787	8469	6318	5488	3960	2456	1485	888	546	188	71	34
					640 mg dose as a 3-h intravenous infusion											
51	ND	8212	14353	21257	15364	13517	8930	7447	5845	3952	2444	1334	663	223	73	42
52	ND	8069	15779	24647	19169	13290	11540	9372	7815	5145	3812	2241	1048	321	109	62
53	ND	8034	14715	22761	14938	13479	12056	7505	6297	4192	2735	1474	837	192	68	44
54	ND	12236	20983	29489	24522	21575	16818	13219	10607	6308	4539	2284	1078	285	107	65
55	ND	9850	16604	22171	16865	13927	10596	9343	6597	4481	2763	1556	679	249	82	46

Legend: ND, not detectable (< 5 ng/mL)

covariance was deemed to be a superior model than the 2-compartment model with unstructured covariance matrix originally used by Yafune and Ishiguro (2002). A proportional residual error model was used. Minimization was successful with this model. Having identified a suitable base model, the parameter estimates and their standard errors were calculated using the following parametric and nonparametric methods:

- First-order approximation with maximum likelihood standard errors (FO);
- First-order conditional estimation with maximum likelihood standard errors (FOCE);
- First-order conditional estimation with interaction with maximum likelihood standard errors (FOCE-I);

- The nonparametric bootstrap using FO-approximation on 1000 bootstrapped data sets; and
- Delete-1 jackknife using FO-approximation.

The default method for all first-order methods used both the gradient and Hessian matrix in the estimation of the standard errors. Standard errors were also calculated using only the gradient (Matrix = S) or only the Hessian (Matrix = R). The results are presented in Table 7.5 and Table 7.6.

In general, all the estimation methods produced roughly equivalent parameter estimates with none of the methods considered to be significantly different from the others. Having the standard errors calculated using only the gradient or Hessian had no effect what-

Table 7.5 Fixed effect parameter estimates and variance components from a 4-compartment model fit using data in Table 7.4.

Parameter	Matrix = R⁻¹ SR⁻¹ (Default) FO	FOCE	FOCE-I	FO jackknife	FO bootstrap	Matrix = R (Hessian) FO	FOCE	FOCE-I	Matrix = S (cross-product gradient) FO	FOCE	FOCE-I
CL	6.06	5.83	6.00	6.03	6.06	6.06	5.83	6.00	6.06	5.83	6.00
V1	5.93	5.88	6.07	5.93	5.94	5.93	5.88	6.07	5.93	5.88	6.07
Q2	1.27	1.26	1.08	1.34	1.26	1.27	1.26	1.08	1.27	1.26	1.08
V2	41.2	42.2	50.2	41.9	41.0	41.2	42.2	50.2	41.2	42.2	50.2
Q3	1.13	1.12	1.12	1.19	1.13	1.13	1.12	1.12	1.13	1.12	1.12
V3	6.56	6.15	6.80	6.89	6.57	6.56	6.15	6.80	6.56	6.15	6.80
Q4	15.0	16.3	15.0	15.2	15.0	15.0	16.3	15.0	15.0	16.3	15.0
V4	6.97	7.01	6.89	6.89	6.96	6.97	7.01	6.89	6.97	7.01	6.89
					Variance components						
CL × 100	2.50	2.99	2.81	2.50	2.47	2.50	2.99	2.81	2.50	2.99	2.81
V1 × 100	4.80	6.08	5.81	4.76	4.74	4.80	6.08	5.81	4.80	6.08	5.81
Q2 × 10	3.79	3.36	3.23	4.00	3.76	3.79	3.36	3.23	3.79	3.36	3.23
V2 × 10	6.58	5.28	4.95	6.22	6.59	6.58	5.28	4.95	6.58	5.28	4.95
Q3 × 100	7.23	8.73	8.28	7.67	7.11	7.23	8.73	8.28	7.23	8.73	8.28
V4 × 1000	1.51	6.72	3.93	1.60	1.50	1.51	6.72	3.93	1.51	6.72	3.93
σ² × 1000	3.89	3.68	3.90	4.00	3.90	3.89	3.68	3.90	3.89	3.68	3.90

Legend: CL, clearance (L/h); V1, central volume of distribution (L); Q2, intercompartmental clearance from central compartment to Compartment 2 (L/h); V2, volume of distribution of Compartment 2 (L); Q3, intercompartmental clearance from central compartment to Compartment 3 (L/h); V3, volume of distribution of Compartment 3 (L); Q4, intercompartmental clearance from central compartment to Compartment 4 (L/h); V4, volume of distribution of Compartment 4 (L); σ², residual error.

soever on the estimation of the parameters, as it should since this option should only affect the calculation of the standard errors. Both the jackknife and bootstrap estimates, which were calculated using FO-approximation, were the same as or near the estimates obtained using the original data set indicating that the parameter estimates have low to zero bias.

Although there was little difference in the standard errors reported by maximum likelihood using the NON-MEM default, bootstrap standard errors were signifi-

Table 7.6 Standard errors of fixed effect parameter estimates and variance components from a 4-compartment model fit using data in Table 7.4.

Parameter	Matrix = R⁻¹ SR⁻¹ (Default) FO	FOCE	FOCE-I	FO jackknife	FO bootstrap	Matrix = R (Hessian) FO	FOCE	FOCE-I	Matrix = S (cross-product gradient) FO	FOCE	FOCE-I
CL × 10	2.23	2.23	2.20	2.47	0.73	1.81	1.98	2.05	3.13	3.02	3.98
V1 × 10	6.23	7.11	6.81	6.19	2.19	5.84	6.78	6.45	12.2	12.9	12.2
Q2 × 10	1.91	2.00	1.49	2.26	0.68	1.30	1.42	1.27	2.81	2.37	1.96
V2	11.5	6.40	10.4	14.2	4.13	7.28	7.57	9.07	12.5	16.7	20.4
Q3 × 100	9.80	10.0	9.47	11.0	3.65	7.50	9.32	8.50	11.7	12.4	12.3
V3 × 10	7.73	8.52	7.37	8.60	2.66	6.46	0.533	4.49	13.4	7.79	5.47
Q4	2.36	2.86	2.70	2.35	0.84	2.42	2.90	2.60	5.20	5.18	4.36
V4 × 10	4.38	4.72	4.50	4.47	1.74	5.00	5.52	5.06	13.9	12.1	10.7
					Variance component standard errors						
CL × 1000	5.91	7.11	6.83	6.32	1.71	7.41	8.95	8.21	17.0	17.7	16.2
V1 × 100	1.77	2.67	2.43	1.89	0.51	1.94	2.43	2.19	4.52	3.12	2.95
Q2 × 100	8.02	7.27	6.11	9.05	2.64	11.6	10.1	9.46	52.3	32.2	29.3
V2 × 10	1.42	1.79	1.84	1.99	0.55	2.63	1.92	1.82	1.38	6.33	4.76
Q3 × 100	3.12	4.20	3.68	3.66	0.99	3.03	3.86	3.14	5.85	5.37	4.26
V4 × 1000	8.12	4.99	3.53	9.03	3.03	8.51	5.88	3.53	24.1	11.4	10.5
σ² × 10000	5.67	5.63	5.31	5.93	2.37	4.66	4.54	3.71	7.16	9.11	5.76

Legend: CL, clearance (L/h); V1, central volume of distribution (L); Q2, intercompartmental clearance from central compartment to Compartment 2 (L/h); V2, volume of distribution of Compartment 2 (L); Q3, intercompartmental clearance from central compartment to Compartment 3 (L/h); V3, volume of distribution of Compartment 3 (L); Q4, intercompartmental clearance from central compartment to Compartment 4 (L/h); V4, volume of distribution of Compartment 4 (L); σ², residual error.

cantly smaller than asymptotic or jackknife estimates. The greater precision observed with the bootstrap may be due to the small sample size. Jackknife estimates were more in line with maximum likelihood estimates than bootstrap estimates. When the Hessian was used to calculate the standard error, instead of the NONMEM default, the standard errors were nearly the same. Some values showed smaller standard errors, while some showed larger standard errors. In all, using the Hessian produced roughly equivalent estimates of the standard errors. However, when the gradient was used to calculate the standard errors, the estimates were decidedly different from default estimates and tended to be larger in general for the model parameters. The variance component standard errors were inconsistent; some were smaller than default estimates, others were larger. Most were larger. These results suggest that if the covariance matrix is unavailable then using the gradient alone to

calculate the standard errors should be avoided whenever possible.

Figure 7.12 presents bootstrap histograms of clearance and its associated variance component calculated using FO-approximation with confidence intervals determined by the percentile method. FO-approximation was needed because to analyze 1000 bootstrap distributions using FOCE-I would have taken weeks of computing power. As it was, 1000 bootstrap distributions using FO-approximation took 3 full days of computing time on a 2.5 GHz personal computer. Shapiro-Wilk's test indicted that both clearance and its variance component were not normally distributed (p < 0.01). An approximate 90% CI using maximum likelihood theory for clearance under FOCE-I was {5.64, 6.36 L/h}, whereas the bootstrap 90% CI was {5.95, 6.19 L/h}. The wider CI observed with maximum likelihood was the result of the larger standard errors observed with this method. Figure 7.13 presents the likelihood profile for clearance using FOCE-I. An approximate 90% CI using this approach was {5.68, 6.34 L/h}, which was very near the maximum likelihood CI. Hence, in this example, maximum likelihood, likelihood profile, and jackknife standard error estimates, produced almost identical results but were larger than bootstrap standard errors.

Others have done similar exercises with other drugs. Gibiansky and Gibiansky (2001) calculated the CIs generated by asymptotic maximum likelihood theory, bootstrap, jackknife, and likelihood profiling for an unidentified, renally cleared drug. Asymptotic approximations were surprisingly similar to bootstrap estimates. When there was a difference between the asymptotic approximation and likelihood profiling, the asymptotic CI tended to be larger. Jackknife and asymptotic

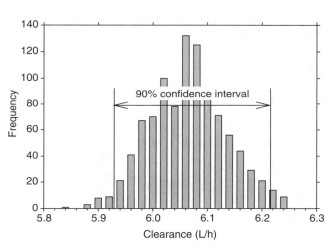

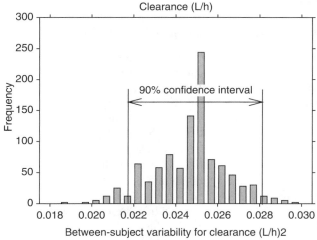

Figure 7.12 Histogram of bootstrap clearance (top) and between-subject variance estimate for clearance (bottom) for 4-compartment model fit to data in Table 7.4. Bootstrap models fit using first-order approximation. Ninety percent confidence intervals using the percentile method are indicated.

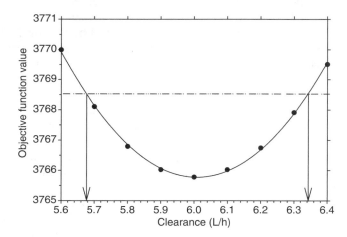

Figure 7.13 Likelihood profile for clearance using the data in Table 7.4. Ninety percent CI is indicated by the arrows. The dotted–dashed line indicates the cut-off at which the change in objective function becomes statistically significant; 2.70 in this case.

estimates were almost always in good agreement, with jackknife CIs slightly larger. Bootstrap CIs were also in good agreement with asymptotic CIs, despite the bootstrap distribution showing nonnormality for many of the parameters examined. Similar results were obtained with two other drugs, aripiprazole (Gibiansky, Gibiansky, and Bramer, 2001) and ISIS 2302 (Gibiansky et al., 2001).

In practice, bootstrapping, although considered the gold standard for standard error and CI estimation, is not always practical owing to the sometimes extensive run times and cannot be recommended (which will surely be debated by others), except for when precise estimates of a particular confidence interval are needed. Gibiansky et al. (2001) reported that for the population pharmacokinetic model for aripiprazole using FOCE-I with 1000 bootstrap data sets, the total run time was about two weeks with only about 500 of 1000 runs converging! Further, the issues of stratification and exchangeability are not always clear and many analysts only bootstrap on subject identification, which can be misleading if the data are nonexchangeable, such as when both healthy volunteers and patients are included in the database, or when the pharmacokinetics are different between individuals. Further, the issue of handling bootstrap runs that do not converge successfully has not been totally resolved. Should these runs be deleted? Should an analyst troubleshoot these runs and re-start them again, perhaps after changing the initial starting values?

Furthermore, it is not always clear how to handle bootstrap runs that do not converge? By only using bootstrap runs that converge successfully, the resulting confidence interval will be overly optimistically biased in favor of the model being bootstrapped and not reflect that perhaps an inappropriate model is being bootstrapped. Also, there are a variety of methods to construct bootstrap CIs (although most modelers use the percentile method, which may not always be appropriate) and it is not immediately clear which one should be used or whether one method should be consistently used over another method.

Statisticians consider jackknifing and likelihood profiling promising techniques, but jackknifing is largely considered an outdated methodology since it has poor properties for nonsmooth estimators, such as the median. This criticism does not apply to pharmacokinetic model parameters and, as such, the jackknife should be considered a viable alternative to ML theory when the covariance matrix is unobtainable. Likelihood profiling also seems to hold promise but needs more experience with other data sets before it can be recommended as standard practice. For most practical problems, the asymptotic results are more than adequate at answering the question "Is the parameter well-defined."

MODEL MISSPECIFICATION AND VIOLATION OF THE MODEL ASSUMPTIONS

Box (1976), in one of the most famous quotes reported in the pharmacokinetic literature, stated "*all models are wrong, some are useful.*" This adage is well accepted. The question then becomes how precise or of what value are the parameter estimates if the model or the model assumptions are wrong. A variety of simulation studies have indicated that population parameter estimates are surprisingly robust to all kinds of misspecifications, but that the variance components are far more sensitive and are often very biased when misspecification of the model or when violations of the model assumptions occur. Some of the more conclusive studies examining the effect of model misspecification or model assumption violations on parameter estimation will now be discussed.

First, however, a key concept in the critique of these studies, and indeed most every simulation study, must be introduced. Simulated data are generated using a model, which is sometimes called a data generating model. Invariably the same model used to generate the data is then used to fit the simulated data. The results are then examined with regards to answering the key questions. The results of these simulations are then overly optimistic because in real life the model used to simulate the data is far more complicated than the model used to analyze the data. What they do provide, however, is an indication of the behavior of the model or study design in the best case scenario. Further, these studies tend to look at how things perform in the long-run, i.e., on-average. For any single case basis, violations of model assumptions can have dramatic and far reaching consequences.

Misspecification of the Structural Model

Wade et al. (1993) simulated concentration data for 100 subjects under a one-compartment steady-state model using either first- or zero-order absorption. Simulated data were then fit using FO-approximation with a first-order absorption model having k_a fixed to 0.25-, 0.5-, 1-, 2-, 3-, and 4 times the true k_a value. Whatever value k_a was fixed equal to, clearance was consistently biased, but was relatively robust with underpredictions of the true value by less than 5% on average. In contrast, volume of distribution was very sensitive to absorption misspecification, but only when there were samples collected in the absorption phase. When there were no concentration data in the absorption phase, significant parameter bias was not observed for any parameter. The variance components were far more sensitive to model misspecification than the parameter estimates with some variance components off by 400%. The authors suggest that if the data cannot support an absorption model, the absorption rate constant should be fixed to a reasonable value, sensitivity analysis be done to assess the impact of the fixed value on the parameter estimates, and a value chosen such that it has little impact on the estimates of the remaining parameters.

The fact that these studies found that k_a cannot be reasonably estimated is not unexpected since it is widely recognized that estimation of k_a is often problematic, even with data rich problems and fitting individual pharmacokinetic data. The poor accuracy in estimation of k_a in real-life may come from the fact that absorption is not a constant throughout the gastrointestinal tract but varies as a function of solubility, contact time, and permeability. However, in all of the simulations just presented, k_a was a constant defined by the user, not a time-dependent parameter. Perhaps the reason that k_a could not be reliably estimated is more a function of the limited number of samples collected in the absorption phase than in some limitation in the estimation algorithms. Nevertheless, most analysts are willing to accept a poor estimate of k_a since steady-state drug concentrations are not dependent on k_a. Indeed, one trick to fitting PopPK models when k_a cannot be reasonable estimated is to use the recommendation of Wade et al (1993) and to fix it at a reasonable value, usually 0.7–1 per h, and then estimate the other model parameters.

Often with sparse pharmacokinetic data, the base model chosen is a simplification of the true pharmacokinetic model (Aarons et al., 1996). For example, the drug may have biexponential kinetics, but samples were collected such that the data only support a 1-compartment model. Kowalski and Hutmacher (2001) used Monte Carlo simulation to examine the impact of fitting a 1-compartment oral model to data that were simulated using a 2-compartment oral model. What they found was that the estimate of the absorption rate constant (k_a) was off by more than two-fold on-average, but that the bias in the estimates of clearance and volume of distribution were all near zero. It should be noted that the volume of distribution reported for the 1-compartment model is really Vss, the sum of the volume of central and peripheral compartments. Surprisingly, although the estimate of k_a was extremely biased, the bias in the estimate of BSV in k_a was near zero. However, the variance estimates for clearance and volume of distribution were biased −20 and −30%, respectively. To compensate, residual variability was off by +35%. The authors also found that the ability to detect a subpopulation in the data was also compromised by fitting the simpler model. They suggest based on their design and data that instead of using the usual value of 3.84 with the LRT to achieve a nominal statis-

tical significance of 0.05, a value closer to nine should be used.

Misspecification of the Distribution of the Random Effects

Hartford and Davidian (2000) studied the effect of covariate submodel misspecification and variance model misspecification on parameter estimates from a 1-compartment model with bolus administration fitted to sparse and rich data using FO-approximation and Laplacian estimation within the NLMIXED macro in SAS, version 6.12[2] (which is not the same Laplacian estimation algorithm used in NONMEM. The SAS version is more akin to NONMEM's FOCE method). Correlated random effects (clearance and volume of distribution) were generated from a normal distribution, bivariate Student's t-distribution, and a mixture of mild and moderately contaminated normal distributions, asymmetric distribution, and a bimodal normal distribution. When the covariate submodel was correctly specified, convergence with FO-approximation was almost always achieved, in contrast to Laplacian estimation which was sensitive to both correct covariate submodel specification and variance model specification. Convergence was always more difficult with sparse data than rich data, regardless of estimation method. When the variance model was misspecified, estimation of the population parameter estimates was little affected, but variance component estimates were. When the true distribution of the random effects was nonnormal, the variability in the parameter estimates across simulations increased and the accuracy of the variance components was greatly affected. Estimates of both the population parameters and the variance components obtained from FO-approximation tended to show more bias than estimates obtained using Laplacian estimation. In summary, the population parameter estimates obtained using Laplacian estimation were relatively unaffected when the random effects were misspecified, although convergence will be problematic. In contrast, variance components were often biased.

Interaction Between the Structural and Covariate Submodel

Wade, Beal, and Sambol (1994) did an interesting study wherein they simulated data from 100 subjects having three samples collected per subject. The pharmacokinetics of the drug was based on digoxin, a drug that

---

[2] More recent versions of SAS use a different, more accurate algorithm than the NLMIXED macro released with earlier versions.

displays biexponential kinetics. After intravenous bolus input, sampling was done only in the beta-phase of the concentration–time curve under four different starting conditions beginning at 3, 6, 12, or 48 h and ending at 120 h. All pharmacokinetic parameters were independent and had no covariance between them. Under the simulation conditions, α-and β-half-life were 35 min and 36 h, respectively, so that even at 3 h the α-phase of drug disposition should have been complete. Both the 1-compartment and 2-compartment models were then fit to the data assuming the clearance and volume of distribution of the central compartment were random effects with no common covariance. Intercompartmental clearance and peripheral volume were modeled as fixed effects.

The percent of data sets that chose the 2-compartment model over the 1-compartment model (using the LRT as the criteria) was near 100% for the 3, 6, and 12 h starting time conditions, but was about 75% when the sampling time began at 48 h. The fact that the 48–120 h sampling time group chose the 1-compartment model only 25% of the time was very surprising given that 48 h after dosing was more than 80 half-lives after the end of the distribution phase.

The authors then reanalyzed the data from the 1-compartment model assuming a common covariance between clearance and central volume. Without the covariance term, the mean decrease in the objective function value between the 1-and 2-compartment model was 272, 99.5, 60.1, and 7.1 for the 3-, 6-, 12-, and 48-h sampling groups, respectively. With the covariance term the mean decrease in the objective function value was 235, 10.9, 0.5, and 0, respectively, indicating that choosing a 1-compartment model was more likely with the covariance term included in the model. Thus, there was an interaction between the ability to detect the correct structural model and the random effects included in the model.

Then using actual data from a pediatric clinical study with netilimicin, the authors found that a 2-compartment model best described the data with no significant covariates affecting central volume. When all the samples prior to 5 h were removed from the data set, a 1-compartment model best described the data. Now, weight and gestational age were important covariates on central volume. Hence, there appeared to be an interaction between identification of important covariates and the structural model. Under all conditions examined, the 2-compartment model consistently identified fewer important covariates than the 1-compartment model.

The authors concluded that the following scheme should be used to build models. First, base models without covariates should be examined with the simplest model chosen as the model to use for covariate inclusion. Second, the influence of the covariates should then be added to the base model. Third, if a more complex structural model appears to be equally plausible then the covariate submodel(s) using the simpler structural model should be tested with the more complicated structural structure. Covariates that were rejected with the simpler model may then need to be reevaluated if the more complex structural model with covariate submodel is the superior model. Lastly, covariates can then be deleted by stepwise deletion.

Misspecification of Sample Times

One assumption made in any analysis is that the sample collection times are recorded without error. In practice, except for perhaps data obtained from Phase 1, this is rarely the case. In any Phase 3 setting, the probability of data collection errors is high despite the best efforts of sponsors. Sun, Ette, and Ludden (1996) used Monte Carlo simulation to study the impact of recording errors in the sample times on the accuracy and precision of model parameter estimates. Concentration data from 100 subjects were simulated using a 2-compartment model with intravenous administration having an α-half-life of 0.065 time units and a β-half-life of 1.0 time units.

They simulated data under three dosing conditions: single dose (Design 1) and multiple dose (Design 2 and 3). Using D-optimality theory, they found that the optimal sample times were as follows: between 0.06 and 0.22, between 0.22 and 0.55, and between 0.55 and 4.0 time units for Design 1; between 0.05 to 0.22, between 1.0 and 5.0, and between 5.0 and 7.0 for Design 2; and between 0.05 and 0.22, between 0.22 and 0.66, and between 5.0 and 7.0 for Design 3.

Two samples from each subject were randomly drawn from each time window for a total of six samples per subject. Uniformly distributed random and systematic errors from 5 to 50% relative error from the true sample times were then introduced into the sample times. For example, if the true time was 5 and the random error was 10% the sampling could occur from 4.5 to 5.5, whereas systematic errors were treated as fixed percentages from the true value. Data was analyzed using FO-approximation using the model used to simulate the data.

After single dose administration, unreliable estimates ($>15\%$ relative error from true value and $>35\%$ standard deviation) of the structural model parameters and most variance components were observed when the degree of random error was more than 30%, whereas biased residual variance was observed when the random error was more than 20% under single dose administration (Design 1). The degree of bias after multiple dose administration depended on the sampling time windows, i.e., bias differed between Designs 2 and 3. Introducing 20% random error into the sampling times into Design 2 yielded unreliable estimates of intercompartmental clearance, residual variance, and the BSV for intercompartmental clearance and peripheral volume. All other model parameters were estimated with low bias and precision. When BSV was less than 45%, a 20% error in the sampling times under Design 3 did not cause more than ±30% bias in the model parameters. In all designs the bias associated with residual variability increased as the error in sampling times increased. Hence, the error in sampling time tended to be aggregated into residual error. The authors conclude that across sampling designs, sampling time error had little or no influence on the estimate of clearance and its variability, although values did tend to be underestimated. This study illustrates how simulation can be used to verify whether a given experimental design can reproduce the data generating mechanism. If, for example, a sampling schedule cannot generate unbiased and precise parameter estimates given a data generating model, how then can it find unbiased estimates to a model of unknown structure?

MODEL VALIDATION

The general topic of validation has already been covered elsewhere in the book and that material will not be represented. This section will focus on the particulars of what currently constitutes a valid PopPK model. Unfortunately, at this time, what constitutes a validated PopPK model is debatable. Different scientists use different methods each claiming afterward that their particular model is validated. One aspect that should always be considered when validating a model is that the validation procedures should test the model for the purposes for which the model was generated (Ette et al., 2003). In other words, if a model is only created to describe the data then validation should focus on how well the data are described and not for how well the model predicts another set of data. The former may rely on simple graphical assessment of the observed versus predicted data, whereas the latter may rely on comparing simulated data to a some other data set. There has yet to be a published PopPK analysis that did not meet its own internal validation criteria.

The approach that will be used here is a three-step validation process:

1. Develop a model with high face validity.
2. Test the assumptions of the model.
3. Determine the quality of the model to a validation data set, either real or simulated.

The first step is to develop a model with high face validity. Recall that face validity, which is a common sense approach to validation, is a model that is superficially valid, i.e., whether the model looks valid. There tends to be an inverse relationship between face validity and model complexity; as the degree of model complexity increases, its face validity decreases. For example, a 6-compartment mammillary model with Michaelis–Menten elimination is highly unlikely and has low face validity since no known drug has such kinetics. Similarly, fitting a 1-compartment model to concentration–time data exhibiting very distinct phases in the concentration–time profile would also have low face validity. Conversely, some pharmacodynamic models are quite complex in order to mimic the biological systems they are describing. To some reviewers and users of models, face validity is the most important component to a validated model.

At the second step, the model assumptions must be examined and confirmed. The reader is referred to the Section on Testing the Model Assumptions for details. Briefly, informative graphics are essential (Ette and Ludden, 1995). Scatter plots of individual versus predicted concentrations, weighted residuals versus predicted concentrations, and weighted residuals versus time provide evidence of the goodness of fit of the model. Histograms and possibly QQ plots of the distribution of the residuals, the ηs (deviations from the mean), and the EBEs of the random effects are used to examine the assumptions of normality. Further, sensitivity analysis can be done to assess the stability of the model.

Once the analyst is satisfied that the model provides an adequate fit to the model building data set, further validation techniques that test the quality of the model may then be applied. Most validation methods are based on a comparison between predictions or simulated data under the observed model and its associated data set to some other set of data. Thus the conclusions drawn from these methods are based on the concept of similarity, i.e., the results are similar between two different data sets. The problem is that no hard criteria exists for what constitutes "similar" and may become almost uninterpretable. This leads to a fundamental difference between the developer of the model and the end user of the model. To the analyst, the definition of validation then becomes one of shades of gray, whereas the user wants a dichotomous outcome, i.e., the model is validated or it is not validated. It then becomes paramount for the modeler to be able to effectively communicate to the user why validation isn't a yes/no outcome, but an outcome of degrees. Usually to a naïve-user, if validation techniques applied at Step 3 cannot be effectively communicated, the user reverts back to face validity as a means to gauge the quality of a model.

In general, validation techniques are comparison strategies based on two types of new or additional data: internal and/or external validation datasets. With external validation the model is compared to an independent data set by two means. One way is to fit the model to the independent data set provided the validation data set has enough data to reliably estimate the model parameters. The model parameters obtained under the independent data set are then compared to the model parameters obtained using the model building data set. For example, Gisleskog et al. (1999) modeled the pharmacokinetics of dutasteride, a 5α-reductase inhibitor, using a 2-compartment model with parallel linear and Michaelis–Menten elimination kinetics based on single dose data from 48 subjects (index data set). They then compared the model to a validation data set of multiple dose data from 53 subjects (validation data set). Table 7.7 presents the population mean parameter estimates for the index and validation data sets.

All model parameters were well estimated by the validation data set, except the *Michaelis constant (Km)*, which had a relative difference of more than 200%. As might be guessed, one problem with this approach is the difficulty in interpreting the results? When do two parameters differ sufficiently in their values so as to render the model invalid? Also, if only one parameter is appreciably different, as in this case, does this mean the whole model is not valid? Because the Michaelis constant was off by 200%, does this mean the whole model was not applicable to the validation data set? In this instance, the authors concluded the pharmacokinetics of dutasteride were similar between the validation data set and index data set and then went on to explain away the difference in Michaelis constants between the data sets.

The second way that an independent data set is used in validation is to fix the parameter estimates under the final model and then obtain summary measures of the goodness of fit under the independent data set (Kimko, 2001). For example, Mandema et al. (1996) generated a PopPK model for immediate release (IR) and controlled-release (CR) oxycodone after single dose administration. The plasma concentrations after four days administration were then compared to model predictions. The log-prediction error (LPE) between observed concentrations (C_p) and model predicted concentrations $\left(\hat{C}_p\right)$ was calculated as

$$LPE = Ln\left(C_p\right) - Ln\left(\hat{C}_p\right). \qquad (7.143)$$

The mean and variance of the LPE were calculated as an estimate of the model bias and the variability of the measured concentrations around the population mean prediction, respectively. In this case the mean and variance of the LPE were -0.0061 and 0.291, respectively, for the IR formulation and 0.0335 and 0.287 for the CR formulation, respectively. In this form, however, interpretation was problematic as it is not clear what -0.0061 means. But, after exponentiation, the model predicted concentrations were on average 0.6% lower and 3.3% higher in the IR and CR formulations, respectively. Two modifications to this approach are often seen. One modification is that instead of using log-transformed concentrations, raw untransformed concentrations are used instead. Bias and variance with untransformed concentrations are directly interpretable and no exponentiation is needed for interpretation. A second modification is to standardize the LPE to the observed concentrations so that a relative LPE is calculated.

Another method is to address validation through the use of simulated data. The simulated data are then compared to the observed data and some judgment

Table 7.7 Population mean parameters for dutasteride under the index and validation data sets as reported by Gisleskog et al. (1999).

Parameter	Units	Single dose data (index data set)	Multiple dose data (validation data set)	Difference (%)
k_a	per h	2.4	1.5	−38
Lag time	h	0.32	0.43	34
Apparent linear clearance	L/h	0.58	0.46	−21
K_m	ng/mL	0.96	2.9	202
V_{max}	μg/h	5.9	5.1	−14
Intercompartmental clearance	L/h	33	36	9
Central volume of distribution	L	173	160	−8
Peripheral volume of distribution	L	338	374	11
Volume of distribution at steady-state	L	511	534	5
Residual variability		0.13	0.13	0

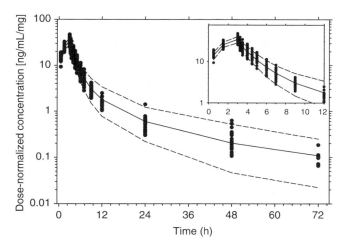

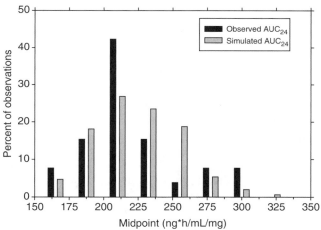

Figure 7.14 Scatter plot of dose-normalized concentrations and 5th and 95th percentiles (dashed lines) from simulated data. Inset is for the first 12 h after dosing. Observed concentration are reported in Table 7.4. Concentration data from 25 subjects at each dose (20–640 mg) were simulated using the final parameters estimates obtained with FOCE-I (Table 7.5). Solid line is the simulated mean concentration.

Figure 7.15 Histogram of observed and simulated dose-normalized area under the curve from time 0 to 24-h postdose based on the observed concentration data (Table 7.4). Concentration data from 25 subjects at each dose (20–640 mg) were simulated using the final parameters estimates in Table 7.5 obtained with FOCE-I.

about the adequacy of the model is made. Obviously this approach is not as rigorous as an independent data set since the validation data set is based on the final model but the method is still useful because model inadequacies can be identified when present. As an example, returning the data set from Yafune and Ishiguro (1999), concentration–time data were simulated under a 4-compartment model with 25 subjects at each dose (20–640 mg) using the same experimental design and parameters estimates obtained with FOCE-I (Table 7.5). The 5th and 95th percentiles (prediction intervals) of the simulated dose-normalized concentrations were calculated and plotted against the observed dose-normalized concentrations. Figure 7.14 presents the results. The model predicts the observed concentrations quite accurately but the simulated concentrations are slightly more variable as would be expected using a larger sample size. But, again, what constitutes failure?

A similar approach called a predictive check is often used. Rather than comparing raw concentration–time profiles, another approach is to simulate data from many individuals, many more than the model development data set, and create a series of summary statistics or functions of the data. The statistics are then compared to the observed data. For example, the concentration–time profile might be simulated and the area under the curve (AUC) calculated. The distribution of the simulated AUCs is then compared to the distribution of the observed AUCs and some measure of similarity or dissimilarity is reported. A high degree of overlap is indicative of a high validity. Figure 7.15 plots the dose-normalized AUC to 24 h (AUC24) for the observed data in Table 7.4 and simulated data from 25 subjects at each

dose (20–640 mg) using the final parameters estimates obtained with FOCE-I (Table 7.5). The observed AUC24 distribution was not normally distributed, whereas the simulated distribution was. A high degree of overlap between observed and simulated data was observed. Analysis of variance on the log-transformed dose-normalized AUC24 values indicated no difference in means (p = 0.51), while a test of equality of variance also indicated no difference. Hence, the simulated AUC24 values were statistically indiscriminate from the observed value.

Another internal validation technique is the posterior predictive check (PPC), which has been used in the Bayesian literature for years, but only recently reported in the PopPK literature by Yano, Beal, and Sheiner (2001). The basic idea is an extension of the predictive check method just described but include hyperparameters on the model parameters. Data are then simulated, some statistic of the data that is not based on the model is calculated, e.g., half-life or AUC by noncompartmental method, and then compared to the observed statistic obtained with real data. The underlying premise is that the simulated data should be similar to the observed data and that any discrepancies between the observed and simulated data are due to chance. With each simulation the statistic of interest is calculated and after all the simulations are complete, a p-value is determined by

$$p = \left(\frac{\text{\# of times the simulated statistics were greater than observed statistic}}{\text{total number of simulations}} \right). \quad (7.144)$$

More typically a histogram of the simulated statistic of interest is plotted and the location of the observed statistic is noted. Unusually small or large values are indicative of poor model validity.

A true PPC requires sampling from the posterior distribution of the fixed and random effects in the model, which is typically not known. A complete solution then usually requires Markov Chain Monte Carlo simulation, which is not easy to implement. Luckily for the analyst, Yano, Sheiner, and Beal (2001) showed that complete implementation of the algorithm does not appear to be necessary since fixing the values of the model parameters to their final values obtained using maximum likelihood resulted in PPC distributions that were as good as the full-blown Bayesian PPC distributions. In other words, using a predictive check resulted in distributions that were similar to PPC distributions. Unfortunately they also showed that the PPC is very conservative and not very powerful at detecting model misspecification.

To illustrate the PPC, the final model under Table 7.4 was analyzed. First, to obtain the model parameters for each simulated data set, a random draw was made from the bootstrap distribution under the final model for each of the model parameters. Concentration–time data were simulated using the same number of subjects, subjects per dose, and sampling times as the original study design. The area under the curve to 12 h and concentration at 6-h postdose were calculated for each subject. The mean of the log-transformed test statistics was then calculated and stored. This process was repeated 250 times and compared to the test statistics under the original data. The results are shown in Figure 7.16. Little difference was seen between the observed test statistics and the PPC distribution suggesting that any discrepancies between the simulated data and observed data were due to chance.

In both the examples just presented, the adequacy of the comparison between observed and simulated data was made by the analyst, the same person who did the simulation, which should not really be done. A more valid approach is the Turning test (1950) wherein data are simulated under the model and given to independent experts for comparison. In this manner, the inherent bias of the analyst is avoided in the comparison process. Ideally, the experts are blinded as to what is real and what is simulated. If the experts cannot determine what is real and what is simulated, the model is validated. Models validated under this method have a high degree of credibility, but to date, no PopPK analyses have been validated using this test.

When an external data set is not available, internal data validation is done instead. This method, usually called data-splitting, splits the available data into two

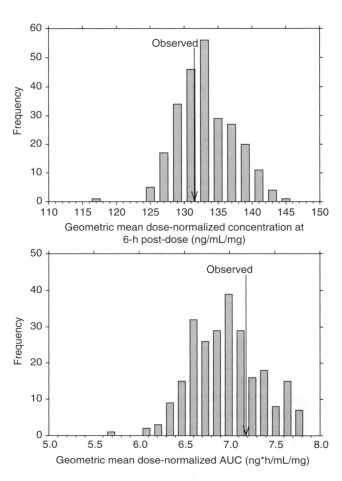

Figure 7.16 Histogram of posterior predictive check based on the observed data in Table 7.4. Concentration data were simulated for 26 subjects under the original experimental design and sampling times at each dose using population values and variance components randomly drawn from the bootstrap distribution of the final model parameter estimates (FOCE-I; Table 7.5). The geometric mean concentration at 6-h postdose (top) and AUC to 12-h postdose (bottom) was calculated. This process was repeated 250 times.

data sets: a model development set and a validation data set. The key here is that the split must be random. What percent of observations to put into the development set and what percent to place into the validation set is not set in stone and varies from investigator to investigator. A rule of thumb is to put 80% of the observations in the development set and 20% in the validation data set. Usually the key splitting element is the subject identifier, and not concentration, although sometimes this is also dependent on studies if the dataset consists of several pooled studies. For instance, 80% of the subjects are placed in the development set, not 80% of the observed concentrations.

An example is found in an analysis of capecitabine and its metabolites in 505 subjects with solid tumors. Gieschke et al. (2003) placed 66% of all data into the model development set and the remainder into the validation data set. They then used the Wilcoxon test for continuous covariates to assess whether the two data sets were different in regards to subject-specific covariates, keeping in mind that with multiple hypothesis testing spurious "statistical significance" is likely to be found due to an inflated Type I error rate (i.e., the multiplicity effect). The development data set was then used to develop the model. Once the final model was obtained, the predicted data from the validation data set was compared to the observed data set and the mean difference and mean squared error of the difference was calculated. Summary statistics of the mean difference were then used to validate the model.

Another internal technique used to validate models, one that is quite commonly seen, is the bootstrap and its various modifications, which has been discussed elsewhere in this book. The nonparametric bootstrap, the most common approach, is to generate a series of data sets of size equal to the original data set by resampling with replacement from the observed data set. The final model is fit to each data set and the distribution of the parameter estimates examined for bias and precision. The parametric bootstrap fixes the parameter estimates under the final model and simulates a series of data sets of size equal to the original data set. The final model is fit to each data set and validation approach per se as it only provides information on how well model parameters were estimated.

The problem with the bootstrap approach is that if an inadequate model is chosen for the final model and if the analyst did not catch the inadequacies with the original data sets will probably not do so with the bootstrap data sets. To illustrate this, consider the model presented by Yafune and Ishiguro (1999) to the data in Table 7.4. They reported that a 2-compartment model was an adequate fit to the data and presented bootstrap distributions of the final model parameters as evidence. Sample bootstrap distributions for clearance and the between-subject variability for clearance under a 2-compartment model are shown in Fig. 7.17. The objective function value using FO-approximation for a 2-, 3-, and 4-compartment model were 4283.1, 3911.6, and 3812.2, respectively. A 4-compartment model was superior to the 2-compartment model since the objective function value was more than 450 points smaller with the 4-compartment model. But comparing Fig. 7.12, the bootstrap distribution under the 4-compartment model, to Fig. 7.17, the bootstrap distribution to clearance under the 2-compartment model, one would not be able to say which model was better since both distributions had small standard deviations. Hence, the bootstrap does not seem a good choice for model selection but more of a tool to judge the stability of the parameter estimates under the final model.

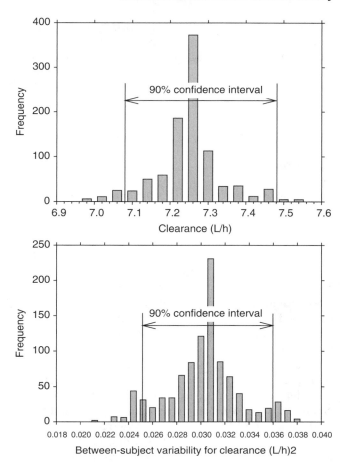

Figure 7.17 Histogram of bootstrap clearance (top) and between-subject variance estimate for clearance (bottom) for 2-compartment model fit to data in Table 7.4. Bootstrap models fit using FO-approximation. Ninety percent confidence intervals indicated based on the percentile method.

Another disadvantage of the bootstrap is given that many different bootstrap data sets must be analyzed, a large commitment in time is needed to obtain a valid bootstrap distribution. The long run times can sometimes limit the choice of estimation algorithm to usually FO-approximation since FOCE algorithms take much longer to complete. Consider a model that takes 10 min to run under FO-approximation and 1 h to run under FOCE. With 500 bootstrap data sets, it would take about 3 days to generate a bootstrap distribution under FO-approximation and almost 3 weeks to run under FOCE. This then leads to a problem because often a final model will be estimated using the best estimation algorithm available, usually FOCE or FOCE-I, but to obtain bootstrap distribution estimates FO-approximation is used. So then how are the model parameter estimates compared if they are estimated using different algorithms? They cannot. One would have to reestimate the model parameters with the original data set under

FO-approximation for the comparison to be valid or analyze all the bootstrap data sets using the same estimation algorithm as the original data set. The latter approach is sometimes seen, regardless of the time needed for such models to be fit. It is this author's opinion that the bootstrap is overrated as a tool for model validation and should not be used as the sole validation method.

A modification to this method is to actually find the best structural model for each bootstrap data set and then using the EBEs from each bootstrap data set perform covariate screening to make sure the same set of covariates is chosen as the original data set. Obviously this modification is extremely time consuming, but quite satisfying if the same models and covariates are chosen using the bootstrap data sets as the original data set. Shen et al. (2002) used this modification in selecting covariates for the PopPK model of carboplatin in 44 subjects with advanced ovarian cancer. Covariate screening suggested an important relationship between serum creatinine and weight for clearance, total bilirubin and weight for central volume of distribution, albumin for intercompartmental clearance, and albumin, serum creatinine, and age for peripheral volume of distribution. The final covariate model included weight and serum creatinine on clearance, weight on central volume of distribution, and albumin on intercompartmental clearance and peripheral volume of distribution. A total of 73 and 64% of the bootstrap data sets associated clearance with serum creatinine and weight, respectively; 67 and 52% of the bootstrap data sets associated central volume of distribution with weight and total bilirubin, respectively; 70% of the bootstrap data sets associated intercompartmental clearance with albumin; and 56, 19, and 22% of the bootstrap data sets associated peripheral volume of distribution with albumin, serum creatinine, and age, respectively. Hence, the bootstrap data sets did not identify any covariates that the original data set did not identify and in some cases showed that the association between a covariate and pharmacokinetic parameter was spurious.

The last internal validation technique that is often seen is cross-validation. The basic idea is to split the data set into two different data sets. One set, called the cross-validation data set, consists of 90% of the observations in the original data set. The other data set, the cross-prediction data set, consists of the remainder of observations. Ten different cross-validation data sets and 10 different sets of cross-prediction data sets are created (for a total of 20 data sets) with each cross-validation data set consisting of unique 90% of observations from

the original data set. So, for instance, if the data set consisted of 50 subjects, the first cross-prediction data set would consist of subjects one to five, while the cross-validation data set would consist of subjects 6–50. The second cross-prediction data set would consist of subjects 6–10, while the cross-validation data set would consist of subjects one to five and 11–50, etc. The final model is fit to each of the cross-validation data sets. The concentrations in the corresponding crossprediction data set are then simulated given the final parameter estimates obtained using the cross-validation data set. The observed and predicted concentrations in the cross prediction data set are compared using either relative difference or relative log-difference. The results from each cross-validation set are then treated as independent estimates of the model parameters and pooled. From the pooled cross-validated parameter estimates, the mean relative error or mean relative log-difference is reported as a measure of accuracy and bias in model predictions. Cross-validation was one method used to validate a ciprofloxacin PopPK model in pediatric patients (Rajagopalan and Gastonguay, 2003).

In summary, there is no one test that "validates" a model. Validation is a matter of degrees and it is the collective validity of all the techniques that lends credibility to a model. Most of the validation techniques do not test whether the model itself is the best model, but test the stability of the parameter estimates under the final model, a subtle but important difference. It is entirely possible that a given model will show good performance with all the validation techniques, but still not be the optimal model, as was illustrated with the Yafune and Ishiguro (1999) data set.

INFLUENCE ANALYSIS

An area related to model validation is influence analysis, which deals with how stable the model parameters are to influential observations (either individual concentration values or individual subjects), and model robustness, which deals with how stable the model parameters are to perturbations in the input data. Influence analysis has been dealt with in previous chapters. The basic idea is to generate a series of new data sets, where each new data set consists of the original data set with one unique subject removed or has a different block of data removed, just like how jackknife data sets are generated. The model is refit to each of the new data sets and how the parameter estimates change with each new data set is determined. Ideally, no subject should show

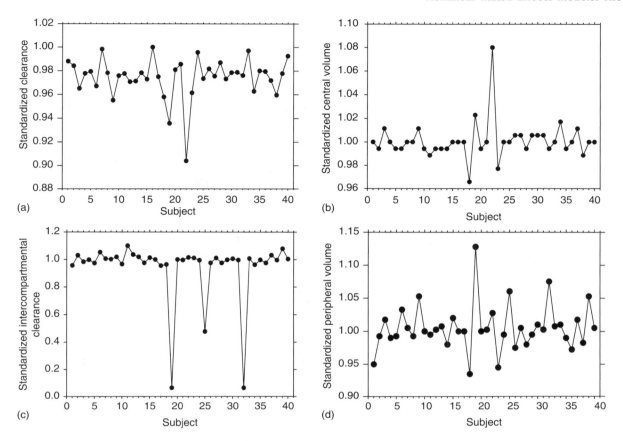

Figure 7.18   Influence analysis on clearance (a), central volume of distribution (b), intercompartmental clearance (c), and peripheral volume of distribution (d) standardized to the original parameter estimate. Forty (40) new data sets were created by removing a unique subject from the original data set and the model refit using the delete n -1 data sets. The results were standardized to the original parameter estimates. Subject 19 appeared to influence clearance, intercompartmental clearance, and peripheral volume of distribution.

profound influence over the parameter estimates in a model. If one does, then how to deal with it is a question not firmly answered in the PopPK literature.

For example, Bonate (2003) in a PopPK analysis of an unnamed drug performed an influence analysis on 40 subjects from a Phase 1 study. Forty (40) new data sets were generated, each one having a different subject removed. The model was refit to each data set and the results were standardized to the original parameter estimates. Figure 7.18 shows the influence of each subject on four of the fixed effect model parameters. Subject 19 appeared to show influence over clearance, intercompartmental clearance, and peripheral volume. Based on this, the subject was removed from the analysis and original model refit; the resultant estimates were considered the final parameter estimates.

This example illustrates some of the issues with influence analysis: which subjects are really important,

what to do with subjects that do show influence, and what to do with a subject that might influence only one parameter? Looking at the standardized parameter plots, the impact of Subject 19 was pretty clear and case deletion seemed a logical choice. However, Subject 32 in Fig. 7.18 appeared to influence intercompartmental clearance and peripheral volume, but none of the other parameters. Should this subject be removed from the analysis?

A useful method to test the overall impact a subject has on the parameters is to first perform principal component analysis (PCA) on the estimated model parameters. PCA is a multivariate statistical method the object of which is to take a set of p-variables, $\{X_1, X_2, \ldots X_n\} = X$ and find linear functions of X to produce a new set of uncorrelated variables $Z_1, Z_2, \ldots Z_n$ such that Z_1 contains the largest amount of variability, Z_2 contains the second largest, etc.

Hopefully, just the first few principal components contain the majority of the variance in X. The outcome of PCA is to take a set of p-variables and reduce it to a set of q-variables (q < p) that contain most of the information within X. It turns out that the solution to PCA is to simply computes the eigenvalues and eigenvectors of X. If the variances of the columns of X are of different scale it is recommended that X be standardized prior to per-

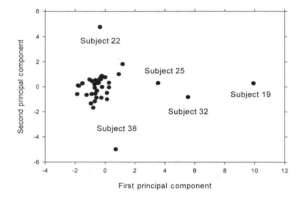

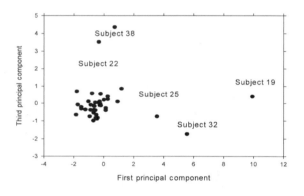

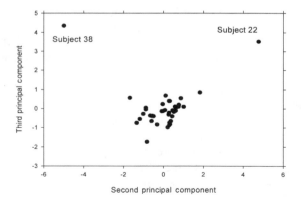

Figure 7.19 Scatter plot of principal component analysis of data in Figure 7.18. The first three principal components are plotted. Subjects that are removed from the bulk of the data represent influential observations that may be influencing the parameter estimates "overall." Potentially influential subjects are noted.

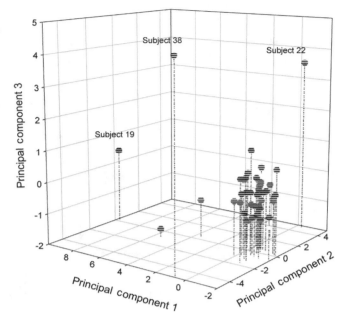

Figure 7.20 Three-dimensional scatter plot of the first three principal components analysis. Subjects that are removed from the bulk of the data represent influential observations that may be influencing the parameter estimates "overall."

forming PCA and that PCA be performed on the correlation matrix rather than the covariance matrix. If X is not standardized then PCA will simply rearrange the original variables in decreasing order of the size of their variances. The reader is referred to Johnson (1991) for details.

It is not necessary for X to be multivariate normal but it is highly desirable for the vectors in X to be correlated. PCA will have little success if the vectors are not correlated. Once the principal components are calculated, a useful rule of thumb is to keep only those that have an eigenvalue greater than 1. A scatter plot of each principal component plotted against the others is then made and examined for outliers. As an example, with the data in Fig. 7.18 there were nine estimable fixed effect parameters in the model. PCA analysis on the standardized parameters revealed three principal components whose eigenvalues were greater than 1 (4.34, 1.73, and 1.11, respectively), which accounted for 80% of the total variability. Scatter plots of the first three principal components are plotted in Fig. 7.19 and a three-dimensional scatter plot is shown in Fig. 7.20. Three subjects appeared to be different from the bulk of subjects: Subject 19, 22, and 38. A cluster analysis using the method of nearest neighbors showed that of the three subjects, Subject 22 was the only one truly different from the others (Fig. 7.21). What to do now, whether to keep or discard this subject, is unclear. One might look at the parameter estimates with and without

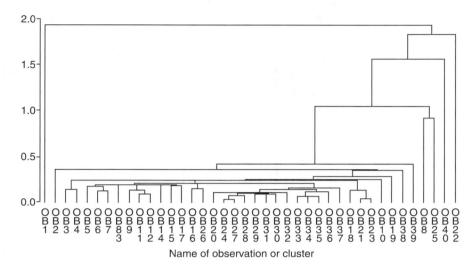

Figure 7.21 Cluster analysis using the method of nearest neighbors with the first three principal components of the data in Figure 7.18. Two main branches are observed, Subject 22 (OB22) and everyone else, suggesting that Subject 22 is different from the bulk of the observations.

this subject to see if a difference is discernible to the eye. If so, then perhaps discarding the subject is in order. Of course, one reason for outliers is model misspecification so removing the subject may bias towards an inadequate model. There are no good answers on what to do with influential subjects in PopPK analysis. Further research is needed before any real guidance can be made in this area.

MORE ON EMPIRICAL BAYES ESTIMATES

As mentioned elsewhere in the chapter, EBEs are conditional estimates of an individual's model parameters given a model and the population parameter estimates. EBEs are useful for a variety of reasons, including:

- They can be used in covariate screening;
- They can be used to derive secondary pharmacokinetic parameters, like α- and β-half-life in a 2-compartment model; and
- They can be used to simulate more complex individual concentration–time profiles.

A natural question that may arise is the quality of the estimate—how close do the EBEs compare to the true model parameters for a subject. That question is data-specific, but some general conclusions can be made which will be shown through example.

Concentration–time data were simulated from a 2-compartment model having a mean systemic clearance of 45 L/h, intercompartmental clearance of 15 L/h, central volume of 125 L, and peripheral volume of 125 L.

Drug administration was intravenous with half the subjects receiving a dose of 100 mg and the other half receiving a dose of 200 mg. Two simulations were done: one with high residual variability and the other with low residual variability. In the simulation with low residual variability, all the pharmacokinetic parameters were treated as random effects having a log-normal distribution with a CV of 40%. Residual variability was log-normal in distribution with 10% CV. In the simulation with high residual variability, the variability was reversed. The pharmacokinetic parameters had a 10% CV but residual error had a 40% CV. A total of 75 or 250 subjects was simulated with each subject having two, four, or eight samples collected per subject. No attempt was made to optimize the sample collection times. Collection times were chosen to capture the relevant portions of the concentration–time profiles so that the entire profile was characterized. A time window approach was used. Subjects having two samples were collected at {0–6 h} and {18–36 h}. Subjects having four samples were collected at {0–2.5 h}, {3–9 h}, {9–18 h}, and {18–36 h}. Subjects having eight samples were collected at {0–0.5 h}, {0.5–1.5 h}, {1.5–3 h}, {3–6 h}, {6–12 h}, {12–18 h}, {18–24 h}, and {24–36 h}. A 2-compartment model was fit to the data using the true model parameters as the initial values. To avoid an infinite objective function value, an additive and proportional error model was used where the additive term was fixed to $0.00001 \ (ng/mL)^2$. Parameters were estimated using FO-approximation and FOCE with interaction.

Figure 7.22 and Fig. 7.23 present scatter plots and box and whisker plots of the true clearance for each individual against their EBE for clearance using

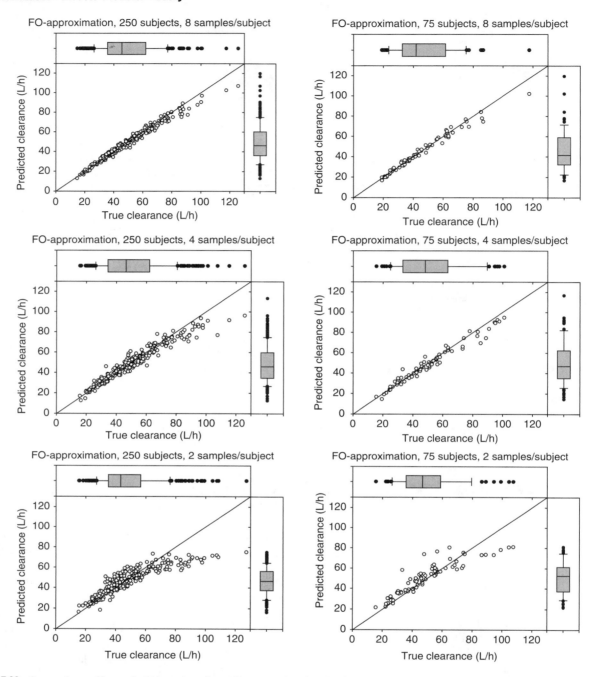

Figure 7.22 Scatter plots and box and whiskers plots of true clearance against the EBE for clearance using FO-approximation. A total of 250 or 75 subjects were simulated with each subject having either 2, 4, or 8 samples collected. In this example, all pharmacokinetic parameters had 40% CV whereas residual error had a 10% CV. A 2-compartment model was fit to the data with all pharmacokinetic parameters treated as log-normal random effects and residual error modeled using an additive and proportional error model where the additive component was fixed to 0.00001 (ng / mL)^2 to avoid infinite objective functions. Solid line is the line of unity.

FO-approximation and FOCE with interaction, respectively, when the data had low residual variability. Figure 7.24 and Fig. 7.25 present scatter plots and box and whisker plots of the true clearance for each individual against their EBE for clearance using FO-approximation and FOCE with interaction, respectively, when the data

had high residual variability. All models minimized successfully, except one. However, the models fit to data having with low residual variability and four or fewer samples needed a lot of tweaking to converge without problems using FOCE with interaction. The model fit using FOCE with interaction to the data set having

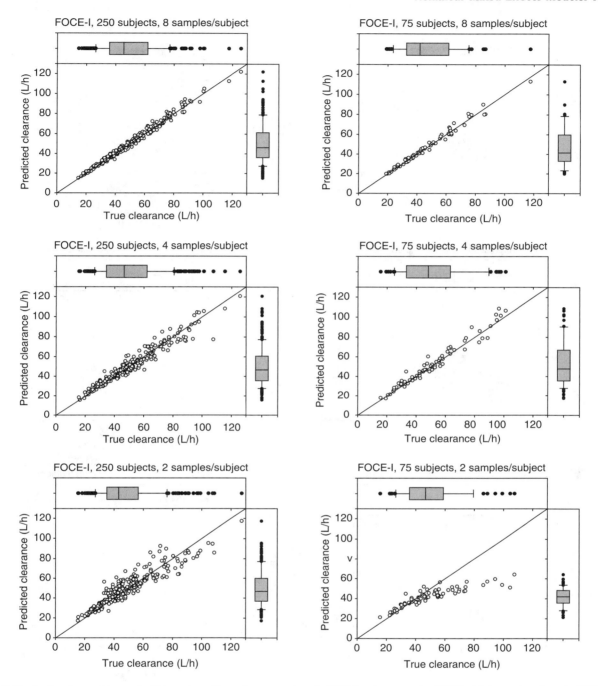

Figure 7.23 Scatter plots and box and whiskers plots of true clearance against the EBE for clearance using FOCE with interaction. A total of 250 or 75 subjects were simulated with each subject having either 2, 4, or 8 samples collected. In this example, all pharmacokinetic parameters had 40% CV whereas residual error had a 10% CV. A 2-compartment model was fit to the data with all pharmacokinetic parameters treated as log-normal random effects and residual error modeled using an additive and proportional error model where the additive component was fixed to 0.00001 (ng / mL)^2 to avoid infinite objective functions. Solid line is the line of unity.

250 subjects with two samples per subject and low residual variability did not minimize successfully and terminated with rounding errors. Examination of the NONMEM output revealed that at the time of termination there were 3.9 significant digits in the parameter estimates and the final parameter estimates themselves were reasonable compared to the true population values. So despite the warning message, the results did appear to be valid and were used in the comparator analysis.

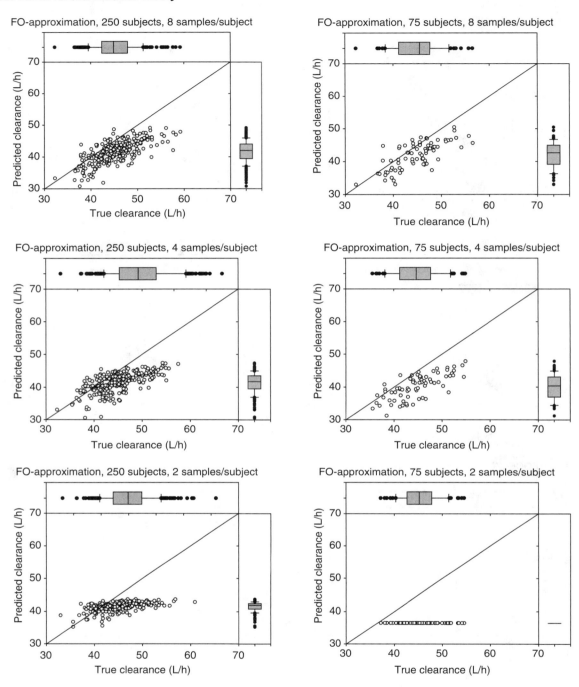

Figure 7.24 Scatter plots and box and whiskers plots of true clearance against the EBE for clearance using FO-approximation. A total of 250 or 75 subjects were simulated with each subject having either 2, 4, or 8 samples collected. In this example, all pharmacokinetic parameters had 10% CV whereas residual error had a 40% CV. A 2-compartment model was fit to the data with all pharmacokinetic parameters treated as log-normal random effects and residual error modeled using an additive and proportional error model where the additive component was fixed to 0.00001 (ng / mL)^2 to avoid infinite objective functions. Solid line is the line of unity.

With low residual variability and with eight samples per subject, the quality of the EBEs was excellent as predicted estimates were very near the true estimates. However, the deviation from the line of unity appeared to increase as clearance increased. This deviation became more pronounced as fewer samples were available from each subject. There did not appear to be much difference in the quality of the estimates when 75 or 250 subjects were used, although better estimates were made when FOCE with interaction was the estimation algorithm

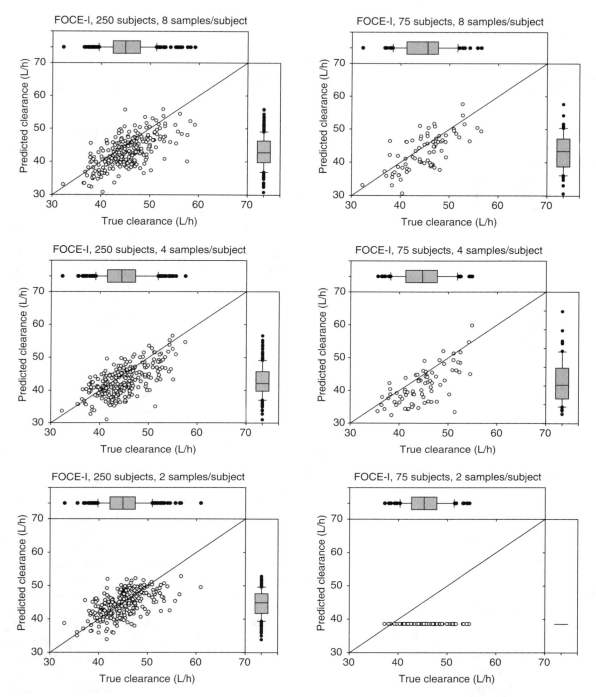

Figure 7.25 Scatter plots and box and whiskers plots of true clearance against the EBE for clearance using FOCE with interaction. A total of 250 or 75 subjects were simulated with each subject having either two, four, or eight samples collected. In this example, all pharmacokinetic parameters had a 10% CV whereas residual error had a 40% CV. A 2-compartment model was fit to the data with all pharmacokinetic parameters treated as log-normal random effects and residual error modeled using an additive and proportional error model where the additive component was fixed to 0.00001 (ng / mL)^2 to avoid infinite objective functions. Solid line is the line of unity.

used. Also, as the number of samples per subject decreased, the range of the EBEs decreased—an effect known as *shrinkage*. When fewer observations are available per subject, the conditional estimates shrink towards the population mean.

When the residual variability was high, the EBEs were of poorer quality than with low residual variability, despite the fact that the BSV in clearance was 10%. With FO-approximation the EBEs tended to be underestimated and the range of the EBEs decreased as the number of samples per subject decreased. With 75 subjects having two samples collected, no BSV in clearance was observed. Again, the quality of the EBEs tended to be better using the FOCE with interaction algorithm than with FO-approximation, but considerable scatter was observed around the line of unity.

This simulation highlights a number of points in regards to the quality of the EBEs. One, the amount of shrinkage depends on the relative magnitude of the BSV and residual variability with the magnitude of shrinkage increasing with increasing residual variability. Best estimates are obtained when BSV is greater than residual variability—the better the model, the better the EBE. Second, the amount of shrinkage depends on the number of observations per subject with more shrinkage occurring with fewer numbers of observations per subject. This makes sense intuitively because less importance should be given to subjects not having a lot of data. Lastly, better estimates are obtained when a more accurate estimation algorithm is used, but the difference in quality is not much and perhaps not even noticeable.

SOFTWARE

Smith (2003) provides an overview of the nonlinear mixed effects model software packages. Two programs designed for pharmacokinetic-pharmacodynamic nonlinear mixed effects models include WinNonmix (Pharsight Corp., Mountain View, CA) and NONMEM (GloboMax Corp., Baltimore, MD). WinNonmix has an advantage in that it was built for a Microsoft Windows environment and has an easy to use graphical user interface. For a first-time user, WinNonmix is highly recommended for its ease of use, although it is not as flexible as other, less user-friendly software packages.

NONMEM was a Fortran program written as a DOS application that requires the user to write a "control stream" that identifies how to read in the data, how the model is defined, and what postprocessor activities should be called, such as building a table. To obtain quality scatter plots requires input into another statistical program, such as SAS, S-Plus, or Xpose (http://xpose.sourceforge.net/). It is difficult to assess what proportion of users use each program. Anecdotal evidence suggests that the industry standard is NONMEM since it was the first software program designed for pharmacokinetic-pharmacodynamic nonlinear mixed effects modeling and because many of the thought leaders in the field use NONMEM exclusively. Because of its dominance in the pharmaceutical industry, in this book the emphasis will be on the use of NONMEM. It should be recognized, however, that although this book refers to and uses NONMEM, this does not imply that only NONMEM can be used.

Nonlinear mixed effects models can also be implemented within SAS (Version 8 or higher, SAS Institute, Cary, NC) or S-Plus (Insightful Corp., Seattle WA). Within SAS, the NLMIXED procedure can be used. Within S-Plus, the NLME routine can be called. Each of these software packages has its own advantages and disadvantages, the primary advantage being that they are both bundled into a general, all-purpose, powerful statistical analysis environment. NLME has the additional advantage in that it can model multilevel random effects, whereas other software packages cannot unless they are "tricked" into doing so. The disadvantage for both packages being that neither routine was designed for pharmacokinetic analysis, although S-Plus does have a library of pharmacokinetic-pharmacodynamic models that the user can now use (steady-state models are not available, however). Modeling of multiple-dose pharmacokinetic data is tedious and difficult with NLMIXED and NLME. Additionally, both NLMIXED and NLME are slow compared to NONMEM. For further details on the use of the NLMIXED procedure in SAS the reader is referred to Littell et al. (1996), while for NLME in S-Plus the reader is referred to Pinheiro and Bates (2000).

It should be pointed out that not all software programs lead to the same model structural model parameter estimates and variance components. Roe (1997) compared the simulated pharmacokinetics of a drug having monoexponential kinetics where clearance was a function of saturable protein binding and renal function and volume of distribution was a function of saturable protein binding only. The basis for the simulated concentrations was a population analysis of 361 quinidine concentration–time measurements from 136 male patients who had experienced cardiac arrhythmia (Verme et al., 1992). The same distribution of simulated observations (e.g., 46 patients had only one sample collected, 33 patients had two samples collected) was used as in the actual study. She and many other participants on the project analyzed the dataset with seven different modeling programs: NONMEM using first-order conditional estimation and Laplacian estimation, NLME within S-Plus, MIXNLIN, NLINMIX within SAS, Gibbs sampling using POPKAN, NLMIX, a semiparametric method developed by Davidian and Gallant (1993), and NPEM, a nonparametric method developed by Schumitsky and colleagues (1991). The results were most illuminating. All datasets gave different results. No two methods produced the same answers. In general, the nonparametric method produced the most accurate results.

A newcomer to the software field is the System for Population Kinetics developed by the Resource Facility for Population Kinetics (RFPK) at the University of Washington. The algorithms in this package were designed to be faster than existing products and produce comparable, if not more accurate results, than existing software programs, including NONMEM. At this time an evaluation of the program is unavailable. Information about the RFPK is available at http://www.rfpk.washington.edu.

Among the other methods, no clearly superior algorithm could be identified. These results indicated that different algorithms produce diverse results, which is not really all that surprising. Even in a nonlinear regression, different algorithms can (Gauss–Newton versus Levenberg–Marquardt for example) produce similar, but not exact, estimates. So it should come as no surprise that given the complexities of the algorithms involved in nonlinear mixed effects models analysis that different algorithms produce different results. What is important is that no algorithm produces results discordant from the other methods. Of course, more complex simulations are needed to make more definitive conclusions, but given the rate at which the estimation algorithms are being improved, once such a simulation study was completed it would be outdated.

SUMMARY

Hopefully, the reader will be able to see the interconnections between nonlinear mixed effects models and linear mixed effects modeling, nonlinear modeling, and linear modeling. The algorithms behind nonlinear mixed effects models are certainly more complex than any of the other model types examined, but the basic ideas behind developing PopPK models are the same as those that were developed using the other classes of models. This chapter has just provided some of the theory behind PopPK models. The next chapter will deal with practical issues in PopPK modeling and the chapter after that will present case studies in PopPK modeling.

Recommended Reading

Bruno, R., Vivier, N., Vergnoid, J.C., De Phillips, S.L., Montay, G., and Sheiner, L.B. A population pharmacokinetic model for docetaxel (Taxotere®): Model building and validation. *Journal of Pharmacokinetics and Pharmacodynamics* 1996; 24: 153–172.

Davidian, M., Giltinan, D.M. Nonlinear models for repeated measurement data. Chapman & Hall, London, 1995.

Ette, E.I., and Ludden, T.M. Population pharmacokinetic modeling: The importance of informative graphics. *Pharmaceutical Research* 1995; 12: 1845–1855.

Karlsson, M.O., Jonsson, E.N., Wiltse, C.G., and Wade, J.R. Assumption testing in population pharmacokinetic models: Illustrated with an analysis of moxonidine data from congestive heart failure. *Journal of Pharmacokinetics and Pharmacodynamics* 1998; 26: 207–246.

Wahlby, U., Jonsson, E.N., and Karlsson, M.O. Assessment of actual significance levels for covariate effects in NONMEM. *Journal of Pharmacokinetics and Pharmacodynamics* 2001; 28: 321–352. With comments and discussion given in 29; 403–412.

Chapter 8

Nonlinear Mixed Effects Models: Practical Issues

In the field of observation, chance favors only the mind that is prepared.

—Louis Pasteur (1822–1895), Chemist and the Father of Stereochemistry

INTRODUCTION

In the last chapter, the theory behind nonlinear mixed effects models was introduced. In this chapter, practical issues related to nonlinear mixed effects modeling will be introduced. Due to space considerations not all topics will be given the coverage they deserve, e.g., handling missing data. What is intended is a broad coverage of problems and issues routinely encountered in actual population pharmacokinetics (PopPK) analyses. The reader is referred to the original source material and references for further details.

THE DATA ANALYSIS PLAN

Today, good modeling practices dictate that a data analysis plan (DAP) be written prior to any modeling being conducted and prior to any unblinding of the data. The reason being that model credibility is increased to outside reviewers when there is impartiality in the model development process. The DAP essentially provides a blueprint for the analysis. It should provide details about how an analysis *will be* conducted (notice the emphasis on future tense) and how the results will be reported. Some companies refer to these as Statistical Analysis Plans (SAPs) based on wording in the International Conference on Harmonisation's (ICH) Guidance on Statistical Principles in Clinical Trials (1998b). Herein, these plans will be referred to as DAPs since modeling is not a statistical activity per se.

The 1999 guidance on Population Pharmacokinetics issued by the Food and Drug Administration (FDA) differentiates two types of DAPs, which they refer to as Study Protocols. The first type is an add-on DAP which is seamlessly interwoven into the clinical protocol from which the pharmacokinetic data will be derived. The other type is a stand-alone DAP, which is independent of any clinical protocols, and can "stand-alone" by itself without reference to other protocols. Stand-alone protocols are useful when data from many different studies will be analyzed. In the guidance issued by the ICH, it is suggested that the essential features of the analysis are included in the clinical protocol, but that the details of the analysis are identified in a stand-alone SAP.

In the stand-alone DAP, the key essential feature is prespecification of the analysis in which the primary analysis variable(s) are defined and methods for dealing with anticipated problems are defined. A DAP differs from the concept of a SAP as defined by the ICH in one important aspect. Modeling is largely an exercise in exploratory data analysis. There are rarely specific hypotheses to be tested. Hence, any PopPK analysis cannot be described in the detail outlined by a SAP under ICH guidelines. Nevertheless, certain elements can be predefined and identified prior to conducting any analysis. But keep in mind that a DAP devoid of detail is essentially meaningless, whereas a DAP that is so detailed will inevitably force the analyst to deviate from the DAP. Hence, there should be a middle ground in the level of detail written into any DAP.

The DAP is usually written by the modeler in conjunction with a physician, a statistician, and, sometimes, someone from data management for analyses of large clinical studies. Some essential elements in a DAP are identified in Table 8.1. The contents of a DAP can be broken down into signature page, objectives, protocol summary, identification of variables to be analyzed, identification of independent variables, model building procedures, and model validation procedures. The title page and signature page should clearly state the authorship of the DAP, date, and version number. As mentioned, the primary analysis variable and the objectives of the analysis should be clearly defined. In the case of pharmacokinetic data this may be easy to do. In the case of pharmacokinetic-pharmacodynamic modeling, where

there may be many possible surrogate markers that may be examined, this may not be easy to do. Particular attention within the DAP should be paid to how the following data types will be dealt with: missing data, censored data, outlier data, time-dependent covariates, and calculation of derived variables. Some DAPs also include detailed "table shells" indicating how all the tables in the report will look when populated with real data. From this, a PopPK report can be easily developed (for example see Table 8.2). Once a DAP is finalized, changes can be made prior to unblinding without penalty. However, once the blind is broken and modeling has commenced, all deviations from the DAP should be noted, along with reason and justification for doing so, in the final report.

CHOOSING AN ESTIMATION METHOD

With NONMEM, the user has a number of available estimation algorithms: first-order (FO) approximation, first-order conditional estimation (FOCE with and without interaction), the hybrid method, and the Laplacian method. The choice of an estimation method is based on a number of factors, including the type of data, the amount of computation time the user is willing to spend on each run, which is dependent on the complexity of the model, and the degree of nonlinearity of the random effects in the model.

Plainly the most accurate algorithm is desired and at this time, the Laplacian algorithm is probably the best. But it is also one of the most computationally expensive, and optimization of a single model on current Pentium-speed computers may take days, which to many would be prohibitive for routine model development. Balanced against speed is the degree to which the random effects enter into the model nonlinearly. Highly nonlinear models require more accurate algorithms, despite the cost due to increased computation time. In general, population models that have nonlinear kinetics, population pharmacodynamic models, and models with multiple dosing tend to be more highly nonlinear than single dose pharmacokinetic models, and may require something other than first-order approximation methods. Pharmacodynamic models of ordinal or categorical data should always use the Laplacian method.

Obviously, the accuracy of FO-approximation is dependent on the accuracy of the Taylor series approximation to the function. FO-approximation has been shown to provide modestly biased parameter estimates under a variety of different models (Rodman and Silverstein, 1990; Sheiner and Beal, 1980), especially when the between-subject and intrasubject variability is high (White et al., 1991). The advantage of

Table 8.1 Sample table of contents of a data analysis plan.

1. Signature page
2. Abbreviations
3. Objectives and rationale
4. Protocol summary
    a. Study design
    b. Sampling design
5. Subject population(s)
    a. Description
    b. Inclusion criteria
    c. Exclusion criteria
6. Data handling
    a. Pharmacokinetic evaluability criteria
        1. Outliers
        2. Missing data
    b. Subject covariates included in the analysis and rationale
    c. Subject accounting
    d. Creation of the NONMEM data file
    e. Data integrity and computer software
7. Data analysis
    a. Exploratory data analysis
    b. Population pharmacokinetic model development
        1. Assumptions
        2. Base model development
        3. Covariate screening
        4. Covariate submodel development
        5. Calculated pharmacokinetic parameters
8. Model performance and stability
    a. Parameter stability
    b. Sensitivity to model inputs
    c. Model predictability
9. Pharmacodynamic correlations (if appropriate)
10. Caveats
11. Representative plots and tables
12. Sample report outline (see Table 8.2)
13. Timelines
14. Miscellaneous considerations
15. References
16. Appendices

Table 8.2 Sample table of contents of a population pharmacokinetic report.

FO-approximation is that it is computationally the simplest estimation algorithm and, hence, the fastest. Whether a conditional estimation method will result in parameter estimates much different from estimates obtained using FO-approximation depends on the degree of between-subject variability (BSV) and the amount of data per subject. When the degree of between-subject variation is small, all methods will produce similar results. Also, the ability of the conditional methods to produce estimates different from FO-ap-

proximation decreases when the amount of data per subject decreases.

In general, a good strategy is to use FO-approximation for developing the structural model. The algorithm is fast, able to detect errors in the data, and can identify gross model departures quickly. In addition, most of the literature to date regarding the accuracy and precision of nonlinear mixed effects model parameter estimates has been done using FO-approximation. However, once a structural model is identified, a more intensive, accurate algorithm is needed. Many studies have now shown that using FO-approximation to develop covariate models may lead to models with many false positive covariates. The speed of most current computers is fast enough that the increase in computation time needed with the conditional estimation algorithms is acceptable for the increase in accuracy.

One reason an estimation method is chosen is that it has a Type I error rate (the probability of rejecting the null hypothesis when true) near nominal values regardless of the experimental design. To examine the Type I error rate using the FO-approximation and FOCE methods, Wahlby, Jonsson, and Karlsson (2001) used Monte Carlo simulation to determine the probability of falsely adding a dichotomous covariate to a model where the covariate was not actually in the model used to generate the data. Pharmacokinetic data were simulated using a default model of a 1-compartment model with no covariates and exponential random error. The number of subjects (10–1000), number of observations per subject (2–19), and size of the residual variance (~ 10 to $\sim 53\%$) was varied. Two nested models were used to analyze the data: one without the covariate (reduced model having p_1 estimable parameters) and one with a dichotomous covariate introduced on clearance (CL) as a fractional change parameter (full model having p_2 estimable parameters). Data sets were simulated and the full and reduced models fit to each data set using FO-approximation, FOCE, and FOCE with interaction (FOCE-I). The change in objective function value (ΔOFV) was calculated for each data set. The proportion of data sets having a ΔOFV greater than 3.84 and 6.63 were determined and deemed the Type I error rate, i.e., the probability of adding another parameter in the model given that the parameter should not be added. Since the OFV produced by NONMEM is proportional to -2 times the log-likelihood, the change in OFVs between two nested models should be chi-squared distributed with $p_2 - p_1$ degrees of freedom; this is the likelihood ratio test (LRT). In this case, with a single degree of freedom, ΔOFV of 3.84 and 6.63 should correspond to a significance of 0.05 and 0.01, respectively.

Based on the results of 10,000 simulations with 50 subjects having two observations per subject and residual error of 10%, FO-approximation had a Type I error rate of 0.004, 0.022, and 0.086 for nominal levels of 0.001, 0.01, and 0.05, respectively. FOCE and the Laplacian method were consistently better than FO-approximation but both also had inflated Type I errors. For both FO-approximation and FOCE, regardless of the number of observations per subject, Type I error rates sharply declined when the number of subjects increased from 10 to 50 but thereafter remained relatively constant to 1000 subjects. In contrast, Type I error rates with both FO-approximation and FOCE sharply increased when the number of observations per subject increased keeping the number of subjects constant. With 19 observations per subject and 1000 subjects, the Type I error rate for FO-approximation and FOCE was about 0.47 and 0.37, respectively. Hence, 47 and 37% of simulations, respectively, declared the covariate was an important influence on CL when in fact it was not important. Increasing the residual error to 42% tended to increase the Type I error rate for FO-approximation. FOCE was not studied using the 42% residual error. Interestingly, the inflated Type I error rate seen with FO-approximation and an exponential residual error was not seen when the residual error was homoscedastic (and hence lacking an $\eta - \varepsilon$ interaction). Also, when the residual variance was modeled using a proportional residual error model, instead of an exponential residual variance model, the Type I error rates decreased with both FO-approximation and FOCE but still remained inflated overall.

Type I error rates with FOCE-I were consistently near nominal values and were unaffected by number of subjects or number of observations per subject. With large residual variability (42%) and two observations per subject, Type I error rates for FOCE-I were higher than nominal, about 0.075 instead of 0.05. But when the number of observations was increased to four, the Type I error rate decreased to the nominal value and remained there as further increases in the number of observations were examined. Also, when the residual variance was modeled using a proportional residual error model, instead of an exponential residual variance model, the Type I error rate decreased. The major conclusion of this analysis was that FOCE-I should be preferred as an estimation method over FO-approximation and FOCE.

Wahlby et al. (2002) later expanded their previous study and used Monte Carlo simulation to examine the Type I error rate under the statistical portion of the model. In all simulations a 1-compartment model was used where both between-subject variability and residual variability were modeled using an exponential model. Various combinations were examined: number of obser-

vations per subject (2–19), number of subjects (25–1000), degree of between-subject variability (BSV) and residual variability, and estimation method (FO-approximation, FOCE, and FOCE-I). In their first simulation they compared using the LRT, a model having a false covariate influencing interindividual variability in clearance

$$CL = CL_\mu \exp\left[COV\eta_1 + (1 - COV)\eta_2\right] \qquad (8.1)$$

to a model without the covariate, where COV was a dichotomous covariate taking values '0' or '1' denoting which group the ith subject was in. The proportion of subjects in each group was 0.5 and both groups were constrained to have the same variance, i.e., $\omega_{CL,1}^2 = \omega_{CL,2}^2 = \omega^2$. In this case, variability was partitioned into two groups. The Type I error rate under FOCE-I remained near the nominal rate of 0.05 as the between-subject variability was increased from 10 to 53% or as the residual error was increased from 10 to 42%. However, the Type I error rate using FO-approximation increased drastically as both between-subject and residual variance increased. For example, the Type I error rate using FO-approximation increased from about 0.06–0.15 when the between-subject variability increased from 10 to 52%. As the number of observations per subject increased from two to 19, the Type I error rate using FO-approximation decreased to nominal values, whereas FOCE-I remained near nominal values throughout.

In their second simulation, they examined the Type I error rate when a covariate influenced residual variability, i.e., residual variability was partitioned into two groups. FOCE-I and FO-approximation had a Type I error rate of about 0.075 and 0.11, respectively, with two observations per subject (collected at 1.75 and 7 h after administration) and a residual error of 10%. When residual error increased to 31%, the Type I error rate for FOCE-I decreased to the nominal value, but increased to 0.16 with FO-approximation. With 19 observations per subject, the Type I error rate for both FO-approximation and FOCE-I was unchanged as residual error increased from 10 to 31%, but FOCE-I remained near 0.05.

In their third simulation, they examined the Type I error rate for inclusion of a false covariance term between CL and V in a 1-compartment model. FOCE-I Type I error rates were dependent on the number of samples collected per subject (more samples tended to decrease the Type I error rate), degree of residual variability (as residual variability increased so did the Type I error rate), and whether the residual error was defined using an exponential or proportional model (exponential residual error models always produced larger Type I errors than proportional error models). With 100 subjects, two observations per subject (at 1.75 and 7 h after dosing), BSV of ~31%, and residual variability of 10%, the Type I error rate was 0.05 using a nominal expected rate of 0.05 under FOCE-I. The Type I error rate increased to 0.08 when the number of subjects were decreased to 25, but deceased to 0.06 when the number of individuals increased to 1000. When the number of observations per subject increased to four (collected at 1, 6, 12, and 18 h) the Type I error rate decreased to the nominal value of 0.05. FO-approximation failed to minimize successfully in most instances with two observations per subject, but with 19 observations per subject, even though minimization was often successful, Type I errors were generally elevated.

In their last simulation, the authors examined the Type I error rate when a false variance term was included in the model. In this instance, the boundary issue related to testing diagonal variance terms would be expected to apply and the LRT would not be expected to follow a chi-squared distribution with a single degree of freedom (Stram and Lee, 1994). The authors generated concentration–time data with volume of distribution fixed to a constant having no variability. They then fit a model having V treated as a log-normal random effect. The Type I error rate with FOCE-I was slightly lower than expected when residual error was ~10%, regardless of how residual error was modeled. But when residual error was increased and the residual error was modeled using an exponential residual error (which was the same error model used to generate the data), Type I error rates increased significantly. In fact, Type I error rates were greater than 0.85 when residual error was ~42% and an exponential residual error model was used. In contrast, Type I error rates remained near their nominal value when a proportional residual error model was used (which was not even how the data were generated). No effect of number of observations per subject, number of subjects, or residual error magnitude was observed when a large number of subjects was combined with a large residual error under FOCE-I, but a significant effect on how the residual error was specified was observed.

In summary, the Type I error rate from using the LRT to test for the inclusion of a covariate in a model was inflated when the data were heteroscedastic and an inappropriate estimation method was used. Type I error rates with FOCE-I were in general near nominal values under most conditions studied and suggest that in most cases FOCE-I should be the estimation method of choice. In contrast, Type I error rates with FO-approximation and FOCE were very dependent on and sensitive to many factors, including number of samples per subject, number of subjects, and how the residual error was defined. The combination of high residual variability with sparse sampling was a particularly disastrous combination using

FO-approximation. Type I error rates for testing the inclusion of a variance component in the model were different depending on how the residual error was modeled. Type I error rates were generally higher, and sometimes considerably higher than expected, when an exponential residual error model was used. Slightly lower Type I error rates were observed when a proportional residual error model was used, an effect possibly due to the boundary issues regarding the use of the LRT and the testing of variance components. The authors conclude that the LRT is not reliable when testing the statistical submodel using FO-approximation, but that FOCE-I is reliable when the data per subject are not too sparse and the residuals are normally distributed.

Besides FO-approximation, FOCE (with and without interaction), and Laplacian estimation there are two other lesser known options available with NONMEM: the hybrid method and centering option. The hybrid method is just a hybrid between FO-approximation and FOCE. In essence, some elements of the random effects are set equal to zero (the FO-approximation algorithm), while the remaining elements are set equal to the Bayes posterior mode of the random effects (the FOCE algorithm). One advantage to the hybrid method is that it may produce estimates as good as the FOCE method but at a fraction of the computation time. There is little experience in the literature concerning the use of this algorithm.

If, after model development is complete and the model still shows systematic bias in the model fit, it may be that the model is misspecified. One assumption of the random effects is that they have zero mean, i.e., they are centered around zero. Whenever one of the conditional estimation algorithms is used within NONMEM, an output of the mean conditional estimate for each random effect, along with a p-value testing the null hypothesis that the mean is zero, is produced. Examination of these p-values may help identify random effects that are not centered. If many of the random effects are significantly different than zero, a centered model may be more appropriate. Caution should be exercised, however, because in testing many independent random effects "p-happens," i.e., with many independent null hypotheses being tested simultaneously the chances of having at least one significant p-value is very high. For example, with a 2-compartment model having five random effects the probability of at least one of those conditional means rejecting the null hypothesis may be as high as 23%. When using FOCE or the Laplacian estimation with centering, the p-values associated with the null hypothesis of the conditional effects may increase. In the worst case, centered models show no difference in their estimates between uncentered models, but may significantly improve a model fit in the best case. Beal and Sheiner (1998) stress that centering should not be used routinely. Like the hybrid method there is little published literature using the centering option. Because there have been no systematic studies comparing these two lesser known methods to the more well known estimation algorithms; their use should be done with great caution.

In summary, the current state of the art is to use FO-approximation for the first few runs to identify and correct any errors in the data set and control streams. Also, FO-approximation provides good initial estimates for more computationally intensive algorithms. Thereafter, conditional estimation (usually FOCE-I) is usually used for method development, unless the model is developed not using the built-in functions within NONMEM. In other words, if the user has to develop the model using user-written differential equations, even a modest size data set with the conditional estimation algorithms may lead to prohibitive run times. Therefore, with these user-written models FO-approximation is usually the algorithm of choice. Perhaps at the final step in model development then a conditional estimation algorithm is used to obtain more accurate parameter estimates.

INCORPORATING CONCOMITANT MEDICATIONS INTO THE MODEL

The goal of including any covariate into a model is to reduce BSV and improve the predictability of the model. Drugs taken in addition to the drug of interest are called concomitant medications (ConMeds) and are considered extrinsic covariates. How ConMeds are dealt with in a PopPK analysis is unique relative to other covariates in that they are often time varying and a ubiquitous part of any Phase 3 study. In most Phase 1 studies, ConMeds are prohibited and PopPK analyses based on this data are not confounded by any potential pharmacokinetic interactions with other medications. In contrast, it is almost impossible to stop a patient from taking a ConMed in a Phase 3 study. It is entirely possible that some yet unidentified ConMed will have a clinically significant drug interaction with the drug of interest. A well designed PopPK study can be used to identify such drug–drug interactions. So, dealing with ConMeds becomes an important issue in any PopPK analysis.

One approach to handling ConMeds is to simply classify whether any ConMed is present or absent, regardless of the drug, and then include this binary covariate in an analysis. Interpreting a significant result then is difficult because what exactly does the result mean. That *any* ConMed affects clearance, for example? Rarely is

this approach successful because all the subjects in a study may take a ConMed at some point in time and the entire database will be coded as 'Yes.' Also this approach suffers from low statistical power at detecting anything real. Hence, simple Yes/No coding of ConMed data cannot be recommended. A modification of this approach may be found in oncology in which ConMeds can be coded based on prior therapy. Subjects are coded as no prior therapy (0), minimally pretreated (1), and heavily pretreated (2). While not specific for any one drug, this approach has some appeal.

If one does decide to test for interactions with Con-Meds, then it must be decided if testing will be done for specific drugs or groups of drugs. Testing for specific drugs is often done by creating a covariate and assigning it a value of '0' until the ConMed is administered, at which point the value is switched to '1' and remains at '1' until the end of study. The covariate can then be treated as a categorical covariate in a PopPK analysis and the inclusion of the covariate in the model is tested for whether it significantly improves the model's goodness of fit. Many drug interactions are identified in this manner. This approach, while successful, is not without its problems due to the time of ConMed administration relative to sample collection. More about this will be discussed shortly. A modification to testing for a specific drug is instead of coding as '0' or '1,' group the ConMed into different dose levels, and attempt to quantify the dose-pharmacokinetic interaction effect.

ConMeds can also be classified into groups by either therapeutic area or by mechanism of interaction. For example, many antiepileptic drugs are known to be metabolic inducers. One could then classify whether the ConMed was an antiepileptic or not and use this as a covariate in an analysis. Using such an approach, Yukawa et al. (2002) classified ConMeds into '0' if the ConMed was phenobarbital, phenytoin, or carbamazepine or '1' if none of the above. PopPK analysis of 218 Japanese subjects revealed that these three ConMeds increased haloperidol clearance by 32%. Of course, this approach assumes that these three inducers all have the same time course and effect on the pharmacokinetic parameter that they affect, which may not be the case.

Alternatively, one could group ConMeds into mechanism of action. If a drug is metabolized by cytochrome p450 (CYP), then one such grouping is by CYP isozyme, metabolic pathway or interaction. For example, doxepin is metabolized by CYP 2C19 to desmethyldoxepin. Meyer-Barner et al. (2002) classified concomitant medications into three groups: substrates of CYP 3A4, CYP 2D6, CYP 2C19, CYP 2C9, CYP 2C8, CYP 1A2, CYP 2A6, CYP 2B6, CYP 1A1 and CYP 1B1; inducers of CYP 2E1, CYP 3A4, CYP 3A1, CYP 3A2, CYP 1A2, and CYP 2B6; and inhibitors of

CYP 3A4, CYP 1A1, CYP 2C9, CUP 2A6, CYP 2D6, and CYP 2C19. PopPK analysis of 114 patients resulted in the identification of CYP inhibitors as significantly reducing doxepin and desmethyldoxepin clearance by about 15%.

Another confounding factor in the inclusion of ConMed data in an analysis is the time when the ConMed was administered relative to administration of the drug of interest. For example, suppose a ConMed was taken days or weeks prior to the collection of a pharmacokinetic sample. Under the coding scheme just discussed, which is one of the more common coding schemes seen in the literature, one would treat the covariate as '0' until the ConMed is taken, at which time the covariate becomes '1' and remains at '1' thereafter. Hence, at the time the pharmacokinetic sample was taken the ConMed would be coded as '1' or present. This coding may be misleading. If the ConMed was a competitive inhibitor of the drug's metabolism and ConMed concentrations were far below the inhibition constant at the time the pharmacokinetic sample was collected, then the effect of the ConMed would be negligible. The ConMed would have no influence on the drug's pharmacokinetics. Clearly, the problem with this approach is that it assumes the ConMed's effect remains in effect forever. What is needed is a modification to switch the covariate back to '0' at some time after the ConMed is taken, unless the ConMed is taken again.

One such approach is to define time windows around drug administration or blood sample collection and only if the ConMed is taken in the time window is the presence of the ConMed noted. For example, if neutralizing antacids, such as Maalox® or Tums®, are known to affect the absorption of the drug, then a window of ±2 h around the time of drug administration is created. If the ConMed is taken within ±2 h of drug administration, the ConMed is coded as '1'; otherwise, the ConMed is coded as '0.' If the ConMed is taken 10 h after drug administration at a time when a blood sample is collected, this sample would be coded as '0' because the drug is already absorbed and the ConMed would have no effect on its kinetics at this point in time. In contrast, suppose the ConMed is phenobarbital, which is a known rapid and long acting enzyme inducer. One might set up a window of a week after the ConMed was taken, so that any blood sample collected in that time is coded as '1'; otherwise, it is coded as '0.'

But this is where it again becomes fuzzy. Taking a single dose of phenobarbital does not instantly cause drug induction nor does a single dose affect metabolic induction to the same degree as repeated administration. So how should these facts be taken into account? One might try to recode the variable into k-levels denoting the various levels of effect. For example, '1' might be

single dose of ConMed, '2' might be multiple dose of ConMed, and '0' might be no ConMed.

Lastly, one other approach to handling ConMeds is to do nothing and not include any ConMeds in an analysis. Many times this is the approach taken by analysts since trying to find important unidentified drug interaction is like trying to find a needle in a haystack. In doing so, however, one accepts that not including an important covariate in a model may lead to larger variance components in the model. Sometimes, in doing an analysis in which ConMeds are not specified as covariates, a subpopulation is identified based on the empirical Bayes estimates (EBEs) of pharmacokinetic parameters or in the concentration–time profiles themselves. In examining those subjects in the subpopulation one may find that they all received the same ConMed. This may cause an analyst to go back, examine all the subjects who received the ConMed, and then include the ConMed in the analysis as a covariate.

But, does lack of a drug interaction in a PopPK analysis mean that the drug interaction does not occur? Of course not. Proving a negative cannot be done. However, by examining the power of the study, one could have some confidence in the conclusion if statistical power was high enough to detect an interaction, but an interaction was not actually detected. More will be discussed on this topic in the section on Experimental Design Issues in Phase 3. In contrast, detecting a drug interaction raises the question, "is the effect real?" Further studies may be required to confirm such an effect or, in the case of a new drug, the sponsor may choose to include the interaction on the label for safety. An example of the latter is the pharmacokinetic interaction between dolasetron and atenolol identified using PopPK analysis which was later reported on the package insert for dolasetron.

On a practical note, extra effort in the collection of the type of ConMed should to be taken for uniformity of spelling or drug name when drug interactions are tested for by specific drug or group. For example, in a Phase 3 study the author participated in, it was found that acetaminophen was coded in the database as acetaminophen, acetominophen, acetamenophen, paracetamol, and Tylenol. Of course, all four were the same thing, but when the database was built, programs like SAS will not recognize this as such, unless specifically coded for by the programmer. Hence, it is good practice to have someone, preferably a pharmacist, review the ConMeds database for consistency and uniformity of drug names prior to database creation so that all ConMeds are accurately accounted for. Second, it should be noted that in reporting analyses involving ConMeds exactly how ConMeds are coded is very important for reproducibility. Many reports in the literature indicate that a

ConMed was tested as a covariate, but does not indicate what time window, if any, was used.

INCORPORATING LABORATORY TESTS INTO THE MODEL

Laboratory tests, which are surrogate markers for physiological status, are intrinsic covariates that can be altered by other intrinsic and extrinsic factors. Incorporating laboratory test values into a model is done the same as any other continuous type covariate. But, there are a number of unique issues involved in dealing with laboratory values in PopPK models. First, laboratory values are not time-invariant. Their value may change during the course of a study due to disease progression, other illnesses, the drug itself, the presence of other drugs, dietary changes, regression towards the mean, or by simple random variation, to list just a few causes. Because the covariate may change with time, covariate screening using regression techniques may not be possible. Recall that most regression-based methods regress the empirical Bayes estimate of a parameter against the covariate, a 1:1 relationship. But when the covariate varies over time, which value of the covariate should be regressed against the EBE? One could use the baseline, the mode, or the median, but this approach may be insensitive at detecting a significant relationship. With time-varying covariates, the best approach is not to use regression-based covariate screening and to test the significance of a time-varying covariate directly in the model by performing the LRT on the full and reduced models or use some other measure to see if the goodness of fit of the model is improved when the covariate is added.

Two often encountered situations are where laboratory tests are not collected at the same time as pharmacokinetic samples or when laboratory tests are collected at the same time as the pharmacokinetic samples but are missing for whatever reason. In both cases, the covariate information is missing. Missing data is a fact of life in any population analysis that regulatory authorities recognize. The FDA Guidance on PopPK (1999) states that "missing data will not automatically invalidate an analysis provided a good-faith effort is made to capture the missing data and adequate documentation is made regarding why the data are unavailable." But unlike age or race, missing laboratory tests are often not completely missing for a subject, rather data are only partially missing. Further, because population studies often have repeated measures in the same individual the usual methods for dealing with missing data, such as those presented in the chapter on Linear Models and Regression, are no longer entirely valid. Handling missing data

in a longitudinal study will be dealt with in a later section in this chapter and the reader is referred there for further discussion on this point.

Laboratory tests may also show a high degree of correlation amongst each other. For example, aspartate aminotransferase (AST) is correlated with alanine aminotransferase (ALT) with a correlation coefficient of about 0.6 and total protein is correlated with albumin, also with a correlation coefficient of about 0.6. Caution needs to be exercised when two or more correlated laboratory values enter in the covariate model simultaneously because of the possible collinearity that may occur (Bonate, 1999). Like in the linear regression case, inclusion of correlated covariates may result in an unstable model leading to inflated standard errors and deflated Type I error rate.

Sometimes, rather than treating the covariate as a continuous variable, the covariate will be categorized and the categorical variable will be used in the model instead of the original value. For example, de Maat et al. (2002) in a population analysis of nevirapine categorized baseline laboratory markers of hepatic function into dichotomous covariates. Patients were coded as '1' if their laboratory value was 1.5 times higher than the upper limit of normal and '0' otherwise. Patients with an aspartate aminotransferase 1.5 times higher than normal had a 13% decrease in nevirapine clearance than patients with normal values.

Another example of categorization might be classifying the covariate into severity of disease state. For example, in a PopPK analysis of quinidine in 60 subjects with arrhythmia, Fattinger et al. (1991) classified subjects having a bilirubin more than 1.8 mg/dL and a prothrombin time less than 60% as having severe liver disease. Subjects who had values outside the normal range and did not meet the criteria for severe liver disease were classified as moderate liver disease. Otherwise, subjects were classified as normal. Classifying subjects in this manner, and including this covariate into the model, resulted in a significant improvement in goodness of fit. Another example along these lines might be classifying creatinine clearance into normal, mild, moderate, or severe renal failure and then using this categorical variable in the covariate model.

In practice, using a normal chemistry panel and complete blood count it is not unusual to have 30 potential covariates, everything from sodium ion concentration to alkaline phosphatase activity. Early in PopPK analyses it was not unusual to screen every single covariate for their impact on the model. But a model might end up having a volume of distribution as a function of chloride ion concentration or clearance that is a function of glucose concentration. Physiologically, these covariates are nonsensical. Ideally at the end of model development you want a model that is interpretable with covariates that make physiologic sense. For example, alkaline phosphatase is a marker of hepatic function and if alkaline phosphatase ends up as a covariate on clearance then the interpretation is easy—hepatic function, as measured by alkaline phosphatase, influences clearance. But if something unusual, like sodium ion concentration influences volume of distribution, then the interpretation is difficult and may make no physiologic sense. Hence, the current state is to test only those covariates that make physiologic sense a priori. So, for example, markers of renal or hepatic function (Table 8.3) will be tested as covariates on clearance, while total protein, albumin, and α_1-acid glycoprotein will be tested as covariates on volume of distribution.

When dealing with time-varying laboratory tests the issue of which value should be modeled often arises. For example, one could use the baseline value, the change from baseline value, or the value itself in the model. Obviously using the baseline value assumes that the value does not change once treatment is initiated, i.e., it removes the time-varying nature of the value. While sometimes it is believed that using change from baseline or percent change from baseline will remove any statistical regression towards the mean; this is not the case (Bonate, 2000). Most analyses use the value itself in the analysis and do not bother with either baseline or change from baseline. While laboratory tests are subject to regression towards the mean, this effect is often ignored in an analysis.

Lastly, one issue that sometimes arises, not during model development, but during development of the data set used for model building, is when multiple studies are combined. First, all medical centers have a clinical chemistry laboratory and, as such, each laboratory establishes their own "normal reference ranges." For example, the normal range for bilirubin may be 0.4–0.7 mg/dL at one lab, but 0.5–0.8 mg/dL at another. Although laboratories attempt to establish a high degree of reliability across other labs, the value obtained at one lab might not be the same as at another. When combining data from many study centers there may be laboratory differences. But is

this difference of significance and what can be done about it? The long and short of it is, there is nothing that can be done. The analyst must accept the data as is. But, and this especially applies to when studies are combined from the United States and outside the United States, the units that laboratories report data may be different. For example, the United States tends to report concentration data as mass/unit volume, e.g., mg/dL, whereas the rest of the world tends to use moles/unit volume. So when combining data from many studies it is imperative that the same units be used throughout. A slightly more subtle difference may be in reporting scientific notation. For example, a typical white blood cell count may be 6.0×10^9 cells/L. Some companies store their laboratory data as two variables, value and unit, each within their own study specific database. In this example, one study database may store the value as '6.0' with units '10^9 cells/L,' whereas another study database may store the value as '6.0×10^9' and the units as 'cells/L.' So, a simple merging of values across databases may result in values ranging from very small to large numbers in the thousands. A quick check of the summary statistics (mean, minimum, maximum, and coefficient of variation) for a lab analyte will often reveal whether there are merging errors as the coefficient of variation and range will be very large. Of course, one way to avoid these issues altogether is to use a central laboratory, i.e., all laboratory measurements are done at one central location, which is often done in Phase 3 studies already, so that units and reporting are kept consistent.

In summary, some general guidelines can be recommended in handling laboratory values. Laboratory tests should be identified a priori based on their physiological relevance attached to certain pharmacokinetic parameters and then systematically tested in the model for actual significance. Any data merging should be checked for consistency of units and values by visual inspection or examination of the summary statistics. The data set should also be examined for any missing data. Any missing data should be imputed and clearly identified in the report. There should be a listing of which values were imputed, the reason for imputation, the method of imputation, and the imputed value. With these guidelines in mind, although some may question the particulars of an analysis, the results will conform to the spirit of regulatory guidelines and be accepted by reviewers.

Table 8.3 Laboratory tests of hepatic and renal function.

Hepatic function	Renal function
• Albumin	• Creatinine clearance
• Prothrombin time	• Serum creatinine
• Bilirubin	• Serum urea (BUN)
• Alkaline phosphatase	• Urine volume
• Gamma glutamyltransferase (GGT)	• Urine urea
• Aspartate aminotransferase (AST)	• Urine sodium
• Alanine aminotransferase (AST)	• Urine protein
	• Urine glucose
	• Hematuria

INCORPORATING WEIGHT AND ITS VARIANTS INTO THE MODEL

Weight, an intrinsic covariate, is probably the most frequently identified covariate in a PopPK analysis. All structural model parameters, except absorption related parameters, may be influenced by a person's weight. That weight is often identified as an important covariate is not surprising. Since many physiological parameters, such as organ size, organ blood flow, and metabolic rate are dependent on body weight, then pharmacokinetic parameters that are dependent on blood flow or organ size should also be a function of body weight. This concept was introduced in previous chapters in regards to allometric scaling.

Weight has many surrogates, such as body surface area (BSA) and body mass index (BMI), any of which may be used in a model. In general, it is best to use a consistent marker for weight throughout an analysis. For example, while modeling clearance as a function of BSA and volume of distribution as a function of actual weight may result in a better model, modeling both clearance and volume of distribution as a function of either weight or BSA alone results in a more harmonious model.

The most frequently used surrogate for weight is BSA and there are many different equations that can be used to calculate a person's BSA. In the absence of height measurements, Livingston and Lee (2001) developed the following equations for BSA

$$\text{BSA} (\text{m}^2) = 0.1173 (\text{Weight in kg})^{0.6466} \quad (8.2)$$

for patients weighing more than 10 kg but less than 250 kg and

$$\text{BSA} (\text{m}^2) = 0.1037 (\text{Weight in kg})^{0.6724} \quad (8.3)$$

for patients weighing less than 10 kg. Given a person's height and weight, more complex equations can be developed, all of which are based on the form

$$\text{BSA} = c(\text{Height})^{a_1} (\text{Weight})^{a_2} \quad (8.4)$$

where c, a_1, and a_2 are constants. There is no evidence to suggest that these more complex equations using both height and weight are more accurate than Livingston and Lee's equation. The rationale for such an equation relates to the area of a sphere or cylinder and although the human body is clearly neither of these, the approximation is a useful one. Equation (8.4) can be linearized by Ln–Ln transformation

$$\text{Ln} (\text{BSA}) = a_0 + a_1 \times \text{Ln}(\text{Height}) + a_2 \times \text{Ln}(\text{Weight}) \quad (8.5)$$

where $a_0 = \text{Ln}(c)$, which will be important later on. Specific equations include DuBois and DuBois (1916)

$$\text{BSA} (\text{m}^2) = 0.007184 (\text{Height in cm})^{0.725} (\text{Weight in kg})^{0.425} \quad (8.6)$$

Gehan and George (1970)

$$\text{BSA} (\text{m}^2) = 0.0235 (\text{Height in cm})^{0.42246} (\text{Weight in kg})^{0.51456} \quad (8.7)$$

Mosteller (1987)

$$\text{BSA} (\text{m}^2) = \sqrt{\frac{(\text{Height in cm}) (\text{Weight in kg})}{3600}} \quad (8.8)$$

and Haycock (1978)

$$\text{BSA} (\text{m}^2) = 0.024265 (\text{Height in cm})^{0.3964} (\text{Weight in kg})^{0.5378}. \quad (8.9)$$

Periodically throughout the literature the validity of the DuBois and DuBois equation, which is the most commonly used predictor in medicinal practice, is challenged since it was based on only nine subjects. Gehan and George (1970) raised this argument and when applied to 401 subjects found that the DuBois and DuBois equation overpredicted BSA by about 15% in about 15% of the cases. Wang, Moss, and Thisted (1992) in an examination of 395 subjects, including neonates and pregnant women, compared the precision of 15 BSA prediction formulas and found that the DuBois and DuBois equation underpredicted BSA by about 5%, slightly more in infants. No differences between age or sex were observed in the study and they concluded that the degree of underprediction with the DuBois and DuBois equation is likely to be clinically irrelevant. The DuBois and DuBois equation continues to be the most commonly used predictor of BSA due to its long history of use, but because of its simplicity the Mosteller equation is being increasingly used instead.

Which equation to use in an analysis is for all practical purposes moot since all methods produce equivalent BSA estimates. Bailey and Briars (1996) asked the question "Why do all these formulas produce equivalent results when their constant terms [i.e., c, a_1, and a_2 in Eq. (8.4)] are so different?" They first analyzed the 401 subjects Gehan and George used to produce their equation and noted that height and weight were highly correlated. Ln-transformed height was a linear function of Ln-transformed weight

$$\text{Ln} (\text{Height}) = 3.489 + 0.396 \times \text{Ln} (\text{Weight}). \quad (8.10)$$

When Eq. (8.10) was inserted into Eq. (8.5), Ln-transformed BSA could be determined solely using weight

$$Ln\,(BSA) = d_0 + d_1 \times Ln\,(Weight) \qquad (8.11)$$

where $d_0 = a_0 + 3.489a_1$ and $d_1 = a_2 + 0.396a_1$. In essence, the relationship linking height and weight to BSA was reduced to a relationship between weight and BSA. Bailey and Briars then computed the estimates of d_0 and d_1 for the various BSA formula. The results are shown in Table 8.4. Despite a large difference in constant terms, the values of d_0 and d_1 were almost exactly the same. The reason then all these equation have such discordant constant terms is parameter instability due to high collinearity between height and weight. When reduced to a more stable model, all these BSA equations are equivalent and any can be used with no difference in the outcome of an analysis.

Other surrogates for weight are lean body weight (LBW), ideal body weight, and BMI. Lean body weight (LBW), which has nothing to do with ideal weight, can be calculated in males using

$$LBW = 1.10\,(Weight\ in\ kg) - \frac{128\,(Weight\ in\ kg)^2}{[100\,(Height\ in\ m)]^2} \qquad (8.12)$$

and in females using

$$LBW = 1.07\,(Weight\ in\ kg) - \frac{148\,(Weight\ in\ kg)^2}{[100\,(Height\ in\ m)]^2}. \qquad (8.13)$$

LBW is the weight of everything in your body except fat. Examples of where LBW was identified as an important covariate in a PopPK analysis can be found with lithium (Jermain, Crismon, and Martin, 1991) and carbamazepine (Martin III, Crismon, and Godley, 1991). Use of LBW as a size descriptor has been criticized when the subject is morbidly obese ($> 30\,kg/m^2$) because such estimates tend to underestimate the subject's true LBW by overestimating the subject's percent body fat (Green and Duffull, 2002).

The second surrogate, ideal body weight (IBW) in kg, can be calculated in males using

$$IBW = 52\,kg + 1.9\,kg\ for\ every\ inch\ 5\,feet \qquad (8.14)$$

and in females using

$$IBW = 49\,kg + 1.7\,kg\ for\ every\ inch\ over\ 5\,feet. \qquad (8.15)$$

Benezet et al. (1997) presented an interesting use of IBW in a PopPK analysis. They showed that using the mean of IBW and actual body weight resulted in better predictability of carboplatin clearance than actual body weight or IBW alone. In fact, IBW alone underpredicted carboplatin clearance while weight alone overpredicted carboplatin clearance. A rationale for this unusual model was not provided suffice to say that others had used similar models (Sawyer et al., 1983). While the combined model may have lead to greater predictability than either weight or IBW alone, this unusual model has credibility problems in the absence of a good physiologic rationale. Lastly, BMI is defined as

$$BMI\left(\frac{kg}{m^2}\right) = \frac{Weight\ in\ kg}{[Height\ in\ m]^2}. \qquad (8.16)$$

Normal ranges are from 20 to $26.99\,kg/m^2$ and apply to both males and females. Rarely is BMI used as a covariate. BSA is more commonly used.

Like laboratory tests, sometimes weight or its surrogates are categorized and the categories used in the model instead. For example, a BMI $\leq 25\,mg/m^2$ would be classified as normal, a BMI between 25 and $29.9\,kg/m^2$ would be "overweight," and a BMI $> 30\,kg/m^2$ would be "obese" (National Institutes of Health, 1998). In this manner, the pharmacokinetics between normal and obese subjects can be compared. Examples of the use of obesity in a PopPK analysis are seen with the neuromuscular blockers, doxacurium, and cisatracurium. Schmith et al. (1997) reported in a PopPD analysis of 408 subjects who were administered doxacurium that obesity, defined as actual body weight $\geq 30\%$ above IBW, significantly affected the sensitivity of individuals to the drug. In a different analysis of 241 surgical subjects who were administered cisatracurium, obesity (using the same definition) was shown to decrease clearance by 12%, a clinically irrelevant change.

Weight is so important a covariate that in models involving children, infants, or neonates weight is often built into the model from the very beginning.

Table 8.4 Values of constant terms for various body surface area formulas.

Equation	a_0	a_1	a_2	d_0	d_1
Du Bois and Du Bois	−4.936	0.725	0.425	−2.41	0.71
Gehan and George	−3.751	0.442	0.515	−2.28	0.68
Haycock	−3.719	0.396	0.538	−2.33	0.69
Mosteller	−4.094	0.500	0.500	−2.35	0.70

Reprinted from Bailey and Briars (1996) with permission.

Weight is treated as an a priori covariate, regardless of whether its inclusion improves the model goodness of fit, for two reasons. First, almost without exception, studies in pediatric populations have shown weight to affect clearance and volume of distribution terms. Second, extrapolations outside the weight range used to develop the model tends to lead to unrealistic predictions.

In pediatric studies, weight is treated like any other continuous variable in a covariate model and can be modeled using either a linear function or power function, although theoretically a power function makes more physiologic sense. Of course, assuming a power of 1 reduces a power function to a linear function. In discussions with experts in this area, the power terms in the model related to weight are typically not treated as estimable parameters. When they are treated as estimable parameters, the values are usually between 0.75 and 1 anyway. Hence, these parameters are usually fixed at 0.75 for clearance terms and 1.0 for volume of distribution terms. As an example, Anderson et al. (2002) presented the PopPK of acetaminophen in premature neonates and infants. Data from six previously published pediatric studies were combined into a single analysis of 238 subjects ranging in age from birth to 64 weeks. A 1-compartment model was used to characterize the data. Clearance (CL) and volume of distribution (V) were modeled as

$$CL = TVCL \left(\frac{Weight}{70 \, kg} \right)^{0.75} \qquad (8.17)$$

$$V = TVV \left(\frac{Weight}{70 \, kg} \right)^{1.0} \qquad (8.18)$$

where TVCL and TVV were the typical clearance and volume of distribution values for the population. What was interesting about this analysis was that weight was scaled to a 70 kg adult, even though all patients weighed less than 7 kg. Once weight was included in the model, age could be reliably examined since models with weight excluded tend to "blur" the age effect (Capparelli, personal communication). Other examples of a priori weight models in pediatric populations include paracetamol (Anderson, Woollard, and Holford, 2000), zidovudine (Mirochnick et al., 1998), amphotericin B (Nath et al., 2001), ciprofloxacin (Schaefer et al., 1996), and acyclovir (Tod et al., 2001).

In summary, weight and its surrogates are important covariates in PopPK analyses. In pediatric studies, weight is often included in the base model as a continuous variable right from the start. In adults, any of the measures of weight can be used as covariates in a model as long as model inclusion improves the goodness of fit and is physiologically plausible. Good modeling practices dictate, however, that whatever variable is used, it is used consistently throughout the model.

INCORPORATING A FOOD EFFECT INTO THE MODEL

Food, an extrinsic covariate, has been shown to affect the pharmacokinetics of many orally administered drugs, both in a positive and negative manner, through its effect on the absorption process (Singh, 1999). In most Phase 1 studies, drug administration is done in the fasted state, whereas drug administration may be in the either fasted or fed state in Phase 2 or 3. Hence, testing of a 'food effect' is commonly done in studies of a mixed nature where the drug can be given either with or without food. As might be surmised, the simplest method for testing of food effect is to create a new covariate (e.g., FOOD) that applies to each dosing interval where samples are collected such that the covariate is coded as either '1' if the drug is administered with food or '0' if the drug is not given with food. The covariate can then be applied to either the absorption rate constant, lag-time, or relative bioavailability (F1), e.g.,

$$F1 = \theta_1(1 + \theta_2 \times FOOD) \qquad (8.19)$$

where θ_1 is the baseline relative bioavailability to the dosing compartment in the absence of food (FOOD = 0) and $1 + \theta_2$ is the proportional multiplier in the presence of food (FOOD = 1).

Of course, like the issue of drug interactions, the timing of when the meal is given is an issue. For solid foodstuff, the half-life of stomach emptying is about 90–120 min (West, 1985). So, one option is to code the covariate as '1' if the drug is taken within 90–120 min of a meal; otherwise the covariate is coded as '0.' For example, suppose for the same subject that pharmacokinetic samples are collected on Day 1 and 5 of a five day dosing regimen and that food was given 1 h prior to drug administration on Day 5, but not on Day 1. Then a new covariate called FOOD can be created which is equal to '1' on Day 1 but '0' on Day 5. In this manner, Van Wart et al. (2004) showed that garenoxacin, a new fluoroquinolone antibiotic, does not exhibit a food effect. Coding is more difficult if food is taken after drug administration, but whatever coding scheme is applied must be consistently applied and specified in the data analysis plan.

The type of meal that is administered may also affect the pharmacokinetics of a drug. For example, a light snack might have no effect but a heavy, fatty meal might. Hence, an alternative coding scheme, instead of '0/1,' would be to use a categorical scheme where '1' might be a light meal or breakfast, '2' might be lunch, and '3' might be dinner. Another method might be to break the meals down into a series of dichotomous variables, one for each meal. Bonate (2003) used such a scheme to quantify the food effect after placebo administration on QTc interval prolongation. He further treated the food effect as not an 'either/or' proposition but as an exponential function

$$QTc = \begin{cases} \theta_1 + \theta_2 \exp(-\theta_5 t) & \text{if breakfast} \\ \theta_1 + \theta_3 \exp(-\theta_5 t) & \text{if lunch} \\ \theta_1 + \theta_4 \exp(-\theta_5 t) & \text{if dinner} \end{cases}. \quad (8.20)$$

In this manner, the food effect increases to its maximal immediately after a meal but then declines in an exponential manner. At baseline (θ_1), QTc intervals were 389 ms but increased by 10.6, 12.5, and 14.7 ms after breakfast (θ_2), lunch (θ_3), and dinner (θ_4). Further the rate of decline in food effect was estimated at 0.4 msec/h (θ_5). Hence, the heavier the meal the larger the increase in QTc intervals.

INCORPORATING PATIENT AGE INTO THE MODEL

Age, an intrinsic covariate, is commonly identified in population analyses as being important since many physiological processes change with age. For example, Gilmore et al. (1992) found that propranolol intrinsic clearance in elderly subjects greater than 62-years-old was 30% lower than in subjects 25–33 years old and that the elimination half-life was two- to three-times longer in the elderly than in the young. The mechanism for difference has been attributed to reduced hepatic blood flow in the elderly. Clearly, understanding age-related changes in pharmacokinetics and pharmacodynamics is important from a therapeutic perspective. For recent reviews on the mechanisms around such age-related changes, the reader is referred to Mangoni and Jackson (2004) who focus on changes in the elderly and Loebstein, Vohra, and Koren (2000) who focus on age-related changes in children.

Often, age is identified as important when the age range in the database is large. Data pooled from Phase 1 studies, where the typical age is from 18 years to the mid-40s, has insufficient signal to identify age as a covariate since the range is so narrow. But, when data from Phase 1 is pooled with data from elderly subjects or pediatric patients, then the signal is usually large enough to detect an age effect, if it is important.

Age can be treated as either a continuous variable in the model, wherein it is typically centered around the mean or median, or it can be treated as a categorical variable. When age is treated as a continuous variable in adults, its value is typically an integer. So if someone was

32 years and 11 months old, they would be treated as simply 32 years old. This truncation is not problematic for adults. But truncation error becomes significant as patients get younger and younger so that age is usually not truncated with pediatric patients. Indeed, for the very young, a few months may have a significant impact on the pharmacokinetics of a drug.

Categorization of age can be done using regulatory documents as guidelines. The (1994) ICH Guidance on studies in pediatric patients (E11) breaks down pediatric patients into four groups:

1. Preterm newborn infants;
2. Term newborn infants (0–27 days);
3. Infant and toddlers (28 days to 23 months);
4. Children (2–11 years);
5. Adolescents (11 years to < 16–18 years, depending on region).

Subjects older than 18 years old are expected to have similar pharmacokinetics—pharmacodynamics as adults. It should be noted that the FDA uses slightly different categories for pediatric patients (United States Department of Health and Human Services et al., 1998). The ICH Guidance on Studies in Support of Special Populations: Geriatrics (E7) FDA Guidance on Drugs Likely to be Used in the Elderly (1994) defines an elderly subject as 65 years or older. Although it may appear reasonable to model pediatric or elderly data using dummy variables based on these categories, this approach may result in loss of information following categorization. Nevertheless, it is common to see this categorization approach used in comparing elderly to young subjects, but it is uncommon in modeling pediatric data. More often, age is treated as a continuous variable after controlling for weight in pediatric studies.

In adults, age is defined based on partpartum age, i.e., time at birth to the date of first dose administration or date of randomization in a study. Normal gestation is defined as 40 weeks with term infants being born after 38–42 weeks gestation. Gestational age is defined as the length of time from conception to delivery. When modeling data from neonates, term newborn infants, and even up to infants and toddlers, postpartum age may not accurately represent the physiological status of the patient if the child was born prematurely (less than 36 weeks gestation) or preterm (36–37 weeks gestation). For this reason, postconceptual age, which is the gestational age plus postpartum age, may be a more accurate reflection of physiological age than postpartum age. Anderson et al. (2002) showed that postconceptual age was an important covariate in predicting acetaminophen apparent volume of distribution and apparent oral clearance in premature neonates and infants. Also, gestational age itself may be a useful covariate in an analysis since premature newborns are more likely to have physiological problems, like respiratory distress, than term newborns. For example, Grimsley and Thomson (1999) found that gestational age, coded as '0' for greater than 35 weeks and '1' for less than 35 weeks, was an important predictor of vancomycin clearance in neonates. Lastly, as an aside, age is typically confounded with weight in a pediatric population and it is difficult to separate the effect of each on a drug's pharmacokinetics. In the modeling of a drug administered to a pediatric population, weight is frequently built into the model a priori (see section on incorporating weight into the model), although this practice is not universally accepted. Once weight is built into the model, age can then usually be added to the model and tested for model improvement.

INCORPORATING FORMULATION EFFECTS AND ROUTE OF ADMINISTRATION INTO THE MODEL

Drug formulation, an extrinsic covariate, plays a major role in the rate and extent of absorption and, hence, in a drug's pharmacokinetic profile. In the development of new orally administered drugs it is not uncommon for the formulation to change during the development process. For example, the first-time-in-man study may administer the drug as a solution, then as a capsule in later Phase 1 studies, and then as a tablet during Phase 2. Perhaps, later, some small change is made in the design of the tablet, like a change in the excipients, which is then the final formulation used throughout Phase 3. The bottom line is that rarely is the marketed formulation used throughout the development process. Yet in a population pharmacokinetic analysis using data across all phases of development, these differences in the formulation must be accounted for. For example, the rate and extent of absorption of the solution formulation may be different than a capsule which may be different than a tablet.

An important concept in the absorption modeling of any extravascular administered drug is that the absorption process is independent of distribution and elimination. Hence, in accounting for these different formulations all that needs to be accounted for is the absorption process because distribution and elimination is usually the same regardless of how the drug is absorbed. Hence, different formulations are usually accorded their own absorption model through a series of IF-THEN statements with one formulation being the reference formulation. Thus, a solution and capsule may be modeled as

$$
\left.
\begin{array}{r}
k_a = \theta_1 \exp(\eta_1) \\
F1 = 1 \\
ALAG = \theta_2 \exp(\eta_2)
\end{array}
\right\} \text{ if solution}
$$

$$
\left.
\begin{array}{r}
k_a = \theta_3 \exp(\eta_3) \\
F1 = \theta_4 \exp(\eta_4) \\
ALAG = \theta_5 \exp(\eta_5)
\end{array}
\right\} \text{ if capsule}
$$

(8.21)

where both the solution and capsule are modeled using a first-order absorption model with different rate constants (defined as k_a), θ_1 and θ_3, and lag-times (defined as $ALAG$), θ_2 and θ_5. Under this model, one formulation must serve as the reference formulation having a bioavailability (defined as F1, where the '1' indicates that bioavailability references compartment number 1) of 1, even though the true bioavailability may not equal one. Hence, θ_4 measures the bioavailability relative to the reference formulation. In this instance, all estimable parameters were treated as random effects, but this is not a requirement. Some, none, or all of the parameters in the model could have been treated as random effects; it depends on the data. BSV associated with absorption is rarely estimable with sparse data and most absorption parameters are treated as fixed effects. It should be noted that other distribution and clearance-related parameters for the drug are then shared between the different formulations. In other words, if the drug follows a 2-compartment model, then clearance, intercompartmental clearance, central volume, and peripheral volume are the same for both routes of distribution.

When a drug is given by two different routes of administration, the same trick is used to model the absorption process. In this case, however, sometimes it is necessary to specify that dosing is into different compartments. For example, suppose the drug follows 1-compartment kinetics and the drug can be administered by the intravenous or oral route of administration. In this case, dosing with the intravenous route is into the central compartment, whereas dosing is into a dosing compartment after oral administration. Which compartment the drug is administered into must be correctly defined for correct identification of model parameters.

INCORPORATING RACE INTO THE MODEL

Decades of research have shown race to be an important determinant of drug effect for some, but not all, drugs (Johnson, 1997). One example is the lower rate of efficacy of β-blockers in Blacks than Whites in the treatment of hypertension. Although it would be easy to conclude that the difference is due to some combination of pharmacokinetic, possibly due to genetic differences in drug metabolizing capability, and pharmacodynamic alterations, the reality is that these differences may also be due to other nonspecific factors like diet, geography, and differences in health care or weight. Nevertheless, it is important to test race as a covariate in a population analysis as it may help to reduce BSV, despite its potential nonspecific causality.

Possibly to avoid the social ramifications of using the word "race," often in the medical literature one sees "race/ethnicity" or simply "ethnicity," as if these were measuring the same thing. They do not. Ethnicity relates to the cultural associations a person belongs to. For example, a person from the Dominican Republic may be classified as 'Hispanic or Latino' on the United States Census but their ethnicity may relate more closely with Blacks. According to the ICH Guideline on Ethnic Factors in the Acceptability of Foreign Clinical Data (1998a), ethnicity has a broader meaning than race as it encompasses cultural as well as genetic constructs; race falsely implies a biological context. How race and ethnicity are used in combination will be discussed shortly.

Although scientists use "race" as if it were a scientific term, race is a social construct—not a biological one. Prior to 1989, a child was classified on its birth certificate in the United States as White only if both parents were White (LaVeist, 1994). A child was classified as Black if the father was Black (regardless of the mother's race) or if the mother was Black (regardless of the father, unless the father was Japanese in which case the child was classified as Japanese). Confusing? Imagine how it is for a child of mixed race ancestry. In contrast, at the same time in Japan, a child was declared Japanese only if the father was Japanese, regardless of the race of the mother. Current standards in the United States still vary from state to state with most states offering a variety of options. In the 2000 United States Census, more than 126 possible racial and ethnic categories were available. Hence, how a person is racially classified is dependent on the country of origin and the current sociopolitical constructs at the time, which can make for problems when pooling racial data from across the globe.

That race is not a biological construct rests on a number of considerations (Williams, 1997). First, the concept of race predates biological attempts at classification; people have always been classified by their skin color and other external features. Second, the phenotypic expression used to classify an individual, like skin color, does not correlate with genetic variability. It is often stated that there is more variability within races than between races. In other words, two individuals from any two races will have about as much genetic variability as any two individuals from within the same

race.[1] While considerable biological variation exists across groups, there is just as much variation within groups. Nevertheless, race is still wrongly viewed as a valid biological construct as it is routinely used for differential medical diagnoses, treatment, and care. And because of this false belief in its biological validity, race has a notorious history for discrimination.

Although the reader may intuitively understand what race is and how to measure it, as it is used ubiquitously throughout the medical literature, there are clear measurement and conceptual issues that must first be resolved before it can be used in an analysis. One problem with race is that many people believe they can define it, usually based on a person's skin color. It's crazy to believe that a person's skin color is a predictor for complex physiological differences, yet this is what scientists do. Further, racial classification is a categorical decision based on a continuous scale. Skin color varies from light to dark. Where is the break-point and who decides? Clearly, race is a surrogate for some other factor: socioeconomic, dietary, genetic, etc. There must be a better way to measure such differences.

External assessment of racial assignment is called physiognomy but is often confounded by ethnocentricity, which means that assessment tends to be in reference to the assigner's own ethnicity. This raises many issues, the least of which is intrarater and interrater consistency and misclassification rate. Boehmer et al. (2002) found a high rate of discordance between internal and external assessment of race in 12,444 patients surveyed for race in a Veterans Administration study of dental outpatients. A total of 14% of Hispanics, 1.5% of Whites, and 5% of Blacks were incorrectly racially classified according to the patient. If such classification is required to be done by external assessment then perhaps a more objective, quantitative measure is needed. Klag et al. (1991) used a light meter to measure the relative lightness or darkness of a person's skin and then used that information to determine the effect of skin color on that person's blood pressure. This approach has not yet been explored in clinical trials to any significant extent.

One approach that has been explored is the use of genetic markers to define race. Given that there are three billion bases in human DNA with 99.9% of these bases exactly the same across individuals, this means that each individual has more than three million unique base pairs. There are too many unique base pairs per individual for classification using all unique base pairs. Hence, the base

---

[1] Current estimates from analysis of variance show that differences among major groups account for at most 5% of the total variability in genetic variation with within-population differences among individuals accounting for the remainder, upwards of 95% (Rosenberg et al., 2002).

pairs are grouped into a few manageable categories or clusters which are then used to define a particular racial group. Wilson et al. (2001) used microsatellite markers to infer genetic clusters from eight racial populations. Using four genetic clusters they found substantial mis-classification; 21% of Afro-Caribbeans were clustered with West Eurasians, while only 24% of Ethiopians were classified with Afro-Caribbeans. A total of 62% of Ethiopians were placed in the same cluster as Jews, Norwegians, and Armenians. Hence, genetic analyses appear to be inadequate to categorizing individuals into groups of sufficient homogeneity to be useful (Risch et al., 2002). Further, *commonly used ethnic labels (such as Black, Caucasian, and Asian) are insufficient and inaccurate descriptions of human genetic variation* (Wilson et al., 2001).

The most common and now recommended approach for identifying race is self-identification. A recent editorial in the *Journal of American Medical Association* (JAMA) states that *individuals should self-designate race to ensure that the designation most closely matches what they believe reflects their personal and cultural background* (Winker, 2004). The International Committee of Medical Journal Editors, of which JAMA belongs, now requires that authors define how race was measured and to justify their relevance in the analysis. Questions may be either open-ended, e.g., race: _____, or closed-ended, e.g., Race: 1.) White, 2.) Black, etc., provided the coding process is transparent. If the questions are closed-ended then the categories should be presented, whether categories were combined, and if so, how they were combined.

This approach, while simple, also appears to be practical. One biotechnology company, NitroMed (Lexington, MA) has recently submitted a New Drug Application with the FDA for BiDil®, a combination tablet containing hydralazine plus isosorbide dinitrate, for the treatment of heart failure in African–Americans. Non African–Americans were specifically excluded from the clinical trial—a first for clinical drug trials (Franciosa et al., 2002). African–Americans were accepted into the trial based on self-designation. In their pivotal trial, a 43% improvement in survival was demonstrated, along with a 33% reduction in first hospitalizations and better quality of life. In 2005, the FDA Cardiac and Renal Advisory Committee recommended approval of the drug, despite concerns by the FDA that the effect observed was based on an *"old-fashioned way of determining race which relies on one's perception of one's race"*. Nevertheless, the medical reviewer at the FDA concluded that *"finally a drug is probably able to efficiently control blood pressure in [African-Americans] and prevent the consequences of both hypertension and [heart failure]"*. Shortly thereafter, the FDA formally approved BiDil for the treatment of *"treatment of heart failure as an adjunct to standard therapy in self-identified black patients to improve survival, to prolong time to hospitalization for heart failure, and to improve patient-reported functional status"*. Interestingly, other races are not listed as special populations in the package insert.

Unfortunately for multiracial studies, blind use of common categories like White, Black, Asian, Hispanic, or Other is too limiting. In 1998 the FDA issued the demographic rule to reflect that some individuals may respond differently to drugs and to make such analyses looking for racial subgroup differences consistent across regulatory submissions (United States Department of Health and Human Services et al., 2003). In their guidance the FDA was required to implement the initiatives published by the Office of Management and Budget (OMB), guidelines that were required of all federal agencies. The following guidelines are suggested:

1. Use a two-question self-reporting format requesting race and ethnicity with ethnicity preceding race to allow for multiracial identities. When self-reporting cannot be done then such information should be provided by a first-degree relative or other knowledgeable source.

2. For ethnicity, the following minimum classes should be offered: 1.) Hispanic or Latino, and 2.) Not Hispanic or Latino.

3. For race the following minimum choices should be made: American–Indian or Alaska Native; Asian; Black or African–American; Native Hawaiian or Other Pacific Islander; and White.

For example, Hispanic or Latino refers to any person of Cuban, Mexican, Puerto Rican, South or Central American, or other Spanish culture or origin, regardless of race. Still, there might be some confusion with their implementation (for example, should a person from Portugal be classified as Spanish or White?), so internal consistency should be stressed. The guideline does allow for more flexibility in the collection of race and ethnicity, e.g., White can be subgrouped to reflect European White or North African White. However, any use of more expansive categories must somehow reflect the original five racial categories suggested. The reader is referred to the guidelines for more details. As an aside, under the new guidelines issued by the OMB, in the 2000 United States Census, the first time individuals were allowed to identify themselves with more than one race, over seven million people said they did in fact belong to more than one race, thus highlighting the need for diversity of racial categorization.

The OMB guidelines were not based in science and this fact is clearly stated; the categories were sociopolitical constructs created for expediency. In a review article on racial categorization, Risch et al. (2002) state that the human race is best categorized into the following groups: Africans, Caucasians, Pacific Islanders, East Asians, and Native Americans. Notice that Hispanics are not included in the list because Hispanics are a mix of Native American, Caucasian, and African/African–American with varying regional proportions. For example, Southwest American Hispanics are a mix of Native American (39%), Caucasian (58%), and African (3%). East Coast Hispanics have a greater proportion of African admixture. Thus, depending on geographic location, Hispanics could coaggregate more similar to Caucasians, Native Americans, or African Americans.

Current guidelines by the FDA and National Institutes of Health mandate that safety data be analyzed by race. Such blanket requirements are unfortunate because they reinforce the impression that race is responsible for possible outcome disparities without regard to cause and effect. Hence, these analyses become "check-box" analyses. Within the context of population analyses, the testing of race as a covariate is not required, thus leaving it to the modeler's discretion. If race is tested as a covariate, its rationale should be justified.

The actual testing of race as a covariate is done using dummy variables. For instance, suppose subjects in a study were either White (coded as "0") or Black (coded as "1") and clearance (CL) was being modeled. Then using the dummy variable approach with a proportional change model, the effect of race on CL could be modeled as

$$CL = \theta_1(1 + RACE \times \theta_2)\exp(\eta) \qquad (8.22)$$

where θ_1 represents the CL in the White participants and $1 + \theta_2$ is the CL multiplier between Whites and Blacks. So, if θ_2 were 0.28 then CL in Blacks would be 28% higher than CL in Whites. It could also be assumed that race, not only affects the population mean, but the variability in CL such that the model could now become

$$CL = \theta_1(1 + RACE \times \theta_2)$$
$$\exp(\eta_2 \times RACE + (1 - RACE)\eta_1) \qquad (8.23)$$

where now θ_1 and θ_2 are defined as before but now η_2 and η_2 define the deviation from the population mean for White and Black subjects, respectively. For more than two categories, IF-THEN statements can be used to define the racial covariate model.

It has been stated that usually at least 80% of participants in clinical trials in the United States are White (Holden, 2003). Hence, nonWhite subjects in other particular groups may have few observations such that it would be almost impossible to detect any significant pharmacokinetic–pharmacodynamic differences among the groups. So as a matter of practice, those subjects with few observations are grouped into

some other group. Immediately, however, the question arises as to which group should another group be placed into. Suppose there were only a handful of Asians in a clinical trial involving hundreds of participants, most of which are White or Black. Should the Asian participants be placed into the White group or Black group? Clearly, this practice has the potential to obscure any real differences among groups.

But does identifying a racial difference imply a biological difference? Not necessarily. Identifying race as a covariate does not imply that there is some underlying genetic or biological difference between groups but that in the absence of other information subjects within one racial category have some characteristics in common allowing them to differ from others in another racial group.

How race will be used in clinical practice raises some interesting problems in their own right. For instance, if a racial difference is identified, its use in clinical practice requires a physician to be aware of the racial difference, make an external assessment of the patient's race, and then identify whether the patient falls into an at-risk category. Further, a patient may not agree with the physician's racial assessment and hence may refuse the differential treatment guidelines. These problems are fortunately outside the modelers realm.

It is important to remember that the finding of race as a covariate carries more political baggage than other covariates, like age or weight, because of its long history as a means to discriminate. It has been argued that emphasizing biological differences will lead to greater discrimination and differences in health care. Others argue that studying racial differences will lead to better health care and improved treatment for patient subgroups. Still, others argue against using race at all in an analysis since it has no proven value for the individual patient (Schwartz, 2001). Although race is fraught with problems in its measurement, its nonbiologic basis, and its implementation it may be a useful surrogate for some other variable, like diet, geography, or environment, and to ignore it is akin to sticking one's head in the sand. A compromise must be achieved that maintains the dignity of those classes affected by the racial model.

INCORPORATING PHARMACOGENETICS INTO THE MODEL

Despite the improvement in goodness of fit when significant covariates are incorporated into a pharmacokinetic model, in reality, the addition of most covariates reduce the unexplained variability in a model by very little. There are very few "silver bullet" covariates where their addition to the model has such an effect that residual variability is reduced by orders of magnitude or all the between-subject variability is explained by the covariate. One example of this might be a drug that is not metabolized and excreted entirely by the kidneys, such as with Org31540/SR90107A, a pentasaccharide, which is eliminated virtually 100% by the kidney as parent drug (Faaji et al., 1998). Creatinine clearance accounts for 90% of the variability in total clearance. Beyond this, most covariates fail to account for the majority of variance, even in the best examples of PopPK analysis.

One potential "silver bullet" that is only now being exploited in PopPK analysis is using genetic information as an intrinsic covariate. Between-subject variability in a drug's pharmacokinetics may be due to a myriad of underlying causes, such as age, sex, and genetic differences. Most genetic differences have focused on differences in metabolism, so called polymorphisms. By definition, a *genetic polymorphism* is a monogenic trait that is caused by the presence of more than one allele at the same locus in the same population having at least one phenotype (usually defective) in the organism wherein the frequency of the least common allele is more than 1% (Meyer, 2001). For example, it is well known that CYP 2D6 has a polymorphic distribution in many different populations, e.g., Caucasians, Asians, etc.

Polymorphisms are usually assessed by either genotyping a subject's DNA or by phenotyping. Genotyping can easily be determined using samples with genomic DNA (tissue, blood luekocytes, buccal swabs, fingernails, or hair) using polymerase chain reaction (PCR)-based assays. Genotyping has the advantage in that it need only be done once (a genotype is a constitutive property of the individual and does not change over time) and is not subject to outside influences. Alternatively, phenotyping may be conducted which measures the functional expression of a genotype. Examples include the debrisoquine metabolite ratio as a test for CYP 2D6 polymorphism and erythromycin breath test as a surrogate for CYP 3A4 activity. However, phenotyping typically requires the administration of another medication prior to therapy and the results are subject to environmental influence, such as when a concomitant medication is administered. However, since phenotyping is under environmental control, its use may be of more value in explaining within-subject variability. In practice, the use of phenotyping is less common in clinical trials than genotyping and is rarely seen in the PopPK literature.

To date, genotyping has been used solely to explain the between-subject variability in clearance with the genotype treated as any other covariate. Kvist et al. (2001) first studied the role CYP 2D6 genotype plays in the clearance of nortriptyline in 20 subjects with depression and 20 healthy volunteers. CYP 2D6 genotype can be classified into four groups based on the number of functional genes:

poor metabolisers (zero genes), heterozygous extensive metabolizers (one gene), homozygous extensive metabolisers (two genes), and ultrametabolisers (three or more genes). Kvist et al. (2001) modeled nortriptyline clearance based on the well stirred model

$$CL = \frac{Q \times CL_{int}}{Q + CL_{int} \exp(\eta)} \qquad (8.24)$$

where Q was hepatic blood flow fixed at 60 L/h and $CL\int$ was intrinsic clearance modeled as a linear function of the number of CYP 2D6 genes (GENE)

$$CL_{int} = \theta_1 + \theta_2 \times GENE. \qquad (8.25)$$

Other functional forms to Eq. (8.25) examining the effect of GENE on intrinsic clearance were studied but none of these models resulted in any improvement in goodness of fit over the linear model. The authors also examined debrisoquine metabolite ratio, a phenotypic marker of CYP 2D6 activity, as a covariate but this, too, resulted in no improvement in goodness of fit. Modeling clearance as a function of number of genes resulted in a significant improvement in goodness of fit compared to a 2-compartment model without covariates. Using variance component analysis, the authors concluded that CYP 2D6 genes explained 21% of the total variability in the oral clearance of nortriptyline.

Mamiya et al. (2000) later studied the role of CYP 2C19 genotype in the clearance of phenytoin, a drug almost exclusively metabolized by cytochrome mediated oxidation, in 134 Japanese adults with epilepsy. Phenytoin clearance was modeled using Michaelis–Menten elimination kinetics with parameters V_{max} (maximal velocity) and K_m (Michaelis constant). Subjects were classified into four groups based on their genotype. Each group was then treated as a categorical variable and V_{max} and K_m were modeled as

$$V_{max} = \begin{cases} \theta_1 & \text{if in Group 1} \\ \theta_1\theta_2 & \text{if in Group 2} \\ \theta_1\theta_3 & \text{if in Group 3} \\ \theta_1\theta_4 & \text{if in Group 4} \end{cases} \qquad (8.26)$$

$$K_m = \begin{cases} \theta_5 & \text{if in Group 1} \\ \theta_5\theta_6 & \text{if in Group 2} \\ \theta_5\theta_7 & \text{if in Group 3} \\ \theta_5\theta_8 & \text{if in Group 4} \end{cases} \qquad (8.27)$$

where θ_1 was the maximal velocity for the wild-type[2] metabolizer. θ_2, θ_3, and θ_4 were the V_{max} multipliers if

---

[2] Wild-type genes are always designated as the ·1 allele and have normal metabolic function.

the subject was in the 2nd, 3rd, or 4th group, respectively. θ_5 was the K_m for the wild-type metabolizer. θ_6, θ_7, and θ_8 were the K_m multipliers if the subject was in the 2nd, 3rd, or 4th group, respectively. In this manner, they showed that subjects in Group 4 had 42% lower V_{max} than the wild type, whereas K_m for Groups 2 and 3 were 22 and 54% higher than Group 1, respectively.

Kirchheiner et al. (2002) used another approach to model the clearance of glyburide, an oral hypoglycemic that is metabolized by CYP 2C9, in 21 healthy volunteers. At the time of the study, the genotype for CYP 2C9 consisted of two inherited functional polymorphisms of three different alleles (denoted *1, *2, and *3) that were known to affect the catalytic efficiency of the CYP 2C9 enzyme. Hence, humans were classified as *1/*1 (wild type), *1/*2, *1/*3, *2/*1, *2/*2, or *2/*3. They could have used a categorical model like Mamiya et al. (2000) but instead chose to model clearance a little differently. The final model for glyburide clearance (CL) was modeled as the sum of the partial clearances

$$CL = CL_{*1} + CL_{*2} + CL_{*3} \qquad (8.28)$$

where CL_{*1}, CL_{*2}, and CL_{*3} were the partial clearances if the subject had the *1, *2, or *3 allele, respectively. For example, if subjects had the *1/*3 alleles their clearance would be modeled as $CL_{*1} + CL_{*3}$. Subjects with the *1/*1 alleles would have their clearance modeled as $CL_{*1} + CL_{*1}$. Under this model, subjects with the wild type *1/*1 alleles had a total clearance of 3.5 L/h, but slow metabolizers having a genotype of *3/*3 had a total clearance of only 1.5 L/h.

To date, the application of genotyping to PopPK modeling has focused on using this information to explain clearance. Genotyping has not been used to explain the variability in other structural model parameters, such as volume of distribution, but this may change. That polymorphisms exist for the two major drug-protein binding sites in plasma, albumin (Takahashi et al., 1987) and α_1-acid glycoprotein (Eap, Cuendet, and Baumann, 1988), has been known for some time. Only lately has it been shown that these protein polymorphisms may result in differential protein binding (Li et al., 2002). Hence, in theory, since volume of distribution is dependent on plasma protein binding, those individuals with different polymorphs may lead to polymorphic volume of distribution, a phenomenon that has not been demonstrated in animals or man (yet). And if this is the case, then genotyping may be useful in explaining the variability of other model parameters as well.

While genotyping may seem useful, the models that are developed may only be applicable until a new nomenclature is used or another defective allele is identified. For example, in 2001, when Kirchheiner et al.

reported their results with glyburide, only two CYP 2C9 alleles, besides the wild type, were known. By mid-2004, about three years later, there were 12 other alleles besides the wildtype, *2 to *13. How the model developed by Kirchheiner et al. applies to the situation today is difficult to determine and may not be applicable at all. For example, what is the clearance for a subject with the *1/*8 or *1/*5 alleles? Under the model by Kirchheiner et al., there is no answer because these wild types were not included in the model.

It is expected that more and more models will include genotype data as a covariate in the model because evidence indicates that drug development will eventually include DNA microarrays as a routine part of Phase 2 and Phase 3 studies in an attempt to identify responders and nonresponders (Roses, 2000). Further, studies are now being done correlating gene expression profiles on gene chips (Affimetrix U95A GeneChip, Santa Clara, CA) to transporter expression in tissue biopsies (Landowski et al., 2003). If during Phase 2 patterns of single nucleotide polymorphisms (SNPs) from DNA microarrays can be found in responders, but not in nonresponders, or gene expression profiles can identify subjects that have abnormal levels of some transporter needed for drug absorption, then the presence of these SNPs can later be used as an inclusion criteria in Phase 3. Hopefully, the probability of "success" for the Phase 3 trial will then be increased compared to had this information not been on-hand. Since, the classification of subjects into groups using gene expression profiles is based on correlative methods, i.e., finding a pattern of SNPs present in responders but not in non nonresponders, there is no reason why similar data cannot be used as covariates in a PopPK analysis. To do so, however, result in two problems: one, the number of covariates that would need to be screened would greatly increase since now there may be many hundreds of genomic variables to analyze; second, many spurious covariates would be added to the model because of multiplicity in hypothesis testing. The benefit of including such genomic covariates in a model, however, is a reduction in the between-subject variability in drug concentrations.

INCORPORATING PRIOR INFORMATION INTO THE MODEL

Pharmacokinetic-pharmacodynamic models are becoming increasingly complex through the incorporation of covariate information, effect mechanisms, and lower quantification limits of assays which reveal compartments not previously known to exist. With sparse data collected during Phase 3 trials it may not be possible to develop and support such complex models because of inadequate information. If such a complex model is used then some parameters may not be estimable, not because they are unidentifiable, but because there is insufficient data to precisely estimate their value. One strategy is to fix these unestimable parameters to values obtained from a previous study or studies where their estimation was possible. An example of this would be the fixing of the absorption rate constant to some reasonable value. But if this value is incorrect then the remaining model parameter estimates may be biased (see Section of Misspecification of the Structural Model in the last chapter for details). Another approach is to include dense data from another study with the sparse data set and fit the more complex model to this combined data set. This approach assumes that the same structural model applies to both studies unless the differences between studies are accounted for in the model. For example, it may be that Phase 1 data is available in healthy volunteers but using a different formulation. Hence, the model needs to account for the different formulations and possible differences in the study populations (healthy volunteer versus patients with the disease).

Gisleskog, Karlsson, and Beal (2003) propose another approach to the problem that is loosely based in Bayesian methodology. Typically θ, the set of model parameters, is estimated based on minimizing some objective function $S(\hat{\theta})$ with respect to the observed data. If data from a dense data set is combined with data from a sparse data set then the total objective function is the sum of the objective functions from the dense data set $S_d(\theta)$ and sparse data set $S_s(\theta)$. If $S_d(\theta)$ is not available then perhaps a numeric representation of $S_d(\theta)$ can be used instead, denoted as $S^d(\theta)$. Then based on the approximation $S^d(\theta)$ and given a sparse data set, an estimate of the total objective function $S(\theta)$ can be made thereby stabilizing the estimation of the model parameters. Gisleskog, Karlsson, and Beal propose approximating $S^d(\theta)$ using what they call a "frequentist prior" equal to -2 times the log-likelihood of the probability density function (pdf) for the model parameters with prior information. The parameters of the pdf are referred to as hyperparameters. So, even though the dense data are not available, given the hyperparameters, an estimate of $S_d(\theta)$ can be made, as can an estimate of the total objective function. In a sense, the approximation $S^d(\theta)$ can be viewed as a penalty function similar to penalty functions described in the chapter on Nonlinear Regression and Modeling to constrain model parameters within certain bounds.

One difficulty with the frequentist prior approach is the choice of the pdf for the model parameters. A common first choice would be to assume that the fixed effects (θ which is of size p) are multivariate normal with mean μ, variance, and pdf

$$\text{pdf}(\theta) = (-2\pi)^{-p/2}||^{-1/2}\exp\left[(\theta - \mu)^{T-1}(\theta - \mu)\right] \tag{8.29}$$

where $||$ is the determinant function. The first choice for independent variance components (Ω of size k) is often an inverse Wishart distribution, which is the multivariate generalization to a gamma distribution, having mean $\bar{\Omega}$ and degrees of freedom v. v quantifies the degree of uncertainty about Ω with decreasing v leading to increasing uncertainty. A noninformative distribution is obtained when $v = 0$. Carlin (1996) suggest using n/20 (n being the number of subjects) as a rule of thumb for the degrees of freedom. Gisleskog, Karlsson, and Beal (2003) propose that v should be n − p so if prior data were available for clearance only in 12 subjects then v would equal 11 (i.e., 12 − 1). The pdf for Ω is given by

$$\left(2^{vk/2}\pi^{k(k-1)/4}\Pi_{i=1}^{k}\Gamma\left(\frac{v+1-i}{2}\right)\right)^{-1}$$
$$\times |\Omega|^{v/2}|\Omega|^{-(v+k+1)/2}\exp\left(-\frac{1}{2}\text{tr}(\Omega\Omega^{-1})\right) \tag{8.30}$$

where $\Gamma(\cdot)$ is the gamma function and tr(.) denotes the trace. Because θ and Ω are independent the joint pdf is the product of the individual pdfs and $-2 \times \text{Ln(pdf)}$ is proportional (up to a constant) to

$$(\theta - \mu)^{T-1}(\theta - \mu) + (v + k + 1)\text{Ln}(|\Omega|) + \text{tr}(\Omega\Omega^{-1}). \tag{8.31}$$

Hence, Eq. (8.31) is the estimate of $S^d(\theta)$. If Ω does not consist of independent elements, i.e., covariance terms exist between the random effects, the penalty term is modified to

$$(\theta - \mu)^{T-1}(\theta - \mu) + (v + k + 1)\sum_{i=1}^{k}\text{Ln}(\Omega_{ii})$$
$$+ \sum_{i=1}^{k}(\Omega_{ii}/\Omega_{ii}). \tag{8.32}$$

If by chance prior information were available on the residual error Σ, a gamma distribution pdf could be used and -2 times the log-likelihood of that pdf added to Eq. (8.30) or (8.32) such that the penalty term includes terms for θ, Ω, and Σ.

One problem with the use of the inverse Wishart distribution is that the distribution does account for correlation among the random effects nor can it express any correlation among θ and Ω. To account for this Gisleskog, Karlsson, and Beal propose using a normal–normal prior where now correlation can be accounted for, although the result may not lead to positive definite covariance matrices. The reader is referred to the original paper for details.

Gisleskog, Karlsson, and Beal compared within NONMEM the various methods (fixing the parameters to estimates obtained with rich data, simultaneously fitting sparse and rich data in combination, and the frequentist prior approach using a normal–inverse Wishart and normal–normal prior) at fitting sparse data that were inadequate to precisely estimate the model parameters. They found little difference between the methods. All three methods were roughly equivalent and led to relatively precise and unbiased estimates of the true parameters. There were some differences in computation times (using a frequentist prior was faster than simultaneous fitting of dense and sparse data) and fixing the parameter estimates to their prior values led to larger standard errors than expected. But overall the simulation results illustrated that the frequentist prior approach shows promise.

To illustrate this approach, concentration–time data were simulated from a 2-compartment model with absorption.[3] All pharmacokinetic variables were log-normal in distribution having a variance of 0.05 (22.4% CV). Residual error was set equal to 0.005 (7.1% CV). The population mean clearance (CL), central volume (V1), intercompartmental clearance (Q), peripheral volume (V2), and absorption rate constant (k_a) were equal to 8 L/h, 20 L, 12 L/h, 125 L, and 0.7 per hour, respectively. A total of 18 subjects were simulated in the dense sampling group having samples collected at 0, 0.25, 0.5, 1, 1.5, 2, 2.5, 3, 4, 6, 8, 12, 24, 48, and 72 h after administration of a single 100 mg dose. Two hundred (200) subjects were simulated in the sparse sampling group where subjects were randomized to one of four doses: 25, 50, 100, or 200 mg. Samples were collected at trough at steady-state in all subjects. Half the subjects were sampled 1 h and the remainder sampled at 6 h after dosing at steady-state. Hence, each subject in the sparse data set had two samples collected on one occasion. A 2-compartment model with absorption was then fit to the dense and sparse data using NONMEM (version 5.1).

The results are presented in Table 8.5. The dense data set resulted in accurate and precise estimates of the fixed effects and the BSV in CL, but overestimated the BSV in V1 and Q. In contrast, the BSV in V2 and k_a was underestimated. The sparse data set resulted in reasonable estimates of all the fixed effects, except V2 which was significantly overestimated (224 L versus a true value of 125 L).

Further, BSV in Q and V2 were also overestimated. Hence, the sparse data set did not reproduce the data

generating model despite having 200 subjects in the data base. When the dense and sparse data sets were combined, all the model parameters were estimated with good accuracy, although BSV in V1 and Q were still overestimated and BSV in V2 and k_a were underestimated. Two models were examined using the frequentist prior. The first model used 13 degrees of freedom (18 subjects with five estimable fixed effects) in the inverse Wishart distribution, while the second used a more noninformative prior with only two degrees of freedom. Using the frequentist prior significantly improved the estimates of the fixed effects and the variance components. When the degree of noninformativeness in the prior increased (as the degrees of freedom decreased from 13 to 2) no change was observed in the estimates of the fixed effects but the estimates of the variance components tended to be larger with smaller degrees of freedom in the inverse Wishart distribution. In this example, a frequentist prior resulted in model parameter estimates not different from the results obtained when the dense and sparse data were combined and analyzed simultaneously and resulted in better estimates of the true model parameters compared to analyzing the sparse data alone.

When applied to real-life problems, however, there is little experience reported using the frequentist prior approach in the literature. Gastonguay et al. (1999) used prior information from adults to estimate the model parameters in a PopPK analysis in children. Simonsen et al. (2000) used prior information to estimate the pharmacokinetics and pharmacodynamics of epirubicin in rats. So, while it appears that using prior information may be useful in certain circumstances, but *caveat emptor* applies at the present time—let the buyer beware. Gisleskog, Karlsson, and Beal conclude that "considerable care must be taken with the use of a frequentist prior." That would seem good advice.

INCORPORATING LAG-TIMES INTO THE MODEL

It is not uncommon after extravascular administration for there to be a delay in observing quantifiable drug concentrations. For instance, for an oral drug to be absorbed it must first dissolve into the fluids in the gastrointestinal tract (GI) and then be absorbed in the splanchnic blood whereupon it will then be distributed by the systemic circulation to the rest of the body. The dissolution step may be slow relative to absorption and in fact may be very slow due to either formulation factors or to food stuffs in the GI tract. Such delays in absorption are modeled using a lag-time between the absorption compartment and the observation compartment. There is a subtle difference in how different programs handle lag-times which is important to understand. Programs like WinNonlin and NONMEM model their pharmaco-

---

[3] The author would like to thank Nick Holford and Mats Karlsson for their help in this example.

Table 8.5 Results of model fitting using prior information.

Parameter	True values	Dense data	Sparse data	Dense and sparse data	Sparse data with normal-inverse Wishart prior (2 df)	Sparse data with normal-inverse Wishart prior (13 df)
CL (L/h)	8.0	7.94 (0.423)	8.47	8.14 (0.135)	8.09 (0.138)	8.13 (0.133)
V1 (L)	20.0	18.4 (2.46)	16.6	19.1 (2.39)	19.4 (2.07)	19.1 (2.09)
Q (L/h)	12.0	11.3 (0.799)	10.1	11.8 (0.669)	11.8 (0.619)	11.9 (0.613)
V2 (L)	125	129 (5.62)	224	134 (5.91)	133 (4.19)	132 (5.03)
k_a (per h)	0.7	0.657 (0.0682)	0.571	0.693 (0.0682)	0.703 (0.0572)	0.693 (0.0572)
ω^2 (CL)	0.05	0.0492	0.0461	0.0415	0.0401	0.0403
ω^2 (V1)	0.05	0.0825	0.0686	0.0736	0.101	0.0813
ω^2 (Q)	0.05	0.0766	0.114	0.0856	0.0911	0.0833
ω^2 (V2)	0.05	0.0215	0.0272	0.0256	0.134	0.0217
$\omega^2(k_a)$	0.05	0.0179	0.113	0.0393	0.0649	0.0188
σ^2	0.005	0.0206	0.00036	0.0213	0.00992	0.0258

Data were simulated from a 2-compartment model with absorption. Dense data were simulated in 18 subjects receiving a single 100 mg dose with repeated samples collected over the dosing interval. Sparse data were simulated from 200 subjects receiving multiple doses of either 25, 50, 100, or 200 mg. At steady-state, a single trough sample was collected from all subjects. Another sample was collected at 1 h after dosing in half the subjects or 6 h later in the remainder of the subjects. Hence, in the sparse design each subject was sampled twice. Fixed effects are reported as estimate (standard error). Standard errors were not available with the sparse data set due to R-matrix singularities. All standard errors were calculated using the R-matrix option in the $COV step.

kinetics as explicit functions, unless otherwise directed by the user. Lag-times (denoted as *lag*) are treated as all-or-none or as a step function. For example, for a drug exhibiting 1-compartment kinetics a lag-time would appear in the function as

$$C = \begin{cases} 0 & \text{if } t < lag \\ \dfrac{FD}{V}\dfrac{k_a}{k_a - k_{el}}[\exp(-k_{el}\Delta t) - \exp(-k_a\Delta t)] & \text{if } t \geq lag \end{cases}$$

(8.33)

where $\Delta t = t - lag$. Hence, if time is less than the lag-time, drug concentrations will be zero. But once time exceeds the lag-time, concentrations will follow the typical profile of a 1-compartment model with absorption but with a shift in the profile to the right. While numerically convenient, the explicit function model is not physiologically realistic.

Another approach to modeling lag-times is to model the kinetic system using differential equations with the lag-time manifested through a series of intermediate or transit compartments between the absorption compartment and observation compartment (Fig. 8.1). For example, the differential equations for Model A in the figure would be written as

$$\frac{dX_1}{dt} = -k_a X_1$$

$$\frac{dX_2}{dt} = k_a X_1 - \frac{1}{lag} X_2$$

$$\frac{dX_3}{dt} = \frac{1}{lag} X_2 - \frac{1}{lag} X_3 \qquad (8.34)$$

$$\frac{dX_4}{dt} = \frac{1}{lag} X_3 - k_{10} X_4$$

$$C(t) = \frac{X_4}{V}$$

It should be noted that 1/lag is sometimes referred to as k_{tr}, the transit rate constant. Such a series of differential equations does not have an all-or-none outcome and is more physiologically plausible. Using a differential equation approach to model lag-compartments the rise in concentration to the maximal concentration is more gradual. But, as the number of intermediate lag-compartments increase so does the sharpness in the rate of rise so that an infinite number of transit compartments would appear as an all-or-none function similar to the explicit function approach (Fig. 8.2). Also, as the number of intermediate compartments increase the peakedness around the maximal concentration increases.

Determining the number of transit compartments can be done through trial and error comparing the AIC with each model and then picking the one with the smallest AIC. Alternatively, the LRT can be used as well. However, the computation time increases as the number of differential equations increase leading to run times that may be prohibitive. Savic et al. (2004) presented a slightly different transit model from Eq. (8.34), but both models lead to exactly the same concentration–time profile (Model B in Fig. 8.1) after single and multiple dose. In the reformulated version however, the amount of drug in the nth transit compartment can be expressed as

$$X_n(t) = D \frac{\left(\frac{1}{lag}t\right)^n}{n!} \exp\left(-\frac{1}{lag}t\right) \qquad (8.35)$$

where n! is the factorial of n. The differential equation for the absorption compartment (X_3 in this case) can then be written as

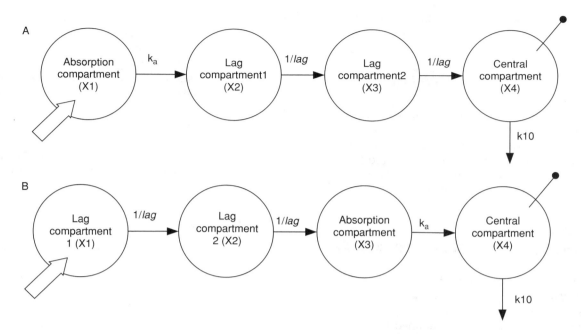

Figure 8.1 Schematic of two different formulations of a 1-compartment model with lag-time using two intermediate lag-compartments to model the lag-time. Model A is the typical model, while Model B is the model used by Savic et al. (2004). Note that $1/lag$ is sometimes referred to as k_{tr}, the transit rate constant. Both models lead to exactly the same concentration–time profile.

$$\frac{dX_3}{dt} = \left[D \frac{\left(\frac{1}{lag} t \right)^n}{n!} \exp\left(-\frac{1}{lag} t \right) \right] \left(\frac{1}{lag} \right) - k_a X_3. \quad (8.36)$$

The mean transit time to the absorption compartment is equal to $lag(n + 1)$. Hence, in Model B in Fig. 8.1 the system of differential equations can be reduced to

$$\frac{dX_1}{dt} = \left[D \frac{\left(\frac{1}{lag} t \right)^n}{n!} \exp\left(-\frac{1}{lag} t \right) \right] \left(\frac{1}{lag} \right) - k_a X_1$$

$$\frac{dX_2}{dt} = k_a X_1 - k_{10} X_2$$

$$C(t) = \frac{X_2}{V}$$

$$(8.37)$$

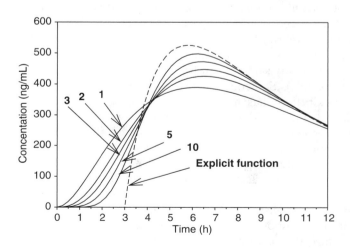

Figure 8.2 Concentration–time profiles illustrating the difference between modeling lag-time using an explicit function [Eq. (8.33)] versus a differential equation approach [Eq. (8.34)] with a variable number of intermediate transit compartments. Concentrations were simulated using a 1-compartment model having a dose of 100 mg, $V = 125\,L$, $k_a = 0.7$ per hour, $k_{10} = 0.15$ per hour and a lag-time of 3 h. The explicit function models lag-times as all-or-none, whereas the differential equation approach models lag-times more gradually.

The only difficulty in this equation is finding n!. NON-MEM in particular does not support the factorial function, so instead Stirling's approximation can be used

$$n! \cong \sqrt{2\pi}(n)^{n+0.5} \exp(-n) \qquad (8.38)$$

which is accurate to at least n = 30. Savic et al. (2004) used this approach to compare the transit model with the explicit function model using glibenclamide, moxonidine, furosemide, and amiloride and found that the transit model resulted in significantly better goodness of fit than the explicit function model in all four cases.

EXPERIMENTAL DESIGN ISSUES IN PHASE 3

It is generally recognized that intensive (also called dense or rich) sampling for pharmacokinetic analysis will occur during Phase 1 and, usually, in Phase 2 as well. Pharmacokinetic models obtained from such data are generally considered to be of better quality than models obtained from Phase 3 since intensive pharmacokinetic sampling is not done routinely within a subject in Phase 3. More often, sparse sampling, as few as one or two samples per subject per dosing interval, is the norm. As one might expect, the ability to obtain accurate and precise parameter estimates in a model derived from sparse data is dependent on the experimental design used to obtain the data. For example, the best times to sample are immediately after dosing and as late as possible thereafter with a 1-compartment model after intravenous administration (Endrenyi, 1981). For a 1-compartment model with absorption it would not be surprising that an accurate estimate of the absorption rate constant cannot be obtained if samples are not collected in the absorption phase. Hence, when samples are collected are of paramount importance. But, balanced against this are usually some restraints on when samples can be collected and how many samples can be collected (usually as few as possible). Sometimes with Phase 3 studies the pharmacokineticist has no say in when samples can be collected and must work with what they are given. It is not uncommon to have Phase 3 studies planned entirely without consultation from a pharmacokineticist and later, at the end of the trial, have the pharmacokineticist analyze the data as part of a regulatory submission.

In cases where the pharmacokineticist has input on when samples can be collected, samples should be obtained at times that maximize the pharmacokinetic "information" about the model parameters while collecting as few as samples as possible. This section will focus on the experimental design considerations to maximize the "information content" obtained during Phase 3 and to survey current practices regarding sample collection times. In order to understand the current state of sample collection and timing for Phase 3 studies it is necessary to first understand the relevant simulation studies on the topic because these are often used to validate clinical decisions on sample times. It must be stated however that many of the conclusions drawn from these studies are study specific and do not necessarily generalize to other conditions. For example, the results from a 1-compartment model may not apply to a 2-compartment model.

Theory Based on Monte Carlo Simulation

Sheiner and Beal (1983) presented the first study on the role of experimental design in one of their seminal papers on nonlinear mixed effects models. They showed that increasing the number of subjects improves parameter estimation accuracy, but that increasing the number of samples per subject subjects does not improve estimation to the same degree when the data were simulated from a 1-compartment model. Hence, it is better to have sparse data from more subjects than intensive pharmacokinetic data with fewer subjects. They also showed that relatively accurate and precise parameter estimates (except for residual variance) can be obtained using FO-approximation with as few as 50 subjects having a single sample collected per subject. Keep in mind, however, this was a very simple pharmacokinetic model with only two estimable parameters.

Al-Banna, Kelman, and Whiting (1990) used Monte Carlo simulation to compare fixed time two and three point designs under a 1-compartment model in 50 subjects for a drug having a half-life of 6.93 h. Recall that at the individual level the best times to estimate the model parameters with a 1-compartment model after intravenous bolus administration are as early and late as possible. In the two point design, one sample was anchored at 0.08 h with the second sample time varying in 2 h intervals up 20 h. In the three point design, one sample was fixed at 0.08 h with another at 20 h. The third sample was varied at 2 h intervals up to 18 h. Although not stated, it is assumed the authors analyzed each data set using FO-approximation.

Acceptable bias and precision in the structural model parameters were observed with two samples per subject across any two time points. However, better precision and accuracy in estimating clearance was obtained when the second sample was collected at later times. Volume of distribution was not as affected by the choice of sample times. Across all time points, the variance components were often significantly underestimated with the range of estimates being quite large.

When the number of samples per individual was increased to three, regardless of where the middle point was collected in time, the structural model parameters remained unbiased but the bias in the variance components was removed. When the number of subjects was increased to 100 and then 150, the bias and precision in the structural model parameters remained unchanged, but improved the estimation of the variance components. Hence, under these conditions, neither more data per subject nor more subjects improved the estimates of the fixed effects in the model. What were affected were the variance components. Both more data within a subject and more subjects resulted in better variance component estimation.

Breant et al. (1996) followed up the work of Al-Banna, Kelman, and Whiting and used Monte Carlo simulation to determine the number of subjects and samples per subject needed to obtain accurate and precise parameter estimates with a drug that showed mono-exponential disposition kinetics. They found that for a 1-compartment model, concentration data from 15 to 20 subjects with two samples per subject produced reasonable parameter estimates. Although the authors did not use NONMEM, their results should be applicable to NONMEM analyses.

Booth and Gobburu (2003) examined whether these conclusions held when a single sample was collected at steady-state compared to when multiple samples were collected after a single dose. With only one sample per subject, the bias and precision in clearance was -16.7 and 22.8% for FO-approximation, but was -28.7 and 32.3% for FOCE-I. Paradoxically, the less accurate estimation algorithm decreased bias and increased precision in estimating clearance. The increased bias and decreased precision using FOCE-I to estimate volume of distribution was in general greater than for clearance. But this was not that unexpected since steady-state data contain more information on clearance than volume of distribution. However, FOCE-I was more accurate and precise than FO-approximation (bias: -6.6% for FO-approximation versus 0.4% for FOCE-I; precision: 6.8% for FO-approximation versus 3.7% for FOCE-I) when the mix of data consisted of 75% sparse data and 25% dense data. The authors conclude that single trough samples do not provide unbiased and precise parameter estimates even when the exact structural model is known a priori. Unbiased and precise parameter estimates can only be obtained when combined with dense data or when some of the other model parameters are fixed to prior values.

Jonsson, Wade, and Karlsson (1996) used Monte Carlo simulation to examine the consequences of collecting two samples per visit instead of one per visit when the drug followed a 1-compartment model with first-order absorption. Samples were collected after the absorption phase was complete. In the modeling process, they fixed the absorption rate constant (k_a) to a constant with all the remaining parameters treated as estimable parameters. Previous studies have shown that for a 1-compartment model when no data are collected during the absorption phase, estimation of k_a is problematic, but when k_a is fixed to a reasonable value then accurate and precise estimates of the remaining model parameters is still obtainable (Wade et al., 1993).

Jonsson, Wade, and Karlsson (1996) concluded, as might be expected, that a design with two samples per visit, regardless of when the samples were collected, resulted in better (less bias and more precise) parameter estimates than a design with one sample per visit. The data herein were simulated using a 1-compartment model. On a log-scale, concentrations decrease linearly during the elimination phase. Hence, it would be expected that irrespective of when the two plasma samples were collected after absorption was complete, roughly equivalent parameter estimates would be obtained. For more complex models, the timing of the second sample would be crucial in estimating the parameters associated with the additional compartment(s).

Jonsson, Wade, and Karlsson's (1996) second conclusion was a logical extension of this argument: two samples are needed to identify more complex models and are especially useful because now interoccasion variability can be estimated, which is not possible from a one sample per visit design. They also concluded that designs in which some fraction of subjects have only samples early after dosing collected with the remainder of subjects having samples collected later after dosing is inferior to one where most subjects have both early and late samples collected. Hence, balance is important in study design.

Ette, Sun, and Ludden (1998) examined the effect of sample size and between-subject variability using balanced study designs wherein an equal number of samples were collected from each subject. In their study, concentration data from 30 to 1000 subjects were simulated using a 2-compartment model with intravenous administration at steady-state. Sample times were chosen based on D-optimality. Once obtained, the concentration–time profile was divided into three windows and two samples per subject were randomly sampled from each time window, i.e., six samples were collected from each subject. Between-subject variability in all the parameters was systematically varied from 30 to 100% with residual variability fixed at 15%. All models were fit using FO-approximation.

In general, accurate and precise estimates of all structural model parameters were obtained across all sample sizes and between-subject variability, except for when the sample size was small (30 subjects) and between-subject variability was large (100%). When between-subject variability was <100%, accurate and precise structural model parameter estimates were obtained irrespective of sample size. In contrast, estimation of the variance components was influenced by both sample size and between-subject variability. Greater numbers of subjects are needed to obtain accurate and precise structural model variance component estimates as between-subject variability increases. However, residual error was always unbiased and imprecise regardless of sample size when between-subject variability was greater than 75%. Hence, any estimates of residual variance with very large between-subject variability should be interpreted with caution.

Review of Current Practice

Returning to current practice, the number of samples collected and their timing depend on many variables, few of which are pharmacokinetically based. First, the primary focus of a Phase 3 study is efficacy and safety. If a drug does not demonstrate efficacy, collecting an adequate pharmacokinetic profile for pharmacokinetic analysis becomes moot (although possibly publishable). Similarly, companies are under tremendous pressure to get new drugs to market as soon as possible. Hence, an unstated goal is to complete the trial forthwith. Factors that hinder recruitment, such as intensive pharmacokinetic sampling, are frowned upon by product team leaders and efforts by the pharmacokineticist to collect many samples per subject are discouraged.

Reviewing the population pharmacokinetic literature, focusing solely on Phase 3 studies, the studies can be broadly grouped into three design types. In the first design, blood samples are collected on each visit with the time of last dose recorded. No attempt is made to control when sampling is done relative to dosing. Hence, blood samples are, in essence, randomly collected. The rationale being that the sheer size in the number of subjects will adequately capture the concentration–time profile. In practice this approach works surprisingly well. For example, Ingwersen et al. (2000) reported this design in the PopPK analysis of 130 epileptic subjects dosed with tiagabine. Subjects were to have a single blood sample collected at eight different visits during an ~1-year period. Sample collection time (relative to dosing) ranged from 0 to 20 h with the bulk of the data obtained within the first 6 h. Visual analysis of the concentration–time profile pooled across subjects clearly showed the data to follow a 1-compartment model with an absorption phase.

A modification to this design is when the samples are not collected at random relative to dosing, but are collected at fixed time points across different visits. One convenient choice is to sample at trough, either one sample per subject total or at multiple visits during the study. The FDA Guidance on PopPK (1999) discourages the single trough design since if only a single sample is collected per subject then between-subject variability and residual variability cannot be isolated. With multiple trough samples, although between-subject variability and residual variability can be separated and there is no stated reason not to use the design, the guidance has a general tone of disdain for this design. Further, Booth and Gobburu (2003) have shown that single trough samples do not provide unbiased and precise parameter estimates even when the exact structural model is known a priori.

Another option, the so-called full pharmacokinetic screen, is to sample at fixed times relative to dosing within a single dosing interval such as with a traditional Phase 1 study. For example, Preston et al. (1998) reported such a design in their PopPK analysis of levofloxacin in 313 subjects with bacterial infections of the respiratory tract, skin, or urinary tract. Therein samples were collected at end of infusion, 2, 6.75, 7.75, and 9.25 h after the third intravenous dose. What made intensive sampling possible in this case was that these subjects were at the hospital already. In general, if the disease state requires hospitalization then intensive sample collection is less a problem than if the subject is treated in an out-patient manner.

The second design is to use a time window wherein blood samples are collected anytime within specified intervals after dosing either within a visit, or more likely, across multiple visits. One recommendation is to collect three samples per subject, one of which is at trough (Aarons et al., 1996). For example, for most orally absorbed drugs the time to maximal concentration is 2–4 h after administration. Assuming that drug concentrations can only be collected during a visit to the physicians office, a three point design may be predose (0 h), 2–4 h, and 4–8 h after dosing once steady-state is reached. To obtain an estimate of interoccasion variability this sampling schedule would be repeated the next time the subject returns to the physician's office.

The pharmacokinetic window design has many variants. One variant is where each subject is sampled twice on each visit. The subject comes to the clinic, has a blood sample drawn at predose, the next dose is taken, the subject remains at the clinic for some time, and then a second sample is collected after a period of time has expired. The disadvantage of this approach is that it requires the subject to remain at the clinic, which places an extra burden both on the subject and on the site in collecting the sample. The advantage of this design is that the quality of the dosing times and sample collection times is usually better than other designs because a third-party (the study nurse or phlebotomist) records the sample and dose times. For example, Jackson et al. (2000) reported such a design in the PopPK analysis of nelfinavir mesylate in human immunodeficiency virus-infected (HIV) patients. Therein, blood samples were to be collected at each visit at trough and at postdose 2 h later, with most samples collected on Weeks 2 and 8 of the study.

Another modification of this design is that on half the visits a blood sample is collected at trough, while the remainder of visits the sample is collected sometime after dosing. Hence, each subject has a single sample collected per subject per visit. For example, Phillips et al. (2001) used such a design in the PopPK analysis of azimilide. Sample times ranged from 0 to 36 h after dosing with two groups of data, one within 0–12 h after dosing and one from 23 to 32 h after dosing. One disadvantage of this approach subjects are required to either keep a dosing diary or to remember the time of their last dose, both of which are often not of the best quality. It is not uncommon to review a diary log on a subject and see that all daily doses were taken at the same time of day, say 8:00 P.M. Were the doses really taken at that time or was this "about" the time the doses were taken and the subject simply rounded to the nearest hour? With a PopPK analysis, often done after the study is complete, it is difficult to go back and reassess the quality of this data. Another disadvantage of this approach is that no estimate of interoccasion variability can be made.

The last design type is where some fraction of subjects undergo intensive pharmacokinetic sampling, usually at a few sites, while the remaining subjects have sparse sampling throughout the study. For example, Moore et al. (1999) reported such a design in their PopPK analysis of lamivudine in subjects infected with HIV. Therein select centers were to collect six samples per subject per visit at fixed times over an 8-h period. The remaining subjects had two samples per visit collected. One sample was taken when the subject arrived at the clinic. If the last dose taken was within the last 6 h, the next sample was taken at least 1 h after the first sample. If the last dose was not taken within the last 6 h, the subject was to take a dose of medication, and have the sample collected at least 1 h later.

One issue that inevitably arises is when to collect the samples in the fixed time point design. One method is to use D-optimality or one of its variants to identify the time points to collect samples. These methods are numerically intensive and beyond the ability of the average pharmacokinetic modeler. The reader is referred to Retout et al. (2002), Ette et al. (1994) and Duffull et al. (2002) for further details. Another method is based on computer simulation. One can simulate data sets having

various design considerations and see which one gives the best estimates of the model parameters (Kowalski and Hutmacher, 2001). Of course, both D-optimality and simulation based approaches assume that previous knowledge of the pharmacokinetics of the drug are known. Sometimes this may not be the case. While D-optimality designs have been used in practice (Karlsson et al., 1998; Nguyen et al., 2002) it is unclear whether these methods offer any practical advantage over pharmacokinetic screens or pharmacokinetic windows.

On the Detection of Subpopulations

Lee (2001) used Monte Carlo simulation to examine the influence of experimental design factors on detecting a pharmacokinetic difference in a subpopulation of individuals having 30% higher clearance than the main population. The factors examined included number of subjects in the subpopulation, sampling scheme, and degree of compliance. Subjects were simulated having twice-a-day dosing with perfect compliance. Concentration–time data were simulated using a 1-compartment model with first-order absorption with two samples per subject collected at steady-state. In most cases the samples were collected 1 h after dosing and 11.5 h after dosing. Lee did not use NONMEM for his analysis but instead used S-Plus's (Insightful Corp., Seattle WA) NLME function, which uses a FOCE algorithm to estimate the model parameters. Clearance was modeled as

$$\text{CL} = \theta_0 + \theta_{\text{slope}}\text{G} \qquad (8.39)$$

where θ_0 is the clearance in the main population, θ_{slope} the shift in clearance in the subpopulation from the main population, and G a dichotomous covariate coding whether a patient is in the main group (G = 0) or subpopulation (G = 1).

In most scenarios, 100 subjects were simulated with the subpopulation having a clearance 30% higher than the main population. One exception was the simulation designed to detect a false subpopulation (Type I error rate) in which θ_{slope} was set equal to zero. The presence of the subpopulation was tested using two different methods. The first method was the LRT comparing the full model [Eq. (8.39)] to the reduced model where the term $\theta_{\text{slope}}\text{G}$ was not included in the covariate model for clearance. The second method was a T-test on θ_{slope}

$$\text{T} = \frac{\theta_{\text{slope}}}{\text{SE}(\theta_{\text{slope}})} \qquad (8.40)$$

where $\text{SE}(\theta_{\text{slope}})$ is the standard error of the estimate for θ_{slope}. For each study design combination, 200 replicates were simulated. The power of each method (LRT and

T-test) was estimated as the number of times the null hypothesis of no subpopulation was rejected using a significance level of 0.01 divided by the total number of simulations.

Under the basic design, the Type I error rate for the T-test and LRT was 2 and 1%, respectively, using a significance level of 1%. The power to detect the subpopulation increased for all methods when the proportion of subjects in the subpopulation increased. A total of 80% power was reached for the LRT when 20% of the population was in the subgroup and never reached 80% for the T-test. Power did not increase much for either method when the percent of subjects in the subpopulation was increased to 30%. The LRT had greater power at detecting a subpopulation than did T-test under all conditions studied.

Many modifications to the basic scenario were also examined. In the first modification, no effect on overall power was observed when the total number of subjects was doubled from 100 to 200 (but keeping the percent of subjects in the subpopulation the same). In the second modification, no difference in power was observed when the sampling times were allowed to vary randomly by ± 10% from their fixed values. In the original design, samples were collected at 1 and 11.5 h on Day 10. In the third modification, an additional sample was collected at 5-h postdose. Power to detect a subpopulation increased dramatically with 80% power being achieved with only 10 subjects in the subpopulation for both the LRT and T-test. Hence, three samples was much better than two samples.

The timing of the samples also appeared critical. When the two steady-state samples were collected at trough, instead of at 1-h postdose, and at 11.5 h postdose, the design resulted in a significant decrease in power. Maximal power reached only ~40% for both the LRT and T-test even with 50% of the population consisting of the subpopulation. But when 25 of 100 subjects had a complete pharmacokinetic profile collected at 1-, 3-, 5-, 8-, and 11.5 h postdose and the remainder of subjects were sampled twice at trough, 80% power was achieved using the T-test when 30% of the population was in the subpopulation. In this instance, the only instance when this was true, power was never more than 40% using the LRT. Interestingly, including the full profiles with trough samples also increased the false positive rate to as much as 25%. This high false positive rate remained near 15% when instead of two troughs one of the samples was collected 1 hour after dosing at steady-state.

Lee's study clearly showed that experimental design factors can have an enormous impact at detecting subpopulations within a population. Increasing the number of subjects in a population from 100 to 200 did not appear to have much impact as long as the size of the main population was much larger than the size of the subpopulation. Much more important was the number of samples collected per subject and the timing of those samples. Good power at detecting a subpopulation and good accuracy at estimating the magnitude of the difference in clearance between the main group and subpopulation could be had with as few as two samples per subject collected at steady-state but was dependent on when those samples were collected. The worst power was obtained if the samples were collected only at trough. Adding complete pharmacokinetic profiles from a proportion of subjects with the remainder having only trough samples did not improve power using the LRT but did so using the T-test. Surprisingly, adding subjects with complete profiles to subjects with only trough data collected also increased the false positive rate to unacceptable high values.

Holford (2002) later repeated Lee's experiment (which used S-Plus's NLME function) with NONMEM using FOCE-I and found that the power to detect a subpopulation was substantially worse for all the designs compared to the results reported by Lee. Like Lee's results, trough samples were the worst design overall. Variable sampling designs where the samples were collected within a time window made the results more stable and less biased but, in contrast to Lee, did not improve the power of the design. It is unclear the reason for the discrepancy between studies, but may have been due to differences between the estimation algorithms within the two software packages.

General Guidelines for Sample Collection

So what are the general guidelines for sample collection in a Phase 3 study? It is better to collect sparse data from more individuals than intensive data from few individuals. Within any dosing interval at least three to four samples per subject should be collected. Whenever possible collect at least three samples on more than one dosing interval to estimate interoccasion variability. Collect samples within a visit in a balanced manner. It is better to have the majority of subjects have samples collected early after dosing and later after dosing than to have some fraction of subjects with all their data early after dosing with the remaining subjects having all their data late after dosing. Whether to use a pharmacokinetic window approach or to use a pharmacokinetic screen where sample times are random is arbitrary and depends on the complexity of the study and the burden to the site and subject. Lastly, in the author's interactions with the regulatory agencies, study designs where a fraction of the subjects have intensive pharmacokinetic sampling and the remainder have sparse sampling are favored over purely sparse sample designs.

In summary, many experimental designs have been used in the collection of Phase 3 pharmacokinetic data. None of them have been proven to be superior in practice. In theory, D-optimal designs offer more efficient parameter estimation over pharmacokinetic screens and windows, but this has not been demonstrated in practice. Clearly, D-optimal designs represent a hardship on a Phase 3 study that few companies are willing to undertake, without perhaps some prodding by regulatory authorities. For example, a D-optimal design may call for a sample to be drawn 6.5-h postdose, which may be a burden on a patient to come in at that particular time or to remain at the clinic after dosing for collection of that sample. Until evidence is provided on the superiority of these designs, pharmacokinetic screens and windows will continue to be commonplace.

TOXICOKINETIC ANALYSES WITH DESTRUCTIVE SAMPLING

As defined by the International Conference on Harmonization (1995), toxicokinetics (TK) is the *"generation of pharmacokinetic data, either as an integral component in the conduct of nonclinical toxicity studies or in specially designed supportive studies, in order to assess systemic exposure."* The usual battery of toxicology studies to support an Investigational New Drug (IND) application include single dose and repeated dose toxicity studies in two species (rodent and nonrodent), at three or more dose levels, in both males and females, by the proposed route of administration. The usual species studied are rat and dog. With dogs, repeated sampling within an animal is not problematic given the typical blood volume in a dog. With rodent species, repeated sampling within an animal is problematic because of the limited blood volume and difficulty in the collection of repeated blood samples. Also, repeated sampling increases the stress of the animal and may confound the toxicologic results. Hence, a typical TK study will employ "satellite" animals, animals that are dosed exactly the same as the other animals in the study, but whose sole purpose is to be used for TK assessment.

Even with satellite animals, repeated sampling within a rodent species is often not performed. Usually, each animal contributes to the data at a single time point. When the animal is sacrificed to obtain the pharmacokinetic data, these animals are said to be destructively sampled. The number of animals in such studies is large and costly since often a study has many different dose levels, are dosed in both males and females, and samples are collected at many time points. As a compromise between cost, number of animals, and manageability, the usual TK study is sparsely designed with concentration data collected at five to seven time points over a dosing interval with three to five animals/sex/dose per time point. As might be expected, due to the sparseness of the design, the choice of sample times in such studies is critical to obtaining valid parameter estimates. Not sampling long enough may miss a phase in the disposition profile of the drug, leading to an underestimate of area under the curve, and an overestimate of clearance. On the other hand, sampling too long may lead to concentrations that are below the lower limit of quantification of the assay and may not be usable. It is beyond the scope of this section to discuss proper sample collection times in TK studies, suffice to say that proper sample times are paramount for accurate parameter estimates. The reader is referred to Smith, Humphrey, and Charuel (1990) and Ette et al. (1995) for further details.

The primary TK endpoints from toxicity studies include measures of exposure, such as area under the curve and maximal concentration, time to maximal concentration, and half-life. Usually, these metrics are obtained by calculating the mean or median concentration at each time point and then using noncompartmental methods to obtain the pharmacokinetic parameter estimates. The problem with this approach is that it ignores between-subject variability. The variability between animals is lumped into a "single" animal and the estimate of the parameter is obtained. In doing so, the error associated with the parameters is biased because of the ignored between-subject variability.

Many simulation studies have shown that nonlinear mixed effects modeling of destructively obtained TK data results in relatively accurate and unbiased estimates of the theoretical pharmacokinetic parameters (Ette et al., 1994; Jones, Sun, and Ette, 1996) that are more accurate than naïve pooling and noncompartmental analysis (Hing et al., 2001b). The phrase "relatively accurate" is used since the sampling times and data are so sparse that very accurate estimation of population parameters is rarely achieved. In a study where more than one sample is collected per subject, the total variability in the concentration data can be isolated into its components: between-subject, intrasubject or interoccasion (if the animal is sampled on more than one dosing occasion), and residual variability. With only one sample per subject, the components of variance cannot be identified. If residual variability is assumed negligible then the only variance component that can be obtained is between-subject variability. This assumption is reasonable since between-subject variability is usually an order of magnitude greater than residual variability (Lindstrom and Birkes, 1984). Another approach is to fix residual variability to some constant, usually the variability of the assay, and allow between-subject variability to remain an estimable parameter. Hing et al. (2001b) showed that setting residual error to near zero, equal to assay error, or twice assay error had little effect on the values of the estimated model parameters.

An early example of this methodology was presented by Burtin et al. (1996) who presented the results of a PopPK analysis from a 13 week toxicology study in male and female rats orally dosed once daily at four dose levels. Each animal provided one sample on the first day of dose administration and one sample after the last dose on Day 92 at one of five possible times (0.5-, 1-, 2-, 7-, and 24-h postdose) at the same time on each occasion. Two animals were sampled at each of the five times. They then compared the results of the PopPK analysis to a traditional noncompartmental approach. Both analysis methods came to similar conclusions, but the PopPK approach, resulted in greater mechanistic interpretations to the data.

TK studies fall under the more broad category of sparse data analysis, which may arise from many different settings, such as when tissues are sampled in addition to blood. For example, Aarons (1991) reported using PopPK methods to characterize the elimination kinetics of flurbiprofen in synovial fluid in 26 rheumatoid arthritis who had only a single synovial fluid sample collected. While it is clear that the use of nonlinear mixed effects modeling of destructively sampled TK data can lead to reliable population estimates and good individual parameter estimates that can be used to generate measures of exposure, the use of this approach in routine drug development has not been implemented, possibly due to the small number of toxicologists who are familiar with the methodology and whether the time invested in the increased complexity of the analysis leads to true benefits in clinical drug development.

HANDLING MISSING AND CENSORED DATA

The reader is advised that before beginning this section to read the section on missing data in the chapter on Linear Models and Regression. The issue of missing data is so complex that entire books have been written on the subject, most notably Little and Rubin (2002) and Schafer (1997). As such it is beyond the scope of this book to cover all aspects of handling missing data. Nevertheless, a brief review of the issues involved and current strategies for dealing with missing data in the longitudinal setting will be discussed. The case where the observations are independent, such as in a linear regression model, has already been covered. What raises the issue again in this chapter is the possibility that observations are correlated within subjects. In other words, all

the observations in a linear regression problem are independent and any of the techniques described in the chapter on Linear Models and Regression may be used. But with a mixed effects model the data are hierarchical and nested within individuals and as such those techniques that are based on the independence of the data are no longer valid.

In a random review of 20 PopPK papers published between 2000 and 2002 in leading journals, e.g., *British Journal of Clinical Pharmacology*, not a single paper even mentioned whether any data were missing, yet alone how missing data were handled. Nevertheless, despite the absence of these techniques in the PopPK literature it is still important to discuss their use and utility so that more widespread use will be seen in the future. It is likely that these techniques are not seen in the PopPK literature simply because most analysts are unfamiliar with them.

When the Dependent Variable is Missing

When the dependent variable is missing, the first question to ask is "why are the data missing?" If the dependent variable is missing completely at random (MCAR) or missing at random (MAR) then the missing data is ignorable and the usual solution is to use a complete case analysis. Neither linear or nonlinear mixed effects models are penalized when the missing dependent variable is simply deleted from the analysis—the resulting model parameters are unbiased but may not be as precise due to a decrease in the sample size.

The real issue with a missing dependent variable is if the dependent variable is missing because of the value of the measurement, in which case the missing data are 'nonignorable.' For example, the concentration of drug in a sample may be below the lower limit of quantification (LLOQ) of the assay in which case the exact value of the measurement is unknown but it is known that its value is less than the LLOQ. Such data are said to be 'left-censored.' One method to handling left-censored data is deleting the censored observation. If the data follow a 1-compartment model, deleting left-censored data from the analysis has little impact on the model parameter estimates (Hing et al., 2001a), which makes sense because the concentration–time profile is declining in a log-linear manner. Linear extrapolation of the observed data to values below the LLOQ on a log-scale would not be expected to be that different from observed data had a lower LLOQ been available. However, omission of left-censored data is not recommended for multiphasic concentration–time profiles. Duval and Karlsson (2002) showed that severe parameter bias can occur when left-censored concentration data are omitted from a pharmacokinetic analysis in the case of a 2-compartment model. Using simulation, Duval and Karlsson showed that clearance tended to be underestimated, peripheral volume was overestimated, and that terminal half-life tended to be overestimated as a consequence. Distributional parameters were not affected to any significant degree since most of the information used in estimating these parameters occurs in the early portion of the concentration–time curve. The degree of bias in the parameter estimates was related to many factors, including the proportion of missingness, the shape of the concentration–time profile, the dosing regimen, and the sampling scheme.

Most often, left-censored data are imputed using some fraction of the LLOQ because of the ease in its implementation. One suggestion to handle missing left-censored data is to replace the first missing value with one-half the LLOQ and then delete all missing values thereafter. Of course, this suggestion assumes that the time distance between the last observed concentration and missing observations is small relative to the drug's half-life. To account for the imputed value the residual error is corrected by the addition of a constant term equal to one-quarter the value of the LLOQ, which assumes that the data around one-half the LLOQ is normally distributed. However, Duval and Karlsson tried this method in their analysis and showed that this method did not improve the model parameter estimates. A modification of this method is to set the missing values to zero, but such a substitution may lead to infinite weights and problems in the optimization process. Hence, zero substitution cannot be recommended. The use of one-half the LLOQ is not tied to any specific theory. Indeed, any value between 0 and the LLOQ could be used, even possibly random draws from a uniform distribution on the interval [0, LLOQ).

To truly account for left-censored data requires a likelihood approach that defines the total likelihood as the sum of the likelihoods for the observed data and the missing data and then maximizes the total censored and uncensored likelihood with respect to the model parameters. In the simplest case with n independent observations that are not longitudinal in nature, m of which are below the LLOQ, the likelihood equals

$$L = \prod_{i=1}^{m} p(Y_i < LLOQ) \prod_{i=m+1}^{n} p(y_i = Y_i). \qquad (8.41)$$

It should be noted that in the case of right-censored data the likelihood is simply

$$L = \prod_{i=1}^{m} p(Y_i > ULOQ) \prod_{i=m+1}^{n} p(y_i = Y_i) \qquad (8.42)$$

where ULOQ is the upper limit of quantification. Lynn (2001) illustrated this approach in modeling the distribution of HIV RNA concentrations with left-censored observations and compared the results with substitution methods using the LLOQ and one-half the LLOQ. Lynn showed that when 15% of the observations were missing, simple substitution methods performed well relative to maximum likelihood (ML) or multiple imputation (MI) methods, but that substitution methods did not perform as well with heavier censoring.

With mixed effects data where the data are longitudinal in nature, the likelihood becomes more complex and difficult to implement. Beal (2001) presents some ML solutions to left-censored missing data within the context of a nonlinear mixed effects model. Using Monte Carlo simulation, Beal examined these ML methods to simple substitution methods and concluded, not surprisingly, that the substitution methods did not perform as well as the ML methods. Under certain conditions, no difference between the substitution methods and ML methods was observed but were situation specific. Under the right conditions, the substitution methods can be shown to fail spectacularly compared to the ML methods. As such, the ML methods are recommended when left-censored data are present. The problem with the ML methods is that they are not implemented in any software package and require the user to write their own likelihood function which then requires access to an optimization routine that can maximize such a function. If a small percentage of the data are missing, substituting one-half the LLOQ is the easiest solution and often seems to result in relatively unbiased estimates. If, however, a large portion of the data are left-censored then ML methods may be required, and the reader is referred to Beal (2001) for details.

When the Independent Variable is Missing

Missing covariate values cannot be ignored in an analysis because many software packages do not allow missing independent values. With some software packages, subjects with missing covariates are either completely ignored, i.e., that subject is not used in the analysis, or the missing values are set equal to zero. One way to handle missing covariate information is to delete the observation from the analysis, the so-called complete case approach. This approach tends to be most useful when the sample size is large and a small fraction of the covariate is missing. Complete case analysis does not result in biased parameter estimates but simply acts to decrease the precision of the estimates by decreasing the sample size. More often, however, substitution methods are used whereby an imputed value is substituted for the missing value and the analysis proceeds as if the data were never missing in the first place. If the missing covariates are static over time, such as if all the covariates are fixed baseline laboratory values, then any of the imputation methods presented in the chapter on Linear Models and Regression can be used. If, however, the covariates change over time within a subject then these methods are no longer valid as they fail to account for correlations within an individual.

In dealing with missing covariate data that are time-dependent, it will be assumed that excluding all subjects with missing data is not an option, that the subject has at least one covariate observation available, and that somehow the missing data must be imputed. Suppose total bilirubin concentration in serum, a marker for hepatic function, was assayed at Weeks 1 and 4, whereas pharmacokinetic samples were collected at Weeks 1, 2, 3, and 4. Hence, there is no total bilirubin concentration available at Weeks 2 and 3. The data are not simply missing. The data were never collected. Since there is some information on the missing values, albeit at different time points, then one option is to impute the missing value based on the observed values. A common imputation method is carry-forward analysis, sometimes called last-observation carried forward (LOCF), where the missing value is set equal to the value of the last observed value. So, in this case the total bilirubin concentration at Weeks 2 and 3 will both be set equal to the concentration observed on Week 1. The data are then analyzed using all the data (observed plus imputed). It is assumed under carry-forward analysis that the distribution of values at the time the data were missing is the same as the last time the value was observed and that the covariate remains constant over time. As the time distance between measurements increases, these assumptions becomes more and more untenable.

Along with carry-forward imputation are a slew of modifications including interpolation, subject-specific mean value imputation, subject-specific regression imputation, and normal value imputation. Suppose that total bilirubin was 0.4 mg/dL on Week 1 but 1.0 mg/dL on Week 4. Should the values on the second and third weeks be the last observation carried forward (LOCF), i.e., 0.4 mg/dL, or should some type of interpolation between 0.4 and 1.0 mg/dL, such as 0.6 mg/dL on Week 3 and 0.8 mg/dL on Week 4, be used? Little or no research has been done examining this issue in the context of PopPK analyses. In this instance, it makes sense that some type of interpolation will be of better predictive value than LOCF, especially when the values drastically change between visits. Albridge, Standish, and Fries (1988) showed that interpolation of missing data when the values are time-dependent generally results in smaller relative errors from true values than other methods, such as LOCF, naively inserting the

subject mean, or linear regression of correlated core-corded covariates (which is what the FDA Guidance on PopPK suggests). In this example, bilirubin values at Week 2 could be linearly interpolated using the two bracketing observed concentrations with the equation

$$\hat{x}_2 = x_1 + \frac{x_4 - x_1}{t_4 - t_1}(t_2 - t_1) \qquad (8.43)$$

where $\hat{x}_2$ is the interpolated value at Week 2, x_1 is the observed bilirubin concentration at Week 1, x_4 and x_1 are the observed bilirubin concentrations at Week 1 and 4, respectively, and t_i is Week i. So the interpolating equation for Week 2 would be

$$\hat{x}_2 = 0.4 + \frac{1.0 - 0.4}{4 - 1}(2 - 1) = 0.6\,\text{mg/dL}. \qquad (8.44)$$

Higher order interpolating polynomials can be developed and should be considered if the covariate changes curvilinearly over time. The reader is referred to Chapra and Canale (1998) for further details on other interpolation methods, such as Lagrange interpolating polynomials. One problem with interpolation is that the interpolation may not accurately reflect the covariate pattern over time and may not be as efficient if only data near the missing value are used (Higgins, Davidian, and Giltinan, 1997).

With subject-specific mean value imputation, the data within an individual are averaged over time (sometimes with weights proportional to the timeinterval between measurements) and then the average value is substituted for the missing value. Again, the average value may not be reflective of the true value if the covariate is changing over time. Subject-specific regression imputation uses a model, either parametric or semiparametric, to predict the value of the missing observation and may be more useful than the other within-subject methods as it uses all the data within an individual and can account for time trends. The predicted value may be model-dependent, however, and a poor model may produce biased imputed estimates. Substituting normal values or disease-specific "normal" values cannot be advocated because the method completely ignores the population of interest and the individual in particular. All the imputation techniques just discussed are useful because they are easy to implement and can be easily communicated to nonmodelers. But, these techniques are all flawed in that they do not take into account the uncertainty in the estimate of the imputed value, a criticism which may be alleviated by using the multiple imputation techniques of Rubin (1987).

The within-subject imputation methods just described tend to be more useful when there is a lot of data within an individual. When the data are sparse, the imputation methods are suspect. A more useful method would be one where the imputation is not only based on within-subject observations but between-subject observations. Thus, although information is used at the individual level, information is also used across individuals. Wu and Wu (2001; 2002) developed such an imputation scheme using the Gibbs sampler to impute missing data in the kinetic modeling of RNA viral load in patients with human immunodeficiency virus (HIV). Using Monte Carlo simulation, Wu and Wu compared their Gibbs sampler approach to within-subject mean value (MV) imputation, LOCF imputation, and complete case (CC) analysis. The Gibbs sampling approach produced the smallest bias and had the greatest precision of the methods studied. The other methods had significantly larger bias and less precision than the Gibbs sampling approach. When these methods were applied to real data, the LOCF and MV approaches produced some parameter estimates with completely different signs than the MI approach. For example, one model parameter produced by CC and MV was positive whereas the MI and LOCF estimate were negative. Because of the large bias produced by the other methods, Wu and Wu proposed that the parameter estimates produced by MI were the most reliable. However, the Gibbs sampling algorithm is not implemented in any software currently and was designed by Wu and Wu for their problem. Hence, routine use of this method cannot be done at this time.

Sometimes, if the missing covariate is censored and not ignorable in the reason for missingness, rather than treating the missing covariate as a continuous variable, the covariate can be categorized and the new categorical variable used in the analysis instead. For example, in a PopPK analysis of gentamicin in 210 subjects with cancer, Rosario et al. (1998) created three new covariates based on serum creatinine concentrations and different "threshold" criteria. With Covariate 1, all creatinine concentrations less than or equal to $60\,\mu\text{mol/L}$ (the lower limit of the reference range used by the hospital) were set equal to $60\,\mu\text{mol/L}$. All other samples were set equal to their original value. With Covariate 2, all creatinine concentrations less than or equal to $70\,\mu\text{mol/L}$ were set equal to $70\,\mu\text{mol/L}$ (an arbitrary intermediate value). All other samples were set equal to their original value. In Covariate 3, all creatinine concentrations less than or equal to $84\,\mu\text{mol/L}$ were set equal to $88.4\,\mu\text{mol/L}$, the equivalent of 1.0 mg/dL. All other samples were set equal to their original value. All three categorical models resulted in a significant improvement in goodness of fit compared to the model treating serum creatinine concentration as a continuous variable.

If the data are collected at fixed time intervals then one trick to generate imputed values that would account for within-subject correlations is to transform the data into a columnar format with one row of data per subject. So if the data were collected at Visits 2, 3, and 4, then three new variables would be generated. Variable 1 would correspond to Visit 2, Variable 2 to Visit 3, etc. In this manner then each row of data would correspond to a single individual. Now any of the imputation techniques introduced in the chapter on Linear Regression and Modeling could be used to impute the missing data based on the new variables. Once the data are imputed, the data set can be reformatted to multiple rows per subject and the analysis proceeds with the imputed data. This approach assumes that all samples are collected at the same time interval for all subjects, i.e., assumes that all samples were assumed at Visits 1–4 in this case.

Because of the need for easy to implement approaches to handling missing data, pharmacokinetic modelers tend to use either simple imputation or a dummy variable approach. An example of the dummy variable approach is given by de Maat et al. (2002). A binary missing value indicator, denoted as MISS, was created which was set equal to '0' if the value was not missing and '1' if the value was missing. Then to model the typical clearance value (TVCL), for example, with a dichotomous covariate x (taking values 0 and 1) having some proportion being missing, the covariate model was defined as

$$\text{TVCL} = \theta_1 \theta_2^{x(1-\text{MISS})} \theta_3^{\text{MISS}}. \qquad (8.45)$$

Under this model are four possible outcomes

x	MISS	TVCL
0	0	θ_1
1	0	$\theta_1\theta_2$
0	1	$\theta_1\theta_3$
1	1	$\theta_1\theta_3$

Thus, θ_1 is the reference value or typical value for a subject with no missing data having $x = 0$. θ_2 is the proportional multiplier for subjects with no missing data having $x = 1$ and θ_3 is the proportional multiplier for any subject with missing data. A similar model was used by Pitsiu et al. (2004) to model apparent oral clearance in an analysis where some subjects did not have creatinine clearance ($\text{CL}_\text{C}\text{R}$) values

$$\text{TVCL} = \theta_1 + \theta_2 \, (1 - \text{MISS}) \, \text{CL}_{\text{CR}} + \theta_3 \text{MISS}. \qquad (8.46)$$

Hence, subjects with missing data (MISS $= 1$) have the model

$$\text{TVCL} = \theta_1 + \theta_3 \qquad (8.47)$$

and subjects without missing data (MISS $= 0$) have the model

$$\text{TVCL} = \theta_1 + \theta_2 \text{CL}_{\text{CR}}. \qquad (8.48)$$

When the proportion of missing data is small and the covariates are static, the dummy variable method seems to work reasonably well, but biased parameter estimates result when the percent of missing data becomes large (Jones, 1996).

Mould et al. (2002), instead of using a conditional model to account for missing covariates, used a joint model that modeled the missing covariate simultaneously within the context of the overall pharmacokinetic model. In their analysis of topotecan pharmacokinetics in subjects with solid tumors, weight was known to be an important covariate but was missing in $\sim$20% of the database. The function for males

$$\text{Weight} = \theta_1 \exp\left(\theta_2[\text{BSA} - 1.73]\right) \exp\left(\theta_3[\text{CL}_{\text{CR}} - 70]\right) \qquad (8.49)$$

and for females

$$\text{Weight} = \theta_1 \exp\left(\theta_2[\text{BSA} - 1.73]\right) \exp\left(\theta_3[\text{CL}_{\text{CR}} - 70]\right)\theta_4 \qquad (8.50)$$

was then used to model weight with the predicted value then fed into the model for clearance. In this manner, the joint function allowed replacement of the missing covariates with reasonable values and still accounted for correlations among the covariates. This approach has the advantage in that it can handle time-dependent covariates in theory. The down-side is that computations times are longer than other imputation approaches.

To illustrate these methods using a data set that does not contain time-dependent covariates, concentration–time data were simulated under a 2-compartment model with intravenous administration after a single dose. Subjects were randomized to one of four dose groups: 25, 50, 100, or 200 mg. Two designs were studied: 75 subjects ($\sim$50:50 males:females) under a dense sampling schedule with samples collected at 0, 0.5, 1, 1.5, 2, 3, 4, 6, 8, 12, 18, 24, 36, 48, and 72 h after dosing and 300 subjects ($\sim$50:50 males:females) under a sparse sampling design where a single sample was randomly drawn from each of the following time intervals: 0.5–1 h, 1–3 h, 22–26 hs, and 72–76 h. Hence, four samples were col-

lected per subject under the sparse design. Clearance was simulated as a function of weight

$$\text{TVCL} = 200\,(\text{Weight})^{0.7} \qquad (8.51)$$

where weight was simulated from a log-normal distribution with a median of 55 kg and CV of 32% for females and a mean of 90 kg with a CV of 27% kg for males. A typical simulated dataset for the dense data had a median of 55 kg with a minimum of 44.6 kg and a maximum of 65.1 kg for females and a simulated median of 90.4 kg with a minimum of 76.3 kg and a maximum of 107.6 kg for males. In addition to weight, height and age were simulated. Height was simulated to be log-normal in distribution with a median of 70 in. and 63 in. males and females, respectively, a CV of 5% in both sexes, and have a correlation with weight of 0.70. Age was simulated independent from height and weight from a normal distribution with a mean of 40 years old and a variance of 4 years. Central volume, intercompartmental clearance, and peripheral volume were all simulated to have a log-normal distribution with a median of 20 L, 12 L/h, and 125 L, respectively. BSV was set at 20% for each pharmacokinetic parameter with all pharmacokinetic parameters being independent of the others. Residual variability was simulated as a log-normal distribution with a CV of 7.5%.

Four data sets were then created where the weight for a subject was randomly set to missing (MCAR) with varying percentages from 0 to 40%. If a subject was chosen to have missing data, all weight information for that subject was set equal to missing. Each data set was analyzed using the following methods: complete case, the indicator method, the joint method, mean imputation, and multiple imputation. A 2-compartment model was then fit to each data set using FOCE-I where clearance was modeled using

$$\text{TVCL} = \theta_1(\text{Weight}/70)^{\theta_2}. \qquad (8.52)$$

For the joint method, weight was modeled using

$$\text{Weight}^* = (\theta_6 + \theta_9\text{Sex})\,(\text{Age}/50)^{\theta_7}\,(\text{Height}/60)^{\theta_8} \qquad (8.53)$$

where Sex was coded as '0' for males and '1' for females. If a patient's weight was missing, then Weight* was used in Eq. (8.52), otherwise the observed weight was used. For the multiple imputation data sets, the MI procedure in SAS was used using monotone imputation with mean drug concentration, sex, age, and height as covariates to impute weight. Five imputation data sets were generated and each were analyzed. The mean parameter values from the multiple imputed data sets were reported as the final parameter values. Mean drug concentration (it could be argued that perhaps geometric mean concentration should have been used instead) was needed in the imputation model because only when the dependent variable is included in the imputation model are the resulting parameter estimates unbiased (Allison, 2002). In fact, leaving out the dependent variable from an imputation model may result in spuriously small parameter estimates for those parameters associated with a covariate having missing data.

The results of the simulation are presented in Tables 8.6–8.10. No difference was observed between any of the imputation methods. Each of the imputation methods resulted in mean parameter estimates that could not be distinguished from the case where no data were missing. Even mean imputation, which is frequently criticized in the literature, did well. A tendency for the variability of the parameter estimates to increase as the percent missing data increased was observed across all methods, although little difference was observed in the variability of the parameter estimates across methods. If anything, multiple imputation performed the worst as the variability in some of the variance components was large compared to the other methods.

In summary, none of the methods were distinguishable from the others under any of the conditions used in the simulation. A key assumption to this conclusion was

that the covariates were not time-dependent. Each covariate was a constant for an individual across all time points. Hence, the results from this simulation, while quite limited, suggest that under the right conditions, even when a large amount of information is missing, appropriate methods may be used to impute the data and recover the parameter estimates. These results also suggest that there may be little to no advantage of using one imputation method over another. But, these results need to be tempered with the fact that the covariates were static and that these results cannot be extrapolated to the case where the covariates are time varying.

There is no one right way to handle missing data. Each data set must be approached on a case-by-case basis. What worked well in one situation may not work well in the next. What is important is being able to justify the method used to handle the missing data and make some evaluation of the impact in how the missing data were handled on the final model. The outcome of an analysis should not depend on the method used to handle the missing data. One way to evaluate the impact of the missing data treatment method is to conduct a sensitivity analysis or, if the proportion of missing data is small, to compare the model with the imputed data to the complete case model with the missing data excluded. Unfortunately, this section was far too brief to cover missing data in its entirety. Handling dropouts in a

Table 8.6 Results from missing data analysis using complete case analysis.

			Dense data sampling		
	True value	No data missing	10% missing	20% missing	40% missing
θ_1 (mL/h)	—	3.97 (0.09)	3.97 (0.10)	3.96 (0.12)	3.97 (0.15)
θ_2	0.7	0.70 (0.10)	0.72 (0.11)	0.69 (0.11)	0.67 (0.14)
V1 (L)	20	20.0 (0.5)	19.9 (0.6)	19.9 (0.6)	19.9 (0.9)
Q (L/h)	12	12.1 (0.3)	12.0 (0.3)	12.0 (0.3)	12.0 (0.4)
V2 (L)	125	124 (2.4)	125 (2.1)	124 (2.6)	125 (3.5)
CV% (CL)	20	20.2 (1.7)	19.9 (1.8)	19.9 (2.0)	19.7 (2.0)
CV% (V1)	20	20.4 (1.8)	20.1 (1.7)	20.3 (1.9)	20.1 (2.1)
CV% (Q)	20	19.3 (1.5)	19.6 (1.3)	19.3 (1.6)	19.4 (2.2)
CV% (V2)	20	19.6 (1.2)	19.6 (1.6)	19.5 (1.8)	19.1 (2.5)
CV% (σ^2)	7.5	7.5 (0.2)	7.5 (0.2)	7.5 (0.2)	7.5 (0.3)

			Sparse data sampling		
	True value	No data missing	10% missing	20% missing	40% missing
θ_1 (mL/h)	—	3.95 (0.04)	3.96 (0.04)	3.96 (0.04)	3.96 (0.05)
θ_2	0.7	0.70 (0.05)	0.70 (0.06)	0.70 (0.06)	0.69 (0.06)
V1 (L)	20	20.2 (0.3)	20.2 (0.2)	20.2 (0.3)	20.1 (0.4)
Q (L/h)	12	12.1 (0.2)	12.1 (0.2)	12.1 (0.2)	12.1 (0.2)
V2 (L)	125	126 (2.1)	126 (2.1)	126 (2.1)	126 (2.2)
CV% (CL)	20	20.0 (0.7)	19.9 (0.7)	19.9 (0.7)	20.2 (0.8)
CV% (V1)	20	19.9 (2.0)	20.1 (1.9)	19.7 (2.1)	19.6 (1.9)
CV% (Q)	20	20.0 (1.3)	20.1 (1.4)	20.0 (1.5)	20.0 (1.8)
CV% (V2)	20	20.0 (1.5)	20.0 (1.6)	19.9 (1.6)	19.1 (1.7)
CV% (σ^2)	7.5	7.2 (0.8)	7.1 (0.9)	7.1 (0.9)	7.1 (0.9)

Table 8.7 Results from missing data analysis using the indicator method.

		Dense data sampling			
	True value	No data missing	10% missing	20% missing	40% missing
θ_1 (mL/h)	—	3.97 (0.09)	3.96 (0.11)	3.97 (0.12)	3.97 (0.15)
θ_2	0.7	0.70 (0.10)	0.71 (0.11)	0.70 (0.12)	0.67 (0.14)
V1 (L)	20	20.0 (0.5)	20.0 (0.5)	20.0 (0.5)	20.0 (0.5)
Q (L/h)	12	12.0 (0.3)	12.0 (0.3)	12.0 (0.3)	12.0 (0.3)
V2 (L)	125	124 (2.4)	124 (2.3)	124 (2.4)	124 (2.4)
CV% (CL)	20	20.2 (1.7)	20.6 (1.8)	21.6 (1.6)	23.3 (2.0)
CV% (V1)	20	20.4 (1.8)	20.3 (1.8)	20.3 (1.8)	20.3 (1.8)
CV% (Q)	20	19.3 (1.5)	19.4 (1.3)	19.4 (1.3)	19.3 (1.3)
CV% (V2)	20	19.6 (1.2)	19.5 (1.6)	19.5 (1.6)	19.8 (1.5)
CV% (σ^2)	7.5	7.5 (0.2)	7.5 (0.2)	7.5 (0.2)	7.5 (0.2)
		Sparse data sampling			
	True value	No data missing	10% missing	20% missing	40% missing
θ_1 (mL/h)	—	3.95 (0.04)	3.96 (0.04)	3.96 (0.04)	3.96 (0.05)
θ_2	0.7	0.70 (0.05)	0.71 (0.06)	0.70 (0.06)	0.69 (0.06)
V1 (L)	20	20.2 (0.3)	20.2 (0.3)	20.2 (0.3)	20.2 (0.3)
Q (L/h)	12	12.1 (0.2)	12.1 (0.2)	12.1 (0.2)	12.1 (0.2)
V2 (L)	125	126 (2.1)	126 (2.1)	126 (2.1)	126 (2.1)
CV% (CL)	20	20.0 (0.7)	20.7 (0.8)	21.6 (0.9)	23.3 (1.1)
CV% (V1)	20	19.9 (2.0)	19.8 (2.0)	19.8 (2.0)	19.8 (2.1)
CV% (Q)	20	20.0 (1.3)	20.0 (1.3)	20.0 (1.3)	20.0 (1.3)
CV% (V2)	20	20.0 (1.5)	20.0 (1.5)	20.0 (1.5)	20.0 (1.5)
CV% (σ^2)	7.5	7.2 (0.8)	7.2 (0.8)	7.2 (0.8)	7.2 (0.8)

Table 8.8 Results from missing data analysis using the joint model.

Dense data sampling					
	True value	No data missing	10% missing	20% missing	40% missing
θ_1 (mL/h)	—	3.97 (0.09)	3.99 (0.09)	3.97 (0.13)	3.99 (0.14)
θ_2	0.7	0.70 (0.10)	0.69 (0.19)	0.70 (0.13)	0.66 (0.20)
V1 (L)	20	20.0 (0.5)	20.1 (0.5)	20.0 (0.6)	20.0 (0.5)
Q (L/h)	12	12.0 (0.3)	12.0 (0.3)	12.0 (0.3)	12.0 (0.3)
V2 (L)	125	124 (2.4)	124 (2.4)	124 (2.6)	124 (2.5)
CV% (CL)	20	20.2 (1.7)	19.9 (2.4)	19.8 (1.7)	20.3 (2.0)
CV% (V1)	20	20.4 (1.8)	20.3 (1.7)	20.5 (1.8)	20.4 (1.8)
CV% (Q)	20	19.3 (1.5)	19.4 (1.2)	19.5 (1.3)	20.0 (1.3)
CV% (V2)	20	19.6 (1.2)	19.4 (1.7)	19.6 (1.3)	19.6 (1.3)
CV% (σ^2)	7.5	7.5 (0.2)	7.5 (0.2)	7.5 (0.2)	7.5 (0.2)
		Sparse data sampling			
	True value	No data missing	10% missing	20% missing	40% missing
θ_1 (mL/h)	—	3.95 (0.04)	3.96 (0.04)	3.96 (0.04)	3.97 (0.04)
θ_2	0.7	0.70 (0.05)	0.70 (0.06)	0.70 (0.06)	0.69 (0.06)
V1 (L)	20	20.2 (0.3)	20.2 (0.2)	20.2 (0.3)	20.2 (0.3)
Q (L/h)	12	12.1 (0.2)	12.1 (0.2)	12.1 (0.2)	12.1 (0.2)
V2 (L)	125	126 (2.1)	127 (2.0)	126 (2.1)	126 (2.2)
CV% (CL)	20	20.0 (0.7)	19.8 (0.7)	20.0 (0.7)	20.2 (0.7)
CV% (V1)	20	19.9 (2.0)	20.0 (2.0)	19.9 (2.0)	19.9 (2.0)
CV% (Q)	20	20.0 (1.3)	20.0 (1.3)	20.0 (1.3)	20.0 (1.4)
CV% (V2)	20	20.0 (1.5)	20.1 (1.4)	20.0 (1.5)	19.9 (1.5)
CV% (σ^2)	7.5	7.2 (0.8)	7.2 (0.8)	7.2 (0.8)	7.3 (0.8)

Table 8.9 Results from missing data analysis using mean imputation.

		Dense data sampling			
	True value	No data missing	10% missing	20% missing	40% missing
θ_1 (mL/h)	—	3.97 (0.09)	3.97 (0.09)	3.97 (0.10)	3.95 (0.09)
θ_2	0.7	0.70 (0.10)	0.70 (0.10)	0.70 (0.10)	0.71 (0.10)
V1 (L)	20	20.0 (0.5)	20.0 (0.5)	20.0 (0.5)	20.0 (0.5)
Q (L/h)	12	12.0 (0.3)	12.0 (0.3)	12.0 (0.3)	12.0 (0.3)
V2 (L)	125	124 (2.4)	124 (2.3)	124 (2.4)	125 (2.3)
CV% (CL)	20	20.2 (1.7)	20.3 (1.7)	20.4 (1.7)	20.5 (1.7)
CV% (V1)	20	20.4 (1.8)	20.3 (1.8)	20.3 (1.8)	20.3 (1.8)
CV% (Q)	20	19.3 (1.5)	19.4 (1.3)	19.4 (1.3)	19.4 (1.3)
CV% (V2)	20	19.6 (1.2)	19.5 (1.6)	19.5 (1.6)	19.4 (1.6)
CV% (σ^2)	7.5	7.5 (0.2)	7.5 (0.2)	7.5 (0.2)	7.5 (0.2)

		Sparse data sampling			
	True value	No data missing	10% missing	20% missing	40% missing
θ_1 (mL/h)	—	3.95 (0.04)	3.95 (0.04)	3.95 (0.04)	3.95 (0.04)
θ_2	0.7	0.70 (0.05)	0.70 (0.05)	0.70 (0.05)	0.70 (0.06)
V1 (L)	20	20.2 (0.3)	20.2 (0.3)	20.2 (0.3)	20.2 (0.3)
Q (L/h)	12	12.1 (0.2)	12.1 (0.2)	12.1 (0.2)	12.1 (0.2)
V2 (L)	125	126 (2.1)	126 (2.1)	126 (2.1)	126 (2.1)
CV% (CL)	20	20.0 (0.7)	20.1 (0.7)	20.2 (0.7)	20.4 (0.7)
CV% (V1)	20	19.9 (2.0)	19.9 (2.0)	19.9 (2.0)	19.8 (2.0)
CV% (Q)	20	20.0 (1.3)	20.0 (1.3)	20.0 (1.3)	20.0 (1.3)
CV% (V2)	20	20.0 (1.5)	20.0 (1.5)	20.0 (1.5)	20.0 (1.5)
CV% (σ^2)	7.5	7.2 (0.8)	7.2 (0.8)	7.2 (0.8)	7.2 (0.8)

Table 8.10 Results from missing data analysis using multiple imputation.

		Dense data sampling			
	True value	No data missing	10% missing	20% missing	40% missing
θ_1 (mL/h)	—	3.97 (0.09)	3.97 (0.10)	3.97 (0.09)	3.97 (0.09)
θ_2	0.7	0.70 (0.10)	0.70 (0.09)	0.69 (0.10)	0.67 (0.10)
V1 (L)	20	20.0 (0.5)	20.0 (0.5)	20.0 (0.5)	20.0 (0.5)
Q (L/h)	12	12.0 (0.3)	12.0 (0.3)	12.0 (0.3)	12.0 (0.3)
V2 (L)	125	124 (2.4)	124 (2.3)	124 (2.4)	124 (2.3)
CV% (CL)	20	20.2 (1.7)	20.3 (1.7)	21.8 (9.8)	20.8 (1.8)
CV% (V1)	20	20.4 (1.7)	20.3 (1.7)	20.4 (2.0)	20.2 (1.9)
CV% (Q)	20	19.3 (1.5)	19.4 (1.3)	19.5 (2.9)	19.4 (1.8)
CV% (V2)	20	19.6 (1.2)	19.4 (1.6)	20.6 (7.0)	19.7 (4.1)
CV% (σ^2)	7.5	7.5 (0.2)	7.5 (0.2)	7.5 (0.2)	7.5 (0.2)

		Sparse data sampling			
	True value	No data missing	10% missing	20% missing	40% missing
θ_1 (mL/h)	—	3.95 (0.04)	3.95 (0.04)	3.95 (0.04)	3.95 (0.04)
θ_2	0.7	0.70 (0.05)	0.69 (0.05)	0.68 (0.05)	0.66 (0.05)
V1 (L)	20	20.2 (0.3)	20.2 (0.3)	20.2 (0.3)	20.2 (0.3)
Q (L/h)	12	12.1 (0.2)	12.1 (0.2)	12.1 (0.2)	12.1 (0.2)
V2 (L)	125	126 (2.0)	126 (2.1)	126 (2.1)	126 (2.0)
CV% (CL)	20	20.0 (0.7)	20.1 (0.7)	20.4 (0.7)	20.7 (0.7)
CV% (V1)	20	19.9 (2.0)	19.9 (2.0)	19.9 (2.0)	19.8 (2.0)
CV% (Q)	20	20.0 (1.3)	20.0 (1.3)	20.0 (1.3)	19.9 (1.3)
CV% (V2)	20	20.0 (1.4)	20.0 (1.4)	20.0 (1.4)	20.0 (1.4)
CV% (σ^2)	7.5	7.2 (0.8)	7.2 (0.8)	7.2 (0.8)	7.2 (0.8)

study was completely ignored. The reader is referred to Allison (2002) for a good overview of handling missing data in general, although he does not cover missing data in the longitudinal case to any great extent. Schafer (1997) and Little and Rubin (2002) are other more extensive, technical references.

INTERNAL VALIDITY CHECKS AND DATA CLEAN-UP

One of the most time consuming tasks in any PopPK analysis is not necessarily model development but developing the datasets used for model building and validation. It is imperative that these datasets are formatted correctly or any analysis will be wasted and possibly incorrect. Prior to any modeling the database should be scrutinized for possible errors. The dates and time of administered doses, reported concentrations, demographic information, and other subject information should be examined for missing data or suspected errors. It is not uncommon for PopPK databases to be merged across many clinical studies which are themselves pooled across many different study centers. For laboratory values in particular, care should be taken that all the variables have the same units. It is not uncommon for sites outside the United States to use the metric system, while sites in the United States do not. Hence, all covariates should be checked for unit consistency. A quick test for consistency is to examine the frequency distribution of the covariate. Multimodal covariate is usually indicative of a units problem. If any data are missing, consistency in handling of missing values or concentration data below the LLOQ should be verified. Details on how these errors and inconsistencies will be corrected should be detailed in the DAP. Any exceptions to the DAP should be documented. Also, any changes or manipulations to the database should be clearly documented. Once all these data set issues have been resolved, model development can proceed.

PROBLEMS AND ERRORS

Abnormal terminations during the optimization process or nonconvergence with nonlinear mixed effects models are usually due to an overparameterized covariance matrix or poor initial estimates and can be overcome by a few approaches (Pinheiro and Bates, 1994). One approach is to treat the variance–covariance matrix as diagonal, treating off-diagonal covariances as zero. By examining the variance components, one or more may be so small so as to be removed from the model. Another approach is to force convergence by setting the maximal number of iterations to some value and then

examine the covariance matrix for elements that can be removed. Sometimes a covariance term may be small enough that the term can be removed. Pinheiro and Bates (1994) suggest examining the eigenvalues of the covariance matrix for overparameterization. If the smallest eigenvalue is small relative to the others or is near zero, this is indicative of overparameterization. Alternatively, one can compute the condition number of the covariance matrix and see how large it is. A large condition number is indicative of an unstable model and should be simplified. If a covariance matrix indicates that some covariance terms are needed but some are not, then perhaps the covariance matrix can be reformulated to a banded matrix where some off-diagonal elements are fixed equal to zero. If the problem is not the covariance matrix, then possibly the initial estimates are poor. Check the magnitude of the starting values to make sure they are the correct scale, e.g., clearance should be in mL/h but the initial estimate is in L/h. Alternatively, a quick user defined grid search can be done to find starting values by setting the maximum number of evaluations equal to zero and looking to see how the objective function value changes. A number of other errors may occur during routine use with NON-MEM which are listed in Table 8.11 along with some solutions.

CONSISTENCY OF MODEL PARAMETER ESTIMATES ACROSS COMPUTER PLATFORMS

NONMEM is provided on either UNIX or DOS platform. Although no formal studies have been done, there is some data to suggest that different platforms may result in different population estimates. Frame et al. (2001) reported that in a population analysis, a particular model could not converge on the DOS platform due to either rounding errors or aborted covariance step, but could do so on the UNIX platform. Curiously, the parameter estimates for both platforms under the final converged model (UNIX) and model at this time of failure (DOS) were almost identical.

Bonate (2002), with the help of many contributors, compared the consistency across users of five different models in NONMEM-reported parameter estimates and their standard errors. All users used NONMEM V on a personal (31/38, 81%), Unix (6/38, 16%), or Macintosh (1/38, 3%) computer. Ten different compilers were tested. In those models that optimized without errors, the estimates of the fixed effects and variance components were 100% consistent across users, although there were some small differences in the estimates of the standard error of the parameter estimates. Different compilers produced small differences in the estimates of the stand-

Table 8.11 Common NONMEM error messages and some solutions.

Example error message	Solution
Minimization terminated due to proximity of last iteration est. to a value at which the obj. func. is infinite (Error = 136)	• This message is telling you that at the point of termination an infinite objective function was encountered, which may have been due to a possible zero concentration in one of the observations. Check and remove. Or add a very small additive error term to the error model, e.g., Y = F* EXP(EPS(1)) + EPS(2), where EPS(2) is fixed to something small (<0.001). Alternatively, try METHOD = HYBRID.
Floating overflow	• This indicates that a division by zero has occurred. Check the control stream for functions that include a division by a variable term and then examine that variable in the data set for any values set equal to zero. It has been reported that when everything else has failed, sometimes a new Fortran compiler can solve the problem.
Occurs during search for ETA at a nonzero value of ETA K21, or K31 is too close to an eigenvalue 0 program terminated by FNLETA message issued from table step	• The error message is the result of running the POSTHOC step. Look at the individual where the error occurs and see if there is something unusual about that person's data. Try using the NOABORT option on the $COV statement. Try changing the starting values.
288 Size of NMPRD4 exceeded; LNP4 is too small in NM-Tran and NONMEM	• Your model may have exceeded the maximum number of fixed effects and variance components. You may need to increase TSIZE and NSIZE within NONMEM.
R-matrix algorithmically singular and algorithmically non-positive-semidefinite covariance step aborted or S-matrix algorithmically singular and algorithmically non-positive-semidefinite covariance step aborted	• This message is not necessarily an error message but a warning. This error is usually due to a model that is overparameterized. Look for parameters, particularly variance components, that are very small, e.g., <1E-6, and remove them from the model. What you are trying to do here is simplify the model.
Minimization terminated due to rounding errors (Error=134) No. of function evaluations used: 672 No. of sig. digits in final est.: 2.8	• Computers are able to retain numbers within their memory only to a certain number of digits. During the computing of a mathematical operation, such as matrix inversion, digits in a number may be lost. This message indicates that a sufficient number of digits were lost resulting in termination of the optimization. One solution is to rerun the model with a new set of starting values and change the number of significant digits to higher than the current value. In this example SIGDIGITS = 3 in the $COV step. One solution would be to set SIGDIGITS = 4. The starting values should then be set equal to the final estimates at the point the algorithm terminated. This process may have to be repeated many times. A second solution is to decrease the number of significant digits, such as to SIGDIGITS = 2 in this example. If the rounding error is a variance component then this is usually an acceptable solution. A third solution is to simplify the model because the model is overparameterized. A fourth solution is to ignore the error or to remove the $COV step. A fifth step is to try the SLOW option on the $COV step.
Program terminated by OBJ error in cels with individual 5 ID= .50000000E+01 weighted sum of "squared" individual residuals is infinite message issued from estimation step at initial Obj. function evaluation	• This indicates that the residual sum of squares for the individual is near zero. Check the initial value of the residual error and see if it is small. If so, increase its value. Alternatively, try fitting the logarithms of the concentration with an additive residual error model.

ard errors. The standard errors were not consistent even with users running the same compiler version.

With one data set, 27 of 38 testers could not minimize the run successfully without abnormal terminations: five due to infinite objective function, 12 due to maximum function evaluations exceeded, and 10 due to rounding errors. Only one user, who used a UNIX computer running HP-UX Fortran 77, reported successful minimization without errors. Interestingly, two other users running the same hardware-software combination reported termination due to maximum number of function evaluations exceeded or termination due to rounding errors. In the 11 testers who could successfully minimize the data set, 10 of 11 reported R-matrix singularity. These results suggest that models that fail to minimize successfully on one platform and compiler may not fail on another, and vice versa. These results are highly suggestive that NONMEM results are machine specific, although the differences across machines may be small enough to be ignored. No such other studies have been done for other software systems, such as the NLMIXED procedure in SAS or with the NLME function in S-PLUS.

REGULATORY REVIEW OF POPULATION ANALYSES

Population analyses are usually targeted to one of three audiences: the medical literature, internal review, or regulatory reviewers. When the objective of an analysis is a publication, model development is usually not as stringent because quite often most medical journals in which population analyses are published are limited in the amount of page space that can be devoted to methods and so often analyses omit the details on method development and focus on the "big picture." The same can be said of analyses conducted for internal review but for different reasons. Often the outcome of an internal analysis is a presentation to project team members or management and a report may never even be written. In contrast, the level of detail in a report can be overwhelming when the audience is regulatory authorities. It is common for a PopPK report, not even including appendices, to total a hundred or more pages with the number of tables and figures in the mid double digits. Already discussed has been a sample report template in this setting (see Table 8.2). What is important with a PopPK report for regulatory authorities is that the report has a clear flow and logic for how model development proceeded and that the conclusions were supported by the analysis. The FDA routinely publishes on the internet their reviews of sponsor's population analyses in support of a New Drug Application (NDA). It is very informative to read some of these to understand how regulatory authorities review these reports. It is not uncommon to see back-seat modeling from regulatory reviewers as they examine the validity of the reported final model. For example, a model may underpredict maximal concentrations. The reviewer then may try to develop better, alternative models that more precisely estimate maximal concentrations. Failing that the reviewer may then examine what impact this underprediction has on the conclusions of the analysis or a pharmacokinetic-pharmacodynamic analysis of the drug.

Reviewers at regulatory agencies now take a question-based approach in reviewing an NDA (Lesko and Williams, 1999). Reviewers develop particular questions and then review the NDA as a means of answering those questions. The particular questions raised might include what are the general attributes of the drug, what are the general clinical pharmacology characteristics of the drug, what intrinsic and extrinsic factors affect drug exposure, what are the particular biopharmaceutical characteristics of the drug, is there a need for all doses the manufacturer will make (for example, the sponsor may market the drug in 5, 10, and 20 mg tablets and the FDA may question whether a 5 mg tablet is necessary), and were the bioanalytical methods sufficiently accurate and precise in quantifying the drug and its metabolites? Many of these questions are answered by a single reviewer, but the review of the population analysis is often done by a different reviewer, one with specific expertise in population analyses. At the FDA this is often the purview of the pharmacometrics group.

Unfortunately there is no standardized policy or procedures guide for reviewing PopPK analyses so these reviews tend to be reviewer-specific. However, pharmacometric reviewers tend to focus on the following areas: data checking (how was the data base developed and examined for outliers or merge errors, what did the data base consist of, how many subjects, how many observations total and per subject overall, did the data base include sufficient numbers of subjects in subpopulations to detect any meaningful relationships with exposure), structural model development (how was the structural model developed, what estimation algorithms were used, what random effects were added and why), covariate models (how were covariates chosen for evaluation, reasonableness of the covariates, any particular obvious covariates not examined, how were covariate models examined, what estimation algorithm was used, which model types were examined, e.g., linear or power, and reasonableness of the final covariate model), validation (what validation techniques were used and how reasonable were the results and conclusions), software (which software was used), and does the analysis contribute to the overall understanding of the drug. Given then the reasonableness of a PopPK model the impact of the model on dosing must be examined. Does the sponsor's dosing recommendations concur with the results of the population analysis? Should some particular groups receive dose reductions, e.g., if creatinine clearance is identified as a covariate should patients with renal impairment be dosed differently than patients with normal renal function?

Every effort should be made to make reports to regulatory agencies as clear and concise as possible with the report written to support the product label and further help in understanding the pharmacology and pharmacokinetics of the drug. In order to facilitate review of these reports, sponsors should provide to the regulatory authorities electronic copies of all data sets and control streams in an ASCII format. A hard copy of the first page of each data set should be included in the report with each individual data column identified. Any SAS programs or programs used to prepare the data sets should be made available. Whatever would be useful for a reviewer to repeat the modeling process from beginning to end should be made available in an easily retrievable format.

SUMMARY

Population pharmacokinetic analyses are fraught with problems. This chapter was meant to explore these issues and present real-world problems and solutions to the reader. Some topics, like missing data, could not be covered in their entirety. Indeed, entire books have been written on some of the topics just briefly covered herein. Obviously the reader is referred to these texts for greater detail. With the topics presented in the last chapter on theory and this chapter on prac-

tical issues, the introduction of real-world PopPK analyses will be made in the next chapter.

Recommended Reading

Aarons, L., Balant, L.P., Mentre, F., Morselli, P.L., Rowland, M., Steimer, J.-L., and Vozeh, S. Practical experience and issues in designing and performing population pharmacokinetic/pharmacodynamic studies. *European Journal of Clinical Pharmacology* 1996; 49: 251–254.

Allison, P. Missing data. Sage, Publications, Thousand Oaks, CA, 2002.

Food and Drug Administration. Guidance for industry: population pharmacokinetics, 1999 (http://www.fda.gov/cder/guidance/1852fnl.pdf).

Kowalski, K. and Hutmacher, K. Design evaluation for a population pharmacokinetic study using clinical trial simulations: A case study. *Statistics in Medicine* 2001; 20: 75–91.

Lee, P.I.D. Design and power of a population pharmacokinetic study. *Pharmaceutical Research* 2001; 18: 75–82.

Wahlby, U., Jonsson, E.N., and Karlsson, M.O. Assessment of actual significance levels for covariate effects in NONMEM. *Journal of Pharmacokinetics and Pharmacodynamics* 2001; 28: 231–252.

Wright, P.M.C. Population based pharmacokinetic analysis: Why do we need it; what is it; and what has it told us about anesthesia. *British Journal of Anesthesia* 1998; 80: 488–501.

Chapter 9

Nonlinear Mixed Effects Models: Case Studies

Materialists and madmen never have doubts.

—G.K. Chesterton (1874–1936), English Author...may be modelers should be added to that list?

INTRODUCTION

This chapter introduces two examples that will be used to explain and illustrate the principles in developing population pharmacokinetic models and nonlinear mixed effects models in general. The first example is the pharmacodynamic modeling of zifrosilone, an acetylcholinesterase inhibitor. This example was chosen because of its simplicity in introducing some of the concepts in model development, in particular, choosing one model over another. The second example is a population analysis of tobramycin in a general population of patients with infection. This example was chosen because the model is not very complex but is sufficient to explain the step-by-step process involved in developing a model, validating the model, and then using the model to answer some "what-if" questions.

PHARMACODYNAMIC MODELING OF ACETYLCHOLINESTERASE INHIBITION

Zifrosilone (MDL 73745) is a potent reversible acetylcholinesterase inhibitor and was studied for the treatment of Alzheimer's disease. Cutler et al. (1995) reported on the pharmacokinetics and pharmacodynamics of zifrosilone in healthy normal volunteers randomized to receive 30–300 mg zifrosilone as a single dose. Blood samples for measurement of zifrosilone concentrations in plasma and RBC cholinesterase inhibition were collected at 0, 0.5, 1, 2, 3, 4, 6, 8, 12, 16, and 24 h after administration. Of particular interest was to develop the exposure–response relationship between zifrosilone plasma concentrations and RBC cholinesterase activity. This analysis was purely exploratory so there was little need for validation. Plasma concentrations were not quantifiable at doses less than 200 mg. Consequently, the exposure–response relationship was based upon complete pharmacokinetic–pharmacodynamic data in the remaining 12 volunteers. A total of 8–11 observations were available per subject (Table 9.1). Figure 9.1 presents a spaghetti plot of percent inhibition over time and a scatter plot of percent inhibition against zifrosilone plasma concentration.

At first glance, the data suggests an E_{max} model might best describe the increase in percent inhibition with increasing concentration, eventually plateauing at a maximal value of ~70% inhibition. See Mager, Wyska, and Jusko (2003) for a useful review of pharmacodynamic models. The first model examined was an E_{max} model with additive (homoscedastic) residual error

Table 9.1   Zifrosilone plasma concentration-and effect-time data as reported in Cutler et al. (1995).

Time (h)	38	39	40	41	43	44	45	46	49	51	53	54
	\multicolumn{12}{Subject identifier and percent of acetylcholinesterase inhibition}										

Time (h)	38	39	40	41	43	44	45	46	49	51	53	54
0	0	0	0	0	0	0	0	0	0	0	0	0
0.5	3	7	12	25	27	7	15	18	40	−12	−8	−4
1	2	27	12	34	53	38	36	38	61	23	3	8
2	44	48	30	33	54	57	51	50	68	53	24	56
3	41	47	28	47	56	51	56	63	72	49	43	49
4	38	49	49	46	45	45	52	64	65	56	60	44
6	29	26	30	21	31	33	44	60	63	45	61	31
8	25	20	22	19	33	16	23	41	35	30	38	16
12	8	10		−4	22	9	13	22	18	3	2	6
16					2				40	7	5	−3
24												−5

Subject identifier and zifrosilone concentration (ng/mL)

Time (h)	38	39	40	41	43	44	45	46	49	51	53	54
0	0.00	0.00	0.00	0.00	0.00	0.00	0.00	0.00	0.00	0.00	0.00	0.00
0.5	0.00	0.14	0.00	1.43	0.68	0.40	0.77	0.27	1.87	0.21	0.00	0.00
1	0.00	0.36	0.16	1.03	0.67	0.60	0.59	0.67	1.46	0.38	0.12	0.18
2	0.64	0.52	0.26	0.81	0.63	0.77	0.47	0.71	3.16	0.57	0.33	0.77
3	0.42	0.51	0.38	0.98	0.68	0.67	0.80	0.83	2.56	0.52	0.80	0.72
4	0.43	0.44	0.46	0.67	0.61	0.51	0.52	0.97	2.24	0.65	1.18	0.64
6	0.28	0.23	0.26	0.37	0.43	0.57	0.45	1.22	2.93	0.41	0.96	0.62
8	0.18	0.14	0.19	0.30	0.27	0.26	0.21	0.64	0.39	0.20	0.43	0.33
12	0.10	0.11		0.20	0.13	0.16	0.11	0.22	0.25	0.10	0.20	0.30
16					0.10			0.10	0.13		0.16	0.13
24												0.13

$$E_{max} = \theta_1 + \eta_1$$
$$IC_{50} = \theta_2 \exp(\eta_2)$$
$$Y = \frac{E_{max}C}{C + IC_{50}} + \varepsilon \qquad (9.1)$$

where C is zifrosilone concentration. Both E_{max} and IC_{50} were treated as random effects. IC_{50} was treated as a log-normal random effect to ensure the parameter remains positive. Model parameters were estimated using Laplacian estimation.

To obtain initial estimates, an E_{max} model was fit to the data set in a naïve-pooled manner, which does not take into account the within-subject correlations and assumes each observation comes from a unique individual. The final estimates from this nonlinear model, 84% maximal inhibition and 0.6 ng/mL as the IC_{50}, were used as the initial values in the nonlinear mixed effects model. The additive variance component and between-subject variability (BSV) on E_{max} was modeled using an additive error models with initial values equal to 10%. BSV in IC_{50} was modeled using an exponential error model with an initial estimate of 10%. The model minimized successfully with R-matrix singularity and an objective function value (OFV) of 648.217. The standard deviation (square root of the variance component) associated with IC_{50} was 6.66E-5 ng/mL and was the likely source of the

singularity. BSV in IC_{50} was removed from the model and the model was refit to the data. Removal of the extraneous variance component resulted in successful minimization with no singularities and had no effect on the OFV. Table 9.2 presents the final model estimates.

The next model examined was a sigmoid E_{max} model

$$E_{max} = \theta_1 + \eta_1$$
$$IC_{50} = \theta_2 \exp(\eta_2)$$
$$n = \theta_3 + \eta_3$$
$$Y = \frac{E_{max}C^n}{C^n + IC_{50}^n} + \varepsilon \qquad (9.2)$$

where the Hill coefficient (n) was treated as a normally distributed random effect. The initial values were the same as before but now the Hill coefficient was initially set to 1.0 with a variance of 0.10. The model minimized successfully with no singularities and an OFV of 637.885. Table 9.2 presents the final model estimates. The likelihood ratio test (LRT) for the full (sigmoid E_{max}) and reduced (E_{max}) model was 10.332 (p = 0.00557 on two degrees of freedom) which indicated the sigmoid E_{max} model was better than the E_{max} model. However, the goodness of fit plots were not

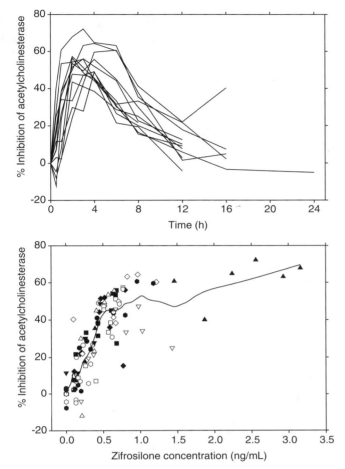

Figure 9.1 Top plot: spaghetti plot of zifrosilone percent inhibition-time profiles. Each line represents a unique individual. Bottom plot: scatter plot of percent inhibition versus zifrosilone concentration (bottom). Each symbol represents a unique individual. Solid line is the LOESS smooth to the data.

Table 9.2 Zifrosilone model development summary.

Parameter	E_{max}	Sigmoid E_{max}	Sigmoid E_{max} with effect compartment	Reduced sigmoid E_{max} with effect compartment
OFV	648.217	637.885	579.174[R]	578.202
E_{max}	100 ± 194	66.2 ± 9.38	74.8	74.9 ± 3.22E-5
$IC_{50} \times 1000$	866 ± 279	404 ± 7.80	432	432 ± 42.0
N	—	1.73 ± 0.406	1.73	1.73 ± 1.47E-4
k_e	—	—	1.30	1.30 ± 1.21E-4
$\omega^2(E_{max})$	156	47.7	7.75E-5	—
$\omega^2(IC_{50})$	—	0.0122	0.0648	0.0646
$\omega^2(n)$	—	0.177	0.162	0.162
$\omega^2(k_e)$	—	—	0.0916	0.0916
σ^2	103	89.1	41.4	41.4

Note: All models with using Laplacian estimation. The symbol "R" denotes R-matrix singularity. —denote that the parameter was not included in the model.

entirely satisfactory (Fig. 9.2). Although the residuals were centered at zero, the residuals were not normally distributed. The same with the weighted residuals. Further, a small trend seemed apparent in the weighted residual over time plot.

To inhibit cholinesterase within the red blood cell (RBC), zifrosilone must first cross the RBC membrane. Hence, there may be a delay in effect. The next model examined was an effect compartment model, which models the effect of a drug based on the drug concentration in a hypothetical effect compartment. In this instance an effect compartment, denoted C_e, with the same first-order rate constant for input and output (k_e) was modeled with the observed drug effect dependent on the effect compartment concentration through an E_{max} model

$$\frac{dC_e}{dt} = k_e C - k_e C_e$$
$$E_{max} = \theta_1 + \eta_1$$
$$IC_{50} = \theta_2 \exp(\eta_2).$$
$$n = \theta_3 + \eta_3 \qquad (9.3)$$
$$k_e = \theta_4 \exp(\eta_4)$$
$$Y = \frac{E_{max} C_e^n}{C_e^n + IC_{50}^n} + \varepsilon$$

Initial values were the final values for the sigmoid E_{max} model with k_e set to 1 per hour. The model minimized successfully with R-matrix singularity and an OFV of 579.174. The source of the singularity was likely the variance component associated with E_{max} since its value was near zero. E_{max} was treated as a fixed effect and the model refit. The resulting model minimized successfully with no singularities and an OFV of 578.202. Table 9.2 presents the final model estimates. The LRT test for this reduced model compared to the sigmoid E_{max} model was 58.711 ($p < 0.0001$ on two degrees of freedom) which indicated that the addition of an effect compartment significantly improved the goodness of fit. Figure 9.3 shows the goodness of fit plots under this model. The residuals were still not normally distributed but the distribution around zero was more symmetric. All the random effects were normally distributed. Further, there was less trend in the residuals over time and better distribution around the line of unity between observed and predicted response.

Hence, based on this analysis, the concentration that inhibited acetylcholinesterase activity by 50% was 0.432 ng/mL with 26% between-subject variability. Zifrosilone also could not completely inhibit acetylcholinesterase activity. Only ~75% of acetylcholinesterase activity appeared to be maximally inhibited with zifrosilone. Further, there was about a half-hour delay between plasma concentrations and acetylcholinesterase inhibition, which was clinically irrelevant. For this type of

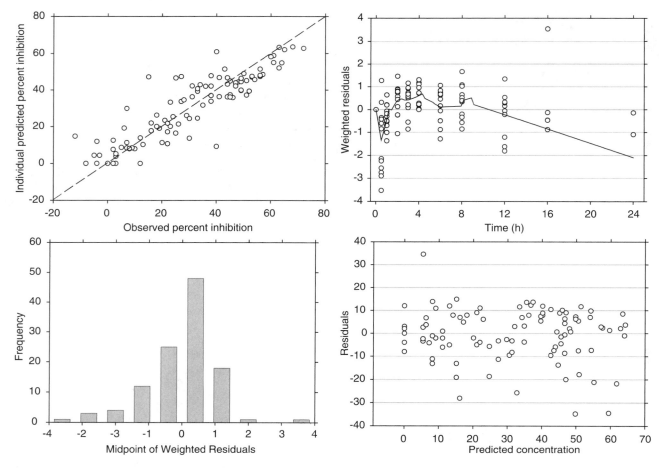

Figure 9.2 Goodness of fit plots for the zifrosilone data under the sigmoid E_{max} model with final values reported in Table 9.2. Dashed line in upper left plot is the line of unity. Solid line in upper right plot is the LOESS smooth to the data with a 0.3 sampling proportion.

drug, it would be reasonable to target concentrations to remain above the IC_{50} throughout the dosing interval. At the zifrosilone doses administered, none resulted in trough concentrations (24-h postdose) above the IC_{50} indicating that twice-daily dosing would be needed. Unfortunately, further zifrosilone clinical development was cancelled so this hypothesis was never tested.

This example was meant to show that the process of developing and evaluating nonlinear mixed effects models is not all that different from developing and evaluating other types of models, like a linear regression model or a linear mixed effects model. Initially a model is postulated, then compared to another model. Using some set of criteria one model is determined to be superior to the other. The superior model is then used until it is repudiated by scientific evidence to the contrary. Hopefully in the next example the modeling process will be further solidified and the interrelationships between nonlinear mixed effect models and other types of modeling will become more obvious.

POPULATION PHARMACOKINETICS OF TOBRAMYCIN

Introduction

Aarons et al. (1989) originally published this analysis in the *British Journal of Clinical Pharmacology*, one of the premier journals publishing population analyses. The authors then graciously provided this data set to the Resource Facility for Population Analysis (RFPK), an academic facility funded by a grant from the National Institutes of Health (EB-01975). This freely accessible data set, along with many others, is found on their web site (http://depts.washington.edu/rfpk/) and can be used for training purposes.

Tobramycin is an aminoglycoside antibiotic used to treat aerobic gram negative infections, such as *Eschericia Coli*, *Enterobacter* species, *Pseudomonas* species, or *Staphylococcus Aureus*. Aminoglycosides are notorious for their narrow therapeutic index and tobramycin is no exception. Prolonged exposure to aminoglycosides may

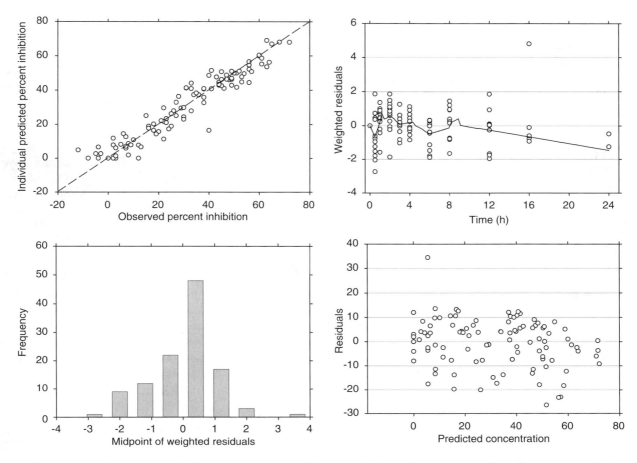

Figure 9.3 Goodness of fit plots for the zifrosilone data under the sigmoid E_{max} model with an effect compartment. Final values are reported in Table 9.2. Solid line in upper left plot is the line of unity. Dashed line in upper right plot is the LOESS smooth to the data with a 0.3 sampling proportion.

result in ototoxicity and nephrotoxicity. On the other hand, aminoglycosides have concentration-dependent bactericidal activity requiring high plasma concentrations for sufficient antibacterial effectiveness. Hence, aminoglycosides are dosed by either short infusions or rapid, intermittent bolus doses. For a drug like tobramycin, reducing the incidence of adverse events and increasing the probability of a successful outcome are desirable goals. Any patient covariates that can be used to reduce BSV in exposure or help develop a suitable dosage regimen would be useful to meet these goals. The purpose of this analysis was to characterize the population pharmacokinetics of tobramycin, determine which patient covariates reduce between-subject variability in dosing, and to explore some "what-if" questions.

Assay Characteristics

Because of its narrow therapeutic index, tobramycin concentrations are frequently monitored. The thera-

peutic range for tobramycin is a steady-state trough concentration in the 0.5–1 mg/L range and a peak concentration in the 4–6 mg/L range. Ototoxicity and nephrotoxicity begin to occur around 12–15 mg/L at peak and with prolonged trough concentrations greater than 2 mg/L. At the time of publication, the state of the art in tobramycin assays was an enzyme immunoassay (EMIT®, Syva Corp., Palo Alto, CA). The assay had a within-and between-assay coefficient of variation (CV%) of 7.4% (at a concentration of 4 mg/L) and 3.6% (at a concentration of 6 mg/L). The lower limit of quantification (LLOQ) was 0.5 mg/L. Of 322 observations in the data base, 27 (8.3%) are listed as below the LLOQ. For purposes of this analysis, these observations were kept in the database even though an argument can be made for their removal. In eight patients not identified in the data set, tobramycin concentrations were followed for 72 h after cessation of therapy using a modified radioimmunoassay having a CV% of 7.3% (at a concentration of 1 mg/L).

Patient and Data Summary

Pharmacokinetic data were available from 97 patients (45 females, 52 males). The following patients covariates were available: age, weight, sex, height, and creatinine clearance (CrCL) estimated using the Cockcroft–Gault (1976) equation. The original data set had CrCL with units of mL/min. In this analysis, CrCL was transformed to L/h to make the units consistent with the units of tobramycin clearance. Table 9.3 presents a summary of available demographic information. All covariate information was complete, except height which was missing in 22% of females and 33% of males. Although only patients with stable renal function were enrolled in the study, according to guidelines presented by the Food and Drug Administration, 12 patients (12%) would be classified as having severe renal failure (a CrCL of <30 mL/min or <1.8 L/h), 32 patients (33%) with moderate renal impairment (CrCL between 30 and 50 mL/min or 1.8–3.0 L/h), and 21 patients (22%) with mild renal impairment (CrCL between 50 and 80 mL/min or 3.0–4.8 L/h),. Only 32 patients (33%) had normal renal function with CrCL greater than 80 mL/min (>4.8 L/h). Patient doses were administered as bolus doses ranging from 20 to 140 mg every 8 h with most patients receiving 80 or 100 mg every 8 h.

Blood samples were collected during therapeutic drug monitoring of routine clinical standard of care. The duration of therapy ranged from 14 to 520 h with most patients receiving ∼6 days of therapy. The time of dosing and sample collection were carefully monitored and recorded. A total of 322 plasma samples were collected with the number of samples per patient ranging from one to nine (median: 2). Observable tobramycin concentrations ranged from 0.09 to 7.55 mg/L with samples collected between 0.5-and 36-h postdose. Figure 9.4 presents a scatter plot of the observed concentrations over time pooled across patients. Most samples were collected between 2-to 6-h postdose (Fig. 9.5).

Data Manipulations and NONMEM Data Base Creation

Because patient height was missing for 28% of the data base, it was decided that only using patients with complete data (complete case analysis) would not be an option as this would decrease the sample size to only 70 patients. Furthermore, the percent missing was rather large and so simple mean imputation did not seem a

Table 9.3 Demographic summary of patients in tobramycin analysis by sex.

	Number missing	Mean	Std Dev	Min	Max
Males (n = 52)					
Weight (kg)	0	69.8	11.9	42	120
Height (cm)	17	174.6	6.5	164	190
Age (years)	0	54.8	18.5	16	85
Creatinine clearance (L/h)	0	4.0	2.1	0.6	10.0
Imputed height (cm)	0	175.1	7.2	156	195
Body surface area (m^2)	17	1.84	0.13	1.56	2.24
Ideal body weight (kg)	17	65.7	4.3	59.0	76.0
Body mass index (kg/m^2)	17	22.8	2.7	18.5	29.7
Lean body weight (kg)	17	50.6	4.5	41	65
Females (n = 45)					
Weight (kg)	0	62.7	12.3	46	103
Height (cm)	10	164.4	6.2	150	178
Age (years)	0	45.8	18.6	16	78
Creatinine clearance (L/h)	0	4.2	1.8	1.2	8.6
Imputed height (cm)	0	164.1	6.2	150	178
Body surface area (m^2)	10	1.69	0.15	1.38	2.11
Ideal body weight (kg)	10	58.8	4.3	49	68
Body mass index (kg/m^2)	10	23.6	4.7	18.1	36.9
Lean body weight (kg)	10	45.1	4.2	35	54
All (included imputed values, n = 97)					
Weight (kg)	0	66.5	12.5	42	120
Age (years)	0	50.6	19.0	16	85
Creatinine clearance (L/h)	0	4.1	2.0	0.6	10.0
Height (cm)	0	170.0	8.7	150	196
Body surface area (m^2)	0	1.77	0.18	1.38	2.52
Ideal body weight (kg)	0	62.6	5.9	49	80
Body mass index (kg/m^2)	0	23.0	3.9	14.4	36.9
Lean body weight (kg)	0	47.9	6.1	35	73

Legend: Std Dev, standard deviation; Min, minimum; Max, maximum.

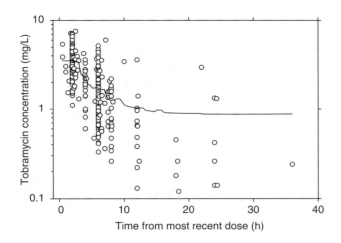

Figure 9.4 Scatter plot of pooled tobramycin concentration–time profiles relative to the most recent dose administered. Solid line is the inverse square kernel smooth to the data using a 0.3 sampling proportion, which suggests that concentrations declined biphasically after dosing.

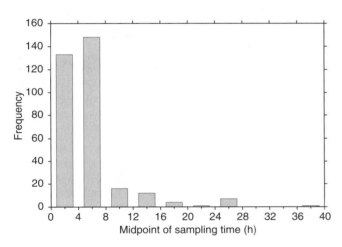

Figure 9.5 Histogram of tobramycin sample collection times.

viable alternative. It was decided that monotonic regression imputation using the multiple imputation procedure (PROC MI) in SAS would be used to impute the missing heights (rounded to the nearest integer) using weight, age, sex, and average tobramycin concentration as covariates. Five imputation data sets were generated but only the first imputed data set was used for model development and validation. The remaining data sets were saved for the final model to obtain the multiple imputation estimates of the population parameters. Once the imputed heights were calculated, the following derived variables were calculated: body surface area using the method of Dubois and Dubois (1916), ideal body weight, body mass index, and lean body weight. Table 9.3 presents the summary statistics for height (observed plus imputed values) and the derived covariates.

Since some subjects were sampled on different occasions, the occasion on which each subject received their dose was determined so that BSV may be further partitioned into interoccasion variability (IOV). Once the data set was created, the first 19 subjects were removed and saved as a validation data set. This represented ~20% of the total data. The remaining subjects were used for model development. Thus, the model development data set consisted of 250 observations from 78 patients, whereas the model validation data set consisted of 72 observations from 19 subjects.

Base Model Development

Base model development proceeded from a 1-compartment model (ADVAN1 TRANS2) estimated using first-order conditional estimation with interaction (FOCE-I) in NONMEM (Version 5.1 with all bug fixes as of April 2005). All pharmacokinetic parameters were treated as random effects and residual error was modeled using an additive and exponential (sometimes called an additive and proportional) error model. Initial values for the fixed effects were obtained from the literature (Xuan et al., 2000): systemic clearance (CL) of 4.53 L/h and volume of distribution (V1) of 27.3 L. Initial values for the variance components was set to 32% for all, except the additive term in the residual error which was set equal to 1 mg/L. The model successfully converged with an OFV of 20.141. The results are shown in Table 9.4.

Table 9.4 Tobramycin 1-, 2-, and 3-compartment model summary.

Parameter	Number of compartments		
	1	2	3
OFV	20.141	-6.280^R	-14.368^R
AIC	32.141	13.720	13.632
CL (L/h)	3.82 (0.263)	3.61	3.53
V1 (L)	21.6 (1.10)	15.0	13.6
Q2 (L/h)	—	2.46	3.42
V2 (L)	—	7.67	5.91
Q3 (L/h)	—	—	0.193
V3 (L)	—	—	6.60
Var (CL)	0.354	0.335	0.334
Var (V1)	0.0149	8.52E–11	4.77E–12
Var (Q)	—	6.35E–11	1.18E–11
Var (V2)	—	0.121	0.257
Var (Q3)	—	—	0.0162
Var (V3)	—	—	2.69E–9
$\sigma^2(E)$	0.0323	0.0321	0.0328
$\sigma^2(A)$	0.00748	0.00302	4.08E–14

All models were fit using FOCE-I. Data are reported as estimate (standard error of the estimate).^{R} denotes model minimized successfully but with R-matrix singularity. (A) denotes additive residual error term. (E) denotes exponential residual error term.

Next, a 2-compartment model (ADVAN3 TRANS4) was then fit to the data. Initial values were taken from the literature (Winslade et al., 1987): 5 L/h for CL, 17 L for V1, 1 L/h for intercompartmental clearance to the peripheral compartment (Q2), and 94 L for the peripheral compartment (V2). BSV was set to 70% for CL and 32% for all remaining pharmacokinetic variance terms. The exponential component of the residual error was set to 23% while the additive component was set to 1 mg/L. Optimization minimized successfully with an OFV of -6.280 (Table 9.4). R-matrix singularity was observed which indicated that the model was overparameterized. The 2-compartment fit was a significant improvement in the goodness of fit compared to the 1-compartment model based on the LRT (26.42 on four degrees of freedom, $p < 0.0001$). Even though the model had R-matrix singularity, near zero variance components were retained in the model since it is better to have an overparameterized covariance matrix than a restrictive, underparameterized one. Hence, model reduction will occur after the covariate model is developed.

Lastly, a 3-compartment model (ADVAN11 TRANS4) was then fit to the data. There were no literature values for fits to a 3-compartment model so initial values were guessed: 4 L/h for CL, 15 L for V1, 2 L/h for Q2, 8 L for V2, 0.01 L/h for intercompartmental clearance to the deep compartment (Q3), and 10 L for the volume of the deep compartment (V3). The model successfully minimized with an OFV of -14.368 but exhibited R-matrix singularity (Table 9.4). The model was not a significant improvement over the 2-compartment model (LRT = 8.09 on 4 degrees of freedom, $p = 0.088$).

Examination of the goodness of fit plots were not very helpful in choosing a suitable base model as all plots were roughly equivalent (Fig. 9.6). All plots showed a few outliers whose weighted residuals were greater than ± 4 and the observed versus individual predicted plots were all roughly the same, although it did seem as if the 2-and 3-compartment models did slightly better at predicting higher concentrations than the 1-compartment model. The 2-and 3-compartment models were virtually indistinguishable in these plots.

The choice for the base model was one between a 2-or 3-compartment model. Even though the 3-compartment model had the smallest AIC, it was decided that a 2-compartment model would be brought forward for further development since the difference in AIC between the 2-and 3-compartment model was small and the LRT testing the additional parameters in the 3-compartment model did not result in a significant improvement. Further, the 2-and 3-compartment models were virtually indistinguishable in the goodness of fit plots. This choice, however, was not clear-cut and another modeler

may have chosen the 3-compartment model as the base model.

Exploration of the 2-compartment model covariance matrix was undertaken to try and find any further improvements in the model. First, an unstructured covariance was examined. Initial values were taken as the final values of the 2-compartment model, except the off-diagonal elements of the covariance matrix which were chosen to have a correlation of 0.5. The model had numerous terminations due to rounding errors in estimating the variance components. Each time the model terminated, the initial values were reset to the estimates at the time of model termination and the number of significant digits was varied between 3 and 5. This approach failed to achieve successful model convergence, so the initial values were reset to their final values at the time of termination and the SLOW option (which uses a different algorithm to estimate the gradient) on the $EST statement was added. As the option suggests, the run time with the SLOW option was considerably slower, but model convergence was achieved, albeit with R-matrix singularity.

The OFV of the final model was -16.688 with an AIC of 15.312. The correlation matrix between the parameters was

$$
r = \begin{bmatrix}
\text{CL} & \text{V1} & \text{Q2} & \text{V2} \\
1.00 & & & \\
1.00 & 1.00 & & \\
0.99 & 1.00 & 1.00 & \\
-0.24 & -0.77 & -0.82 & 1.00
\end{bmatrix} \quad (9.4)
$$

which indicated that the correlation between most of the random effects was high. A review of the scatter plot matrix between the random effects under the model using only a diagonal covariance matrix confirmed this result (data not shown).

Because of the very high correlation between CL and V1 and between CL and Q2 it was decided that a reduced covariance matrix should be developed. Hence, the model was modified to

$$
\begin{aligned}
\text{CL} &= \theta_1 \exp(\eta_1) \\
\text{V1} &= \theta_2 \exp(\theta_5 \eta_1) \\
\text{Q2} &= \theta_3 \exp(\theta_6 \eta_1) \\
\text{V2} &= \theta_4 \exp(\eta_2)
\end{aligned} \quad (9.5)
$$

where η_1 and η_2 were correlated. In this model, the variance of V1 and Q2 was a function of CL. The model minimized successfully with no singularities, an OFV of -16.205, and an AIC of 5.795. The reduced covariance model had an OFV almost near the unstructured covariance model but had a much smaller AIC.

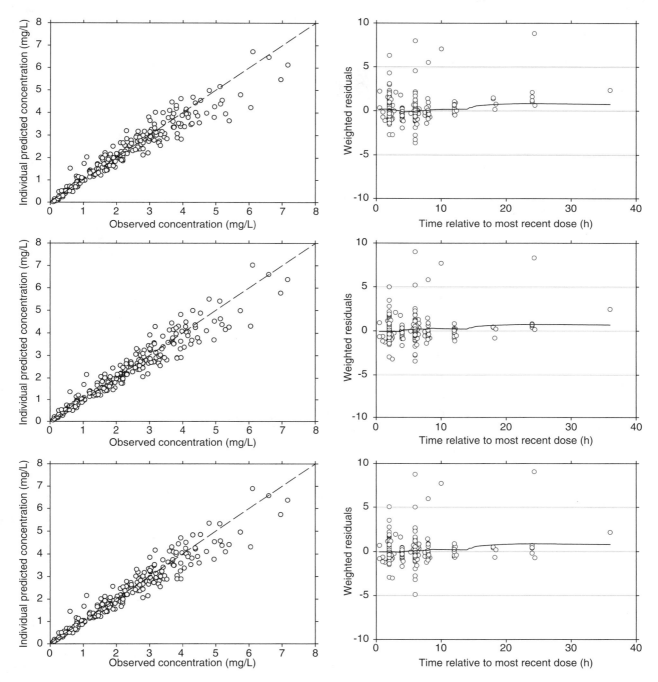

Figure 9.6   Goodness of fit plots for the 1-compartment (top), 2-compartment (middle), and 3-compartment (bottom) tobramycin models with no covariates. Solid line in the weighted residual plot is an inverse square kernel smoother with 0.4 sampling proportion. Dashed line in observed versus predicted plot is the line of unity. Clearly, judging model superiority based on graphical assessment is difficult.

Figure 9.7 presents the goodness of fit plots, residual plot, and histograms of the distribution of the weighted residuals and random effects for the 2-compartment model with reduced covariance matrix. Under this model there were seven observations with weighted residuals greater than ±5 (Patients 28, 33, 45, 54, 69, 81, and 104). Also, η_1 was decidedly nonnormal in distribu-

tion. Examination of these patient's covariates showed that they all had moderate or severe renal impairment with CrCL values less than 2.7 L/h (45 mL/min). Also, a scatter plot of CrCL against each patient's empirical Bayes estimate (EBE) of tobramycin systemic clearance (Fig. 9.8) showed an unusually strong relationship between the two variables.

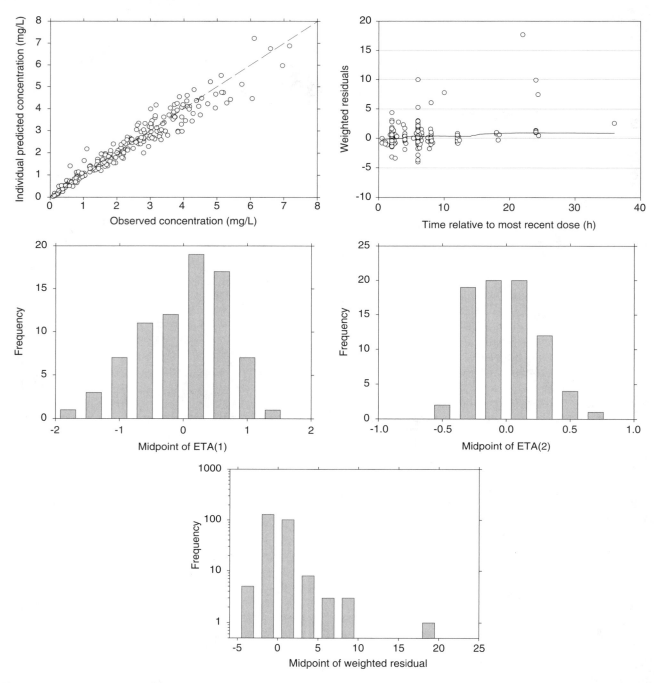

Figure 9.7 Goodness of fit plot, residual plot, and histograms of random effects and weighted residuals under the 2-compartment model with reduced unstructured covariance matrix. Dashed line in observed versus predicted plot is the line of unity. Solid line in the weighted residual plot is an inverse square kernel smoother with 0.4 sampling proportion.

Hence, it was decided that CrCL should be included in the base model at the outset. Three functions (linear, power, and exponential) were examined treating CrCL as a covariate on CL

$$CL = [\theta_1 + \theta_7(CrCL - 7.2)]\exp(\eta_1) \quad (9.6)$$

$$CL = \theta_1(CrCL/7.2)^{\theta_7}\exp(\eta_1) \quad (9.7)$$

$$CL = [\theta_1 \exp(\theta_7 \times CrCL/7.2)]\exp(\eta_1) \quad (9.8)$$

where each model was either scaled or centered for numerical stability to a normal reference CrCL value of 7.2 L/h. Starting values for all parameters were the

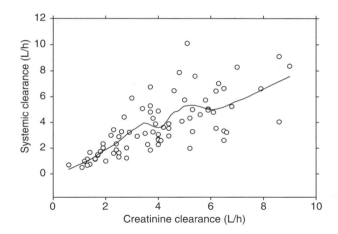

Figure 9.8 Scatter plot of creatinine clearance against the empirical Bayes estimate for tobramycin systemic clearance under the 2-compartment model with reduced unstructured covariance matrix. Solid line is the LOESS smoother with 0.3 sampling proportion.

final estimates under the 2-compartment model with reduced covariance matrix, except for θ_7 which was set to 1.0 for the power model and 0.001 for the linear and exponential models. The SLOW option was also removed.

Table 9.5 presents the results of the model fitting. All models minimized successfully, although the linear and power functions had R-matrix singularities. All models resulted in a significant improvement in the goodness of fit as indicated by the LRT (p < 0.0001 in all cases) against the equivalent model without CrCL as a covariate. But the two best models were the linear and power functions with the power function having a slight

edge over the linear function. Also, the addition of CrCL into the model reduced the BSV in Q2 to essentially zero with all three functions. Hence, CrCL was a very powerful explanatory variable. Whether to choose the linear or power function for further development was not clear. The power function had a slight advantage based on OFV and theoretical considerations. But the value of θ_7 in the power function was 0.892, which was probably not significantly different from the value 1.0 and would suggest that the power function was in fact the linear function without an intercept. In other words, the power function reduces to the no-intercept linear function when θ_7 equals 1.0, which may be the case here. Hence, the two functions may in fact be equivalent

Figure 9.9 presents goodness of fit plots, residual plots, and histograms of the weighted residuals and random effects under the 2-compartment reduced model with tobramycin clearance modeled using a power function of CrCL. The power function resulted in better distribution of predicted values around the line of unit in the goodness of fit plot and less trend in the residuals over time. The range of the weighted residuals was decreased with all values less than ±5 and most values within ±2. Also, while the distribution of the weighted residuals was not normally distributed, the distribution of both random effects were normally distributed. Overall, adding CrCL to the model resulted in a significant and sizable improvement in goodness of fit. For now, further model development will focus on the power function, but in later development may change to a linear function without intercept.

At this point, a model was tested including IOV on CL and V2. While most patients had samples collected on a single occasion, some patients had samples collected on up to four different occasions. Hence, an attempt was made to model the variability in pharmacokinetics on these different occasions. The new model tested was then

$$CL = \theta_1 \left(\frac{CrCL}{7.2\ \text{L/h}} \right)^{\theta_7} \exp\left(\eta_1 + \eta_{1i} OCC_i \right)$$
$$V1 = \theta_2 \exp\left(\theta_5 \eta_1 \right)$$
$$Q2 = \theta_3 \exp\left(\theta_6 \eta_1 \right) \tag{9.9}$$
$$V2 = \theta_4$$

where OCC_i was a dichotomous covariate set equal to '1' to denote the ith occasion and '0' otherwise and $\eta_{11} = \eta_{12} = \eta_{13} = \eta_{14}$ and $\eta_{21} = \eta_{22} = \eta_{23} = \eta_{24}$. η_1 and η_2 denote the random effect in the absence of IOV. The resulting model minimized successfully with R-matrix singularity and had an OFV of -139.624, a significant improvement over the model without IOV

Table 9.5. Tobramycin 2-compartment model summary using creatinine clearance as a covariate on clearance.

| Parameter | Function type on clearance | | |
	Linear	Power	Exponential
OFV	-96.219^R	-98.327^R	-79.958
AIC	-72.219	-74.327	-55.958
θ_1 (L/h)	0.522	6.32	1.63 (0.170)
V1 (L)	12.8	12.4	11.9 (1.59)
Q2 (L/h)	3.94	3.98	4.25 (0.593)
V2 (L)	6.48	6.74	6.45 (1.45)
θ_5	0.782	0.838	0.802 (0.129)
θ_6	7.47E−8	7.80E−9	5.29E−7 (6.31E−3)
θ_7	6.15	0.792	1.41 (0.171)
Var(CL)	0.145	0.143	0.194
Corr(CL, V2)	-0.62	-0.61	-0.73
Var(V2)	0.504	0.492	0.425
σ^2(E)	0.0255	0.0254	0.0250
σ^2(A)	0.00541	0.00534	0.00592

All models were fit using FOCE-I with an unstructured covariance matrix. The models for clearance are given in Eqs. (9.6)–(9.8). ^{R} denotes R-matrix singularity. Data are reported as estimate (standard error of the estimate). (A) denotes additive residual error term. (E) denotes exponential residual error term.

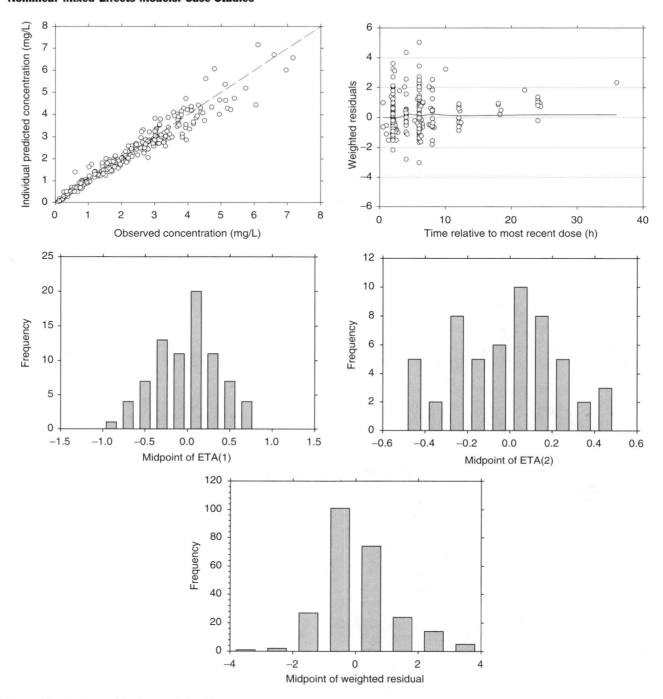

Figure 9.9 Goodness of fit plots, residual plots, and histograms of weighted residuals and random effects under the reduced 2-compartment model with tobramycin clearance modeled using a power function of CrCL. Dashed line in observed versus predicted plot is the line of unity. Solid line in the weighted residual plot is an inverse square kernel smoother with 0.4 sampling proportion.

(LRT = 41.387, p < 0.0001 on two degrees of freedom). IOV associated with CL and V2 was estimated at 31% and <1%, respectively. Hence, the model was simplified by removing IOV from V2 and refit.

The resulting modeling minimized successfully, again with R-matrix singularity, and an OFV of −139.627. However, with this model the correlation between V2 and CL was ~1.00. Hence, the model was simplified further to

$$CL = \theta_1 \left(\frac{CrCL}{7.2\,L/h} \right)^{\theta_8} \exp\left(\eta_1 + \eta_{1i}OCC_i\right)$$

$$V1 = \theta_2 \exp(\theta_5 \eta_1)$$
$$Q2 = \theta_3 \exp(\theta_6 \eta_1) \qquad (9.10)$$
$$V2 = \theta_4 \exp(\theta_7 \eta_1)$$

and refit. The resulting model minimized successfully with R-matrix singularity and an OFV of −139.627.

Notice how the model is becoming simpler but the OFV is changing very little. In this model the additive term in the residual error variance was estimated at 1.58E-7(mg/L)^2, a very small value. Hence, the model was reduced again, this time simplifying the residual error to an exponential error model. The model was refit and this time minimized successfully with no singularities and an OFV of −139.627 (Table 9.6). Figure 9.10 presents the goodness of fit plots, which showed a more concise random distribution around the line of unity compared to the model without IOV. Further, the weighted residual plots showed no trend over time. Although the weighted residuals were not normally distributed, they were symmetrically distributed around zero

Table 9.6 Tobramycin reduced 2-compartment model with clearance modeled using IOV and a power function of creatinine clearance (base model).

Parameters	Estimate
θ_1(L/h)	6.78 ± 0.368
V1 (L)	17.9 ± 1.43
Q2 (L/h)	0.961 ± 0.649
V2 (L)	7.00 ± 1.39
θ_5	0.00804 ± 0.268
θ_6	1.91 ± 1.04
θ_7	0.728 ± 0.364
θ_8	0.845 ± 0.0611
Var(CL)	0.0945 (31%)
IOV(CL)	0.0169 (13%)
σ^2(E)	0.0219 (15%)

Model was fit using FOCE-I. CL was modeled using a power function of CrCL [Eq. (9.7)]. (E) denotes exponential residual error term. The OFV was −139.627.

with no values exceeding ± 3. Importantly, comparing Fig. 9 to Fig. 10, the random effect associated with CL was normally distributed around zero, which was not observed when IOV was not included in the model. The

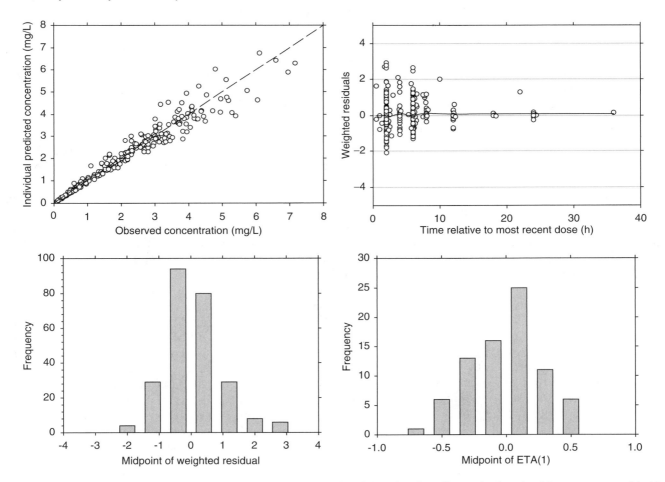

Figure 9.10 Goodness of fit plots, residual plots, and histograms of weighted residuals and random effects under the reduced 2-compartment model with tobramycin clearance modeled using a power function of CrCL and interoccasion variability on CL. Dashed line in observed versus predicted plot is the line of unity. Solid line in the weighted residual plot is an inverse square kernel smoother with 0.4 sampling proportion.

model showed that the BSV for CL was 31% with 13% IOV. This model was deemed the final base model.

Covariate Screening

Once the base model was determined, the role of additional covariates was examined. In a typical modeling effort, covariate screening would be done through direct screening using NONMEM or by regression-based analysis of either the EBE of the pharmacokinetic parameters or the random effects. All approaches will be done herein for comparison purposes. After including CrCL in the model, the following covariates were available: age, sex, weight, BSA, IBW, BMI, and LBW. It should be noted one apparent outlier was in the data set. Patient 100 was a 23 year old male weighing 120 kg. The next closest individual weighed 103 kg. It was decided to keep this individual in the data base but attention would be paid to how this individual might influence the results when weight-related covariates were included in the model.

The first covariate screening approach is graphical assessment. For simplicity only CL will be examined. At the outset, using graphical assessment and regression-based methods to screen for covariates is problematic because CL was time-dependent due to CrCL changing over time in some individuals. So which CL value should be plotted? The average? The baseline value? There are no guidelines for which value to use so for purposes herein, the baseline value was used as the dependent variable in the analysis. Figure 9.11 presents scatter plots of each continuous covariate against the EBE for baseline CL under the base model as shown in Table 9.6. Figure 9.12 presents scatter plots of each continuous covariate against the EBE for η_1 under the base model. Also shown in the figures is a box and whisker plot of the EBE for baseline CL and η_1 against patient sex. The graphs suggested that two covariates might be important predictors of CL: age and sex. None of the weight-based metrics appeared to be predictive of CL as the LOESS smooths to the data were essentially flat lines. Hence, age and sex would be brought forward for further model development under this approach.

The next covariate screening approach would be to use a regression-based method and take a more rigorous statistical approach to the problem. Using the generalized additive model (GAM) procedure in SAS, a LOESS smooth was applied to the continuous covariates wherein the procedure was allowed to identify the optimal smoothing parameter for each covariate tested. Two dependent variables were examined: η_1 and the EBE for CL. To avoid possible skewness in the residuals,

the EBE for CL was log-transformed prior to analysis. A second approach was to use simple linear regression and test for the significance of the covariate using Wald's test. Lastly, Spearman's rank correlation coefficient was calculated between the covariate and the dependent variable. A p-value less then 0.05 was considered significant for each test. The results are shown in Table 9.7.

Clearly different methods lead to different covariates to take forward. Using CL as the dependent variable under a GAM analysis showed that only age was an important covariate. But using η_1 as the dependent variable in a GAM analysis showed BMI, but not age, to be an important covariate. Patient sex, which was a categorical variable, was tested using analysis of variance wherein log-transformed clearance and η_1 were the dependent variables and sex was a fixed effect. The p-values for the F-test were 0.0293 for the EBE of CL and 0.1564 for η_1. Hence, one variable showed a significant difference between sexes, while the other did not. One reason for the conflicting results may be the presence of the outlier in the data set that may have exerted undue influence on the results of the analysis. These results highlight that regression-based approaches to covariate selection must use the same criteria and meet the same assumptions in choosing a model as any other regression model—residuals should be examined for normality and heteroscedasticity and influence analysis should be conducted for identifying and controlling influential observations.

For direct screening in NONMEM, continuous covariates were tested using linear, power, and exponential functions. Covariates were standardized to their mean values listed in Table 9.3. Sex was modeled using a proportional change model. The importance of each covariate was tested using the LRT with a significance level of 0.05 using the reference model given in Table 9.6. Tables 9.8–9.11 present the results of direct covariate screening within NONMEM. None of the covariates tested had the magnitude of effect CrCL did when it was included in the model as a covariate. BSA, weight, LBW, and IBW appeared to be important predictors of CL. The importance of BMI depended on the functional form used. Age and sex did not appear to be important covariates, which was in direct contrast to the GAM analysis. All the weight-based metrics and patient sex were important predictors of V1 with BSA being the most important. Patient age was not an important predictor of V1. The weight-based metrics were mixed in their importance on Q2. BSA, LBW, and weight were all important predictors of Q2, but patient sex, BMI, and age were not. The importance of IBW depended on the

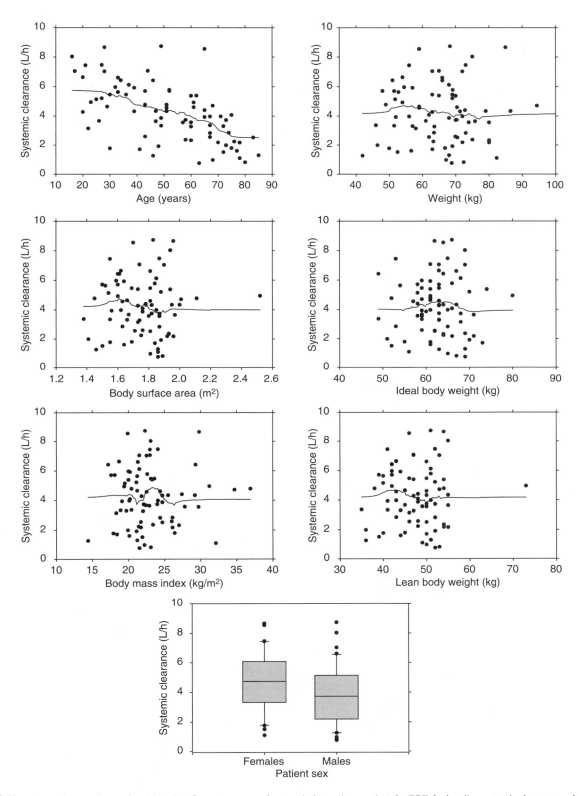

Figure 9.11   Scatter plots and box and whisker plots for continuous and categorical covariates against the EBE for baseline systemic clearance under the base model. Solid lines in the scatter plots are the LOESS smooth the data using a 0.3 sampling proportion.

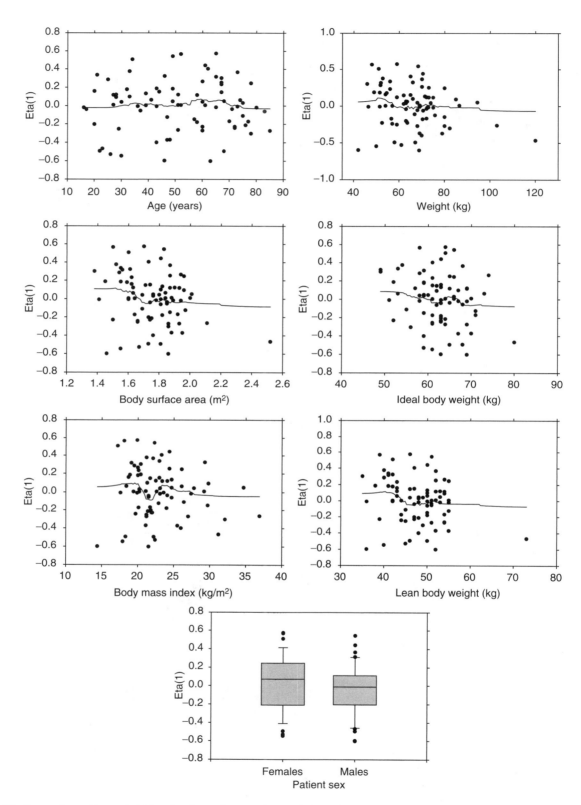

Figure 9.12 Scatter plots and box and whisker plots for continuous and categorical covariates against η_1 under the base model. Solid lines in the scatter plots are the LOESS smooth the data using a 0.3 sampling proportion.

Table 9.7 Results of covariate screening using regression-based approaches.

Parameter	Covariate	GAM	Linear regression	Spearman's correlation
Clearance	Age	<0.0001	<0.0001	<0.0001
	Weight	0.2164	0.8085	0.7433
	BSA	0.1221	0.9508	0.7304
	IBW	0.4988	0.7021	0.8058
	BMI	0.1883	0.7020	0.9348
	LBW	0.2286	0.9185	0.8715
η_1	Age	0.3575	0.9086	0.7354
	Weight	0.0676	0.0507	0.0725
	BSA	0.1300	0.0297	0.0394
	IBW	0.1652	0.0450	0.0786
	BMI	0.0151	0.3257	0.3053
	LBW	0.0892	0.0520	0.0616

Values represent the p-value from the analysis. Legend: GAM, generalized additive model; BSA, body surface area; IBW, ideal body weight; BMI, body mass index; and LBW, lean body weight.

functional form used. Lastly, only BMI was an important predictor of V2.

What is interesting is the covariates identified through graphical analysis and regression-based methods as being an important covariates when they were actually included in the model did not result in a significant improvement as indicated by the LRT. Hence, the NONMEM approach identified a different set of covariates than the regression-based and graphical approaches. Because of this disconnect between the

Table 9.8 Summary of covariate screening for clearance using NONMEM sorted from smallest to largest p-value.

Covariate	Function	Objective function value	Likelihood ratio test	p-value
BSA	Linear	−157.195	17.57	<0.0001
Weight	Linear	−155.768	16.14	<0.0001
BSA	Power	−155.077	15.45	<0.0001
LBW	Linear	−155.004	15.38	<0.0001
BSA	Exponential	−153.215	13.59	0.0002
Weight	Power	−152.789	13.16	0.0003
LBW	Power	−152.068	12.44	0.0004
Weight	Exponential	−150.830	11.20	0.0008
LBW	Linear	−150.300	10.67	0.0011
IBW	Linear	−147.008	7.38	0.0066
IBW	Power	−146.482	6.86	0.0088
IBW	Exponential	−146.313	6.69	0.0097
BMI	Linear	−143.928	4.30	0.0381
BMI	Power	−142.855	3.23	0.0723
BMI	Exponential	−142.414	2.79	0.0949
Sex	Proportional	−141.563	1.94	0.1637
Age	Power	−140.994	1.37	0.2418
Age	Exponential	−140.873	1.25	0.2636
Age	Linear	−140.173	0.55	0.4583

All models were fit using FOCE-I. The reference model was the reduced 2-compartment model where clearance was modeled using a power function of CrCL and IOV was included (OFV of −139.627). The LRT for each model had one degree of freedom.

Table 9.9 Summary of covariate screening for central volume using NONMEM sorted from smallest to largest p-value.

Covariate	Function	Objective function value	Likelihood ratio test	p-value
BSA	Exponential	−169.009	29.38	<0.0001
BSA	Power	−168.660	29.03	<0.0001
Weight	Power	−168.584	28.96	<0.0001
Weight	Linear	−168.512	28.89	<0.0001
Weight	Exponential	−168.363	28.74	<0.0001
LBW	Linear	−167.725	28.10	<0.0001
BSA	Linear	−167.662	28.04	<0.0001
LBW	Power	−166.635	27.01	<0.0001
LBW	Linear	−165.754	26.13	<0.0001
BMI	Power	−154.823	15.20	<0.0001
BMI	Linear	−154.815	15.19	<0.0001
BMI	Exponential	−154.357	14.73	0.0001
IBW	Exponential	−150.031	10.40	0.0013
IBW	Power	−148.818	9.19	0.0024
IBW	Linear	−148.687	9.06	0.0026
Sex	Proportional	−145.777	6.15	0.0131
Age	Linear	−139.669	0.04	0.8415
Age	Power	−139.629	0.00	1.0000
Age	Exponential	−139.629	0.00	1.0000

All models were fit using FOCE-I. The reference model was the reduced 2-compartment model where clearance was modeled using a power function of CrCL and IOV was included (OFV of −139.627). The LRT for each model had one degree of freedom.

Table 9.10 Summary of covariate screening for intercompartmental clearance using NONMEM sorted from smallest to largest p-value.

Covariate	Function	Objective function value	Likelihood ratio test	p-Value
BSA	Exponential	−150.327	10.70	0.0011
LBW	Linear	−150.090	10.46	0.0012
Weight	Exponential	−149.920	10.29	0.0013
BSA	Power	−149.420	9.79	0.0018
Weight	Power	−148.477	8.85	0.0029
LBW	Power	−148.455	8.83	0.0030
IBW	Exponential	−145.846	6.22	0.0126
BSA	Linear	−144.116	4.49	0.0341
LBW	Linear	−143.781 (I)	4.15	0.0416
Weight	Linear	−143.637 (I)	4.01	0.0452
IBW	Power	−143.622	4.00	0.0455
Age	Exponential	−143.003	3.38	0.0660
Age	Power	−142.233	2.61	0.1062
IBW	Linear	−141.313	1.69	0.1936
BMI	Power	−141.069	1.44	0.2301
BMI	Linear	−141.006	1.38	0.2401
BMI	Exponential	−140.980	1.35	0.2453
Age	Linear	−140.777	1.15	0.2835
Sex	Proportional	−139.829	0.20	0.6547

All models were fit using FOCE-I. The reference model was the reduced 2-compartment model where clearance was modeled using a power function of CrCL and IOV was included (OFV of −139.627). The LRT for each model had one degree of freedom. Legend: (I) denotes that model terminated due to infinite objective function.

Table 9.11 Summary of covariate screening for peripheral volume using NONMEM sorted from smallest to largest p-value.

Covariate	Function	Objective function value	Likelihood ratio test	p-Value
BMI	Exponential	−143.905	4.28	0.0386
BMI	Power	−143.799	4.17	0.0411
BMI	Linear	−143.756	4.13	0.0421
Weight	Exponential	−143.191	3.56	0.0592
Weight	Power	−143.127	3.50	0.0614
Weight	Linear	−143.115	3.49	0.0617
LBW	Power	−142.689	3.06	0.0802
LBW	Linear	−142.676	3.05	0.0807
LBW	Linear	−142.665	3.04	0.0812
BSA	Exponential	−142.578	2.95	0.0859
BSA	Power	−142.566	2.94	0.0864
BSA	Linear	−142.507	2.88	0.0897
IBW	Exponential	−139.994	0.37	0.5430
IBW	Power	−139.936	0.31	0.5777
IBW	Linear	−139.893	0.27	0.6033
Sex	Proportional	−139.739	0.11	0.7401
Age	Power	−139.634	0.01	0.9203
Age	Exponential	−139.634	0.01	0.9203
Age	Linear	−139.629	0.00	1.000

All models were fit using FOCE-I. The reference model was the reduced 2-compartment model where clearance was modeled using a power function of CrCL and IOV was included (OFV of −139.627). The LRT for each model had one degree of freedom.

different approaches and because computers are so much faster today than they were even just a few years ago, the regression-based approaches and graphical approaches have fallen out of favor in recent years and most covariate screening is done directly within NONMEM.

Covariate Model Development

Of all the covariates studied, BSA on V1 tended to have the greatest impact as indicated by the largest LRT. Followed closely behind was weight on V1. In the absence of other information, BSA on V1 would be brought forward for further model development. However, physicians as a matter of practice dose antiinfectives on a weight-basis, much like oncologists as a matter of practice dose oncolytics on a body surface area basis. Thus, physicians would be more comfortable if weight were used as a covariate in the model rather than BSA. Since there was very little difference in the OFVs using either weight or BSA this change seems acceptable. Further, BSA is a derived variable that is sometimes difficult to calculate and is more susceptible to calculation error than the measurement of a person's weight. Hence, it was decided that V1 modeled using a power function of weight would be the next step in the covariate model. Now the model had CrCL on CL and weight on V1, both modeled using a power function scaled to their respective means

$$CL = \theta_1 \left(\frac{CrCL}{7.2\,L/h} \right)^{\theta_8} \exp\left(\eta_1 + \eta_{1i} OCC_i \right)$$

$$V1 = \theta_2 \left(\frac{Weight}{67\,kg} \right)^{\theta_9} \exp\left(\theta_5 \eta_1 \right). \tag{9.11}$$

$$Q2 = \theta_3 \exp\left(\theta_6 \eta_1 \right)$$

$$V2 = \theta_4 \exp\left(\theta_7 \eta_1 \right)$$

Next, model development tested the remaining covariates for their significance. Since it would not be logical to include other weight-based covariates on V1 due to collinearity and theoretical concerns, no other weight-based covariates were tested on V1.

The results of the first round of forward stepwise covariate development are shown in Table 9.12. Weight as a predictor of Q2 using a power function showed the best improvement in the model. The next round of covariate development would then include weight in the model on Q2

Table 9.12 Tobramycin forward stepwise covariate model development (Round 1).

Covariate	Parameter	Function	OFV	LRT	p-Value
Weight	Q2	Power	−174.086	5.50	0.0190
Weight	Q2	Exponential	−173.773	5.19	0.0227
BMI	V2	Exponential	−173.384	4.80	0.0285
BMI	V2	Power	−173.091	4.51	0.0337
BMI	V2	Linear	−173.043	4.46	0.0347
Weight	Q2	Linear	−172.814	4.23	0.0397
LBW	Q2	Power	−172.611	4.03	0.0447
LBW	Q2	Linear	−172.399	3.82	0.0506
LBW	Q2	Exponential	−172.187	3.60	0.0578
Weight	Q2	Linear	−172.096	3.51	0.0610
Weight	Q2	Power	−172.041	3.46	0.0629
Weight	Q2	Exponential	−171.643	3.06	0.0802
IBW	CL	Exponential	−170.893	2.31	0.1285
IBW	CL	Power	−170.864	2.28	0.1311
IBW	CL	Linear	−170.801	2.22	0.1362
Sex	V1	Proportional	−170.360	1.78	0.1821
Weight	CL	Linear	−170.275	1.69	0.1936
Weight	CL	Power	−169.997	1.41	0.2351
Weight	CL	Exponential	−169.929	1.35	0.2453
LBW	CL	Linear	−169.682	1.10	0.2943
Weight	CL	Linear	−169.633	1.05	0.3055
LBW	CL	Power	−169.392	0.81	0.3681
LBW	CL	Exponential	−169.344	0.76	0.3833
Weight	CL	Power	−169.162	0.58	0.4463
Weight	CL	Exponential	−169.113	0.53	0.4666
IBW	Q2	Power	−168.700	0.12	0.7290
IBW	Q2	Exponential	−168.690	0.11	0.7401
BMI	CL	Linear	−168.585	0.00	1.000

All models fit using FOCE-I. The reference model was the reduced 2-compartment model where V1 was a power function of weight and CL was modeled as a power function of CrCL with IOV included. The OFV of the reduced model was −168.584. Weight and CrCL were modeled using power functions scaled to a reference value of 67 kg and 7.2 L/h, respectively. Sex was modeled using a proportional change model. The LRT for each model had one degree of freedom.

$$CL = \theta_1 \left(\frac{CrCL}{7.2\,L/h}\right)^{\theta_8} \exp(\eta_1 + \eta_{1i}OCC_i)$$

$$V1 = \theta_2 \left(\frac{BSA}{1.77\,m^2}\right)^{\theta_9} \exp(\theta_5\eta_1). \qquad (9.12)$$

$$Q2 = \theta_3 \left(\frac{Weight}{67\,kg}\right)^{\theta_{10}} \exp(\theta_6\eta_1)$$

$$V2 = \theta_4 \exp(\theta_7\eta_1)$$

Since all the weight-based metrics measure essentially the same thing it would not make sense to include these covariates on Q2. Hence, the only remaining covariate to examine would be BMI on V2. No other covariates were significant at the 0.05 level. Round 2 of forward stepwise model development is shown in Table 9.13. BMI did not improve the model. Hence, Eq. (9.12) represents the end of forward stepwise model building.

The next step in the process is pruning the tree or backwards stepwise development where a more stringent p-value is required to stay in the model. In this case, a p-value of 0.01 was required to remain in the model. θ_5 to θ_{10} were fixed to zero one by one and the change in OFV calculated. Only those parameters whose change in OFV was greater than the critical value based on the LRT and a p-value of 0.01 were retained in the model, e.g., 6.635 with one degree of freedom. The results are shown in Table 9.14. With the first round of pruning θ_5,θ_6, and θ_7 appear to be superfluous as their p-values were 0.1771, 0.0900, and 0.0133, respectively. In the next step, θ_5 was fixed to zero (since it appeared to be the most insignificant parameter) and then θ_6 to θ_{10} were fixed to zero one by one. The LRT was then calculated for each model using two degrees of freedom. This time θ_{10} appeared to be insignificant having a p-value of 0.0462. In the next step θ_{10} was fixed to zero and then θ_6 to θ_9 were fixed to zero one by one. The LRT was then calculated for each model using three degrees of freedom. Now all model parameters were significant at the 0.01 level and no further pruning appeared to be necessary. Hence, the best model after backwards stepwise model development was

Table 9.13 Tobramycin forward stepwise covariate model development (Round 2).

Covariate	Parameter	Function	OFV	LRT	p-Value
BMI	V2	Exponential	−174.992	0.91	0.3401
BMI	V2	Linear	−174.968	0.88	0.3482
BMI	V2	Power	−174.958	0.87	0.3510

All models fit using FOCE-I. The reference model was the reduced 2-compartment model where CL was modeled as a power function of CrCL scaled to a reference value of 7.2 L/h with IOV included. V1 and Q2 were modeled using a power function scaled to a reference value of 67 kg. The OFV of the reduced model was −174.086. The LRT for each model had one degree of freedom.

$$CL = \theta_1 \left(\frac{CrCL}{7.2\,L/h}\right)^{\theta_7} \exp(\eta_1 + \eta_{1i}OCC_i)$$

$$V1 = \theta_2 \left(\frac{Weight}{67\,kg}\right)^{\theta_8} \qquad (9.13)$$

$$Q2 = \theta_3 \exp(\theta_5\eta_1)$$

$$V2 = \theta_4 \exp(\theta_6\eta_1)$$

with an OFV of −167.935.

Examination of the model parameter estimates showed that θ_7 was 0.868 ± 0.0641. Previous model efforts with tobramycin have shown that CL was proportional to CrCL, i.e., $\theta_7 = 1$ (Aarons et al., 1989; Xuan et al., 2000). A Z-test testing the null hypothesis that $\theta_7 = 1$ versus the alternative hypothesis that $\theta_7 \neq 1$ was equal to $|0.868 - 1|/0.0641 = 2.07$ with a p-value of 0.0395. Hence, θ_7 was not equal to 1.0 at the 0.05 level. To further test the impact of making CL proportional to CrCL, θ_7 was fixed to 1.0 and the model was refit. The resulting model had an OFV of −167.858. The LRT comparing the model with θ_7 as an estimable parameter against θ_7 as a fixed value was 0.077 on one degree of freedom ($p = 0.7814$). Hence, there did not appear to be any advantage in allowing θ_7 to be treated as an estimable parameter and that θ_7 could be fixed to a value of 1.0 without any decrement in goodness of fit.

Also, in Eq. (9.13) the estimate of θ_8 was 1.13 ± 0.295. Previous model efforts with tobramycin have shown that V1 was proportional to weight, i.e., $\theta_8 = 1$ (Aarons et al., 1989; Xuan et al., 2000). A Z-test testing the null hypothesis that $\theta_8 = 1$ versus the alternative hypothesis that $\theta_8 \neq 1$ was equal to $|1.13-1|/0.295 = 0.44$ with a p-value of 0.6703. Hence, θ_8 was equal to 1.0 at the 0.05 level. To further test the impact of making V1 proportional to weight, θ_8 was fixed to 1.0 and the model was refit. The resulting model had an OFV of −167.590. The LRT comparing the model with θ_8 as an estimable parameter against θ_8 as a fixed value was 0.345 on one degree of freedom ($p = 0.557$). Treating θ_8 as an estimable parameter did not result in any improvement in goodness of fit and could be considered to be directly proportional to weight. Thus, the model at this point was

$$CL = \theta_1 \left(\frac{CrCL}{7.2L/h}\right) \exp(\eta_1 + \eta_{1i}OCC_i)$$

$$V1 = \theta_2 \left(\frac{Weight}{67\,kg}\right) \qquad (9.14)$$

$$Q2 = \theta_3 \exp(\theta_5\eta_1)$$

$$V2 = \theta_4 \exp(\theta_6\eta_1)$$

with the model parameter estimates shown in Table 9.15.

Table 9.14 Tobramycin backwards model development summary.

Model	df	θ_5	θ_6	θ_7	θ_8	θ_9	θ_{10}	OFV	LRT	p-Value
				Parameters removed from model						
0								−174.086		
1	1	X						−172.264	1.82	0.1771
2	1		X					−171.212	2.87	0.0900
3	1			X				−167.957	6.13	0.0133
4	1				X			−67.793	106.29	0.0000
5	1					X		−148.477	25.61	0.0000
6	1						X	−168.584	5.50	0.0190
7	2	X	X					−163.492	10.59	0.0050
8	2	X		X				−164.522	9.56	0.0084
9	2	X			X			−67.794	106.29	0.0000
10	2	X				X		−147.310	26.78	0.0000
11	2	X					X	−167.935	6.15	0.0462
12	3	X	X				X	−156.803	17.28	0.0006
13	3	X		X			X	−162.146	11.94	0.0076
14	3	X			X		X	−61.914	112.17	0.0000
15	3	X				X	X	−139.625	34.46	0.0000

All models fit using FOCE-I. The reference model (Model 0) was is given in Eq. (9.12) and had an OFV of −174.086. Legend: df, degrees of freedom compared to reference model.

Two last models were examined. In the first model, V1 was modeled using a simple linear model with weight as a covariate

$$V1 = \theta_7 + \theta_2 \left(\frac{\text{Weight}}{67\,\text{kg}} \right). \quad (9.15)$$

While the second modeled CL using a simple linear model with CrCL as a covariate

Table 9.15 Tobramycin parameter estimates after backwards stepwise model development under the model presented in Eq. (9.14).

Parameter	All data	Outliers removed	No outliers and no influential observations
Number of observations	250	248	223
Number of patients	78	78	74
OFV	−162.898	−168.249	−131.972
AIC	−144.9	−150.2	−114.0
Condition number	102	89	35
θ_1 (L/h)	7.48 (0.288)	7.50 (0.283)	7.48 (0.293)
θ_2 (L)	17.2 (1.14)	17.1 (1.10)	17.1 (0.995)
θ_3 (L/h)	1.44 (0.485)	1.44 (0.459)	1.35 (0.296)
θ_4 (L)	7.83 (1.24)	7.83 (1.20)	8.61 (1.13)
θ_5	1.67 (0.622)	1.72 (0.580)	1.74 (0.319)
θ_6	1.02 (0.366)	1.04 (0.358)	1.69 (0.430)
Var(CL)	0.0862 (30%)	0.0813 (29%)	0.0839 (30%)
IOV(CL)	0.0206 (14%)	0.0195 (14%)	0.0175 (13%)
Var(Q2)	0.240 (52%)	0.241 (52%)	0.254 (54%)
Var(V2)	0.0896 (31%)	0.0879 (30%)	0.239 (52%)
Residual variance	0.0183 (14%)	0.0185 (14%)	0.0165 (13%)

All models fit using FOCE-I. The final model is presented in Eq. (9.14). Estimable parameters are reported as estimate (standard error of the estimate), except for the variance components which are reported as estimate (estimate expressed as %CV).

$$CL = \left[\theta_7 + \theta_1 \left(\frac{CrCL}{7.2\,\text{L/h}} \right) \right] \exp(\eta_1 + \eta_{1i} OCC_i). \quad (9.16)$$

The first model resulted in successful minimization but with R-matrix singularity and had an OFV of −133.282, a difference of 1.31 (p = 0.2522), which was not considered a significant improvement in the model. The second model resulted in successful minimization with no singularities and had an OFV of −134.073, a difference of 2.101 (p = 0.1472), which was also not considered a significant improvement over the model presented in Eq. (9.14). Hence, this concluded model development with the model given by Eq. (9.14) being considered the final covariate model with the final parameter estimates given in Table 9.15 (all data).

Outlier and Influence Analysis

Once a suitable covariate model is identified and no further model development will be done, the next step is to examine the dataset for outliers and influential observations. It may be that a few subjects are driving the inclusion of a covariate in a model or that a few observations are biasing the parameter estimates. Examination of the weighted residuals under Eq. (9.14) with the model estimates given in Table 9.15 showed that the distribution was skewed with two observations outside the acceptable limits of ± 5. Patient 54 had an observable concentration of 4.05 mg/L 6-h postdose but had a predicted concentration of 1.22 mg/L, a difference of 2.83 mg/L and a corresponding weighted residual of +5.4. Patient 84 had an observable concentration of 1.57 mg/L 7.5-h postdose but had a predicted concentration of 0.34 mg/L, a difference of 1.23 mg/L with corresponding weighted residual of +7.8. Both these observations represent questionable values. Some modelers might then remove these observations as outliers, others might not.

To see what impact these observations might have on the parameter estimates, these observations were removed and the best model after backwards stepwise model development was refit. The results are shown in Table 9.15. Removal of these observations resulted in a decrease in the OFV, AIC, and condition number with little to no change in the parameter estimates. Although to be fair, direct comparison of the OFVs and AICs is not valid because of the unequal number of observations in the data sets. More importantly, although the distribution of weighted residuals was not normally distributed, the distribution was no longer skewed. Also, the standard error of the estimates all decreased. Whether to remove these observations from the data set is not immediately clear and if removal of observations was not specified a priori in the data analysis plan then their removal should probably not be made. In this case, it was decided to remove the observations in the data set.

Every patient was then assigned a unique index number ranging from 1 to 78. Each patient was then singularly removed from the data set and 78 new data sets were created, each one having a single patient missing. Every one of the new delete-1 data sets was then refit using the model in Eq. (9.14) with FOCE-I. The two questionable observations seen with the final model (Patients 54 and 84) were removed prior to creating the delete-1 data sets. The percent change in the parameter estimates from each data set was then calculated relative to the parameter estimates presented in Table 9.15. An index plot of the structural model parameters and variance components is shown in Fig. 9.13 and Fig. 9.14, respectively. Generally, when a patient is removed from a data set and the parameter estimates change by more than $\pm 20\%$ then that subject may considered to be influential. θ_3, θ_5, θ_6, and IOV showed sensitivities greater than $\pm 20\%$. Removal of Patient 114 (Index number 74) resulted in a change in θ_3 of -25.0%. Removal of Patient 117 (Index number 77) resulted in a change of 21.5% in θ_5. Removal of Patient 113 (Index number 73) and Patient 115 (Index number 75) resulted in a change in θ_6 of greater than $\pm 20\%$. Removal of Patient 114 (Index number 74) resulted in a change in IOV of -27.2%.

With a data set consisting of many patients, some patients may show influence over a single parameter. That is to be expected. The more important question is are there any patients that exert profound influence over a single parameter or are there a few patients that might exert influence "overall" on the parameter estimates? None of the patients identified in the index plots seem to exert *profound* influence over a single parameter.

To get at the question of overall influence, the matrix of structural model parameters and variance components was subjected to principal component analysis. Principal component analysis (PCA) was introduced in the chapter on Nonlinear Mixed Effects Model Theory and transforms a matrix of values to another matrix such that the columns of the transformed matrix are uncorrelated and the first column contains the largest amount of variability, the second column contains the second largest, etc. Hopefully, just the first few principal components contain the majority of the variance in the original matrix. The outcome of PCA is to take X, a matrix of p-variables, and reduce it to a matrix of q-variables ($q < p$) that contain most of the information within X. In this PCA of the standardized parameters (fixed effects and all variance components), the first three principal components contained 74% of the total variability in the original matrix, so PCA was largely successfully. PCA works best when a high correlation exists between the variables in the original data set. Usually more than 80% variability in the first few components is considered a success.

Figure 9.15 plots the first three principal components. In these plots, one looks for observations that stand out from the bulk of the data. In a plot of the first versus second principal component, four such observations were noted: Patient 57 (Index number 31), 114, 115, and 117. Three of these patients (Patients 114, 115, and 117) were identified in the index plot as potentially influential. In the plot of the first versus third principal component, Patients 114, 115, and 117 were again identified as outside the bulk of data, as were Patients 57 and 115 in a plot of the second versus third principal component. A review of these patient's demographics failed to reveal anything unusual. It was decided that Patients 57, 114, 115, and 117 were too influential in the overall estimation of the model parameters and that they should be removed from the data set.

Earlier it was noted that Patient 100 (Index number 65) was an obese male whose BMI was $31.2 \, \mathrm{kg/m^2}$ with a corresponding BSA of $2.52 \, \mathrm{m^2}$. This patient may represent an influential patient or outlier as this patient's set of weight covariates was far removed from the bulk of the data. However, examination of this subject's principal components (Fig. 9.15) revealed him to have no influence on the final parameter estimates so there appeared to be no need to remove him from the data set. Thus, it was decided that Patients 57, 114, 115, and 117 would be removed from the data set. After removal of the three influential patients and the two questionable

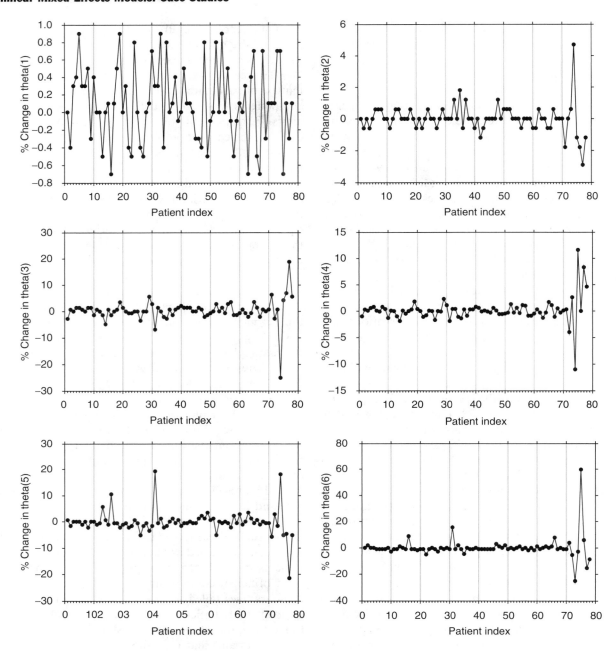

Figure 9.13 Index plots of structural model parameter estimates expressed as percent change from baseline using the delete-1 jackknife. Each patient was assigned an index number ranging from 1 to 78 and then singularly removed from the data set. The delete-1 data set was then used to fit the model in Eq. (9.14) using FOCE-I.

observations, the data set consisted of 223 observations (89% of the original) from 74 patients (95% of the complete data set).

In the original data set, some of the values for height were missing. Multiple imputation was used to impute the missing data which were then used in the analysis as though they were never missing in the first place. Since the final model has only CrCL and weight as covariates in the model, none of which were missing, no

further analysis needs to be done with the imputation data sets. Hence, Eq. (9.14) was fit using the original data set with no missing data, the results of which are presented in Table 9.15. Goodness of fit plots using the model development data set with the two questionable observations and four influential patients removed are shown in Fig. 9.16. Individual predicted concentrations showed good distribution around the line of unity. No trend in the residuals was observed over time. Although

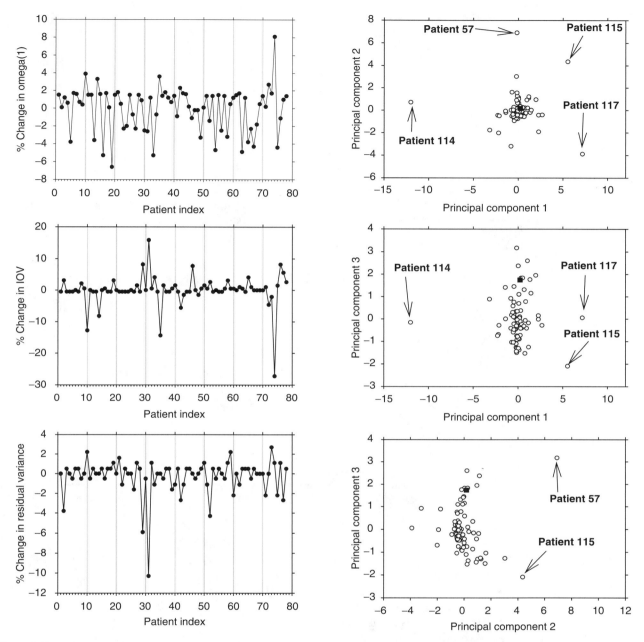

Figure 9.14 Index plots of variance components expressed as percent change from baseline using the delete-1 jackknife. Each patient was assigned an index number ranging from 1 to 78 and then singularly removed from the data set. The delete-1 data set was then used to fit the model in Eq. (9.14) using FOCE-I.

Figure 9.15 Scatter plots of the first three principal components of all structural parameters and variance components. Each index patient was singularly removed from the data set and the model in Eq. (9.14) was refit using FOCE-I. The resulting matrix of structural parameters and variance components was then analyzed using principal components analysis. Influential observations are noted in the figures. Patient 100, who had a BSA of $2.52\,m^2$ and a BMI of $31.2\,kg/m^2$, is denoted as a solid square.

the weighted residuals were not normally distributed, the values were symmetrical, centered at zero, and no value was greater than $\pm\,5$. The largest weighted residual was 3.67. Further, the distribution of η_1, the only random effect in the model, was normally distributed and centered at zero. Hence, the resulting model appeared to adequately characterize the observed concentrations.

Model Validation

The next step in the analysis is validating the model. As a first step, 1000 bootstrap data sets were created from the data set, excluding influential observations and patients. The best model as presented in Eq. (9.14) was then fit to each bootstrap distribution. Of the 1000

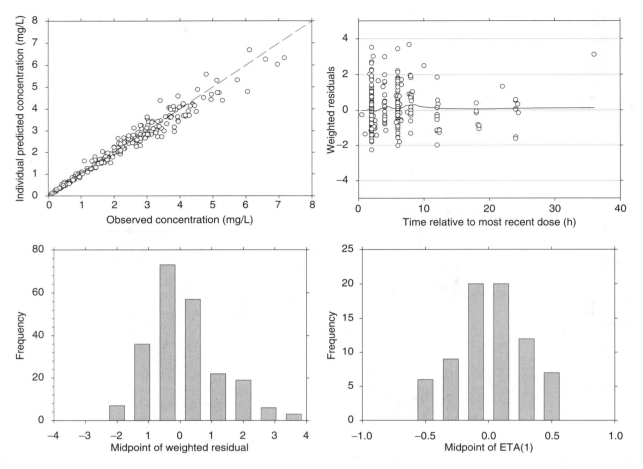

Figure 9.16 Goodness of fit plots, residual plots, and histograms of weighted residuals and random effects under Eq. (9.14) after removal of two outlier observations and four influential patients. Solid line in the residual plot is the inverse square kernel smooth to the data using a sampling proportion of 0.3. Solid line in the upper left plot is the line of unity. Solid line in the upper right plot is the LOESS smooth to the data using a 0.3 sampling proportion.

bootstrap data sets, 987 minimized successfully and 13 terminated due to rounding errors. Table 9.16 presents summary statistics for the bootstrap distributions for each model parameter. Confidence intervals were determined using the bias-corrected bootstrap (see Book Appendix for details). The bootstrap estimates for θ_1 to θ_4 were precisely estimated, as were the variance components, as the relative bias for these parameters was small. However, the relative bias for θ_5 and θ_6 was more than $\pm 20\%$ indicating a high degree of bias in these estimates. The 90% confidence interval (CI) for θ_6 contained zero indicating that this parameter was not needed in the model. Also, even though the 90% CI for θ_5 did not include zero, there were many values that were near zero. In fact, the smallest observed θ_5 was 3.58E−14 which would tend to suggest that θ_5 was not needed in the model either. Hence, it is one step forward two steps back. Based on bootstrapping, the model was further reduced to

$$CL = \theta_1 \left(\frac{CrCL}{7.2\,L/h} \right) \exp\left(\eta_1 + \eta_{1i} OCC_i \right)$$

$$V1 = \theta_2 \left(\frac{Weight}{67\,kg} \right)$$

$$Q2 = \theta_3$$

$$V2 = \theta_4$$

(9.17)

The same bootstrap data sets were then used to fit Eq. (9.17). Of the 1000 bootstrap data sets, all 1000 converged successfully. The results are presented in Table 9.17 and shown graphically in Figure 9.17. All the random effects were normally distributed, except θ_4 which showed right skewness. The relative bias of the parameters was less than $\pm 3\%$ and the confidence intervals for CL and V1 were precise (<10% CV). The CIs for Q2 and V2 were not as precise which was expected because the data set consisted of sparse data. Examination of the concentration–time profile showed there were few sam-

Table 9.16 Results of bootstrap analysis of tobramycin model presented in Eq. (9.14) with questionable observations and influential patients removed.

Parameter	Final model estimate	Bootstrap mean	Relative bias (%)	Bias-corrected Lower 90% CI	Bias-corrected Upper 90% CI
θ_1 (L/h)	7.48	7.48	<0.1	6.98	7.96
θ_2 (L)	17.1	17.1	<0.1	15.3	18.7
θ_3 (L/h)	1.35	1.32	−1.9	0.69	1.85
θ_4 (L)	8.61	8.55	−0.6	6.07	11.20
θ_5	1.74	2.18	25.5	1.55	4.69
θ_6	1.69	1.35	−20.4	0.00	2.19
Var(CL)	0.0839	0.0850	1.5	0.0612	0.117
IOV(CL)	0.0175	0.0168	−3.6	0.00830	0.0390
σ^2	0.0165	0.0158	−3.9	0.0126	0.0198

ples collected in the β-phase and, as such, precise estimation of the parameters related to the peripheral compartment might not be expected. Also, the precision of the variance components was not unusually large and was about what was expected. Hence, bootstrap analysis indicated little bias in the model estimates and supported the model presented in Eq. (9.17) as the best model.

Little difference was observed in the goodness of fit and residual plots under Eq. (9.17) (shown in Fig. 9.18) compared to the more complex model presented in Eq. (9.14). Individual predicted concentrations showed good distribution around the line of unity. No trend in the residuals was observed. Although the weighted residuals were not normally distributed, the values were symmetrical, centered at zero, and no value was greater than ± 4. The largest weighted residual was 3.65. Further, the distribution of η_1, the only random effect in the model, was normally distributed and centered at zero. Predicted concentrations based on Eq. (9.17) overlaid with observed concentrations for four patients randomly selected from each of the renal function groups is shown in Fig. 9.19. The model appeared to be a good representation of what was happening in each individual pharmacokinetically. Hence, Eq. (9.17) appeared to ad-

equately characterize the observed concentrations both overall and within individual subjects.

No external databases were available for comparison, so validation in this analysis used internal methods where the complete database was divided into a model development data set and a validation data set. The goodness of fit plot, residual plot, and histograms for the validation data set under Eq. (9.17) are shown in Fig. 9.20.

Good distribution around the line of unity was observed in the observed versus predicted plot and no trend was observed in the residuals. Further, although the weighted residuals were not normally distributed, they were symmetrical and centered around zero. One observation was poorly predicted showing a weighted residual of +4.9. Patient 3 at 6-h postdose had an observed concentration of 1.67 mg/L but had a predicted concentration of 0.63 mg/L, a difference of 1.04 mg/L. η_1 was normally distributed and centered at zero. The mean error (individual predicted concentration − observed concentration) was <0.001 mg/L (not significantly different than zero) and ranged from −1.42 to 1.73 mg/L (the range of observed concentrations was 0.36–7.55 mg/dL), which corresponded to a mean relative error of 1.5% (not significantly different than zero)

Table 9.17 Results of bootstrap analysis of tobramycin model presented in Eq. (9.17) with questionable observations and influential patients removed.

Parameter	Final model estimate	Bootstrap mean	Relative bias (%)	Bias-corrected Lower 90% CI	Bias-corrected Upper 90% CI
θ_1 (L/h)	7.47	7.46	−0.1	6.96	7.94
θ_2 (L)	17.4	17.3	−0.4	15.0	20.0
θ_3 (L/h)	1.50	1.50	0.2	0.60	2.33
θ_4 (L)	7.73	7.96	2.9	6.20	11.30
Var(CL)	0.0833	0.0821	−1.4	0.0595	0.110
IOV(CL)	0.0166	0.0165	−0.4	0.00913	0.0284
σ^2	0.0191	0.0187	−1.9	0.0156	0.0235

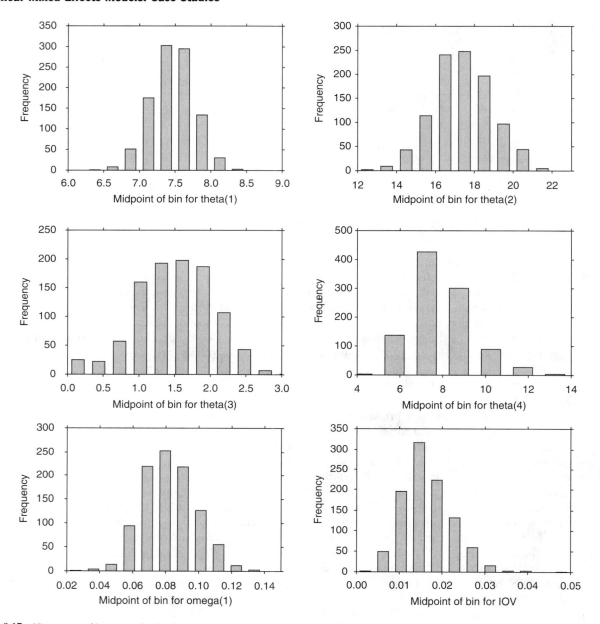

Figure 9.17 Histograms of bootstrap distributions under the model presented in Eq. (9.17).

with a range of −20 to 75%. Hence, using an internal data set for validation the model showed good predictive properties and did not seem to show any bias outside a single poorly predicted observation.

The model estimates were obtained using FOCE-I. Of interest was how these values would compare using a different estimation algorithm. Hence, the model was estimated using FO-approximation, FOCE, Laplacian, and generalized least-squares (GLS). The results are shown in Table 9.18. FOCE and Laplacian produced essentially the same results. Similarly, FOCE-I and GLS produced essentially the same results as well. Conditional methods tend to produce different results from

FO-approximation as the amount of data per subject decreases. This data set was fairly sparse with most subjects having about two samples per subject. It would be expected that the methods would produce fairly different estimates but this was not the case. All methods generated roughly the same parameter estimates indicating that the model was fairly robust to choice of estimation algorithm.

As a last measure of validation, the plausibility of the covariates was examined. The covariates identified in this analysis have a high degree of face validity. A 2-compartment model was identified as the best model. An examination of the observed concentration–time

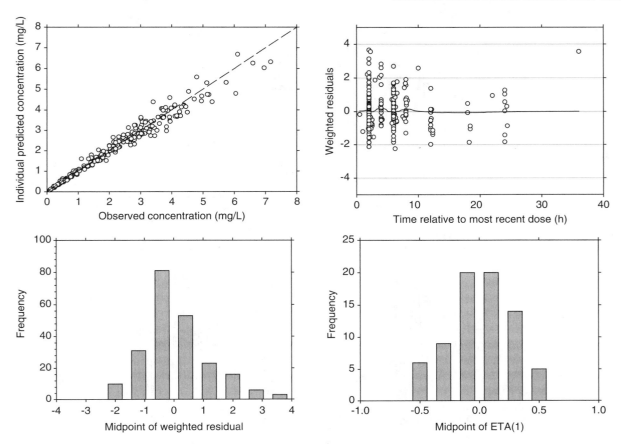

Figure 9.18 Goodness of fit plots, residual plots, and histograms of weighted residuals and random effects under the model presented in Eq. (9.17) using the parameter estimates reported in Table 9.18 (FOCE-I) after removal of two outlier observations and four influential patients. Solid line in the residual plot is the inverse square kernel smooth to the data using a sampling proportion of 0.3. Dashed line in the upper right plot is the LOESS smooth to the data using a 0.3 sampling proportion.

data on a log-scale revealed a multiphasic decline in concentrations over time (Fig. 9.4) so a 2-compartment model was consistent with this observation. Tobramycin is a large compound with a molecular weight of 468 Da that is almost exclusively cleared by glomerular filtration (Naber, Westenfelder, and Madsen, 1973). A common marker of the glomerular filtration rate is CrCL and, hence, that CrCL was identified as a covariate was expected. Tobramycin is an aminoglycoside that is extremely polar having a calculated log-octanol-to-water partition coefficient (cLog P) of -5.5 with 10 amine and hydroxyl groups. For a drug this polar would not be expected to cross membranes readily and would be expected to have a volume of distribution near extracellular fluid volume of $\sim$14 L. The volume of distribution for a 67 kg person was estimated at $\sim$26 L based on this analysis, which was consistent with expectations. In summary, the covariates identified in this analysis and the model structure had good face validity. The model appeared to be plausible without any serious concerns.

So how does the model generated herein compare to other tobramycin population analyses? This data set was

originally published by Aarons et al. (1989). They proposed that tobramycin kinetics were consistent with the following 2-compartment model:

$$CL(L/h) = 0.059 \times (\text{CrCL in mL/min}) \exp(\eta_1)$$
$$V1(L/kg) = [0.327 + 0.014 \times \text{Weight in kg}] \exp(\eta_2).$$
$$k_{12} = 0.012 \text{ per h}$$
$$k_{21} = 0.027 \text{per h}$$

$$(9.18)$$

BSV in CL was estimated at 32% with a residual error of 21%. The only covariates examined by Aarons et al. were weight, BSA, sex, CrCL, and age. Not examined were other weight-based metrics: BSA, LBW, IBW, or BMI. The model by Aarons et al. and the model in Eq. (9.17) were similar but different in that in the model by Aarons et al. did not account for IOV. Further, the model by Aarons et al. included an intercept on V1. In this analysis, the goodness of fit when the intercept was added did not improve. The net effect of these differences was that residual variability in the

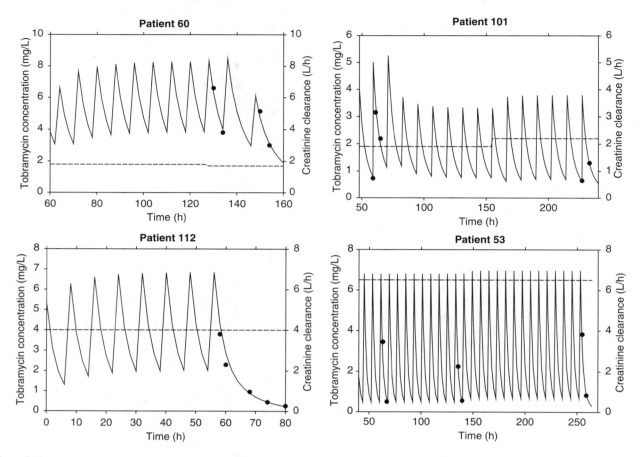

Figure 9.19 Scatter plots of observed tobramycin concentrations (●) overlaid with predicted concentrations (solid line) in four patients randomly selected from each of the renal function groups. Patient 60, severe renal impairment; patient 101, moderate renal impairment; patient 112, mild renal impairment; patient 53, normal renal function. Each patient's CrCL is plotted as a dashed line. The model predicted concentrations were based on Eq. (9.17) using the final estimates reported in Table 9.18 (FOCE-I) after removal of two outlier observations and four influential patients.

model by Aarons et al. was estimated at 21% but was reduced to 14% in this model. Hence, the model generated herein had slightly better goodness of fit.

Xuan et al. (2000) reported on the pharmacokinetics of tobramycin in 327 adult hospitalized patients. The pharmacokinetics of tobramycin were consistent with the following 1-compartment model

$$CL(L/h) = 0.066 \times (CrCL \text{ in mL/min}) \exp(\eta_1)$$
$$V1(L/kg) = [0.40 \times Weight \text{ in kg}] \exp(\eta_2)$$

$$(9.19)$$

BSV in CL and V1 were estimated at 37 and 29%, respectively. The covariates identified in this model were the same as those identified by Aarons et al. (1989). However, Xuan et al. used a 1-compartment model despite the fact that the 2-compartment model in their own analysis resulted in a lower OFV (how

much different was not reported). The variance estimate for CL was the same as Aarons et al., but the BSV in V1 was much higher, 29% by Xuan et al. and 3% for Aarons et al. The only covariates examined by Xuan et al. were serum creatinine, CrCL, age, and weight. No other weight-based metrics were examined. Hence, the results of this analysis were similar to but not the same as those reported by others and act to further reinforce the validity of the analysis.

In summary, tobramycin pharmacokinetics were best characterized with a 2-compartment model where CL was proportional to CrCL and V1 was proportional to body weight. BSV in CL was 29% with 13% variability across occasions. Residual variability was small, 14%, which compares well to assay variability of <7.5%. The model was robust to estimation algorithm and was shown to accurately predict an internally derived validation data set not used in the model development process.

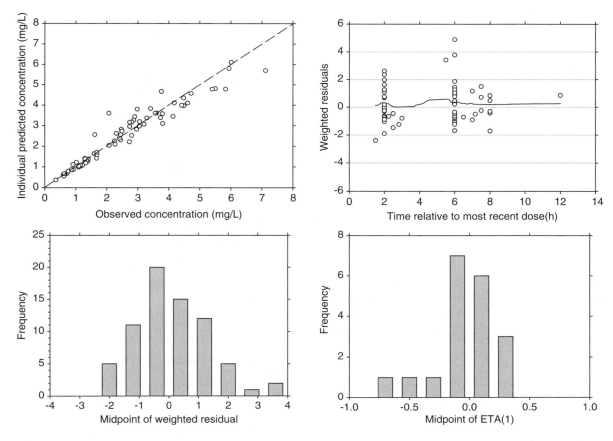

Figure 9.20 Goodness of fit plots, residual plots, and histograms of weighted residuals and random effects for the validation data set under the model presented in Eq. (9.17) using the parameter estimates reported in Table 9.18 (FOCE-I) after removal of two outlier observations and four influential patients. Solid line in the upper left plot is the line of unity. Solid line in the upper right plot is the LOESS smooth to the data using a 0.3 sampling proportion.

Simulation of Dosing Regimens and Dosing Recommendations

Simulations are useful to understand the system under consideration and to answer "what if" questions. Indeed, without simulations a model is like a bicycle without a rider. In the absence of simulations, the model simply exists and can only be used for characterizing or summarizing a system. A few simple examples will be developed herein to illustrate how simulation may be useful.

The first simulation is to show how half-life, a pharmacokinetic parameter physicians are particularly interested in, varies as function of patient covariates. Many times when a modeler shows nonscientists an equation, some of them cannot understand how the variables interact or how the dependent variable might change when the one of the predictor variables is

Table 9.18 Tobramycin parameter estimates with questionable observations and influential patients removed using different estimation algorithms under the model presented in Eq. (9.17).

Parameter	FOCE-I	FO	FOCE	Laplacian	GLS
OFV	−115.492	−78.029	−88.482	−88.171	−119.903
θ_1 (L/h)	7.47 (0.290)	7.46 (0.273)	7.44 (0.294)	7.46 (0.296)	7.48 (0.292)
θ_2 (L)	17.4 (1.54)	19.3 (1.54)	18.9 (1.24)	18.9 (0.411)	17.4 (1.52)
θ_3 (L/h)	1.50 (0.555)	0.637 (0.546)	0.539 (0.415)	0.533 (0.411)	1.56 (0.518)
θ_4 (L)	7.73 (1.35)	5.98 (1.10)	5.60 (0.805)	5.59 (0.789)	7.79 (1.30)
Var(CL)	0.0833	0.0900	0.0823	0.0832	0.0827
IOV(CL)	0.0166	0.0201	0.0165	0.0165	0.0159
σ^2	0.0191	0.0238	0.0234	0.0235	0.0199

GLS was performed using FOCE-I with one iteration. Values in parentheses are the standard error of the estimate.

changed. A graph is an easy way to present data, even to the mathematically challenged. As the old adage goes, "A picture is worth a thousand words." This deterministic simulation can be done by using the equation for a 2-compartment model

$$C(t) = A \exp(-\alpha t) + B \exp(-\beta t). \qquad (9.20)$$

The α-half-life and β-half-life are given by

$$\alpha\text{-half-life} = \frac{Ln(2)}{\alpha} \qquad (9.21)$$

$$\beta\text{-half-life} = \frac{Ln(2)}{\beta}, \qquad (9.22)$$

where

$$\alpha = 0.5\left(k_{12} + k_{21} + k_{10} + \sqrt{(k_{12} + k_{21} + k_{10})^2 - 4k_{21}k_{10}}\right)$$

$$\beta = 0.5\left(k_{12} + k_{21} + k_{10} - \sqrt{(k_{12} + k_{21} + k_{10})^2 - 4k_{21}k_{10}}\right).$$

$$k_{10} = CL/V1$$
$$k_{21} = Q2/V2$$
$$k_{12} = Q2/V1$$

$$(9.23)$$

Hence, by varying weight from 40 to 120 kg by 10 kg increments and varying CrCL from 2 to 10 L/h by 0.5 L/h increments, α- and β-half-life can be easily calculated and then plotted as a response surface. The results are shown in Fig. 9.21. α- and β-half-life were positively related to weight and negatively related CrCL. As weight increased so did α- and β-half-life, but α- and β-half-life decreased as CrCL increased. Further, the plots showed that the relationship between weight and CrCL with α-half-life was linear, but was curvilinear with β-half-life. Hence, as renal function deteriorates in a patient, reducing the dose or dosing frequency may be required to maintain concentrations within the therapeutic window. Conversely, in patients with low body weight the dosing interval may need to be increased to achieve and maintain therapeutic concentrations.

Dosing with tobramycin is guided by its therapeutic window. Recommended guidelines are to have peak concentrations at steady-state in the range of 4–6 mg/L with trough concentrations in the range of 0.5–1 mg/L for patients with life-threatening infections. The upper range of the window is driven by the incidence of nephrotoxicity, which is observed in patients with consistently elevated concentrations greater than 12 mg/L. The lower range of the window is driven by the concentration needed for microorganism inhibition in vitro and

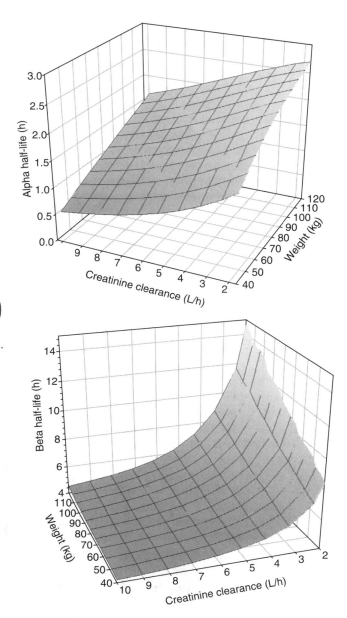

Figure 9.21 Response surface for tobramycin α-half-life (top) and β-half-life (bottom) as a function of weight and CrCL under the final model given in Eq. (9.17) and final parameter values as given in Table 9.18 (FOCE-I).

reduced tissue accumulation. The recommended tobramycin dose for adult patients having normal renal function is 3 mg/kg/day in three equal doses every 8 h in patients with serious infections. An interesting simulation is to examine what percent of the population will be within the therapeutic window at steady-state under the current recommended labeling guidelines assuming they have normal renal function and have a life-threatening infection.

Assuming that the demographics of the patients in this analysis were representative of the population as a whole, the simulation begins by first simulating patient weight and CrCL. In the patient population, weight and CrCL had a marginal correlation (Pearson's r: 0.23, p = 0.0208). To generate bivariate normally distribute random variables (X, Y) with correlation ρ the following procedure can be used. If Z_1 and Z_2 are bivariate standard normal random deviates with mean 0 and variance 1 then let

$$X = \mu_X + Z_1\sigma_X$$
$$Y = \mu_Y + \sigma_Y\left(\rho Z_1 + Z_2\sqrt{1 - \rho^2}\right) \tag{9.24}$$

where μ_X and σ_X are the mean and standard deviation for X and μ_Y and σ_Y are the mean and standard deviation for Y. For simplicity, it will be assumed that the normal range for CrCL is approximately 4.8–9.6 L/h with a mean of 7.2 L/h pooled across the sexes. This corresponds to an approximate standard deviation of 0.4 L/h. It will also be assumed that weight is normally distributed with a mean of 70 kg and a standard deviation of 6 kg. Substituting the appropriate estimators then CrCL (X) and weight (Y) can be simulated using

$$CrCL \text{ in } L/h = 7.2 + Z_1 \times 0.4$$
$$\text{Weight in kg} = 70 + 6\left(0.23 \times Z_1 + Z_2\sqrt{1 - (0.23)^2}\right) \tag{9.25}$$

A total of 10,000 patients were simulated. The simulated mean weight was 70 kg with a range of 45–90 kg. The simulated mean CrCL was 7.2 L/h with a range of 5.7–8.7 L/h. The correlation between weight and CrCL was 0.23. The means, covariance, and correlation for the simulated data were acceptable in simulating a patient with normal renal function.

The next step in the simulation was to simulate concentrations at steady-state after a infusion of 1 mg/kg (3 mg/kg/day divided into three equal doses) over a 30 min period, collecting samples at the end of infusion and at trough (8 h later). The average simulated maximal concentration was 3.7 mg/L with a range of 2.7–5.9 mg/L. A total of 8% of patients attained the maximal concentration within the therapeutic window of 4–6 mg/L and no patients attained toxic concentrations greater than 12 mg/L. The average simulated concentration at trough was 0.3 mg/L with a range of 0.01–2.3 mg/L. Only 9% of patients had trough concentrations greater than 1 mg/L. While this dosage regimen meets the trough requirement in most subjects, it fails to attain the peak concentrations required for maximal inhibitory activity.

The last simulation will be to simulate the pharmacokinetics given by a different route of administration. For instance, suppose a central venous line could not be established in an elderly 50 kg female patient, which is not that uncommon an occurrence. A physician then asks whether they could give the dose by intramuscular injection and whether this would impact the drug's pharmacokinetics. To simulate the pharmacokinetics after intramuscular administration requires an absorption model, which is unknown. Some guesses can be made, however, after a review of the published literature.

Jernigan, Hatch, and Wilson (1988) studied the pharmacokinetics of tobramycin after intramuscular administration in cats. Bioavailability was estimated at 102.5% with maximal concentrations occurring within about an hour. Hence, tobramycin absorption appears rapid and complete. There are few papers modeling the intramuscular absorption of drugs. Swabb et al. (1983) modeled the intramuscular administration of aztreonam, another antibiotic, in humans and found that a simple first-order absorption was adequate to explain the rapid (time to maximal concentrations was 0.88 h) and complete (101% bioavailability) absorption. Similarly, Krishna et al. (2001) also found that first-order absorption was sufficient to model the pharmacokinetics of quinine after intramuscular administration. In both cases, the drugs were formulated in water.

Applying these results to this simulation, it can be assumed that bioavailability would be 100% and that a first-order absorption model would apply such that the time to maximal concentrations was ~1 h (which corresponds to an absorption rate constant of 1.2 per hour). Under these assumptions, the simulated concentration-time profile after repeated administration of 1 mg/kg every 8 h is shown in Fig. 9.22. Maximal concentrations were attained ~1.1 h. after intramuscular administration and were about half the maximal concentration attained after intravenous administration. Trough concentrations at steady-state after intramuscular administration were very near trough concentrations after intravenous administration. Hence, based on this simulation, the physician could either keep the dose as is or increase the dose to more attain the concentrations seen after intravenous administration.

This example in population pharmacokinetics illustrates the process of starting with a data set and then moving through model development, ultimately leading to a model that can explain the data in terms of a few pharmacokinetic parameters and patient covariates. Once a model is developed, it can be used for many purposes, including answering questions to which no answer might be readily available or to just explain data.

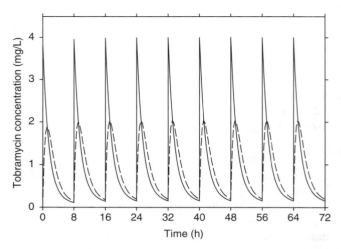

Figure 9.22 Simulated concentration–time profile in a 50 kg patient after repeated intravenous administration (solid line) and intramuscular administration (dashed line) of 1 mg/kg every 8 h assuming the final model given in Eq. (9.17). Parameter values are given in Table 9.18. Absorption after intramuscular administration was modeled assuming first-order absorption with a rate constant of 1.2 per hour and complete bioavailability.

SUMMARY

These examples were meant to illustrate the process that modelers go through in developing models: data clean-up, model building, model evaluation, how to use a model once one is developed, etc. Some models can be developed quite simply. Others are quite complex. Are these the best models? Probably not. But the models that were developed were adequate to reach the desired goal. It is important before a project is tackled to identify the goal and see what is the quickest way to get there. It does no one any good for a modeler who presents too complex a model when a simpler one can be used instead.

Recommended Reading

De Alwis, D.P., Aarons, L., and Palmer, J.L. Population pharmacokinetics of ondansetron: A covariate analysis. *British Journal of Clinical Pharmacology* 1998; 46: 117–125.

Gieschke, R., Burger, H.-U., Reigner, B., Blesch, K.S., and Steimer, J.-L. Population pharmacokinetics and concentration–effect relationships of capecitabine metabolites in colorectal cancer patients. *British Journal of Clinical Pharmacology* 2003; 55: 252–263.

Gisleskog, P.O., Hermann, D., Hammarlund-Adenaes, M., and Karlsson, M.O. Validation of a population pharmacokinetic/pharmacodynamic model for 5α-reductase inhibitors. *European Journal of Pharmaceutical Sciences* 1999; 8: 291–299.

Kerbusch, T., Wahlby, U., Milligan, P.A., and Karlsson, M.O. Population pharmacokinetic modelling of darifenacin and its hydroxylated metabolite using pooled data, incorporating saturable first-pass metabolism, CYP2D6 genotype and formulation-dependent bioavailability. *British Journal of Clinical Pharmacology* 2003; 56: 639–652.

Appendix

INTRODUCTION

A number of topics figure prominently in this book. This appendix is intended to present the relevant background for this material. While not meant to be a comprehensive coverage of the topics, it is meant as a high-level overview of the following material: matrix theory relevant to modeling, Taylor series approximation, elements of probability relevant to modeling, maximum likelihood, and computer intensive statistical methods, such as bootstrapping and jackknifing.

MATRIX THEORY RELEVANT TO MODELING

Matrices are central to this book. In order to completely understand much of the material contained herein, a basic understanding of vectors, matrices, and linear algebra is required. There are a number of introductory texts on this material—every undergraduate school in the world probably offers a class in linear algebra, so local university bookstores are a good source for more definitive references. In particular, the books by Harville (1998) and Gentle et al. (1998) present the material from a statistics point of view and may be more applicable than a general linear algebra book.

A scalar is a single number like '2' or '3.' A column vector is a single column with n-rows, e.g.,

$$X = \begin{bmatrix} 1 \\ 2 \\ 3 \\ 4 \end{bmatrix}. \tag{A.1}$$

A row vector is a single row of numbers with p-columns, e.g.,

$$X = [1 \ 2 \ 3 \ 4]. \tag{A.2}$$

If X is a row vector of size n then

$$X^T X = \sum_{i=1}^{n} X^2. \tag{A.3}$$

Hence, if X were the residuals from a linear model then $X^T X$ could be used to compute the residual sum of squares. A matrix is a group of columns all having the same number of rows. The number of rows in a matrix does not have to equal the number of columns, e.g., the matrix below has 4 rows and 5 columns

$$X = \begin{bmatrix} 1 & 2 & 3 & 4 & 5 \\ 6 & 7 & 8 & 9 & 10 \\ 11 & 12 & 13 & 14 & 15 \\ 16 & 17 & 18 & 19 & 20 \end{bmatrix}. \tag{A.4}$$

The size of a matrix is the number of rows and columns; hence, X in Eq. (A.4) is 4×5 (4 rows by 5 columns). The rank of a matrix is the number of linearly independent rows or columns (since the row and column rank of a matrix are the same). A matrix of size $n \times p$ that has rank less than p cannot be inverted (matrix inversion is discussed later). Similarly, a matrix of size $n \times n$ cannot be inverted if its rank is less than n.

The values of a vector or matrix are typically enclosed by brackets, parentheses, or braces. Elements within a vector are identified by the matrix name followed by the row or column number in subscript. For example, X_2 denotes the number '2' in Eq. (A.1). Identification of matrix elements are based on subscripts but, in this case, two subscripted integers are used: the first integer in the subscript denotes the row while the second integer denotes the column. So, for example, X_{11} in Eq. (A.4) refers to the number '1,' X_{32} refers to the number '12,' etc. To refer to an entire row, the '.' notation is often used. To refer to the entire second row in X, then X_2 is used. To refer to the entire third column of X then $X_{.3}$ is used.

The transpose of a matrix, denoted with a superscript 'T,' basically turns a matrix on its side such that the first row of the old matrix becomes the first column of the transposed matrix, e.g., in Eq. (A.4)

$$X^T = \begin{bmatrix} 1 & 6 & 11 & 16 \\ 2 & 7 & 12 & 17 \\ 3 & 8 & 13 & 18 \\ 4 & 9 & 14 & 19 \\ 5 & 10 & 15 & 20 \end{bmatrix}. \tag{A.5}$$

An $n \times p$ matrix becomes a $p \times n$ matrix after transposition.

Some matrices have specific names. A square matrix is a matrix with the same number of rows and columns, e.g.,

$$X = \begin{bmatrix} 1 & 2 & 3 \\ 4 & 5 & 6 \\ 7 & 8 & 9 \end{bmatrix}. \tag{A.6}$$

Note that Eq. (A.4) is not a square matrix. The diagonal elements of matrix are those along the diagonal, e.g., X_{11}, X_{22}, X_{33}, etc. So, in Eq. (A.6) the diagonal elements are {1, 5, 9}. The trace of a matrix is the sum of all the diagonal elements. In Eq. (A.6) the trace is 15. The remaining elements are called the off-diagonal elements.

An upper triangular matrix consists of a square matrix whose elements below the main diagonal are zero, e.g.,

$$X = \begin{bmatrix} 1 & 2 & 3 \\ 0 & 5 & 6 \\ 0 & 0 & 9 \end{bmatrix}. \tag{A.7}$$

A lower triangular matrix is the opposite of an upper triangular matrix, e.g.,

$$X = \begin{bmatrix} 1 & 0 & 0 \\ 4 & 5 & 0 \\ 7 & 8 & 9 \end{bmatrix}. \tag{A.8}$$

A square matrix whose off-diagonal elements are zero is referred to as a diagonal matrix

$$X = \begin{bmatrix} 1 & 0 & 0 \\ 0 & 5 & 0 \\ 0 & 0 & 9 \end{bmatrix}. \tag{A.9}$$

A diagonal matrix whose diagonal elements are all '1' is referred to as the identity matrix (I or I_n).

In algebra, a number multiplied by its inverse results in a value of '1.' In matrix algebra, the inverse of a square matrix (denoted by a superscript '−1') multiplied by itself results in the identity matrix. In other words, the inverse of X is the matrix X^{-1} such that $XX^{-1} = X^{-1}X = I$. Two matrices are said to be orthogonal or independent if $XY^T = I$. The inverse of an orthogonal matrix is its transpose. Not all matrices can be inverted. However, one condition for inversion is that the matrix must be square. Sometimes an inverse to a matrix cannot be found, particularly if the matrix has a number of linearly dependent column. In such a case, a generalized estimate of inverted matrix can be estimated using a Moore–Penrose inverse (denoted as superscript '−', e.g., X^-).

A symmetric matrix is one whose elements are mirror images of each other, i.e., $X_{11} = X_{11}$, $X_{12} = X_{21}$, $X_{22} = X_{22}$, $X_{23} = X_{32}$, etc., e.g.,

$$X = \begin{bmatrix} 1 & 2 & 3 \\ 2 & 5 & 6 \\ 3 & 6 & 9 \end{bmatrix}. \tag{A.10}$$

Symmetric matrices have the property that $XX^T = I$ or $X^T = X$. For simplicity, sometimes elements in the lower triangle are not shown, thereby implying the matrix is symmetric, e.g.,

$$X = \begin{bmatrix} 1 & 2 & 3 \\ & 5 & 6 \\ & & 9 \end{bmatrix} = \begin{bmatrix} 1 & 2 & 3 \\ 2 & 5 & 6 \\ 3 & 6 & 9 \end{bmatrix}. \tag{A.11}$$

Notice that for a symmetric matrix, the corresponding lower off-diagonal elements are defined by defining any of the upper off-diagonal elements and vice versa. Covariance and correlation matrices are symmetric.

Two matrices may be added, element by element, provided both matrices have the same number of rows and columns, e.g.,

$$\begin{bmatrix} 1 & 0 & 0 \\ 4 & 5 & 0 \\ 7 & 8 & 9 \end{bmatrix} + \begin{bmatrix} 2 & 3 & 4 \\ 0 & 3 & 1 \\ 1 & 2 & 3 \end{bmatrix} = \begin{bmatrix} 3 & 3 & 4 \\ 4 & 8 & 1 \\ 8 & 10 & 12 \end{bmatrix}. \quad (A.12)$$

Matrix addition with a scalar is done in a similar manner, e.g.,

$$\begin{bmatrix} 1 & 0 & 0 \\ 4 & 5 & 0 \\ 7 & 8 & 9 \end{bmatrix} + 3 = \begin{bmatrix} 4 & 3 & 3 \\ 7 & 8 & 3 \\ 10 & 11 & 12 \end{bmatrix}. \quad (A.13)$$

If X is an $n \times p$ matrix, Y is an $n \times p$ matrix or a scalar, and Z is either an $n \times p$ matrix or a scalar then the following properties hold:

1. $X + Y = Y + X$ (commutative property);
2. $(X + Y) + Z = X + (Y + Z)$ (associative property) ; and
3. $X + Y$ or $X + Z$ is an $n \times p$ matrix (closure property).

Multiplication of a matrix by a scalar results in element-wise multiplication by the scalar and is commutative. For example, if y is a scalar equal to two and X is the matrix given in Eq. (A.10) then $2X = X2$ and numerically

$$2\begin{bmatrix} 1 & 2 & 3 \\ 2 & 5 & 6 \\ 3 & 6 & 9 \end{bmatrix} = \begin{bmatrix} 1 & 2 & 3 \\ 2 & 5 & 6 \\ 3 & 6 & 9 \end{bmatrix} 2 = \begin{bmatrix} 2 & 4 & 6 \\ 4 & 10 & 12 \\ 6 & 12 & 18 \end{bmatrix}. \quad (A.14)$$

Matrices can be multiplied providing the matrix being multiplied has the same number of columns as the multiplying matrix has columns. In other words, if one wishes to multiply matrix X by matrix Y and X is of size $n \times p$, then Y must be of size $p \times q$. The resulting size matrix will be the number of rows in X by the number of columns of Y, i.e., $n \times q$. For example,

$$\begin{bmatrix} 4 \\ 5 \\ 6 \end{bmatrix} [1\ 2\ 3] \quad (A.15)$$

is legal with the resulting matrix being a square 3×3 matrix. But

$$[1\ 2\ 3] \begin{bmatrix} 4 \\ 5 \\ 6 \\ 7 \end{bmatrix} \quad (A.16)$$

is not legal because the first matrix is 1×3 while the second matrix is 4×1. In the case where vectors are being multiplied, the resulting matrix is calculated by multiplying each row by each column element by element, so for example, in Eq. (A.15) the result would be

$$\begin{bmatrix} 4 \\ 5 \\ 6 \end{bmatrix} [1\ 2\ 3] = \begin{bmatrix} 4 \times 1 & 4 \times 2 & 4 \times 3 \\ 5 \times 1 & 5 \times 2 & 5 \times 3 \\ 6 \times 1 & 6 \times 2 & 6 \times 3 \end{bmatrix} = \begin{bmatrix} 4 & 8 & 12 \\ 5 & 10 & 15 \\ 6 & 12 & 18 \end{bmatrix}. \quad (A.17)$$

For actual matrix multiplication, the resulting matrix is more difficult to calculate and best illustrated by example. If X and Y were square 2×2 matrices then multiplying the two matrices leads to

$$\begin{aligned} XY &= \begin{bmatrix} a & b \\ c & d \end{bmatrix} \begin{bmatrix} A & B \\ C & D \end{bmatrix} \\ &= \begin{bmatrix} aA + bC & aB + bD \\ cA + dC & cB + dD \end{bmatrix}. \end{aligned} \quad (A.18)$$

If

$$X = \begin{bmatrix} 1 & 2 \\ 3 & 4 \end{bmatrix}, Y = \begin{bmatrix} 5 & 6 \\ 7 & 8 \end{bmatrix} \quad (A.19)$$

then

$$XY = \begin{bmatrix} 19 & 22 \\ 43 & 50 \end{bmatrix}, \quad (A.20)$$

but notice that the converse is not true

$$YX = \begin{bmatrix} 23 & 34 \\ 31 & 46 \end{bmatrix}. \quad (A.21)$$

Hence, matrix multiplication is not commutative, i.e., XY does not necessarily equal YX. Matrix multiplication is difficult to do by hand and is prone to error.

The determinant of a matrix, denoted $|x|$, is a scalar measure of the overall "volume" of a matrix. For variance–covariance matrices, the determinant sometimes expresses the "generalized variance" of a matrix. In the simplest case, a 2×2 matrix, the determinant is calculated by

$$|X| = \begin{bmatrix} X_{11} & X_{12} \\ X_{21} & X_{22} \end{bmatrix} = X_{22}X_{11} - X_{12}X_{21}. \quad (A.22)$$

So if X is a covariance matrix and X_1 and X_2 are highly correlated then the determinant or "volume" will be smaller than if X and Y were independent. For higher-order matrices, calculating the determinant is difficult and will not be shown.

Eigenvalues, which are also sometimes called latent roots or characteristic roots, are important in determining the stability of a matrix to inversion and eigenvalues/eigenvectors play an important role in many aspects of multivariate statistical analysis like principal component analysis. If X is a square symmetrical matrix then X can be decomposed into

$$X = ADA^{-1} \qquad (A.23)$$

where A is a square matrix of eigenvectors whose columns are orthogonal and D is a diagonal matrix of eigenvalues whose sum will equal the trace of X. If X has n rows then A and D will be size n. It should be noted that each eigenvector is associated with the corresponding eigenvalue, so for example, A_1 corresponds to D_{11}, etc.

A matrix that has all eigenvalues greater than zero is called positive definite and when all the eigenvalues are nonnegative the matrix is called positive semidefinite. If X is a square matrix that is positive definite then X can be decomposed into $X = C^T C$ where C is an upper triangular matrix that is called the Cholesky decomposition of X. The Cholesky decomposition of a matrix can be thought of as the square root function for a scalar, but in matrix form. The Cholesky decomposition is important for decomposing covariance matrices and using the result to simulate random variables.

It is useful for any modeler to have access to both a symbolic calculation engine, like MathCad or Maple (Mathsoft, Inc., Cambridge, MA) and a higher-order programming language like Gauss (Aptech Systems, Inc., Maple Valley, WA), MATLAB (The Mathworks, Natick, MA), O-Matrix (Harmonic Software, Breckenridge, CO), S-Plus (Insightful Corp., Seattle, WA), or the IML procedure within SAS (SAS Institute, Cary, NC). Symbolic calculation is useful for determining general expressions, such as finding the equations for the first and second derivatives of the 1-compartment model with first-order absorption. Numeric calculations are then needed to implement the equations in practice. Higher-order programming languages are more useful than languages like C++ or Basic, since functions like matrix multiplication are built-in to the program already, so that if, for example, two matrices need to be multiplied then typing 'A*B' may be all that is needed. Which of these programs to choose depends upon their cost and the level of functionality required by the user.

TAYLOR SERIES APPROXIMATION

Taylor's theorem, published in 1715, and its accompanying series, which was not developed until more than a century later, has a variety of uses in the numerical analysis of functions, including:

- They provide information about $f(x; \theta)$ when all of its derivatives are zero at the evaluation point.
- They can be used estimate accuracy bounds of lower approximations.
- They are easier to manipulate than the function itself since the approximations themselves are often low-level polynomials.
- They allow for evaluation of difficult to evaluate definite integrals.
- They allow for understanding asymptotic behavior in important parts of the function's domain.
- They allow solving of differential equations.
- They can be used for function optimization.

A Taylor series, which is essentially a high-order polynomial, approximates a function at a new point (x) given the function value and its derivatives at another point (x_0). The Taylor series approximation to a function f(x) expanded around x_0 can be written as

$$f(x) \cong f(x_0) + \frac{df}{dx}(x - x_0) + \frac{1}{2!}\frac{d^2 f}{dx^2}(x - x_0)^2 \\ + \dots \frac{1}{n!}\frac{d^n f}{dx^n}(x - x_0)^n. \qquad (A.24)$$

If the series is expanded around zero, the expansion is known as a MacLaurin series. The approximation consists of a linear combination of the function evaluated at x_0 and derivatives of increasing degree.

The best way to understand the series is to examine how each term contributes to the series. The first term in the series is the zero-order approximation

$$f(x) \cong f(x_0) \qquad (A.25)$$

which means that the value of x is approximately equal to the function evaluated at x_0. Intuitively this makes sense because if x and x_0 are near each other, then the new function value should be equal to the current function value. The next term in the series is the first-order approximation

$$f(x) \cong f(x_0) + \frac{df}{dx}(x - x_0), \qquad (A.26)$$

where the second term on the right hand side is essentially the slope (df/dx) multiplied by the distance between x and x_0, i.e., $(x - x_0)$. Equation (A.26) is basically a linear regression model and is useful for linear functions that have little or no curvature. To capture curvature in a function, higher order terms are added

$$f(x) \cong f(x_0) + \frac{df}{dx}(x - x_0) + \frac{1}{2!}\frac{d^2f}{dx^2}(x - x_0)^2. \quad (A.27)$$

Additional terms can be added to complete the series

$$f(x) \cong$$
$$f(x_0) + \frac{df}{dx}(x - x_0) + \frac{1}{2!}\frac{d^2f}{dx^2}(x - x_0)^2 + \dots \frac{1}{n!}\frac{d^nf}{dx^n}(x - x_0)^n \quad (A.28)$$

which is called a nth-order Taylor series approximation. Only with infinite terms is the '$\cong$' sign in Eq. (A.28) replaced with an '$=$' sign. Usually only one or two terms order are used in practice and are called first- and second-order approximations, respectively. However, as more terms are used, the approximation to the function becomes more precise.

For example, given the function for a 1-compartment model with first-order absorption

$$C = \frac{D}{V}\left(\frac{k_a}{k_a - k_{el}}\right)(e^{-k_{10}t} - e^{-k_at}) \quad (A.29)$$

a fourth-order Taylor series approximation to f(t) at $t = 0$ is

$$f(t) = 0 + \left[\frac{D}{V}\left(\frac{k_a}{k_a - k_{10}}\right)(-k_{el}e^{-k_{10}t} + k_ae^{-k_at})\right](t - 0) +$$
$$\frac{1}{2!}\left[\frac{D}{V}\left(\frac{k_a}{k_a - k_{10}}\right)(k_{10}^2e^{-k_{10}t} - k_a^2e^{-k_at})\right](t - 0)^2 +$$
$$\frac{1}{3!}\left[\frac{D}{V}\left(\frac{k_a}{k_a - k_{10}}\right)(-k_{10}^3e^{-k_{10}t} + k_a^3e^{-k_at})\right](t - 0)^3 +$$
$$\frac{1}{4!}\left[\frac{D}{V}\left(\frac{k_a}{k_a - k_{10}}\right)(k_{10}^4e^{-k_{10}t} - k_a^4e^{-k_at})\right](t - 0)^4 \quad (A.30)$$

which simplifies to

$$f(t) = t\left[\frac{D}{V}\left(\frac{k_a}{k_a - k_{10}}\right)(k_a - k_{10})\right]$$
$$+ \frac{t^2}{2}\left[\frac{D}{V}\left(\frac{k_a}{k_a - k_{10}}\right)(k_{10}^2 - k_a^2)\right]$$
$$+ \frac{t^3}{6}\left[\frac{D}{V}\left(\frac{k_a}{k_a - k_{10}}\right)(k_a^3 - k_{10}^3)\right]$$
$$+ \frac{t^4}{24}\left[\frac{D}{V}\left(\frac{k_a}{k_a - k_{10}}\right)(k_{10}^4 - k_a^4)\right] \quad (A.31)$$

As mentioned, the function reduces to a 4th degree polynomial in t. Figure A.1 plots the function and the 1st through 4th-order approximations to the function. As the number of terms in the function increases, the approximation is accurate over a greater range of the function. However, for all approximations, eventually the function fails as it moves away from the origin.

For multivariate functions the Taylor series approximation to a function evaluated at (x_0, y_0) is given by

$$f(x, y) = f(x_0, y_0) + \frac{\partial f}{\partial x}(x - x_0) + \frac{\partial f}{\partial y}(y - y_0)$$
$$+ \frac{1}{2!}\left[\frac{\partial^2 f}{\partial x^2}(x - x_0)^2 + 2\frac{\partial^2 f}{\partial x \partial y}(x - x_0)(y - x_0) + \right.$$
$$\left. \frac{\partial^2 f}{\partial y^2}(y - y_0)^2\right] + \dots \quad (A.32)$$

where all the partial derivatives are evaluated around (x_0, y_0). Because of the difficulty in evaluating the higher order partial derivatives, most often a first-order multivariate Taylor series approximation to a function is used

$$f(x, y) = f(x_0, y_0) + \frac{\partial f}{\partial x}(x - x_0) + \frac{\partial f}{\partial y}(y - y_0). \quad (A.33)$$

As an example, consider the function,

$$Z = \exp(xy). \quad (A.34)$$

over the range 0 to 1 for both x and y. The function surface is plotted in Fig. A.2. The partial derivatives evaluated at $\{x_0, y_0\} = \{0, 0\}$ are

$$\frac{\partial f}{\partial x} = y\exp(xy) \Rightarrow f(0, 0) = 0 \quad (A.35)$$

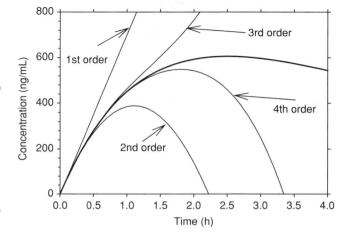

Figure A.1 Plot of Taylor-series approximations at $t = 0$ up to 4th order for a 1 compartment model with first-order absorption up to 4 h post dose. Heavy black line is the function line given $D = 100$ mg, $V = 100$ L, $k_{10} = 0.2$ per h, and $k_a = 0.7$ per h.

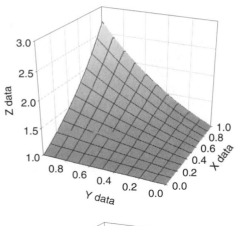

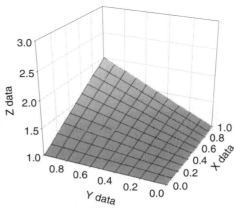

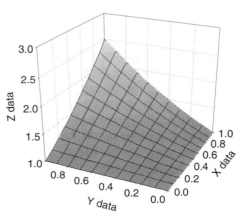

Figure A.2 Plot of the function exp(xy) (top plot), its second-order Taylor series approximation (middle plot), and third-order Taylor-series approximation (bottom plot).

$$\frac{\partial f}{\partial y} = x \exp(xy) \Rightarrow f(0, 0) = 0 \qquad (A.36)$$

$$\frac{\partial^2 f}{\partial x^2} = y^2 \exp(xy) \Rightarrow f(0, 0) = 0 \qquad (A.37)$$

$$\frac{\partial^2 f}{\partial y^2} = x^2 \exp(xy) \Rightarrow f(0, 0) = 0. \qquad (A.38)$$

$$\frac{\partial f}{\partial y \partial x} = xy \exp(xy) + \exp(xy) \Rightarrow f(0, 0) = 1 \qquad (A.39)$$

Hence, the second-order Taylor series approximation would be

$$z \cong e^{x_0 y_0} + (y_0 e^{x_0 y_0})(x - x_0) + (x_0 e^{x_0 y_0})(y - y_0)$$
$$+ \frac{1}{2} y_0^2 e^{x_0 y_0}(x - x_0)^2 + \frac{1}{2}(x_0^2 e^{x_0 y_0})(y - y_0)^2.$$
$$+ [x_0 y_0 e^{x_0 y_0} + e^{x_0 y_0}](y - y_0)(x - x_0) \qquad (A.40)$$

which evaluated at $\{0, 0\}$ would be

$$z \cong 1 + (0)(x) + (0)(y) + \frac{1}{2}(0)(x^2) + \frac{1}{2}(0)(y^2) + (xy)(1)$$
$$\cong 1 + xy$$

$$(A.41)$$

The series is a linear model with no accounting for curvature. A plot of this surface is shown in Fig. A.2. Notice that the series is a quite good approximation to the true response surface near the evaluation point and up to around $\{x, y\} = \{0.8, 0.8\}$. At this point, the function begins to fail because the true function begins to grow exponentially whereas the linear approximation remains linear in its growth. Figure A.2 presents a third-order approximation

$$z \cong 1 + xy + \frac{1}{2} x^2 y^2 \qquad (A.42)$$

which has a quadratic term in the model, the approximation produces excellent results over the entire range of the function since now the curvature in the function is accounted for. In this book, Taylor series will have two primary uses. First, Taylor series play an important role in the first-order estimation methods of nonlinear mixed effect models, and second, they play an important role in function optimization using the Newton–Raphson algorithm.

ELEMENTS OF PROBABILITY RELEVANT TO MODELING

Random Variables and Probability Densities

In its most simplest form, a random variable is a variable that changes unpredictably or randomly. If some variable is repeatedly measured and every time a new observation is obtained, that variable is random or stochastic. If the same value is obtained every time, the variable is fixed or deterministic. Mathematically, a random variable is a function defined over some sample space that associates a real number to every possible outcome in the sample space. For notation, capital letters A, B, C... will denote the random variables, whereas lower case letters will denote the possible values that the random variable can obtain. If the set of all possible values for random variable X is countable or finite then X is a discrete random variable. However, if the set of all possible X values is not countable and X is continuous over the real line, then X is a continuous random variable. For example, age, weight, height, and drug clearance are all continuous random variables, whereas sex is a discrete random variable. Study subjects can be fixed or random. If an analysis is interested in those particular subjects, i.e., if the discussion is going to be limited to the subjects in a subject and interest does not lie with the more general population from which the subjects in the study were sampled from, then subjects are treated as fixed; otherwise, subjects are considered random. For purposes herein, continuous random variables will be focused on, although everything discussed here applies to the discrete case as well.

Every possible outcome of a random variable is associated with a probability for that event occurring. Two functions map outcome to probability for continuous random variables: the probability density function (pdf) and cumulative distribution function (cdf). In the discrete case, the pdf and cdf are referred to as the probability mass function and cumulative mass function, respectively. A function f(x) is a pdf for some continuous random variable X if and only if

$$f(x) \geq 0 \qquad (A.43)$$

for all real-values of x and

$$\int_{-\infty}^{\infty} f(x) \, dx = 1. \qquad (A.44)$$

If X is a random variable with pdf f(x) then the cumulative probability of an event x occurring, denoted F(x), is

$$F(x) = p(X \leq x) = \int_{-\infty}^{x} f(u) \, du. \qquad (A.45)$$

F(x) is called the cdf and it is the integral of the pdf evaluated from $-\infty$ to x. For random variables that cannot take on negative values, then the integral is evaluated from 0 to x. Clearly, if F(x) is a cdf then dF(x)/dx is the pdf. The cdf is a monotonically increasing function with limits equal to 0 as x approaches $-\infty$ and 1 as x approaches $+\infty$. By changing the limits of

integration, the probability that x lies between a and b(a < b) is

$$p(a < x < b) = \int_{a}^{b} f(x) \, dx \qquad (A.46)$$
$$= F(b) - F(a)$$

Notice that in Eq. (A.45) the probability that x is less than or equal to some value is being evaluated. A question that is sometimes asked is what is the probability the event of interest was observed. In other words, suppose that weight was being measured. One question that might be asked is "what is the probability that this person's weight is exactly 75 kg?" This question is unanswerable from Eq. (A.46). Continuous random variables can take on an infinite number of values and as the limits of integration in Eq. (A.46) get smaller and smaller, the probability that x lies between (a, b) approaches zero. Hence, the probability that weight equals exactly 75 kg is zero. However, the probability that weight is less than or equal to 75 kg, greater than or equal to 75 kg, or greater than 30 mg but smaller than 150 kg, for example, can be integrated and is answerable.

Knowing the pdf of a distribution is useful because then the expected value and variance of the distribution may be derived. The expected value of a pdf is its mean and can be thought of as the "center of mass" of the density. If X is a continuous random with domain $\{-\infty, \infty\}$ variable then its expected value is

$$E(X) = \int_{-\infty}^{\infty} xf(x) \, dx \qquad (A.47)$$

provided that $\int |x| \, f(x)dx < \infty$. The variance of X is

$$Var(X) = E[(X - \mu)^2] = E(X^2) - \mu^2. \qquad (A.48)$$

As an aside, it should be noted that E(X) and E(X²) are referred to as the first and second moments of a distribution and that $E(X^k)$ is referred to as the kth moment of a pdf. Returning to the mean and variance, the mean of an exponential distribution (which is useful for modeling the time to some event occurring) having pdf

$$f(X) = \lambda \exp(-\lambda x), \lambda > 0, x > 0 \qquad (A.49)$$

has mean

$$f(x) = \int_0^\infty x\lambda \exp(-\lambda x)dx$$

$$= \left[\frac{-x\lambda\exp(-\lambda x) - \exp(-\lambda x)}{\lambda}\right]\Big|_\infty$$

$$- \left[\frac{-x\lambda\exp(-\lambda x) - \exp(-\lambda x)}{\lambda}\right]\Big|_0$$

$$= [0-0] - \left[0 - \frac{1}{\lambda}\right] = \frac{1}{\lambda} \tag{A.50}$$

and variance

$$\text{var}(x) = \int_0^\infty x^2\lambda\exp(-\lambda x)dx - \left(\frac{1}{\lambda}\right)^2$$

$$= -\left[x^2\exp(-\lambda x) + \frac{2x\lambda\exp(-\lambda x)}{\lambda^2} + \frac{2\exp(-\lambda x)}{\lambda^2}\right]_\infty$$

$$+ \left[-x^2\exp(-\lambda x) + \frac{2x\lambda\exp(-\lambda x)}{\lambda^2} + \frac{2\exp(-\lambda x)}{\lambda^2}\right]_0$$

$$- \left(\frac{1}{\lambda}\right)^2 = \frac{2}{\lambda^2} - \left(\frac{1}{\lambda}\right)^2 = \frac{1}{\lambda^2}. \tag{A.51}$$

A useful property is the expected value of a linear combination of random variables. If $X_1, X_2, \ldots X_n$ are random variables with expectation $E(X_1), E(X_2), \ldots E(X_n)$ and

$$Z = a + \sum_{i=1}^n b_i X_i \tag{A.52}$$

then the expected value of Z is

$$E(Z) = a + \sum_{i=1}^n b_i E(X_i) \tag{A.53}$$

with variance

$$\text{Var}(Z) = \sum_{i=1}^n b_i^2 E(X_i). \tag{A.54}$$

For continuous variables, the most common pdf is the normal or Gaussian distribution, which is written as

$$f(x;\mu;\sigma^2) = \frac{1}{\sqrt{2\pi\sigma^2}}\exp\left[\frac{-(x-\mu)^2}{2\sigma^2}\right] \tag{A.55}$$

where μ is the population mean ($-\infty < \mu < \infty$) and σ^2 the variance ($\sigma^2 > 0$). The short-hand notation for the statement "X has a normal distribution with mean μ and variance σ^2" is $X \sim N(\mu, \sigma^2)$. If $\mu = 1$ and $\sigma = 1$, this distribution is a special case of the normal distribution called the standard normal distribution. The cdf of the normal distribution cannot be expressed in a closed-form solution, i.e., the integral cannot be expressed analytically and must be evaluated numerically. Figure A3 shows three representative pdfs for the normal distribution and their cdfs. As is well known, the normal distribution is useful in practice when the distribution of X is symmetrical about its mean. Other distributions, such as the gamma or log-normal distribution, may be useful when the distribution is skewed. Normal distributions have another useful property, besides symmetry. If $X \sim N(\mu, \sigma^2)$ and $Z = aX + b$ then $Z \sim N(a\mu + b, a^2\sigma^2)$. In other words, a linear function of a normally distributed random variable is itself normally

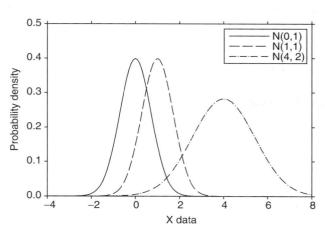

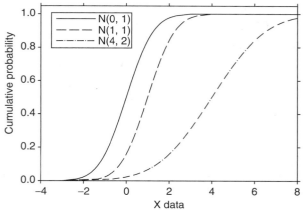

Figure A.3 Representative probability density functions (top) and cumulative distribution functions (bottom) for the normal distribution.

distributed. This property will become important in determining the expected value and variance of normally distributed random variables.

Joint Distributions

In many experiments there will be more than a single random variable of interest, say X_1, X_2, X_3, ... etc. These variables can be conceptualized as a k-dimensional vector that can assume values (x_1, x_2, x_3, ... etc). For example, age, height, weight, sex, and drug clearance may be measured for each subject in a study or drug concentrations may be measured on many different occasions in the same subject. Joint distributions arise when there are two or more random variables on the same probability space. Like the one-dimensional case, a joint pdf is valid if

$$f(x_1, x_1, \ldots x_p) \geq 0 \qquad (A.56)$$

for all real value x_1, x_2, x_3, ... x_p and

$$F(x_1 \ldots x_p) = \int_{-\infty}^{x_p} \ldots \int_{-\infty}^{x_2} \int_{-\infty}^{x_1} f(y_1 \ldots y_p) \, dy_1 dy_2 \ldots dy_p = 1. \qquad (A.57)$$

If all the random variables are independent then

$$f(x_1, x_1, \ldots x_p) = f(x_1)f(x_1) \ldots f(x_p). \qquad (A.58)$$

In other words, if all the random variables are independent, the joint pdf can be factored into the product of the individual pdfs. For two random variables, X_1 and X_2, their joint distribution is determined from their joint cdf

$$F(x_1, x_2) = p(X_1 \leq x_1, X_2 \leq x_2) = \int_{-\infty}^{x_1} \int_{-\infty}^{x_2} f(u, v) \, du \, dv. \qquad (A.59)$$

As in the one-dimensional case, their joint pdf can be obtained by

$$f(x_1, x_2) = \frac{\partial}{\partial X_1 \partial X_2} F(x_1, x_2). \qquad (A.60)$$

Many times, the density of only one of the random variates in a joint pdf is of interest, while the other variables are considered nuisance variables. The density of one random variable alone is called the marginal pdf and is obtained by integrating out (or averaging out) the remaining pdfs. For example, the marginal pdf of the random variable X_1

$$f_{x_1}(x_1, x_2, \ldots x_p) = \int_{-\infty}^{x_p} \ldots \int_{-\infty}^{x_3} \int_{-\infty}^{x_2} f(y_1, y_2, \ldots y_p) dy_2 \ldots dy_p \qquad (A.61)$$

is obtained by integrating out the random variables X_2, X_3, ... X_p from their joint pdf. A related concept is conditional probability, which provides the answer to the question "What is the probability of an outcome given some other event?" For example, suppose the random variables X_1 and X_2 are jointly distributed, an example of conditional probability relates to "what is the probability of x_1 given x_2 has already occurred?" The conditional density of X_1 given X_2, denoted $f_{X_1|X_2}(x_1, x_2)$ is defined by

$$f_{X_1|X_2}(x_1, x_2) = \frac{f(x_1, x_2)}{f(x_2)} \qquad (A.62)$$

where $f(x_1, x_2)$ is the joint pdf between X_1 and X_2 and $f(x_2)$ is the pdf of X_2 alone. Alternatively, the conditional density of X_2 given X_1 is

$$f_{X_2|X_1}(x_1, x_2) = \frac{f(x_1, x_2)}{f(x_1)} \qquad (A.63)$$

where $f(x_1)$ is the pdf of X_1. If X_1 and X_2 are independent, then $p(x_1|x_2) = p(x_1)$ and $p(x_2|x_1) = p(x_2)$.

Assume that X and Y are random variables that have a joint distribution that is bivariate normal. The joint pdf between X and Y is

$$f(x,y) = \frac{1}{2\pi\sigma_x\sigma_y\sqrt{1-\rho^2}} \exp\left\{ -\frac{1}{2(1-\rho^2)} \left[\left(\frac{x-\mu_x}{\sigma_x}\right)^2 -2\rho\left(\frac{x-\mu_x}{\sigma_x}\right)\left(\frac{y-\mu_y}{\sigma_y}\right) + \left(\frac{y-\mu_y}{\sigma_y}\right)^2 \right] \right\} \qquad (A.64)$$

where ρ is the correlation between X and Y. The marginal distributions are themselves normally distributed: $X \sim N(\mu_x, \sigma_x^2)$ and $Y \sim N(\mu_y, \sigma_y^2)$. This is illustrated in Fig. A.4. In contrast, the conditional pdf of Y given X is

$$f_{Y|X}(x,y) = \frac{f(x,y)}{f(x)}$$

$$= \frac{1}{\sqrt{2\pi\sigma_y^2(1-\rho^2)}} \exp\left\{ \frac{-\left(y-\mu_y-\rho\frac{\sigma_y}{\sigma_x}(x-\mu_x)\right)^2}{2\sigma_y^2(1-\rho^2)} \right\} \qquad (A.65)$$

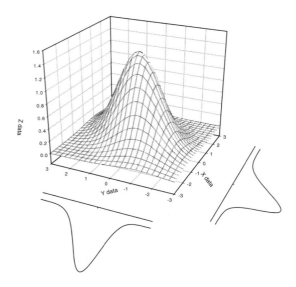

Figure A.4 Joint pdf of the bivariate normal distribution and the marginal distributions for X and Y. In this example, both X and Y have a standard normal distribution with a correlation between variables of 0.6.

which is the pdf for a normal distribution with mean $\mu_y + \rho(x - \mu_x)\sigma_y/\sigma_x$ and variance $\sigma_y^2(1 - \rho^2)$. The conditional pdf for Y given X is illustrated in Fig. A.5.

What the conditional pdf does is "slice" the joint pdf at X and evaluate the pdf at that point in space.

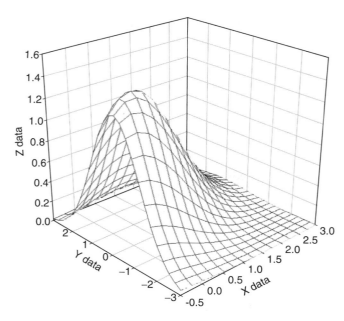

Figure A.5 Conditional pdf of Y given X from the joint distribution shown in Fig. 4. Here, X equals -0.5.

Notice that the conditional pdf is normally distributed wherever the joint pdf is sliced parallel to X. In contrast, the marginal distribution of Y or X evaluates the pdf across all of X or Y, respectively. Hence, the mean and variance of the marginal and condition distribution from a bivariate normal distribution can be expressed as:

Distribution	Mean	Variance
• Marginal (Y)	μ_y	σ_y^2
• Conditional (Y|X)	$\mu_y + \rho(x - \mu_x)\sigma_y\sigma_x$	$\sigma_y^2(1 - \rho^2)$

Without any information about Y or X, the best guess of what Y will be is μ_y and the variance will be σ_y^2. Now suppose x is observed. In this case the data in-hand allows refinement in the estimation of the pdf of Y. The variance then becomes $\sigma_y^2(1 - \rho^2)$, which is smaller than the variance when nothing is known about X. Hence, conditional distributions increase the precision of an estimator of one random variable by knowing something about the other random variable.

An extension to the bivariate normal distribution is when there are more than two random variables under consideration and their joint distribution follows a multivariate normal (MVN) distribution. The pdf for the MVN distribution with p random variables can be written as

$$f(x_1, x_2, \ldots x_p) =$$
$$\frac{1}{2\pi^{p/2}|\Sigma|^{1/2}} \exp\left[-\frac{1}{2}(x - \mu)^T\Sigma^{-1}(x - \mu)\right] \quad (A.66)$$

where x is an $n \times p$ matrix of observations $\{x_1, x_2, \ldots x_p\}$, μ is a p-size vector of population means, Σ is a $p \times p$ variance–covariance matrix, and $|.|$ is the determinant function. Eq. (A.66) is no different than Eq. (A.64), except that now the joint pdf is expressed in matrix notation. A set of random variables having a MVN distribution have the following properties:

1. The multivariate normal distribution is completely defined by the mean and covariance of X.
2. All of the marginal densities are themselves normally distributed.
3. Any conditional density is normally distributed.
4. Linear combinations of the random variables are also MVN.

The scalar variable $|\Sigma|$ is sometimes called the generalized variance and represents the overall "volume" of the variance–covariance matrix. Practically, it allows the variance–covariance matrix to be represented as a single number. The larger the number, the larger the "volume" of the variance–covariance matrix.

MAXIMUM LIKELIHOOD

One-Dimensional Case

Many families of probability distributions depend on only a few parameters. Collectively, these parameters will be referred to as θ, the population parameters, because they describe the distribution. For example, the exponential distribution depends only on the parameter λ as the population mean is equal to $1/\lambda$ and the variance is equal to $1/\lambda^2$ [see Eqs. (A.50) and (A.51)]. Most probability distributions are summarized by the first two moments of the distribution. The first moment is a measure of central tendency, the mean, which is also called the expected value or location parameter. The second moment is a measure of the dispersion around the mean and is called the variance of the distribution or scale parameter. Given a random variable Y, the expected value and variance of Y will be written as E(Y) and Var(Y), respectively. Unless there is some a priori knowledge of these values, they must be estimated from observed data.

Maximal likelihood was first presented by R.A. Fisher (1921) (when he was 22 years old!) and is the backbone of statistical estimation. The object of maximum likelihood is to make inferences about the parameters of a distribution θ given a set of observed data. Maximum likelihood is an estimation procedure that finds an estimate of θ (an estimator called $\hat{\theta}$) such that the likelihood of actually observing the data is maximal. The Likelihood Principle holds that all the information contained in the data can be summarized by a likelihood function. The standard approach (when a closed form solution can be obtained) is to derive the likelihood function, differentiate it with respect to the model parameters, set the resulting equations equal to zero, and then solve for the model parameters. Often, however, a closed form solution cannot be obtained, in which case optimization is done to find the set of parameter values that maximize the likelihood (hence the name).

When observations are sampled independently from a pdf, the joint distribution may be written as the product of the individual or marginal distributions. This joint distribution for Y having pdf $f(Y_i|\theta)$ is called the likelihood function

$$L(\theta) = \prod_{i=1}^{n} f(Y_i|\theta) \qquad (A.67)$$

which is a joint distribution conditional on some θ. By definition, the likelihood $L(\theta)$ is the probability of observing Y as a function of θ. This is important because maximum likelihood maximizes the likelihood of observing the data assuming θ is the true parameter, even though this is not what is really wanted. What is really wanted is maximizing the likelihood of θ given Y, which falls into the realm of Bayesian statistics and is outside the scope of this book.

For the normal distribution, the likelihood function for n-independent normally, distributed samples is denoted as

$$L(\theta) = \prod_{i=1}^{n} \frac{1}{\sqrt{2\pi\sigma^2}} \exp\left[\frac{-(Y_i - \mu)^2}{2\sigma^2}\right]. \qquad (A.68)$$

Maximum likelihood finds the set of θ that maximizes the likelihood function given a set of data Y. If $L(\theta)$ is differentiable and assumes a maximum at $\hat{\theta}$ then a maximum likelihood estimate will be found at

$$\frac{d}{d\theta} L(\theta) = 0. \qquad (A.69)$$

In other words, a maximum likelihood estimate will be found at that value of θ where the derivative is zero. Notice that the phrase "a maximum likelihood estimate will be found" was used, not the phrase "*the* maximum likelihood estimate will be found." It is possible for more than one maximum likelihood solution to exist since the derivative can also be at a minimum when it is equal to zero. Technically, $\hat{\theta}$ should be verified for a maximum by checking the second derivatives, but this is rarely done.

One problem with using the likelihood function directly is that it often involves multiplying many different numbers together which may lead to numerical overflow or underflow. For this reason, the log of the likelihood, which is called the log-likelihood function, is often used instead. Taking the logarithm of a likelihood function leads to a summation function, which is much easier for computers to handle. For example, the log-likelihood function for Eq. (A.68) is

$$\text{Ln}[L(\theta)] = LL(\theta) = \sum_{i=1}^{n} \text{Ln}\left(\frac{1}{\sqrt{2\pi\sigma^2}} \exp\left[\frac{-(Y_i - \mu)^2}{2\sigma^2}\right]\right)$$

$$= -\frac{n}{2}\text{Ln}(2\pi) - n\text{Ln}(\sigma^2) - \frac{1}{2\sigma^2}\sum_{i=1}^{n}(Y_i - \mu)^2$$

$$(A.70)$$

Still, most optimization routines do not find function maxima, they are concerned with finding function minima. For this reason the log-likelihood function is often multiplied by a negative constant (usually -1 or -2) to obtain the negative log-likelihood. The maximum likelihood estimate of θ is then the values of θ that minimize the negative log-likelihood and where

$$\frac{d}{d\theta} LL(\theta) = 0. \qquad (A.71)$$

As an example, consider the data set $Y = \{-2.1, -1.6, -1.4, -0.25, 0, 0.33, 0.5, 1, 2, 3\}$. The likelihood function and log-likelihood function, assuming the variance is known to be equal to 1, are shown in Fig. A.6. As μ increases from negative to positive, the likelihood increases, reaches a maximum, and then decreases. This is a property of likelihood functions. Also note that both functions parallel each other and the maxima occur at the same point on the x-axis. Intuitively one can then see how maximum likelihood estimation works. Eyeballing the plot shows that the maximum likelihood estimate (MLE) for μ is about 0.2.

Going back to Eq. (A.70), the first two terms on the right hand side contribute nothing to the log-likelihood except as a constant. Similarly, the denominator $(2\sigma^2)$ of the third term in the equations behaves as a constant since in this case the variance is a constant. Hence, the only thing in Eq. (A.70) that contributes to the likelihood function that is data-dependent is

$$\sum_{i=1}^{n} (Y_i - \mu)^2 \qquad (A.72)$$

which is often called the kernel and may be familiar to the reader as the sum of squares. The MLE is obtained when the sum of squares is minimized.

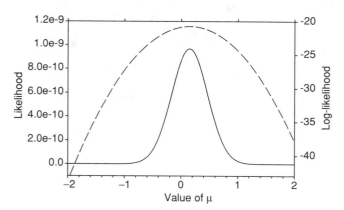

Figure A.6 Line plot of likelihood function (solid line) and log-likelihood function (dashed line) assuming a normal distribution with a known variance equal to 1 and given the data $Y = \{-2.0, -1.6, -1.4, 0.25, 0, 0.33, 0.5, 1, 2,$ and $3\}$.

Maximum likelihood estimates (MLEs) have a number of useful properties when the sample size is large, which is why they are used so often in parameter estimation. These include:

1. Under reasonable conditions, if $\hat{\theta}$ are MLEs then $\hat{\theta}$ converges in probability to θ as $n \to \infty$. Thus, $\hat{\theta}$ is said to be a consistent estimator for θ. In plain terms, $\hat{\theta}$ will be get closer and closer to the true values of θ for large sample sizes.
2. MLEs are unbiased, i.e., $E(\hat{\theta}) = \theta$.
3. $\hat{\theta}$ is normally distributed with mean θ and variance

$$\frac{1}{nE\left(\frac{\partial}{\partial\theta} LL(\theta)\right)^2}. \qquad (A.73)$$

4. In general, MLEs have smaller confidence intervals than other estimation procedures.
5. $g(\hat{\theta})$ is a MLE of $g(\theta)$ if is the MLE of θ and if $g(\theta)$ is a function of θ. This is called the invariance property of MLEs.
6. Log-likelihood functions are additive. For example, if $LL_X(\theta)$ is the log-likelihood function for X and $LL_Y(\theta)$ is the log-likelihood function for Y, then the total log-likelihood is $LL_X(\theta) + LL_Y(\theta)$. Similarly, likelihood functions are multiplicative.

Multidimensional Case

Most real world models often require multiparameter solutions. So, to characterize a normal distribution an estimate of the mean μ and variance σ^2 is needed. In some instances, only a subset of parameters in the model may be of interest, e.g., only the mean of the distribution may be of interest, in which case the other parameters are considered nuisance parameters. In fitting a likelihood function, however, maximization is done relative to all model parameters. But, if only a subset of model parameters are of interest, a method needs to be available to 'concentrate' the likelihood on the model parameters of interest and eliminate the nuisance parameters.

Nuisance parameters are generally eliminated by computing the marginal likelihood. In the two-dimensional case, with random variables X and Y, the marginal likelihood can be obtained by integrating out the nuisance parameter from the joint likelihood. For example,

$$L(X) = \int L(X,Y) \, dY \qquad (A.74)$$

or

$$L(Y) = \int L(X,Y)\ dX \qquad (A.75)$$

where L(X, Y) is the joint likelihood for X and Y defined as the product of the marginal likelihoods

$$L(X,Y) = L(X)L(Y). \qquad (A.76)$$

A marginal likelihood can also be derived from the conditional distribution of joint random variables. If f(X) is the pdf of X and f(Y) is the pdf of Y then the conditional pdf of X given Y is

$$f(X|Y) = \frac{f(X,Y)}{f(Y)}. \qquad (A.77)$$

Rearranging Eq. (A.77), solving for the joint likelihood, and expressing the pdf as a likelihood gives

$$L(X) = \int f(X|Y)f(Y)\ dY. \qquad (A.78)$$

Marginal likelihoods can easily be extended to more than two-dimensions. Suppose that L(X), L(Y), and L(Z) are the likelihood functions for random variables X, Y, and Z, respectively. Then the joint likelihood is

$$L(X,Y,Z) = L(X)L(Y)L(Z) \qquad (A.79)$$

and the marginal likelihood for X is

$$L(X) = \int_Y \int_Z L(X,Y,Z)\ dZ\ dY. \qquad (A.80)$$

As an example, consider a linear mixed effect model that has two random effects: between-subject variability (U) and residual variability (ε). The model can be written as

$$Y = x\beta + zU + \varepsilon \qquad (A.81)$$

where $\varepsilon \sim N(0,R)$ and U is a nuisance variable of no interest with distribution N(0, G). The joint likelihood is the product of the individual likelihoods

$$L(\beta,R,U,G) = L(\beta,R)L(U,G) \qquad (A.82)$$

$$L(\beta,R,U,G) =$$

$$\left\{ \frac{1}{2\pi^{n/2}|R|^{1/2}} \exp\left[-\frac{1}{2}(Y - x\beta - zU)^T R^{-1}(Y - x\beta - zU) \right] \right.$$

$$\left. \times \left\{ \frac{1}{2\pi^{p/2}|G|^{1/2}} \exp\left[-\frac{1}{2} U^T G^{-1} U \right] \right\} \right\} \qquad (A.83)$$

with the marginal likelihood obtained by integrating out the nuisance variable

$$L(\beta,G,R) = \int L(\beta,R,U,G)\ dU. \qquad (A.84)$$

If $V = Z^T GZ + R$, then after a lot of algebraic manipulation (see Davidian and Giltinan (1995) for details), the marginal likelihood can be expressed as

$$L(\beta,G,R) =$$

$$\left\{ \frac{1}{2\pi^{n/2}|V|^{1/2}} \exp\left[-\frac{1}{2}(Y - x\beta - zU)^T V^{-1}(Y - x\beta - zU) \right] \right\}.$$

$$(A.85)$$

which has as its MLE solution for β the usual weighted least-squares solution

$$\hat{\beta} = \min\left[(Y - x\beta)TV^{-1}(Y - x\beta) \right]. \qquad (A.86)$$

Because the individual likelihoods were normally distributed and ε was independent of U, the resulting marginal likelihood was solvable and itself normally distributed. For nonlinear mixed effect models or when ε is not independent of U, the evaluation of the marginal likelihood cannot be computed analytically and must be evaluated numerically. It is how the individual software packages evaluate the marginal likelihood function that differentiates them.

COMPUTER INTENSIVE STATISTICAL METHODS

Background

Estimation of any statistic, like a model parameter or sample mean for example, has some degree of uncertainty associated with it. Little confidence is placed in statistics with a high degree of uncertainty. This uncertainty, called the standard error of the statistic, is usually expressed in terms of a confidence interval (CI) which has a different interpretation depending on whether you are a Bayesian (who believe that the CI is the interval a true parameter lies within with probability $1-\alpha$) or frequentist (who believe that if the experiment could be repeated over and over again and a $(1-\alpha)100\%$ CI were generated each time, then $(1-\alpha)100\%$ of those intervals would contain the true parameter.)[1]

Parametric methods for estimating the CI of a statistic require the assumption of a sampling distribution for the statistic and then some way to calculate the parameters of that distribution. For example, the sampling distribution for the sample mean is a normal distribution having mean μ, which is estimated by the sample mean $\bar{x}$, and standard deviation equal to the standard error of the mean SE $(\bar{x})$, which is calculated using

$$SE(x) = \frac{s}{\sqrt{n}} \qquad (A.87)$$

where s is the sample standard deviation and n is the sample size. The $(1-\alpha)\%$ CI for the sample mean is then given by

$$x \pm Z_{\alpha/2} \times SE(x) \qquad (A.88)$$

where Z is the $\alpha/2$-tail from a standard normal distribution.

Sometimes, the distribution of the statistic must be derived under asymptotic or best case conditions, which assume an infinite number of observations, like the sampling distribution for a regression parameter which assumes a normal distribution. However, the asymptotic assumption of normality is not always valid. Further, sometimes the distribution of the statistic may not be known at all. For example, what is the sampling distribution for the ratio of the largest to smallest value in some distribution? Parametric theory is not entirely forthcoming with an answer. The bootstrap and jackknife, which are two types of computer intensive analysis methods, could be used to assess the precision of a sample-derived statistic when its sampling distribution is unknown or when asymptotic theory may not be appropriate.

As might be surmised, computer intensive statistical analysis methods have become more popular and useful with the advent of modern personal computers having faster speeds and greater computing capability. The two most popular among these methods, the bootstrap and the jackknife, have funny names but have proven to be incredibly useful. In fact, this is how the jackknife got its name; it was meant as a useful tool in the statistician's armament (Tukey, 1977). The bootstrap, which is a generalization of the jackknife, was so named to allow one to pull themselves "up by their bootstraps" (Efron, personal communication). These two methods, as well as resampling methods, will be discussed.

The Jackknife

For simplicity θ will be assumed to be one dimensional, but what will be discussed below applies to multivariate θ as well. First, define θ and θ_{-i} as the statistic of interest with and without the ith observation, respectively. Then, define the ith pseudo value for θ as

$$P_i = n\theta - (n-1)\theta_{-i}. \qquad (A.89)$$

The average of all pseudovalues

$$P = \frac{\sum_{i=1}^{n} P_i}{n} \qquad (A.90)$$

is called the jackknife estimate of θ with variance

$$\sum = \frac{1}{n(n-1)} \sum_{i=1}^{n} (P_i - P)^2. \qquad (A.91)$$

The square root of Σ is the jackknife standard error of the estimate. This method is called the "delete-1" jackknife because a single observation is removed at a time. A modification of this method, called the "delete-n" jackknife, is to delete "chunks" of data at a time and then create the pseudovalues after removal of these chunks.

The jackknife has a number of advantages. First, the jackknife is a nonparametric approach to parameter inference that does not rely on asymptotic methods to be accurate. A major disadvantage is that a batch or script file will need to be needed to delete the ith observation, recompute the test statistic, compute the pseudovalues, and then calculate the jackknife statistics; of course, this disadvantage applies to all other computer intensive methods as well, so it might not be a disadvantage after all. Also, if θ is a "nonsmooth" parameter, where the sampling distribution may be discontinuous, e.g., the median, the jackknife estimate of the variance may be quite poor (Pigeot, 2001). For example, data were simulated from a normal distribution with mean 100 and

---

[1] Many texts often define the CI using some blend of the Bayesian and frequentist interpretation, although most people in practice use a Bayesian interpretation despite having used a frequentist method to calculate the CI.

standard deviation 20. Three sample sizes were simulated: 12, 24, and 36 observations. The median was calculated, the data were jackknifed, and the 95% CI based on the jackknife estimate of the standard error (SE_{median}) was calculated for the sample median using the equation

$$95\% \text{ CI} = \text{Median} \pm SE_{median} \times t_{\alpha/2, n-1} \qquad (A.92)$$

where t is value of Student's t-distribution with n-1 degrees of freedom and $\alpha/2$ degrees of freedom. This process was repeated 2000 times. The percent of CIs that contained the true median of 100 was calculated. Approximately 95% of the observed CIs from the 2000 simulation iterations should contain the true median to have nominal coverage.[2] The coverage was 72, 70, and 72 with 12, 24, and 36 observations, respectively, nowhere near the required nominal coverage. Because of the perceived problems with the jackknife about non-smooth estimators and the generally poorer coverage of jackknife CIs, the use of the jackknife has declined in recent years and has been largely supplanted by the bootstrap.

The Bootstrap

The bootstrap comes in many flavors, both with parametric and nonparametric options, and can be used to assess the precision of a statistic without making strong distributional assumptions. The basic idea behind the bootstrap is to use Monte Carlo simulation to repeatedly sample from the observed data with replacement, thus generating a new set of data the same size as the original data set. From the resampled data set, the statistic of interest can be recomputed, thus generating a bootstrap estimate of the statistic of interest. If this bootstrap process is repeated many times, a distribution of bootstrapped statistics can then be used to empirically estimate the observed statistic's sampling distribution. In its parametric form, distributional assumptions are placed on the bootstrap distribution, but more interesting and useful is the nonparametric form which places no such strong assumptions on the bootstrap distribution.

Consider the univariate case where a random variable X is measured n-times and some statistic f(x) is calculated from the sample vector X. In its most basic form, the nonparametric bootstrap is done as follows:

---

[2] Coverage is the proportion or percent of times a CI contains the true parameter of interest. A 95% CI should contain the true parameter 95% of the time—this is its nominal coverage.

1. Sample from X with replacement n-times to obtain a bootstrap data set and call these samples X.
2. Calculate the bootstrap estimate of the sample statistic using the bootstrap data set f(X*).
3. Repeat Steps 1 and 2 B-times (where B is large) to estimate the bootstrap distribution.

For example, suppose $x = \{1, 2, 3, 4, 5, 6, 7\}$ with sample mean 4. The first bootstrap data set may consist of $\{1, 1, 4, 5, 3, 5, 3\}$ with sample mean 3.14. The second bootstrap data set may consist of $\{1, 4, 1, 3, 4, 2, 3\}$ with sample mean 2.57. The bootstrap means, 3.14, 2.57, etc., can then be used to estimate the standard error of the observed sample mean and its corresponding CI. Notice that not every number is represented in the bootstrap data set and that sometimes an observation is repeated; these are properties of resampling *with replacement*. By resampling with replacement, an observation can be repeated or excluded. A key assumption of the bootstrap is that resampling (the simulation process) mimics the experimental procedure that gave rise to the observed data as closely as possible. In other words, as Fox (2002) has stated: "*The population is to the sample as the sample is to the bootstrap sample.*" For example, if the data were correlated then resampling should mimic that correlation—it would not be valid to simulate assuming independence of the observations.

If the bootstrap estimate of the statistic is estimated B-times (i.e., Steps 1 to 3 are repeated B-times) then the bias and variance of the observed statistic can be calculated by

$$\text{Bias} = f(x) - \frac{\sum_{i=1}^{B} f(x^*)}{B} \qquad (A.93)$$

$$\text{Variance} = \frac{\sum_{i=1}^{B} \left[f(x_i^*) - \frac{\sum_{i=1}^{B} f(x_i^*)}{B} \right]^2}{B-1}. \qquad (A.94)$$

The square root of the bootstrap variance is the estimate for the standard error of the observed statistic.

A key question that often arises is how large should B be to be valid. There are no hard and fast rules here and often ad hoc choices are made. In the case of estimating the bias, 50–100 bootstrap estimates will suffice. To estimate the variance, more is better but often B = 100 will suffice. To estimate the CI, which is often based on estimating the tails of the bootstrap distribution, B should be at least 1000, although 1000 is the usual choice.

The real difference in the bootstrap methods is in how the CIs are calculated. Three different classes for generating CIs exist: nonpivotal, pivotal, and test-inversion. Test inversion methods are not seen frequently and will not be discussed here; the reader is referred to Carpenter and Bithell (2000) for a summary and Carpenter (1999) for a more complete exposition. Nonpivotal methods, which are the simplest, most common form were the first methods examined by Efron and colleagues (1979; 1982). The percentile method simply involves sorting the bootstrap estimates of the statistic from smallest to largest and then finding the $B(\alpha/2)$th and $B(1 - \alpha/2)$th observation. These values are declared the lower and upper CI. For example, if B is 1000 then the lower and upper 95% CI is the 25th and 975th observation. An advantage of this method is that the CI holds if the bootstrap distribution were transformed. For example, suppose the rate constant of elimination (λ) from a concentration–time profile were bootstrapped with lower and upper CI $\{L_\lambda, U_\lambda\}$. The half-life would be $Ln(2)/\lambda$ with lower and upper CI $\{Ln(2)/L_\lambda, Ln(2)/U_\lambda\}$. This method has been criticized, however, for a heavy reliance on symmetry and poor coverage error when the bootstrap distribution is asymmetrical (Carpenter and Bithell, 2000). Still, this is perhaps the most common method used to estimate the CI for a statistic.

To overcome some of the shortcomings of the percentile method the bias-corrected (BC) method was developed (Efron, 1987). With this method:

1. The number of bootstrap estimates of the statistic less than the observed test statistic is calculated and called p. Set $b = \Phi^{-1}(p/B)$ where $\Phi^{-1}(\cdot)$ is the inverse of the standard normal distribution.
2. Calculate the upper endpoint of the bias-corrected CI as $B \times \Phi(2b + Z_{\alpha/2})$.
3. Calculate the lower endpoint of the bias-corrected CI as $B \times \Phi(2b - Z_{\alpha/2})$.

So for example, if $p = 0.60$ and $B = 1000$ then the lower and upper 95% CI shifts from the 25th and 975th observation to the 73rd and 993rd observation, respectively. The nonlinear transformation of the Z-distribution affects the upper and lower values differentially. The bias-corrected method offers the same advantages as the percentile method but offers better coverage if the bootstrap distribution is asymmetrical. The bias-corrected method is not a true nonparametric method because it makes use of a monotonic transformation that results in a normal distribution centered on f(x). If $b = 0$ then the bias-corrected method results are the same as the percentile method.

While the bias-corrected method corrects for asymmetry, it does not correct for skewness and this in turn led to the accelerated bias-corrected (BCa) method (Efron, 1992). Under this method, b is calculated as in the bias-corrected method. Now a new factor, called the acceleration constant (a), is calculated based on jackknifing the original data set. Let $\bar\theta_{-i}$ be the average of the pseudovalues of the jackknife statistic θ_{-i} then

$$a = \frac{\sum\limits_{i=1}^{n} [\theta_{-i} - \overline{\theta}_{-i}]^3}{6\left[\sum\limits_{i=1}^{n} (\theta_{-i} - \overline{\theta}_{-i})^2\right]^{3/2}} \qquad (A.95)$$

and the lower and upper CI is given by the integer part of

$$B \times \Phi\left(b \pm \frac{Z_{\alpha/2} + b}{1 - a(Z_{\alpha/2} + b)}\right). \qquad (A.96)$$

Accelerated bias-corrected CIs are generally smaller than percentile and bias-corrected CIs.

All the percentile-like methods just presented are predicated on the assumption that the mean of the bootstrap estimators are asymptotically normally distributed around their mean. The percentile t-method is one of a class of pivot methods that transform the bootstrap estimators into a standardized t-variable t^*

$$t_i^* = \frac{f(x_i^*) - f(x)}{\sigma_{x_j^*}} \qquad (A.97)$$

where the variable $\sigma_{x_j^*}$ denotes the standard error of $f(x_i^*)$, $j = 1$ to B, which must be calculated either parametrically or nonparametrically. If the latter, a double-bootstrap is needed wherein within each main bootstrap iteration a second bootstrap, albeit much smaller with 50 to 100 iterations, is done to estimate the standard error of $f(x^*)$. Hence, for a bootstrap with 1000 iterations using a percentile t-method, 50,000 to 100,000 iterations total may be needed. Once the set of t^*s are calculated they are sorted from smallest to largest and the $\alpha/2$ and $1-\alpha/2$ percentile values of t^* are found. The lower and upper CI is then

$$\begin{aligned} &\text{Lower: } f(x) - SE[f(x)] \times t^*_{-\alpha/2} \\ &\text{Upper: } f(x) + SE[f(x)] \times t^*_{1-\alpha/2} \end{aligned} \qquad (A.98)$$

where SE[f(x)] is the standard error of the observed test statistic calculated using either the original data or estimated from the bootstrap. The advantage of percentile-t

CIs is that they are very accurate when $\sigma_{x_j^*}$ is independent of $f(x^*)$. The disadvantage, besides the obvious calculation cost, is that the intervals are not transformation respecting. Percentile-t CIs are very similar to the other methods when the distribution of the data is normal, but tend to be much wider, but more accurate, when the distribution is skewed.

Davison, Hinkley, and Schechtman (1986) showed how "balanced bootstrapping" can be done to improve the precision of the bootstrap bias and standard error. Bootstrapping with replacement may result in some observations being selected more often or less often than other observations purely by chance. Balanced bootstrapping controls the number of times an observation occurs so that each observation occurs an equal number of times albeit in different bootstrap data sets. So for example, suppose two bootstrap data sets were created. In one bootstrap data set an observation occurs twice, but another observation occurs once. In the next bootstrap data set the first observation cannot occur while the second observation can only occur once. The simplest way to achieve a balanced bootstrap is to generate a vector with all the observations strung together B-times. The vector is permutated to randomize the observations and then cut B-times to generate the bootstrap data sets. If the data set consisted of {1, 2, 3} and three bootstrap datasets were to be generated, the first step is to generate the bootstrap vector {1, 2, 3, 1, 2, 3, 1, 2, 3}. The vector is randomized, say to {3, 1, 1, 2, 3, 1, 3, 2, 2}, and then split into the three bootstrap data sets {3, 1, 1}, {2, 3, 1}, and {3, 2, 2}. When the number of bootstrap replications is large, balanced and unbalanced bootstrapping CIs are often comparable. But when the number of bootstrap replications is small, then balanced bootstrapping tends to be more efficient.

Obviously to estimate many of these CIs some kind of computer software is needed. The problem is that often the bootstrap solutions are problem-specific making a generalized software program difficult to develop. To truly solve most classes of problems, access to a vectorized computer language, like MATLAB or the IML procedure within SAS, is needed, but for some relatively simple problems, SAS does have some built-in procedures. Which CI to ultimately calculate is largely chosen based on the time to compute the bootstrap estimate, the ease of programming, and the familiarity of the analyst to the different methods. Carpenter and Bickel (2000) present some more objective guidelines for method selection but one most typically sees the percentile method used in the literature. Indeed, whether the various other methods offer any significant improvement over the percentile method remains to be seen. What an analyst is most often interested in is the preci-

sion of an estimate, which should be determinable regardless of the CI method chosen.

To illustrate the methods, Jiang et al. (2004) reported the steady-state clearance of 5-fluorouracil (5-FU) in 20 patients having gestational trophoblastic tumors. The data are presented in Table A.1. Jiang et al. reported a mean clearance of 4.74 L/min. A Kolmogorov–Smirnoff test for normality indicated that the data were normally distributed. The parametric 95% CI using the usual formula given by Eq. was 3.69–5.80 L/min. In this case, it is not necessary to use the bootstrap to calculate the CI because parametric theory provides a solution. However, the bootstrap will be used to compare the nonparametric to the parametric CIs. Figure A.7 presents the unbalanced bootstrap distribution for the mean 5-FU clearance based on 1000 bootstrap replicates. The bootstrap distribution was normally distributed as might be expected under the central limit theorem. The nonparametric bootstrap CIs were 3.89–5.76 L/min, 3.93–5.81 L/min, 3.90–5.80 L/min, and 3.57–5.69 L/min for the percentile, BC, BCa, and percentile-t methods, respectively; all of which were very near the parametric CI. Even the jackknife distribution had the same CI as the parametric CI: 3.69–5.80 L/min. Using a balanced bootstrap the CIs were 3.77–5.76 L/min, 3.80–5.78 L/min, 3.76–5.79 L/min, and 3.39–5.78 L/min for the percentile, BC, BCa, and percentile-t methods, respectively. In this case, the balanced bootstraps were slightly larger than the unbalanced bootstrap CIs, as would be expected when the number

Table A.1 Pharmacokinetic parameters for patients receiving 5-FU as reported in Jiang et al. (2004).

Patient number	Dihydrouracil/ uracil ratio (DUUR)	5-FU CL (L/min)
1	1.27	1.29
2	3.25	3.90
3	9.61	6.54
4	3.94	3.94
5	1.29	1.55
6	11.24	10.18
7	2.65	3.39
8	2.23	2.99
9	6.07	4.90
10	2.51	4.92
11	3.44	3.66
12	7.80	7.27
13	3.49	5.60
14	8.13	5.06
15	3.16	3.78
16	2.50	2.90
17	8.36	8.29
18	6.56	7.55
19	2.90	3.29
20	4.95	3.89

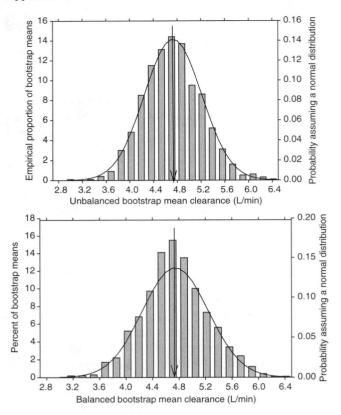

Figure 7. Bootstrap distribution for the mean 5-FU clearance data reported in Table 1 using unbalanced (top) and balanced bootstrapping (bottom) based on 1000 bootstrap replications. The solid line is the theoretical probability assuming a normal distribution. The unbalanced bootstrap distribution was normally distributed but the balanced bootstrap was slightly nonnormal. The arrow shows the observed mean clearance.

of bootstrap replications was this large. However, when the number of bootstrap replications was decreased to 100 the balanced and unbalanced percentile-t CIs were 3.57–5.58 L/min and 3.29–5.41 L/min. Hence, more precise CIs can be obtained using a balanced approach when the number of bootstrap replications is small.

One particular criticism of the bootstrap is that the CIs are not reproducible—that because of the simulation step and the stochastic nature of the analysis, the results will change depending on the seed used in the simulation and the number of bootstrap replications used. Returning to the 5-FU example, the seed was changed and the CIs reestimated. This time the 95% bootstrap CIs for the mean clearance were 3.81–5.70 L/min, 3.89–5.72 L/min, 3.83–5.72 L/min, and 3.39–5.65 L/min for the percentile, BC, BCa, and percentile t-methods, respectively. The CIs the second time were similar but were not exactly the same as the first time. Often the variability due to the simulation step can be decreased by increasing the number of bootstrap iterations.

To understand how the bootstrap methods compare, an empirical simulation was conducted. Data

were simulated from a normal, log-normal, and Student's t-distribution with mean 100 and 20% coefficient of variation. The data were similar in mean and range but differed in the shape of their distribution. Two sets of sample sizes were simulated: 15 and 30 observations. The mean was calculated and the 95% CI for the mean was calculated using parametric theory, bootstrap using the percentile method, bootstrap using the bias-corrected percentile method, bootstrap using the accelerated bias-corrected percentile method, and bootstrap method using the percentile-t method. For calculating the CI for the log-normal distribution, the data were Ln-transformed, the CI calculated, and then exponentiated back to the original domain. A total of 1000 bootstrap samples were drawn for each bootstrap method with 100 bootstrap samples drawn for the double bootstrap with the percentile-t method. The width of each CI was calculated and stored. This simulation was repeated 2000 times and the percent of CIs that contained the true value of 100 was determined; this is called the percent coverage, which should be 95%.

Table A.2 presents the percent coverage. Figure 8 presents box and whiskers plots of the width of the CIs across simulations after trimming the upper 1% to avoid any possible outliers in the results. As expected, when the sample size increased, the width of the CIs decreased. When the distribution was normal, parametric CI and percentile-t bootstrap CIs had coverage near 95% but also tended to have wider confidence intervals than the other methods. The percentile, BC, and BCa bootstrap methods had lower than expected coverage because the 95% CIs were closer to 92% CIs. When the distribution was log-normal (right skewed), parametric CIs, BCa bootstrap CIs, and percentile-t bootstrap methods had coverage near 95%, but again the percentile and BC bootstrap methods had too small of coverage. Interestingly, the BCa bootstrap method had larger CI width than the other methods. When the distribution was Student's t-distribution (heavy tailed), the parametric CIs and percentile-t bootstrap CIs had slightly higher coverage than 95%, but again the percentile, BC, and BCa bootstrap methods had too low coverage. The width of the CIs were all near the same when the sample size was 15, but the width of the percentile-t bootstrap CI was larger than the others when the sample size was 30. These results indicate that the percentile-t distribution, under these conditions, while leading to larger CIs than the other bootstrap methods (but with mostly comparable widths to the CI based on parametric theory) had the best coverage compared to the other bootstrap methods. Indeed, although the percentile bootstrap is the most widely used method, the percentile-t method is preferred when computing the second level bootstrap is a viable option. When the second level bootstrap is not

Table 2 Percent coverage of parametric and bootstrap confidence intervals using various distributions and sample sizes.

Distribution	Sample size	Parametric	Percentile	BC	BCa	Percentile-t
Normal	15	94.9	92.9	92.1	92.4	95.4
	30	95.4	93.6	93.6	93.8	95.2
Log-normal	15	94.4	90.2	90.6	95.0	94.7
	30	95.7	90.6	91.2	98.3	94.0
Student's t	15	96.5	91.7	90.7	91.1	97.9
	30	96.1	93.4	92.6	93.0	97.9

Note: Coverage was based on 2000 simulation iterations and represent the percent of times the CI contained the true mean of the distribution.

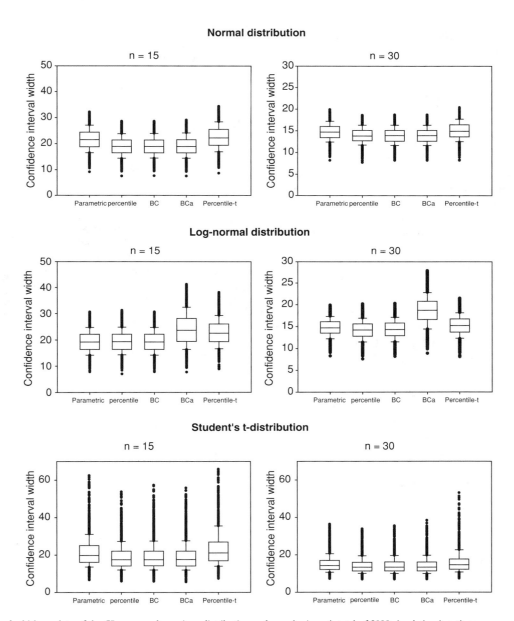

Figure 8 Box and whiskers plots of the CI range under various distribution and sample sizes. A total of 2000 simulation iterations were used with the upper 1% of the data trimmed.

a viable option because of long computing times, the BCa method is the preferred method for generating nonparametric CIs. The percentile and BC bootstrap method should be used cautiously, particularly with complex problems (Schenker, 1985).

The bootstrap cannot just be applied to any problem. There do exist situations where the bootstrap will fail, particularly those situations where the statistic *"depends on a very narrow feature of the original sampling process"* (Stine, 1990), such as the sample maximum. For instance, the bootstrap may have poor coverage in estimating the CI associated with maximal drug concentrations (C_{max}). The bootstrap will also have trouble when the sample size is small although what constitutes "small" is debatable. The number of possible combinations drawn from an n-size sample with replacement is

$$\binom{2n-1}{n} = \frac{(2n-1)!}{n!(n-1)!}. \qquad (A.99)$$

So for a sample with 8, 9, and 10 observations there are 6,435, 24,310, and 92,378 possible combinations, respectively. With 2000 bootstrap resamples and 20 observations, the probability is greater than 0.95 that no bootstrap sample will repeat (Chernick, 1999). As a practical rule, bootstrapping would not be advised with less than 10 observations, although Chernick (1999) suggests that no fewer than 50 be used. With eight or fewer observations an exact bootstrap estimate can be developed using all possible bootstrap combinations (Fisher and Hall, 1991).

Up to now it has been assumed that the distribution to be bootstrapped is univariate and that the statistic of interest is some function of the data. In pharmacokinetics it may be of more interest to bootstrap some regression model, either linear or nonlinear in nature, to obtain the bootstrap CI or standard error of the model parameters. In general, two methods exist for bootstrap resampling of regression models. Suppose that $Y = f(x;\theta) + \varepsilon$ where the residuals are independent, identically distributed from a normal distribution with mean 0 and variance σ^2. If the predictor variables are random and not under control of the experimenter, then bootstrapping proceeds using the paired combination (Y, X) and not just X. So the algorithm for this case would be:

1. Let $Z = (Y, X)$. Resample Z. From Z form the bootstrapped dependent variable Y^* and dependent variable X^*.
2. Fit the model to the bootstrapped dependent variable to obtain the bootstrap estimate of the model parameters (denoted $\hat{\theta}^*$).

3. Repeat Steps 2 to 3 B-times to obtain the bootstrap distribution of the parameter estimates.
4. Use any of the CI methods presented in the univariate case to obtain the bootstrap CIs for the parameter estimates.

Under this algorithm the response is kept with the observed value X. This method is illustrated by again using the 5-FU example of Jiang et al. (2004). In their analysis they found that the baseline ratio of dihydrouracil to uracil (DUUR) was a significant predictor of 5-FU clearance (Fig. A.9). Using linear regression they found that 79% of the variability in 5-FU clearance could be explained by DUUR. The slope of the regression line was 0.69 L/min with a standard error of 0.084. Under a linear model where the residuals are normally distributed, the CI for the slope (θ_1) is given by

$$\hat{\theta}_1 \pm SE(\hat{\theta}_1) \times t_{n-2,\alpha/2} \qquad (A.100)$$

where

$$SE(\hat{\theta}) = \sqrt{\frac{MSE}{\sum_{i=1}^{n}(x_i - \bar{x})^2}} \qquad (A.101)$$

and MSE is mean square error.

The 95% CI for the slope was 0.51–0.87 L/min. Figure A.10 shows the bootstrap distribution for the slope after resampling cases. The bootstrap distribution was normally distributed, as parametric theory suggested. The 95% bootstrap CIs were 0.48–0.87 L/min, 0.47–0.86 L/min, 0.48–0.87 L/min, and 0.56–0.77 L/min for the percentile, BC, BCa, and percentile-t method,

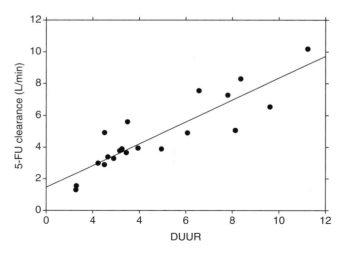

Figure 9 Scatter plot of 5-FU clearance versus dihydrouracil to uracil ratio (DUUR) as reported in Table 1. The solid line is the linear regression line.

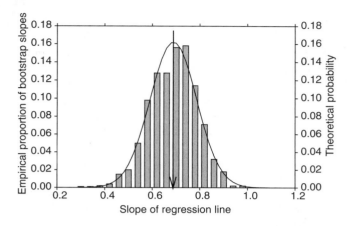

Figure 10 Bootstrap distribution for the linear regression (slope) of 5-FU clearance versus dihydrouracil to uracil ratio as reported in Table 1. The solid line is the theoretical probability assuming a normal distribution. The bootstrap distribution was normally distributed using Kolmogorov–Smirnoff's test for normality. The arrow shows the observed slope.

respectively. The nonparametric CIs were very near the parametric CI.

If, however, the predictor variables in an experiment are fixed, such as in a designed experiment where the predictor variables are under the experimenter's control, then bootstrapping of the residuals is done to preserve the fixed nature of the predictor variables. So the method would be as follows:

1. Fit the model $f(x;\theta)$ to obtain the maximum likelihood or least-squares estimate of θ (denoted $\hat{\theta}$) and the residuals (denoted e).
2. Resample the modified residuals (denoted e*) and holding the predictor variables as fixed, generate the bootstrap dependent variable as $Y^* = f(x;\hat{\theta}) + e^*$. Sometimes instead of resampling the modified residuals, e* is resampled from $e_1 - e, e_2 - e, \ldots e_n - e$ instead. In the linear model the mean residual is zero so this is equivalent to bootstrapping the modified residuals. But, the mean residual is not necessarily equal to zero in the nonlinear case so correcting for the mean is necessary.
3. Fit the model to the bootstrapped dependent variable to obtain the bootstrap estimate of the model parameters (denoted $\hat{\theta}^*$).
4. Repeat Steps 2 to 3 B-times to obtain the bootstrap distribution of the parameter estimates.
5. Use any of the CI methods presented in the univariate case to obtain the bootstrap CIs for the parameter estimates.

Bootstrapping residuals is not without its own problems. Particularly, that an appropriate model has been chosen and that $e \rightarrow \varepsilon$ at least asymptotically (in fact, OLS residuals typically underestimate ε). For this latter reason, sometimes residuals corrected for leverage are used

$$e^* = \frac{Y - f(x;\hat{\theta})}{(1 - h)^{0.5}} \quad (A.102)$$

where h is the HAT value (the diagonal elements of $x(x^Tx)^{-1}x^T$) associated with the predictor variable x. Since the average HAT value in a linear model is equal to p/n, where p is the number of estimable model parameters and n is the sample size, another alternative is to use

$$e^* = \frac{Y - f(x;\hat{\theta})}{(1 - p/n)^{0.5}}. \quad (A.103).$$

In both cases, the correction factor (the denominator) "fattens" the residuals (Stine, 1990). Such modifications are necessary in developing bootstrapped prediction intervals (Stine, 1985).

When the variance model is heteroscedastic, the algorithm for bootstrapping the residuals will not be valid because the bootstrapped data set might not have the same variance model as the original data. In fact, more than likely, bootstrapping heteroscedastic residuals will lead to a homoscedastic model. Heteroscedasticity is not a problem for the random case because heteroscedasticity will be preserved after bootstrapping. In the heteroscedastic case, the modified residuals need to be corrected for their variance so that Eq. (A.102) becomes

$$e^* = \frac{Y - f(x; \hat{\theta})}{V(x;\hat{\theta};\hat{\Phi})(1 - h)^{0.5}} \quad (A.104)$$

where $\hat{\Phi}$ is the set of variance function parameters and V(.) is the variance function that defines how the residual variability changes as a function of x and $\hat{\theta}$. Bootstrapping then proceeds as before but now in Step 2 the bootstrapped dependent variable is generated from

$$Y^* = f(x;\hat{\theta}) + \sqrt{V(x;\hat{\theta};\hat{\Phi})}(e^*). \quad (A.105)$$

In this manner the modified bootstrapped residuals will maintain the variance model of the original data. It should be noted that bootstrapping nonlinear models is done in the same manner as bootstrapping linear models.

The bootstrap has been used in pharmacokinetics sporadically on a largely theoretical basis and has not really been implemented on a routine basis, except in the case of "validating" population models. Bonate (1993), which was later improved upon by Jones et al. (1996), showed how the bootstrap can be applied to obtain CIs for individual drug concentrations, which could be of importance in therapeutic drug monitoring. Bonate later

(1998) illustrated how the bootstrap can be used to obtain nonparametric estimates of the standard error for area under the curve in a toxicokinetic experiment. Dilleen, Hiemann, and Hirsch (2003) showed how the bootstrap can be used to assess the precision of dose-response curves. The bootstrap has also been applied to assess bioequivalence, particularly in the case of individual bioequivalence (Kimanani, Lavigne, and Potvin, 2000; Shao, Chow, and Wang, 2000). However, bootstrapping may not be entirely valid because of the small numbers of subjects typically enrolled in bioequivalence studies. Pigeot (2001) discuss other instances where bootstrapping bioequivalence problems may not result in valid answers, while Chow and Liu (2000) discuss bootstrapping bioequivalence data more generally.

Bootstrapping has found its greatest application in the field of PopPK, where it is usually implemented by resampling cases with replacement. The method was first advocated by Ette (1996) and has been used for many population models including clofarabine (Bonate et al., 2004) and ciprofloxacin (Rajagopalan and Gastonguay, 2003), to name a few. But, in every case reviewed in the literature, bootstrap CIs were computed using the percentile method—in no instance (that the author could find) were more accurate bootstrap CI methods, like the BCa or percentile-t method, used.

Resampling and Permutation Tests

Resampling methods, which are also called randomization tests or permutation tests, are an extension of bootstrap methods but are used primarily for hypothesis testing. The idea behind resampling is as follows: Suppose there are two groups of data with n_1 and n_2 observations, respectively, and some function of the data (a statistic) between the two groups, like the difference in means, is determined. Of interest is estimating the probability of observing the statistic by chance alone. Now suppose each observation is written on a set of index cards which are then shuffled and sorted into two piles with n_1 and n_2 cards each. The piles represent the two groups. Based on the shuffled piles, the test statistic is recalculated. If there is no difference between the groups then the recalculated statistic should be similar to the original test statistic. If this reshuffling process is done over and over again each time recalculating the test statistic, the distribution of the reshuffled test statistics can be determined. Based on this distribution the probability of observing the original test statistic can be calculated as the number of times the recalculated test statistic was equal to or greater than the original test statistic divided by the number of reshuffling iterations. So if the data were shuffled 1000 times and 32 of those times the reshuffled test statistic was greater than the

observed test statistic, then the probability of observing the original test statistic by chance is 0.032.

Reshuffling or resampling becomes a little more complicated with repeated measures data in which case shuffling must occur within the same relative time interval. So, if samples were collected on Days 1, 2, and 3, resampling would have to be done within Day 1, and then within Day 2, and then within Day 3—not by pooling across days and then reshuffling. Also, if the number of observations is small then resampling should be done using exact methods. The shuffling method just described results in an asymptotically approximate p-value. An exact p-value can be derived for small sample sizes (in which all possible combinations can be determined) by first defining all possible combinations, computing the test statistic, then determining the number of combinations whose test statistic was greater than the observed test statistic divided by the total number of combinations. For example, suppose that in the previous example, the first group had four observations and the second group had five observations, for a total of nine observations. The total number of possible combinations is

$$\text{total combinations} = \frac{(n_1 + n_2)!}{n_1! n_2!} \qquad (A.106)$$

which in this case is $9!/(5!4!) = 126$. If 14 of the combinations resulted in test statistics greater than the original value, the probability of observing the original test statistic by chance is $14/126$ or 0.11. Hence, by determining all possible 126 combinations of observations an exact p-value can be determined. Some software packages, like Resampling Stats (Resampling Stats, Inc., Arlington, VA), are designed to compute these exact tests for many common statistics.

Randomization tests are not commonly seen in pharmacokinetics, although their use has been used in the analysis of population data as a means to determine whether a covariate is statistically significant. Wahlby et al. (2001) used simulation to see how randomization tests compare to parametric tests under a population model using NONMEM. Under the parametric model, the likelihood ratio test (LRT) is computed as the change in objective function value (OFV) between a population model containing the covariate of interest (full model) and a model without the covariate of interest (reduced model). In the randomization test, randomization is based on shuffling the covariate among subjects, thereby breaking any association between the covariate and the pharmacokinetic parameter of interest. The reduced model is fit to original data while the full model is fit to the randomized data. The LRT is then computed as the difference in OFVs between the models.

The randomization process is done many times with the LRT computed for each randomized data set. The p-value for the original data set is the number of randomized LRT values greater than or equal to the original LRT value divided by the number of randomized data sets.

Wahlby et al. showed that the type of covariate, dichotomous or continuous, and covariate distribution did not influence the p-value using a randomization test. They also showed that FO-approximation overestimated the significance of a covariate based on the LRT without randomization. In other words, for a full and reduced model having one degree of freedom difference, a change in objective function value (i.e., LRT) of 3.84 or greater is required for statistical significance at the 0.05 level assuming a chi-squared distribution. But the randomization test showed that this cutoff value was too liberal and that a cutoff value closer to 10–15 should be used. However, the LRT required for significance under the randomization test was very near the theoretical value (4.03 versus 3.84 for 0.05 level significance) when the models were fit using first-order conditional estimation with interaction (FOCE-I). Lastly, their research showed that the significance level changes depending on the covariate model. For example, when sex was treated as a covariate for clearance a change in OFV of 13.84 was required for 0.05 level of significance, but was 9.43 when sex was treated as a covariate for volume of distribution.

One difficulty with this approach is if other covariates are included in the model and they are correlated with the randomized covariate of interest. In this case, care must be taken to maintain the correlation among covariates as much as possible. The method is further complicated when the covariates vary over time. Gobburu and Lawrence (2002) illustrate a method for reshuffling when the covariates are correlated. In their study, age and weight were correlated covariates where weight affected clearance (CL) and age affected volume of distribution (V) in a 1-compartment model. Randomizing age without regard to weight could result in considerable bias in the covariates, like a 1-year-old patient weighing 100 kg. In testing the first covariate in the model, weight on CL in this instance, randomization of the first covariate across subjects can be done as has been discussed. However, when the second covariate is included in the model, given the first covariate is already included in the model, a different permutation must be done. Gobburu and Lawrence treated the first covariate as fixed for a subject and then developed a linear regres-

sion model between the first covariate and the second covariate. It should be stressed that it is not necessary to always use a linear regression model—any appropriate model, linear or nonlinear, could be used. The residuals under the linear regression model between covariates are saved and then used in the randomization. In other words, randomization of the second covariate is not done directly, but done indirectly through the residuals. The residuals are then added to the linear regression model to generate the randomized second covariate. So, for example, suppose the linear regression model was Age $= 14 + 0.3 \times$ Weight where weight was the first covariate included in the model and age is the second covariate being tested in the model. Now suppose that patient has a weight of 70 kg and randomized residual of -7. Then that patient's randomized age would be $14 + 0.3 \times 70 - 7$ or 28 years old.

Randomization tests clearly have their advantages. As Noreen (1989) points out: "... *the randomization test is valid for situations in which the conventional parametric tests are valid*" with essentially no loss in power. Further, "... *the parametric tests are not always valid in situations in which the randomization test is valid.*" However, like any computer intensive method, their utility is limited by the speed of the computer doing the randomization and analysis.

Summary

Computer intensive methods like the bootstrap and randomization tests are extremely useful and it can be expected that their use will increase as computers become faster and faster. Carpenter and Bitthel (2000) suggest that bootstrapping be done whenever there is reason to doubt the assumptions underlying parametric confidence intervals or whether no such parametric solution exists. However, they cannot be used indiscriminately as they do require some assumptions, like mild smoothness in the statistic of interest, and have some minimal sample size requirements. In most instances in PopPK, however, many of these assumptions are easily met and should not be of any great concern. However, the empirical bootstrap distribution must also mimic the distribution of interest (at least weakly), and if outliers are present in the data then this assumption will not be met. Do not forget, bootstrap estimators themselves have an estimated variance associated with their measurement due to sample variability and bootstrap resampling variability. There are many good books on bootstrapping and the jackknife that the reader should refer to for further details. Mooney and Duval (1993) present a good introduction to the topic although the examples are geared towards the social sciences. Chernick (1999) presents a good broad overview without a lot of mathematics and has over 1600 references. Efron and Tibshirani (1994) is comparable to Chernick but more mathematical in nature. Davison and Hinkley (1997) is very comprehensive but highly technical. An excellent introductory book on permutation tests is Good (2000).

Recommended Reading

Carpenter, J. and Bithell, J. Bootstrap confidence intervals: When, which, what? A practical guide for medical statisticians. *Statistics in Medicine* 2000; 19: 1141–1164.

Harville, D.A. Matrix algebra from a statistician's perspective. Springer-Verlag, New York, 1998.

References

Aarons, L. The kinetics of flurbiprofen in synovial fluid. *Journal of Pharmacokinetics and Biopharmaceutics* 1991; 19: 265–269.

Aarons, L., Balant, L.P., Mentre, F., Morsellu, P.L., Rowland, M., Steimer, J.L., and Vozeh, S. Practical experience and issues in designing and performing population pharmacokinetic/pharmacodynamic studies. *European Journal of Clinical Pharmacology* 1996; 49: 251–254.

Aarons, L., Karlsson, M.O., Mentre, F., Rombout, F., Steimer, J.L., Van Peer, A., and invited COST B Experts. Role of modelling and simulation in Phase I drug development. *European Journal of Pharmaceutical Sciences* 2001; 13: 115–122.

Aarons, L., Vozeh, S., Wenk, M., Weiss, P., and Follath, F. Population pharmacokinetics of tobramycin. *British Journal of Clinical Pharmacology* 1989; 38: 305–314.

Acton, F. *Real computing made real: Preventing errors in scientific engineering calculations.* Princeton University Press, Princeton, NJ, 1996.

Adolph, E.F. Quantitative relations in the physiological constitutions of mammals. *Science* 1949; 109: 579–585.

Agranat, I., Caner, H., and Caldwell, J. Putting chirality to work: The strategy of chiral switches. *Nature Reviews Drug Discovery* 2002; 1: 753–768.

Akaike, H. Information theory as an extension of the maximum likelihood principle. In: *Second International Symposium on Information Theory.* (Petrov, B.N. and Csaki, F. Eds.). Akademiai Kiado, Budapest, 1973, pp. 267–281.

Al-Banna, M.K., Kelman, A.W., and Whiting, B. Experimental design and efficient parameter estimation in population pharmacokinetics. *Journal of Pharmacokinetics and Biopharmaceutics* 1990; 18: 347–360.

Albridge, K.M., Standish, J., and Fries, J.F. Hierarchical time-oriented approaches to missing data inference. *Computers and Biomedical Research* 1988; 21: 349–366.

Allison, P.D. Multiple imputation for missing data: A cautionary tale. *Sociological Methods and Research* 2000; 28: 301–309.

Allison, P.D. *Missing data.* Sage, Thousand Oaks, CA, 2002.

Altham, P.M.E. Improving the precision of estimation by fitting a model. *Journal of the Royal Statistical Society, Series B* 1984; 46: 118–119.

Altman, D.G. Categorising continuous variables. *British Journal of Cancer* 1991; 64: 975.

Analytical Methods Committee, Royal Society of Chemistry. Uses (proper and improper) of correlation coefficients. *Analyst* 1988; 113: 1469–1471.

Anderson, B., Woollard, G.A., and Holford, N.H.G. A model for size and age changes in the pharmacokinetics of paracetamol in neonates, infants, and children. *British Journal of Clinical Pharmacology* 2000; 50: 125–134.

Anderson, B.J., van Lingen, R.A., Hansen, T.G., Lin, Y.C., and Holford, N.H. Acetaminophen developmental pharmacokinetics in premature neonates and infants: A pooled population analysis. *Anesthesiology* 2002; 96: 1336–1345.

Asai, G., Ando, Y., Saka, H., Ando, M., Sugiura, S., Sakai, S., Hasagawa, Y., and Shimokata, K. Estimation of the area under the concentration–time curve of carboplatin following irinotecan using a limited sampling model. *European Journal of Clinical Pharmacology* 1998; 54: 725–727.

Ascione, F.J., Kirking, D.M., Gaither, C.A., and Welage, L.S. Historical overview of generic medication policy. *Journal of the American Pharmacists Association* 2001; 41: 567–577.

Atkinson, A.C. Two graphical displays for outlying and influential observations in regression. *Biometrika* 1981; 68: 13–20.

Atkinson, A.C. *Plots, transformations, and regression: An introduction to graphical methods of diagnostic regression analysis.* Oxford Science Publications, Oxford, UK, 1985.

Audoly, S., D'Angio, L., Saccomani, M.P., and Cobelli, C. Global identifiability of linear compartmental models— A computer algebra algorithm. *IEEE Transactions on Biomedical Engineering* 1998; 45: 36–47.

Bailey, B.J.R., and Briars, G.L. Estimating the surface area of the human body. *Statistics in Medicine* 1996; 15: 1325–1332.

Baille, T.A., Cayen, M.N., Fouda, H., Gerson, R.J., Green, J.D., Grossman, S.J., Klunk, L.J., LeBlanc, B., Perkins, D.G., and Shipley, L.A. Drug metabolites in safety testing. *Toxicology and Applied Pharmacology* 2002; 182: 188–196.

Bain, L.J., and Engelhardt, M. *Introduction to probability and mathematical statistics.* Duxbury Press, Boston, 1987.

Balant, L.P., and Gex-Fabry, M. Modelling during drug development. *European Journal of Pharmaceutics and Biopharmaceutics* 2000; 50: 13–26.

Bartholomew, M.J. Foundation for nonlinear models with thresholds for longitudinal data. *Journal of Biopharmaceutical Statistics* 2000; 10: 469–480.

Bates, D.M., and Watts, D.G. Relative curvature measures of nonlinearity. *Journal of the Royal Statistical Society, Series B* 1980; 42: 1–25.

Bates, D.M., and Watts, D.G. *Nonlinear regression analysis and its applications.* Wiley, New York, 1988.

Bayles, M.D. *Professional ethics.* Wadsworth, Belmont, CA, 1989.

Bazunga, M., Tran, H.T., Kertland, H., Chow, M.S.S., and Massarella, J. The effects of renal impairment on the pharmacokinetics of zalcitabine. *Journal of Clinical Pharmacology* 1998; 38: 28–33.

Beal, S.L., and Sheiner, L.B. *NONMEM users guide - Part VII: conditional estimation methods.* Globomax, Hanover, MD, 1998.

Beal, S.L. Ways to fit a PK model with some data below the quantification limit. *Journal of Pharmacokinetics and Pharmacodynamics* 2001; 28: 481–504.

Beal, S.L., and Sheiner, L.B. Methodology of population pharmacokinetics. In: *Drug fate and metabolism: Methods and techniques*, Vol. 5. (Garrett, E.R. and Hirtz, J.L. Eds.). Marcel Dekker, New York, 1985, pp. 135–183.

Beal, S.L., and Sheiner, L.B. Heteroscedastic nonlinear regression. *Technometrics* 1988; 30: 327–338.

Begg, C.B., and Gray, R. Calculation of polychotomous logistic regression parameters using individualized regressions. *Biometrika* 1984; 71: 11–18.

Belanger, B.A., Davidian, M., and Giltinan, D.M. The effect of variance function estimation on nonlinear calibration inference in immunoassay data. *Biometrics* 1996; 52: 158–175.

Bellman, R., and Astrom, K.J. On structural identifiability. *Mathematical Biosciences* 1970; 7: 329–339.

Belsley, D.A., Kuh, E., and Welsch, R.E. *Regression diagnostics: Identifying influential data and sources of collinearity.* Wiley, New York, 1980.

Benezet, S., Guimbaud, R., Catelut, E., Chevreau, C., Bugat, R., and Canal, P. How to predict carboplatin clearance from standard morphological and biological characteristics in obese patients. *Annals of Oncology* 1997; 6: 607–609.

Berry, D.A. Logarithmic transformations in ANOVA. *Biometrics* 1987; 43: 439–456.

Bies, R.R., Sale, M.E., Smith, G., Muldoon, M., Lotrich, F., and Pollack, B.G. Outcome of NONMEM analysis depends on modeling strategy. Presented at the American Society for Clinical Pharmacology and Toxicology Annual Meeting, Washington, D.C., 2–5 April, 2003.

Boeckmann, A.J., Sheiner, L.B., and Beal, S.L. *NONMEM users guide - Parts I–V.* NONMEM Project Group, San Francisco, 1994.

Boehmer, U., Kressin, N.R., Berlowitz, D.R., Christiansen, C.L., Kazis, L.E., and Jones, J.A. Self-reported versus administrative race/ethnicity data and study results. *American Journal of Public Health* 2002; 92: 1471–1472.

Bogumil, R.J. Sensitivity analysis of biosystem models. *Federation Proceedings* 1980; 39: 97–103.

Bonate, P.L. Approximate confidence intervals in calibration using the bootstrap. *Analytical Chemistry* 1993; 65: 1367–1372.

Bonate, P.L. Coverage and precision of parametric and nonparametric confidence intervals for area under the curve in a toxicokinetic experimental design. *Pharmaceutical Research* 1998; 15: 405–410.

Bonate, P.L. The effect of collinearity on parameter estimates in nonlinear mixed effect models. *Pharmaceutical Research* 1999; 16: 709–717.

Bonate, P.L. *Analysis of pretest-posttest designs.* Chapman & Hall/CRC Press, Boca Raton, FL, 2000.

Bonate, P.L. Consistency of NONMEM parameter estimates across platforms and compilers. Presented at American Association of Pharmaceutical Scientists Annual Meeting, Toronto Canada, 2002.

Bonate, P.L. Assessment of QTc interval prolongation in a Phase I study using Monte Carlo simulation. In: *Simulation for designing clinical trials: A pharmacokinetic-pharmacodynamic modeling perspective.* (Kimko, H.C. and Duffull, S., Eds.). New York, 2003

Bonate, P.L. Covariate detection in population pharmacokinetics using partially linear mixed effects models. *Pharmaceutical Research* 2005; 22: 541–549.

Bonate, P.L., Craig, A., Gaynon, P., Gandhi, V., Jeha, S., Kadota, R., Lam, G.N., Plunkett, W., Razzouk, B., Rytting, M., Steinherz, P., and Weitman, S. Population pharmacokinetics of clofarabine, a second-generation nucleoside analog, in pediatric patients with acute leukemia. *Journal of Clinical Pharmacology* 2004; 44: 1309–1322.

Bonate, P.L., and Howard, D. Prospective allometric scaling: Does the emperor have clothes? *Journal of Clinical Pharmacology* 2000; 40: 335–340.

Bonate, P.L., Swann, A., and Silverman, P.B. A preliminary physiological based pharmacokinetic model for cocaine in the rat: Model development and scale-up to humans. *Journal of Pharmaceutical Sciences* 1996; 85: 878–883.

Booth, B.P. and Gobburu, J. Considerations in analyzing single-trough concentrations using mixed-effects modeling. *Journal of Clinical Pharmacology* 2003; 43: 1307–1315.

Box, G.E.P. Science and statistics. *Journal of the American Statistical Association* 1976; 71: 791–799.

Box, G.E.P. and Cox, D.R. An analysis of transformations. *Journal of the Royal Statistical Society, Series B* 1964; 26: 211–243.

Box, G.E.P. and Hill, W.J. Discrimination among mechanistic models. *Technometrics* 1967; 9: 57–71.

Boxenbaum, H. Pharmacokinetic tricks and traps: Flip-flip models. *Journal of Pharmacy and Pharmaceutical Sciences* 1999; 1: 90–91.

Boxenbaum, H. and Dilea, C. First-time-in-human dose selection: Allometric thoughts and perspectives. *Journal of Clinical Pharmacology* 1995; 35: 957–966.

Breant, V., Charpiat, B., Sab, J.M., Maire, P., and Jelliffe, R.W. How many patients and blood levels are necessary for population pharmacokinetic analysis? A study of a one compartment model applied to cyclosporine. *European Journal of Clinical Pharmacology* 1996; 51: 283–288.

Breen, R. *Regression models: Censored, sample selected, and truncated data.* Sage, Thousand Oaks, CA, 1996.

Breiman, L. Statistical modeling: The two cultures (with commentary). *Statistical Science* 2002; 16: 199–231.

Breusch, T.S. and Pagan, A.R. A simple test for heteroscedasticity and random coefficient of variation. *Econometrica* 1979; 47: 1287–1294.

Brown, T., Havlin, K., Weiss, G., Cagnola, J., Koeller, J., Kuhn, J., Rizzo, J., Craig, J., Phillips, J., and Von Hoff, D. A phase I trial of taxol given by a 6-h intravenous infusion. *Journal of Clinical Oncology* 1991; 9: 1261–1267.

Bruno, R., Vivier, N., Vergniol, J.C., De Phillips, S.L., Montay, G., and Shiener, L.B. A population pharmacokinetic model for docetaxel (Taxotere): Model building and validation. *Journal of Pharmacokinetics and Biopharmaceutics* 1996; 24: 153–172.

Buonaccorsi, J.P. Prediction in the presence of measurement error: General discussion and an example predicting defoliation. *Biometrics* 1995; 51: 1562–1569.

Burnham, K.P. and Anderson, D.R. *Model selection and multimodel inference: A practical information-theoretic approach.* Springer-Verlag, New York, 2002.

Burtin, P., Mentre, F., Van Bree, J., and Steimer, J.-L. Sparse sampling for assessment of drug exposure in toxicological studies. *European Journal of Drug Metabolism and Pharmacokinetics* 1996; 21: 105–111.

Buse, A. The likelihood ratio, Wald, and Lagrange multiplier tests: An expository note. *American Statistician* 1982; 36: 153–157.

Butler, S.M. and Louis, T.A. Random effects models with nonparametric priors. *Statistics in Medicine* 1992; 11: 1981–2000.

Byers, V.S., Rodvien, R., Grant, K., Durrant, L.G., Hudson, K.H., Baldwin, R.W., and Scannon, P.J. Phase I study of monoclonal antibody-Ricin A chain immunotoxin Xomazyme-791 in patients with metastatic colon cancer. *Cancer Research* 1989; 49: 6153–6160.

Carlin, B.P. Hierarchical longitudinal modelling. In: *Markov Chain Monte Carlo in practice.* (Gilks, W.R., Richardson, S., and Spiegelhalter, D.J., Eds.). Chapman & Hall, London, 1996, pp. 303–319.

Carlin, B.P. and Louis, T.A. *Bayes and empirical Bayes methods for data analysis.* Chapman & Hall, New York, 1996.

Carpenter, J. and Bithell, J. Bootstrap confidence intervals: When, which, what? A practical guide for medical statisticians. *Statistics in Medicine* 2000; 19: 1141–1164.

Carpenter, J.R. Test-inversion bootstrap confidence intervals. *Journal of the Royal Statistical Society, Series B* 1999; 61: 159–172.

Carroll, R.J., Juchenhodd, H., Lombard, F., and Stefanki, L.A. Asymptotics for the SIMEX estimator in nonlinear measurement error models. *Journal of the American Statistical Association* 1996; 91: 242–250.

Carroll, R.J. and Ruppert, D. *Transformation and weighting in regression.* Chapman & Hall, New York, 1988.

Carroll, R.J., Ruppert, D., and Stefanski, L.A. *Measurement error in nonlinear models.* Chapman & Hall, New York, 1995.

Carroll, R.J. and Ruppert, D.J. Power transformations when fitting theoretical models to data. *Journal of the Institute of Mathematical Applications* 1984; 79: 321–328.

Carter, W.H., Jones, D.E., and Carchman, R.A. Application of response surface methods for evaluating the interactions of soman, atropine, and pralidoxime chloride. *Fundamental and Applied Toxicology* 1985; 5: S232–S241.

Chambers, H.E. *Effective communication skills for scientific and technical professionals.* Perseus, Cambridge, MA, 2001.

Chan, K.K.H. and Gibaldi, M. Assessment of drug absorption after oral administration. *Journal of Pharmaceutical Sciences* 1985; 74: 388–393.

Chappell, M.J., Godfrey, K., and Vajda, S. Global identifiability of the parameters of nonlinear systems with specified inputs: A comparison of methods. *Mathematical Biosciences* 1990; 102: 41–73.

Chappell, W.R. and Mordenti, J. Extrapolation of toxicological and pharmacological data from animals to humans. In: *Advances in drug research.* (Testa, B., Ed.). Academic, New York, 1990, pp. 1–116.

Chapra, S.C. and Canale, R.P. *Numerical methods for engineers: With programming and software applications.* McGraw-Hill, New York, 1998.

Chatfield, C. *Problem solving: A statistician's guide.* Chapman & Hall, London, 1988.

Chatfield, C. Model uncertainty, data mining, and statistical inference. *Journal of the Royal Statistical Society, Series A* 1995; 158: 419–466.

Chernick, M.R. *Bootstrap methods: A practitioner's guide.* Wiley, New York, 1999.

Chow, S.C. and Liu, J.P. *Design and analysis of bioavailability and bioequivalence studies.* Marcel Dekker, New York, 2000.

Cleveland, W.S. Graphs in scientific publications. *American Statistician* 1984a; 38: 261–269.

Cleveland, W.S. *The elements of graphing data.* Hobart, Summit, NJ, 1984b.

Cleveland, W.S., Diaconis, P., and McGill, R. Variables on scatter plots look more highly correlated when the scales are increased. *Science* 1982; 216: 1138–1141.

Cleveland, W.S. and McGill, R. Graphical perception: Theory, experimentation, and application to the development of graphical methods. *Journal of the American Statistical Association* 1984a; 79: 531–554.

Cleveland, W.S. and McGill, R. The many faces of a scatterplot. *Journal of the American Statistical Association* 1984b; 79: 807–822.

Cleveland, W.S. and McGill, R. Graphical perception and graphical methods for analyzing scientific data. *Science* 1985; 229: 828–833.

Cobelli, C. Carson, E.R., Finkelstein, L., and Leaning, M.S. Validation of simple and complex models in physiology and medicine. *American Journal of Physiology* 1984; 246: R259–R266.

Cobelli, C., and DeStefano, J.J. Parameter and structural identifiability concepts and ambiguities: A critical review and analysis. *American Journal of Physiology* 1980; 239: R7–R24.

Cockcroft, D.W. and Gault, M.H. Prediction of creatinine clearance from serum creatinine. *Nephron* 1976; 16: 31–41.

Colburn, W. and Lee, J.W. Biomarkers, validation, and pharmacokinetic-pharmacodynamic modeling. *Journal of Clinical Pharmacology* 2003; 42: 997–1022.

Cone, E. Pharmacokinetics and pharmacodynamics of cocaine. *Journal of Analytical Toxicology* 1995; 19: 459–478.

Congdon, P. *Bayesian statistical modeling.* Wiley, New York, 2001.

Cook, J.R. and Stefanski, L.A. Simulation-extrapolation estimation in parametric measurement error models. *Journal of the American Statistical Association* 1994; 89: 1314–1328.

Cook, R.D. and Weisberg, S. *Residuals and influence in regression.* Chapman & Hall, New York, 1982.

Covey, S.R. *The 7 habits of highly effective people.* Fireside, New York, 1989.

Cox, D.S., Kleiman, N.S., Boyle, D.A., Aluri, J., Parchman, L.G., Holdbrook, F., and Fossler, M.J. Pharmacokinetics and pharmacodynamics of argatroban in combination with a platelet glycoprotein IIB/IIIA receptor antagonist in patients undergoing percutaneous coronary intervention. *Journal of Clinical Pharmacology* 2004; 44: 981–990.

Cross, M. and Moscardini, A.O. *Learning the art of mathematical modeling.* Ellis Horwood, Chichester, 1985.

Cutler, N.R., Seifert, R.D., Schleman, M.M., Sramek, J.J., Szylleyko, O.J., Howard, D.R., Barchowsky, A., Wardle, T.S., and Brass, E.P. Acetylcholinesterase inhibition by zifrosilone: Pharmacokinetics and pharmacodynamics. *Clinical Pharmacology and Therapeutics* 1995; 58: 54–61.

D'Agostino, R.B. An omnibus test of normality for moderate and large sizes. *Biometrika* 1971; 58: 341–348.

D'Agostino, R.B., Belanger, A., D'Agostino, J.R, R.B. A suggestion for using powerful and informative tests of normality. *American Statistician* 1990; 44: 316–321.

D'Arcy, J. *Technicall speaking: A guide for communicating complex information.* Battelle Press, Columbus, OH, 1998.

Davidian, M. and Carroll, R.J. Variance function estimation. *Journal of the American Statistical Association* 1987; 82: 1079–1091.

Davidian, M. and Gallant, A.R. The nonlinear mixed effects model with smooth random effects density. *Biometrika* 1993; 80: 475–488.

Davidian, M. and Giltinan, D.M. *Nonlinear models for repeated measures data.* Chapman & Hall, New York, 1995.

Davidian, M. and Haaland, P.D. Regression and calibration with nonconstant error variance. *Chemometrics and Intelligent Laboratory Systems* 1990; 9: 231–248.

Davies, M. and Whitting, I.J. A modified form of Levenberg's correction. In: *Numerical methods for non-linear optimization.* (Lootsma, F.A. Ed.). Academic, New York, 1972, pp. 191–201.

Davison, A.C. and Hinkley, D.V. *Bootstrap methods and their application.* Cambridge University Press, Cambridge, UK, 1997.

Davison, A.C., Hinkley, D.V., and Schechtman, E. Efficient bootstrap simulation. *Biometrika* 1986; 73: 555–566.

de Maat, M.M.R., Huitema, A.D.R., Mujlder, J.W., Meenhorst, P.L., van Gorp, E.C.M., and Beijnen, J.H. Population pharmacokinetics of nevirapine in an unselected cohort of HIV-I infected individuals. *British Journal of Clinical Pharmacology* 2002; 54: 378–385.

Demidenko, E. and Stukel, T.A. Influence analysis in linear mixed-effects models. *Statistics in Medicine* 2005; 24: 893–909.

Dennis, J.E. Nonlinear least squares and equations. In: *The state of the art in numerical analysis.* (Jacobs, D.A.H., Ed.). Academic, London, 1977, pp. 269–312.

Derendorf, H. and Meibohm, B. Modeling of pharmacokinetic/pharmacodynamic (PK/PD) relationships: Concepts and perspectives. *Pharmaceutical Research* 1999; 16: 176–185.

Diggle, P.J. An approach to the analysis of repeated measures. *Biometrics* 1988; 44: 959–971.

Diggle, P.J. and Kenward, M.G. Informative drop-out in longitudinal data analysis (with discussion). *Applied Statistics* 1994; 43: 49–93.

Dilleen, M., Heimann, G., and Hirsch, I. Non-parametric estimators of a monotonic dose–response curve and bootstrap confidence intervals. *Statistics in Medicine* 2003; 22: 869–882.

DiMasi, J.A., Hansen, R.W., and Grabowski, H.G. The price of innovation: New estimates of drug development costs. *Journal of Health Economics* 2003; 835: 1–35.

DiStefano, J.J. and Landaw, E.M. Multiexponential, multicompartmental, and noncompartmental modeling. I. Methodological limitations and physiological interpretations. *American Journal of Physiology* 1984; 246: R651–R664.

Doane, D.P. Aesthetic frequency classification. *American Statistician* 1976; 30: 181–183.

Domingos, P. The role of Occam's razor in knowledge discovery. *Data mining and knowledge discovery* 1999; 3: 409–425.

Donaldson, J.R. and Schnabel, R.B. Computational experience with confidence regions and confidence intervals for nonlinear least squares. *Technometrics* 1987; 29: 67–82.

du Toit, S.H.C., Steyn, A.G.W., and Stumpf, R.H. *Graphical exploratory data analysis.* Springer-Verlag, New York, 1986.

DuBois, D. and DuBois, E.F. A formula to estimate the approximate surface area if height and weight be known. *Archives of Internal Medicine* 1916; 17: 863–871.

Duffull, S.B., Retout, S., and Mentre, F. The use of simulated annealing for finding optimal population designs. *Computer Methods and Programs in Biomedicine* 2002; 69: 25–35.

Dutta, S., Matsumoto, Y., and Ebling, W.F. Is it possible to estimate the parameters of the sigmoid E_{max} model with truncated data typical of clinical studies? *Journal of Pharmaceutical Sciences* 1996; 85: 232–239.

Duval, V. and Karlsson, M.O. Impact of omission or replacement of data below the limit of quantification on parameter estimates in a 2-compartment model. *Pharmaceutical Research* 2002; 19: 1835–1840.

Eap, C.B., Cuendet, C., and Baumann, P. Orosomucoid (alpha-1 acid glycoprotein) phenotyping by use of immobilized pH gradients with 8 M urea and immunoblotting. A new variant encountered in a population study. *Human Genetics* 1988; 80: 183–185.

Efron, B. Bootstrap methods: Another look at the jackknife. *Annals of Statistics* 1979; 7: 1–26.

Efron, B. *The jackknife, the bootstrap, and other resampling plans.* Society for Industrial and Applied Mathematics, Philadelphia, PA, 1982.

Efron, B. Better bootstrap confidence intervals. *Journal of the American Statistical Association* 1987; 82: 171–200.

Efron, B. More accurate confidence intervals in exponential family. *Biometrika* 1992; 79: 231–245.

Efron, B. and Tibshirani, R.J. *An introduction to the bootstrap.* CRC Press/Chapman & Hall, Boca Raton, FL, 1994.

Eisenhauer, E.A., ten Bakkel Huinink, W.W., Swenerton, K.D., Gianni, L., Myles, J., van der Burg, M.E.L., Kerr, I., Vermorken, J.B., Buser, K., Colombo, N., Bacon, M., Santa Barbara, P., Onetto, N., Winograd, B., and Canetta, R. European–Canadian randomized trial of paclitaxel in relapsed ovarian cancer: High-dose versus low-dose and long versus short infusion. *Journal of Clinical Oncology* 1994; 12: 2654–2666.

Endrenyi, L. Design of experiments for estimating enzyme and pharmacokinetic experiments. In: *Kinetic data analysis: Design and analysis of enzyme and pharmacokinetic experiments.* (Endrenyi, L., Ed.). Plenum, New York, 1981, pp. 137–167.

Epstein, M.A.F. Winds of change: Current focus of the modeling in physiology department. *American Journal of Physiology* 1994; 267: E628.

Ette, E., Howie, C.A., Kelman, A.W., and Whiting, B. Experimental design and efficient parameter estimation in preclinical pharmacokinetic studies. *Pharmaceutical Research* 1995; 12: 729–737.

Ette, E., Sun, H., and Ludden, T.M. Balanced designs in longitudinal population pharmacokinetic studies. *Journal of Clinical Pharmacology* 1998; 38: 417–423.

Ette, E., Williams, P.J., Kim, Y.H., Lane, J.R., Liu, M.-J., and Capparelli, E.V. Model appropriateness and population pharmacokinetic modeling. *Journal of Clinical Pharmacology* 2003;43: 610–623.

Ette, E.I. Comparing nonhierarchical models: Application to nonlinear mixed effects modeling. *Computers in Biology and Medicine* 1996; 6: 505–512.

Ette, E.I., Kelman, A.W., Howie, C.A., and Whiting, B. Influence of interanimal variability on the estimation of population pharmacokinetic parameters in preclinical studies. *Clinical Research and Regulatory Affairs* 1994; 11: 121–139.

Ette, E.I. and Ludden, T.M. Population pharmacokinetic modeling: The importance of informative graphics. *Pharmaceutical Research* 1995; 12: 1845–1855.

Ette, E.I., Sun, H., and Ludden, T.M. Design of population pharmacokinetic studies. In: *Proceedings of the American Statistical Association (Biopharmaceutics Section).* American Statistical Association, Alexandria, VA, 1994, pp. 487–492.

Eubank, R.L. and Webster, J.T. The singular value decomposition as a tool for problem solving estimability problems. *American Statistician* 1985; 39: 64–66.

European Agency for the Evaluation of Medicinal Products and Committee for Proprietary Medicinal Products. *Points to Consider on Missing Data,* 2001.

Evans, N.D., Godfrey, K.R., Chapman, M.J., Chappell, M.J., Aarons, L., and Duffull, S. An identifiability analysis of parent-metabolite pharmacokinetic model for ivabradine. *Journal of Pharmacokinetics and Pharmacodynamics* 2001; 28: 93–105.

Everitt, B.S. An introduction to finite mixture distributions. *Statistical Methods in Medical Research* 1996; 5: 107–127.

Faaji, R.A., Burgaaf, J., Schoemaker, H.C., Stiekema, J.C.J., Siegert, C., and Cohen, A.F. The influence of renal function on the pharmacokinetics (PK) and pharmacodynamics of the novel antithrombotic agent Org31540/SR90107A. *British Journal of Clinical Pharmacology* 1998; 45: 211P.

Fattinger, K., Vozeh, S., Ha, H.R., Borner, M., and Follath, F. Population pharmacokinetics of quinidine. *British Journal of Clinical Pharmacology* 1991; 31: 279–286.

Fisher, N.I., and Hall, P. Bootstrap algorithms for small samples. *Journal of Statistical Inference and Planning* 1991; 27: 157–169.

Fisher, R.A. On the mathematical foundations of theoretical statistics. *Philosophy and Transactions of the Royal Society* 1921; 222: 309–368.

Fitzmaurice, G.M., Laird, N.M., and Ware, J.H. *Applied longitudinal analysis.* Wiley, New York, 2004.

Fowlkes, E.B. Some methods for studying the mixture of two normal (log-normal) distributions. *Journal of the American Statistical Association* 1979; 74: 561–575.

Fox, J. *An R and S-PLUS companion to applied regression.* Sage, Newbury Park, CA, 2002.

Frame, B., Koup, J., Miller, R., and Lalonde, R. Population pharmacokinetics of clinafloxacin in healthy volunteers and patients with infections: Experience with heterogeneous pharmacokinetic data. *Clinical Pharmacokinetics* 2001; 40: 307–315.

Frame, B., Miller, R., and Lalonde, R.L. Evaluation of mixture modeling with count data using NONMEM. *Journal of Pharmacokinetics and Biopharmaceutics* 2003; 30: 167–183.

Franciosa, J.A., Taylor, A.L., Cohn, J.N., Yancy, C.W., Ziesche, S., Olukotun, A., Ofili, E., Ferdinand, K., Loscalzo, J., Worcel, M., and the A-HEFT Investigators. African–American heart failure trial (A-HeFT): Rationale, design, and metholology. *Journal of Cardiac Failure* 2002; 8: 128–135.

Freedman, D. and Diaconis, P. On the histogram as a density estimator: L2 theory. *Zeitschrift für Wahrscheinlichkeitstheorie und verwandte Gebiete* 2003; 57: 453–476.

Friberg, L.E., Henningsson, A., Mace, K., Nguyen, L., and Karlsson, M.O. Model of chemotherapy-induced myelosuppression with parameter consistency across drugs. *Journal of Clinical Oncology* 2002; 20: 4713–4721.

Fuller, W.A. *Measurement error models.* Wiley, New York, 1987.

Gabrielsson, J. and Weiner, D. *Pharmacokinetic and pharmacodynamic data analysis: Concepts and applications.* Swedish Pharmaceutical Press, Stockholm, 2000.

Garden, J.S., Mitchell, D.G., and Mills, W.N. Nonconstant variance regression techniques for calibration-curve-based analysis. *Analytical Chemistry* 1980; 52: 2310–2315.

Garfinkel, D. and Fegley, K.A. Fitting physiological models to data. *American Journal of Physiology* 1984; 15: R641–R650.

Gastonguay, M.R., Gibiansky, L., Gillespie, W.R., Khoo, K.-C., and the PPRU Network. Population pharmacokinetics in pediatric patients using Bayesian approaches with informative prior distributions based on adults. Presented at East Coast Population Analysis Group (ECPAG), 1999.

Gehan, E.A. and George, S.L. Estimation of human body surface area from height and weight. *Cancer Chemotherapy Reports* 1970; 54: 225–235.

Gelman, A., Carlin, J.B., Stern, H.S., and Rubin, D.B. *Bayesian data analysis.* Chapman & Hall, London, 1995.

Gentle, J.E. *Numerical linear algebra for applications in statistics.* Springer-Verlag, New York, 1998.

Gianni, L., Kearns, C.M., Giani, A., Capri, G., Vigano, L., Lacatelli, A., Bonadonna, G., and Egorin, M.J. Nonlinear pharmacokinetics and metabolism of paclitaxel and its pharmacokinetic/pharmacodynamic relationships in humans. *Journal of Clinical Oncology* 1995; 13: 180–190.

Gibaldi, M. and Perrier, D. *Pharmacokinetics.* Marcel Dekker, New York, 1982.

Gibiansky, E., Gibiansky, L., and Bramer, S. Comparison of NONMEM, bootstrap, jackknife, and profiling parameter estimates and confidence intervals for the aripiprazole population pharmacokinetic model. Presented at American Association of Pharmaceutical Scientists Annual Meeting, Boston MA, 2001.

Gibiansky, L. and Gibiansky, E. Parameter estimates and confidence intervals for a population pharmacokinetic model. Presented at American Association of Pharmaceutical Scientists Annual Meeting, Boston MA, 2001.

Gibiansky, L., Gibiansky, E., Yu, R.Z., and Geary, R.S. ISIS 2302: Validation of the population pharmacokinetic model and PK/PD analysis. Presented at American Association of Pharmaceutical Scientists Annual Meeting, Boston MA, 2001.

Gieschke, R., Burger, H.-U., Reigner, B., Blesch, K.S., and Steimer, J.-L. Population pharmacokinetics and concentration–effect relationships of capecitabine metabolites in colorectal cancer patients. *British Journal of Clinical Pharmacology* 2003; 55: 252–263.

Gilmore, D.A., Gal, J., Gerber, J.G., and Nies, A.S. Age and gender influence the stereoselective pharmacokinetics of propranolol. *Journal of Pharmacology and Experimental Therapeutics* 1992; 261: 1181–1186.

Giltinan, D.M. and Ruppert, D. Fitting heteroscedastic regression models to individual pharmacokinetic data using standard statistical software. *Journal of Pharmacokinetics and Biopharmaceutics* 1989; 17: 601–614.

Gisleskog, P.O., Hermann, D., Hammarlund-Udenaes, M., and Karlsson, M.O. Validation of a population pharmacokinetic/pharmacodynamic model for 5a-reductase inhibitors. *European Journal of Clinical Pharmacology* 1999; 8: 291–299.

Gisleskog, P.O., Karlsson, M.O., and Beal, S.L. Use of prior information to stabilize a population data analysis. *Journal of Pharmacokinetics and Pharmacodynamics* 2003; 29: 473–505.

Gobburu, J. and Lawrence, J. Application of resampling techniques to estimate exact significance levels for covariate selection during nonlinear mixed effects model building: Some inferences. *Pharmaceutical Research* 2002; 19: 92–98.

Godfrey, K.R. and Chapman, M.J. The problem of model indistinguishability in pharmacokinetics. *Journal of Pharmacokinetics and Biopharmaceutics* 1989; 17: 229–267.

Godfrey, K.R., Chapman, M.J., and Vajda, S. Identifiability and indistinguishability of nonlinear pharmacokinetic models. *Journal of Pharmacokinetics and Biopharmaceutics* 1994; 22: 229–251.

Godfrey, K.R., Jones, P.R., and Brown, R.G. Identifiable pharmacokinetic models: The role of extra inputs and measurements. *Journal of Pharmacokinetics and Biopharmaceutics* 1980; 8: 633.

Goldfeld, S.M. and Quandt, R.E. Some tests for homoscedasticity. *Journal of the American Statistical Association* 1965; 60: 539–547.

Goldfeld, S.M. and Quandt, R.E. *Nonlinear methods in econometrics.* North Holland, Amsterdam, 1972.

Good, P. Permutation tests: A *practical guide to resampling methods for testing hypotheses.* Springer-Verlag, New York, 2000.

Goodman, B. Multiple investigations. *The Statistician* 1996; 10: 1.

Gough, K., Hutchison, M., Keene, O., Byrom, B., Ellis, S., Lacey, L., and McKellar, J. Assessment of dose proportionality: Report from the statisticians in the pharmaceutical industry/pharmacokinetics UK joint working party. *Drug Information Journal* 1995; 29: 1039–1048.

Gray, J.B. A simple graphic for assessing influence in regression. *Journal of Statistical Computing and Simulation* 1986; 24: 121–134.

Gray, J.B., and Woodall, W.H. The maximum size of standardized and internally studentized residuals in regression analysis. *American Statistician* 1994; 48: 111–113.

Greco, W.R., Bravo, G., and Parsons, J.C. The search for synergy: A critical review from a response surface perspective. *Pharmacological Reviews* 1995; 47: 331–385.

Green, B. and Duffull, S. Caution when lean body weight is used as a size descriptor for obese subjects. *Clinical Pharmacology and Therapeutics* 2002; 72: 743–744.

Grem, J.L. Tutsch, K.D., Simon, K.J., Alberti, D.B., Willson, J.K., Tormey, D.C., Swaminathan, S. and Trump, D.L. Phase I study of taxol administered as a short i.v. infusion daily for 5 days. *Cancer Treatment Reports* 1987; 71: 1179–1184.

Grimsley, C. and Thomson, A.H. Pharmacokinetics and dose requirements of vancomycin in neonates. *Archives of Disease in Children: Fetal and Neonatal Edition* 1999; 81: F221–F227.

Haegle, K.D., Alkan, R., Grove, J., Schecter, P.J. and Koch-Weser, J. Kinetics of a-difluoromethylornithine: An irreversible inhibitor of ornithine decarboxylase. *Clinical Pharmacology and Therapeutics* 1981; 30: 210–217.

Harmatz, J.S. and Greenblatt, D.J. Falling off the straight line: Some hazards of correlation and regression. *Journal of Clinical Psychopharmacology* 1992; 12: 75–78.

Harrison, M.J. and McCabe, B.P.M. A test for heteroscedasticity based on ordinary least squares residuals. *Journal of the American Statistical Association* 1979; 74: 494–499.

Hartford, A. and Davidian, M. Consequences of misspecifying assumptions in nonlinear mixed effects models. *Computational Statistics & Data Analysis* 2000; 34: 139–164.

Hartley, H.O. The modified Gauss–Newton method for the fitting of nonlinear regression functions. *Technometrics* 1961; 3: 269–280.

Harville, D.A. Maximum likelihood approaches to variance component estimation and to related problems. *Journal of the American Statistical Association* 1977; 72: 320–340.

Harville, D.A. *Matrix algebra from a statistician's perspective.* Springer-Verlag, New York, 1998.

Haycock, G.B., Schwartz, G.J. and Wisotsky, D.H. Geometric method for measuring body surface area: A height weight formula validated in infants, children and adults. *Journal of Pediatrics* 1978; 93: 62–66.

Healy, M.J.R. The use of R^2 as a measure of goodness of fit. *Journal of the Royal Statistical Society, Series A* 1984; 147: 608–609.

Heatherington, A., Vicini, P. and Golde, H. A pharmacokinetic/pharmacodynamic comparison of SAAM II and PC/WinNonlin modeling software. *Journal of Pharmaceutical Sciences* 1998; 87: 1255–1263.

Helland, I.S. On the interpretation and use of R^2 in regression analysis. *Biometrics* 1987; 43: 61–69.

Henderson, C.R. *Applications of linear models in animal breeding.* University of Guelph Press, Guelph, Canada, 1985.

Henningsson, A., Karlsson, M.O., Vigano, L., Gianni, L., Verweij, J. and Sparreboom, A. Mechanism-based pharmacokinetic model for paclitaxel. *Journal of Clinical Oncology* 2001; 19: 4065–4073.

Higgins, K.M., Davidian, M. and Giltinan, D.M. A two-step approach to measurement error in time-dependent covariates in nonlinear mixed-effects models, with application to IGF-1 pharmacokinetics. *Journal of the American Statistical Association* 1997; 93: 436–448.

Hill, A.B. The environment and disease: Association or causality? *Proceedings of the Royal Society of Medicine* 1965; 58: 295–300.

Hing, J.P., Woolfrey, S.G., Greenslade, D. and Wright, P.M. Analysis of toxicokinetic data using NONMEM: Impact of quantification limit and replacement strategies for censored data. *Journal of Pharmacokinetics and Pharmacodynamics* 2001a; 28: 465–479.

Hing, J.P., Woolfrey, S.G., Greenslade, D. and Wright, P.M.C. Is mixed effects modeling or naive pooled data analysis preferred for the interpretation of single sample per subject toxicokinetic data. *Journal of Pharmacokinetics and Pharmacodynamics* 2001b; 28: 193–210.

Hinkley, D.V. Jackknifing in unbalanced situations. *Technometrics* 1977; 19: 285–292.

Hodges, J.S. Six (or so) things you can do with a bad model. *Operations Research* 1991; 39: 355–365.

Hodges, S.D. and Moore, P.G. Data uncertainties and least squares regression. *Applied Statistics* 1972; 21: 185–195.

Hoeting, J.A., Madigan, D., Raftery, A.E. and Volinsky, C.T. Bayesian model averaging: A tutorial. *Statistical Science* 1999; 14: 382–401.

Holden, C. Race and medicine. *Science* 2003; 302: 594–596.

Holford, N.H.G. A size standard for pharmacokinetics. *Clinical Pharmacokinetics* 1996; 30: 329–332.

Holford, N.H.G. The population pharmacokinetic screen—How well does it work? Presented at 3rd Annual Clinical Trial Simulation in Drug Development: Best Practices for Creating Cost Effective Modeling and Simulation Practices, 2002.

Holford, N.H.G., Gobburu, J. and Mould, D. Implications of including and excluding correlation of random effects in hierarchical mixed effects pharmacokinetic models. Presented at Population Approach Group in Europe, Verona, Italy, 2003.

Hollander, M. and Wolfe, D.A. *Nonparametric statistical methods.* Wiley, New York, 1999.

Hosmer, D.W. and Lemeshow, S. *Applied logistic regression.* Wiley, New York, 1989.

Hossain, M., Wright, E., Baweja, R., Ludden, T. and Miller, R. Nonlinear mixed effects modeling of single dose and multiple dose data for immediate release (IR) and a controlled release (CR) dosage form of alprazolam. *Pharmaceutical Research* 1997; 14: 309–315.

Huber, P.J. *Robust statistics.* Wiley, New York, 1981.

Huff, D. *How to lie with statistics.* Norton, New York, 1954.

Huizing, M.T., Keung, A.C., Rosing, H., van der Kuij, V., ten Bokkel Huinink, W.W., Mandjes, I.M., Dubbelman, A.C., Pinedo, H.M. and Beijnen, J.H. Pharmacokinetics of paclitaxel and metabolites in a randomized comparative study in platinum-pretreated ovarian cancer patients. *Journal of Clinical Oncology* 1993; 11: 2127–2135.

Hurvich, C.M. and Tsai, C.-L. Regression and time series model selection in small samples. *Biometrics* 1989; 76: 297–307.

Hussein, R., Charles, B.G., Morris, R.G. and Rasiah, R.L. Population pharmacokinetics of perhexiline from very sparse, routine monitoring data. *Therapeutic Drug Monitoring* 2001; 23: 636–643.

IBM Business Consulting Services. *Pharma 2010: The threshold of innovation.* International Business Consulting Services, London, UK, 2003.

Iman, R.L., Helton, J.C. and Campbell, J.E. An approach to sensitivity analysis of computer models: Part I—Introduction, input variable selection and preliminary variable assessment. *Journal of Quality Technology* 1981; 13: 174–183.

Ingwersen, S.H. Population pharmacokinetics of tiagabine in epileptic patients on monotherapy. *European Journal of Pharmaceutical Sciences* 2000; 11: 247–254.

International Conference on Harmonization of Technical Requirements for Registration of Pharmaceuticals for Human Use. *Studies in Support of Special Populations: Geriatric (E7)*, 1994.

International Conference on Harmonization of Technical Requirements for Registration of Pharmaceuticals for Human Use. *Toxicokinetics: The Assessment of Systemic Exposure in Toxicity Studies (S3A)*, 1995.

International Conference on Harmonization of Technical Requirements for Registration of Pharmaceuticals for Human Use. *General Considerations for Clinical Trials (E8)*, 1997.

International Conference on Harmonization of Technical Requirements for Registration of Pharmaceuticals for Human Use. *Ethnic Factors in the Acceptability of Foreign Clinical Data (E5)*, 1998a.

International Conference on Harmonization of Technical Requirements for Registration of Pharmaceuticals for Human Use. *Statistical Principles for Clinical Trials (E9)*, 1998b.

Iwatsubo, T., Hirota, N., Ooie, T., Suzuki, H., Shimada, N., Chiba, K., Ishizaki, T., Green, C.E., Tyson, C.A. and Sugiyama, Y. Prediction of in vivo drug metabolism in the human liver from in vitro metabolism data. *Pharmacology Therapeutics* 1997; 73: 147–171.

Iwatsubo, T., Hirota, N., Ooie, T., Suzuki, H. and Sugiyama, Y. Prediction of in vivo drug disposition from in vitro data based on physiological pharmacokinetics. *Biopharmaceutics and Drug Disposition* 1996; 17: 273–310.

Jackson, J.E. *A user's guide to principal components.* Wiley, New York, 1991.

Jackson, K.A., Rosenbaum, S.E., Kerr, B.M., Pithavala, Y.K., Yuen, G. and Dudley, M.N. A population pharmacokinetic analysis of nelfinavir mesylate in human immunodeficiency virus-infected patients enrolled in a Phase III clinical trial. *Antimicrobial Agents and Chemotherapy* 2000; 44: 1832–1837.

Jacquez, J.A. *Compartmental analysis in biology and medicine.* BioMedware, Ann Arbor, MI, 1996.

Jacquez, J.A. and Perry, T. Parameter estimation: Local identifiability of parameters. *American Journal of Physiology* 1990; 258: E727–E736.

James, W. and Stein, C. Estimation with quadratic loss. In: *Proceedings of the Fourth Berkeley Symposium on Mathematical Statistics and Probability, vol. 1.* (Neyman, J., Ed.). University of California Press, Berkeley, CA, 1960, pp. 361–380.

Jeffcoat, R.A., Perez-Reyes, M., Hill, J.M., Sadler, B.M., and Cook, C.E. Cocaine disposition in humans after intravenous injection, nasal insufflation (snorting), or smoking. *Drug Metabolism and Disposition* 1989; 17: 153–159.

Jermain, D.M., Crismon, M.L., and Martin, E.S. Population pharmacokinetics of lithium. *Clinical Pharmacy* 1991; 10: 376–381.

Jernigan, A.D., Hatch, R.C., and Wilson, R.C. Pharmacokinetics of tobramycin in cats. *American Journal of Veterinary Research* 1988; 49: 608–612.

Jiang, H., Jing, L., Jiang, J., and Hu, P. Important role of the dihydrouracil/uracil ratio in marked interpatient variations of fluoropyrimidine pharmacokinetics and pharmacodynamics. *Journal of Clinical Pharmacology* 2004; 44: 1260–1272.

John, J.A., and Draper, N.R. An alternative family of transformations. *Applied Statistics* 1980; 29: 190–197.

Johnson, D.E., Braeckman, R.A., and Wolfgang, G.H.I. Practical aspects of assessing toxicokinetics and toxicodynamics. *Current Opinion in Drug Discovery and Development* 1999; 2: 49–57.

Johnson, J.A. Influence of race and ethnicity on pharmacokinetics of drugs. *Journal of Pharmaceutical Sciences* 1997; 86: 1328–1333.

Johnston, J. *Econometric methods*. McGraw-Hill, New York, 1972.

Jones, C.D., Sun, H., and Ette, E.I. Designing cross-sectional population pharmacokinetic studies: Implications for pediatric and animal studies. *Clinical Research and Regulatory Affairs* 1996; 13: 133–165.

Jones, G., Wortberg, M., Kreissig, S.B., Hammock, B.D., and Rocke, D.M. Application of the bootstrap to calibration experiments. *Analytical Chemistry* 1996; 68: 763–770.

Jones, P.D. Indicator and stratification methods for missing explanatory variables in multiple linear regression. *Journal of the American Statistical Association* 1996; 91: 222–230.

Jonsson, E.N. and Karlsson, M.O. Automated covariate model building in NONMEM. *Pharmaceutical Research* 1998; 15: 1463–1468.

Jonsson, E.N. Wade, J.R., and Karlsson, M.O. Comparison of some practical sampling strategies for population pharmacokinetic studies. *Journal of Pharmacokinetics and Biopharmaceutics* 1996; 24: 245–263.

Judge, G.G., Hill, R.C., Griffiths, W.E., Lutkepohl, H., and Lee, T.C. *Introduction to the theory and practice of econometrics*. Wiley, New York, 1982.

Karlsson, M.O., Beal, S.L., and Sheiner, L.B. Three new residual error models for population PK/PD analyses. *Journal of Pharmacokinetics and Biopharmaceutics* 1995; 23: 651–672.

Karlsson, M.O., Jonsson, E.N., Wiltse, C.G., and Wade, J.R. Assumption testing in population pharmacokinetic models: Illustrated with an analysis of moxonidine data from congestive heart failure patients. *Journal of Pharmacokinetics and Biopharmaceutics* 1998a; 26: 207–246.

Karlsson, M.O., Molnar, V., Bergh, J., Freijs, A., and Larsson, R. A general model for time-dissociated pharmacokinetic-pharmacodynamic relationships exemplified by paclitaxel myelosuppression. *Clinical Pharmacology and Therapeutics* 1998b; 63: 11–25.

Karlsson, M.O. Molnar, V., Freijs, A., Nygren, P., Berghm, J., and Larson, R. Pharmacokinetic models for the saturable distribution of paclitaxel. *Drug Metabolism and Disposition* 1997; 27: 1220–1223.

Karlsson, M.O. and Sheiner, L.B. The importance of modeling interoccassion variability in population pharmacokinetic analyses. *Journal of Pharmacokinetics and Biopharmaceutics* 1993; 21: 735–750.

Kaul, S. and Ritschel, W.A. Quantitative structure-pharmacokinetic relationship of a series of sulfonamides in the rat. *European Journal of Drug Metabolism and Pharmacokinetics* 1990; 15: 211–217.

Keene, O.N. The log transformation is special. *Statistics in Medicine* 1995; 14: 811–819.

Kerbusch, T., Milligan, P.A., and Karlsson, M.O. Assessment of the relative in vivo potency of the hydroxylated metabolite of darifenacin in its ability to decrease salivary flow using pooled population pharmacokinetic-pharmacodynamic data. *British Journal of Clinical Pharmacology* 2003; 57: 170–180.

Khorasheh, F., Ahmadi, A., and Gerayeli, A. Application of direct search optimization for pharmacokinetic parameter estimation. *Journal of Pharmacy and Pharmaceutical Sciences* 1999; 2: 92–98.

Kimanani, E.K., Lavigne, J., and Potvin, D. Numerical methods for the evaluation of individual bioequivalence criteria. *Statistics in Medicine* 2000; 19: 2775–2795.

Kimko, H. Qualifying models for simulation: Model evaluation methods. Presented at the American Association of Pharmaceutical Scientists Annual Meeting, Denver, CO, 2001.

Kirchheiner, J., Brockmoller, J., Meineke, I., Bauer, S., Rohde, W., Meisel, C., and Roots, I. Impact of CYP2C9 amino acid polymorphisms on glyburide kinetics and on the insulin and glucose response in healthy volunteers. *Clinical Pharmacology and Therapeutics* 2002; 71: 286–296.

Klag, M.J., Whelton, P.K., Coresh, J., Grim, C.E., and Kuller, L.H. The association of skin color with blood pressure in US blacks with low socioeconomic status. *Journal of the American Medical Association* 1991; 265: 599–602.

Kowalski, K.G. and Hutmacher, M. Design evaluation for a population pharmacokinetic study using clinical trial simulations: A case study. *Statistics in Medicine* 2001; 20: 75–91.

Kowalski, K.G. and Hutmacher, M. Efficient screening of covariates in population models using Wald's approximation to the likelihood ratio test. *Journal of Pharmacokinetics and Pharmacodynamics* 2002; 28: 253–275.

Kowalski, K.G. Screening covariate models using Wald's approximation: An evaluation of the WAM algorithm on several data sets. Presented at the 9th Annual Midwest User's Forum: Population Data Analysis (MUFPADA), 2001.

Krishna, S., Nagaraja, N.V., Planche, T., Agbenyega, T., Bedo-Addo, G., Ansong, A., Owusu-Ofori, A., Shroads, A.L., Henderson, G., Hutson, A., Derendorf, H., and Stacpoole, P.W. Population pharmacokinetics of intramuscular quinine in children with severe malaria. *Antimicrobial Agents and Chemotherapy* 2001; 45: 1803–1809.

Kullback, S. The Kullback–Leibler distance. *American Statistician* 1987; 41: 340–341.

Kvalseth, T.O. Cautionary note about R^2. *American Statistician* 1985; 39: 279–285.

Kvist, E.E., Al Shurbaji, A., Dahl, M.L., Nordin, C., Alvan, G., and Stahle, L. Quantitative pharmacogenetics of nortriptyline: A novel approach. *Clinical Pharmacokinetics* 2001; 40: 869–877.

Lacey, L.F., O'Keene, O.N., Pritchard, J.F., and Bye, A. Common noncompartmental pharmacokinetic variables: Are they normally and log-normally distributed? *Journal of Biopharmaceutical Statistics* 1997; 7: 171–178.

Landowski, C.P., Sun, D., Foster, D.R., Menon, S.S., Barnett, J.L., Welage, L.S., Ramachandran, C., and Amidon, G.L. Gene expression in the human intestine and correlation with oral valacyclovir pharmacokinetic parameters. *Journal of Pharmacology and Experimental Therapeutics* 2003; 306: 778–786.

Laporte-Simitsidis, S., Girard, P., Mismetti, P., Chabaud, S., Decousus, H., and Boissel, J.P. Interstudy variability in population pharmacokinetic analysis: When and how to estimate it? *Journal of Pharmaceutical Sciences* 2000; 89: 155–166.

LaVeist, T.A. Beyond dummy variables and sample selection: What health services researchers ought to know about race as a variable. *Human Services Research* 1994; 29: 1–16.

Lee, P.I.D. Design and power of a population pharmacokinetic study. *Pharmaceutical Research* 2001; 18: 75–82.

Lee, P.M. *Bayesian statistics: An introduction*. Arnold, London, 1997.

Lefevre, F., Duval, M., Gauron, S., Brookman, L.J., Rolan, P.E., Morris, T.M., Piraino, A.J., Morgan, J.M., Palmisano, M., and Close, P. Effect of renal impairment on the pharmacokinetics and pharmacodynamics of desirudin. *Clinical Pharmacology and Therapeutics* 1997; 62: 50–59.

Lesko, L.J. Rowland, M., Peck, C.C., and Blaschke, T.F. Optimizing the science of drug development: Opportunities for better candidate selection and accelerated evaluation in humans. *Pharmaceutical Research* 2000; 17: 1335–1344.

Lesko, L.J. and Williams, R.J. The question based review (QRB): A conceptual framework for clinical pharmacology and biopharmaceutics. *Applied Clinical Trials* 1999; 8: 56–62.

Lewandowsky, S. and Spence, I. Discriminating strata in scatterplots. *Journal of the American Statistical Association* 1989; 84: 682–688.

Li, J.H., Xu, J.Q., Cao, X.M., Ni, L., Li, Y., Zhuang, Y.Y., and Gong, J.B. Influence of the ORM1 phenotypes on serum unbound concentration and protein binding of quinidine. *Clinical Chimica Acta* 2002; 317: 85–92.

Liang, E. and Derendorf, H. Pitfalls in pharmacokinetic multicompartmental analysis. *Journal of Pharmacokinetics and Biopharmaceutics* 1998; 26: 247–260.

Lin, L.I. A concordance correlation coefficient to evaluate reproducibility. *Biometrics* 1989; 45: 255–268.

Lindsey, J.K. Some statistical heresies. *The Statistician* 1999; 48: 1–40.

Lindsey, J.K. *Nonlinear models in medical statistics*. Oxford University Press, 2001.

Lindsey, J.K., Byrom, W.D., Wang, J., Jarvis, P., and Jones, B. Generalized nonlinear models for pharmacokinetic data. *Biometrics* 2000; 56: 81–88.

Lindstrom, F.T. and Birkes, D.S. Estimation of population pharmacokinetic parameters using destructively obtained experimental data: A simulation study of the 1-compartment open model. *Drug Metabolism Reviews* 1984; 15: 195–264.

Lindstrom, M.J. and Bates, D.M. Nonlinear mixed-effects models for repeated measures data. *Biometrics* 1990; 46: 673–687.

Littell, R.C., Milliken, G.A., Stroup, W.W., and Wolfinger, R.D. *SAS system for mixed models*. SAS Institute, Inc., Cary, NC, 1996.

Little, R.J. Regression with missing X's: A review. *Journal of the American Statistical Association* 1992; 87: 1227–1237.

Little, R.J. Modeling the drop-out mechanism in repeated measures studies. *Journal of the American Statistical Association* 1995; 90: 1112–1121.

Little, R.J. and Rubin, D.B. *Statistical analysis with missing data*. Wiley, New York, 2002.

Livingston, E.H. and Lee, S. Body surface area prediction in normal-weight and obese patients. *American Journal of Physiology* 2001; E586: E591.

Loebstein, R., Vohra, S., and Koren, G. Drug therapy in pediatric patients. In: *Melmon and Morelli's clinical pharmacology*. (Carruthers, S.G., Hoffman, B.B., Melmon, K.L., Nierenberg, D.W., Eds.). McGraw-Hill, New York, 2000, pp. 1143–1149.

Long, J.S. and Ervin, L.H. Using heteroscedasticity consistent standard errors in the linear regression model. *American Statistician* 2000; 54: 217–224.

Longford, N. *Random coefficient models*. Oxford University Press, Oxford, 1993.

Longnecker, S.M., Donehower, R.C., Cates, A.E., Chen, T.L., Brundrett, R.B., Grochow, L.B., Ettinger, D.S., and Colvin, M. High-performance liquid chromatographic assay for taxol in human plasma and urine and pharmacokinetics in a phase I trial. *Cancer Treatment Reports* 1987; 71: 53–59.

Looney, S.W. and Gulledge, T.R., Jr. Use of the correlation coefficient with normal probability plots. *American Statistician* 1985; 39: 75–79.

Ludden, T.M., Beal, S.L., and Sheiner, L.B. Comparison of the Akaike Information Criterion, the Schwarz criterion, and the F-test as guides to model selection. *Journal of Pharmacokinetics and Biopharmaceutics* 1994; 22: 431–445.

Lynn, H.S. Maximum likelihood inference for left-censored HIV RNA data. *Statistics in Medicine* 2001; 21: 33–45.

MacKinnon, J.G. and White, H. Some heteroskedasticity consistent covariance matrix estimators with improved finite sample properties. *Journal of Econometrics* 1985; 29: 53–57.

Mager, D.E., Wyska, E., and Jusko, W.J. Diversity of mechanism-based pharmacodynamic models. *Drug Metabolism and Disposition* 2003; 31: 510–519.

Mahmood, I. Interspecies pharmacokinetic scaling: Principles, applications, and limitations. In: *Pharmacokinetics in drug development: Clinical study design and analysis*. (Bonate, P.L., and Howard, D., Eds.). AAPS Press, Alexandria, VA, 2004, pp. 423–444.

Mahmood, I. and Balian, J.D. Interspecies scaling: Predicting clearance of drugs in humans. Three different approaches. *Xenobiotica* 1996; 26: 887–895.

Mahmood, I. and Balian, J.D. The pharmacokinetic principles behind scaling from preclinical to Phase I protocols. *Clinical Pharmacokinetics* 1999; 36: 1–11.

Maitre, P.O., Buhrer, M., Thomson, D., and Stanski, D.R. A three-step approach combining Bayesian regression and NONMEM population analysis: Application to midazolam. *Journal of Pharmacokinetics and Biopharmaceutics* 1991; 19: 377–384.

Mallows, C.L. Some comments on Cp. *Technometrics* 1973; 15: 661–675.

Mamiya, K., Hadama, A., Yukawa, E., Ieiri, I., Otsubo, K., Ninomiya, H., Tashiro, N., and Higuchi, S. CYP2C19 polymorphism effect on phenobarbitone. Pharmacokinetics in Japanese patients with epilepsy: Analysis by population pharmacokinetics. *European Journal of Clinical Pharmacology* 2000; 55: 821–825.

Mandel, J. Use of the singular value decomposition in regression analysis. *American Statistician* 1982; 36: 15–24.

Mandema, J.W., Verotta, D., and Sheiner, L.B. Building population pharmacokinetic-pharmacodynamic models. I. Models for covariate effects. *Journal of Pharmacokinetics and Biopharmaceutics* 1992; 20: 511–528.

Mandema, J., Kaiko, R.F., Oshlack, B., Reder, R.F., and Stanski, D.R. Characterization and validation of a pharmacokinetic model for controlled-release oxycodone. *British Journal of Clinical Pharmacology* 1996; 42: 747–756.

Mangoni, A.A., and Jackson, S.H. Age-related changes in pharmacokinetics and pharmacodynamics: Basic principles and practical applications. *British Journal of Clinical Pharmacology* 2004; 57: 6–14.

Manley, B.F. Exponential data transformation. *The Statistician* 2002; 25: 37–42.

Marquardt, D.W. An algorithm for least-squares estimation of nonlinear parameters. *Journal of the Society for Industrial and Applied Mathematics* 1963; 11: 431–441.

Marroum, P.J. and Gobburu, J. The product label: How pharmacokinetics and pharmacodynamics reach the practitioner. *Clinical Pharmacokinetics* 2002; 41: 161–169.

Martin, III, E.S., Crismon, M.L., and Godley, P.J. Postinduction carbamazepine clearance in an adult psychiatric population. *Pharmacotherapy* 1991; 11: 296–302.

Maurer, R. *Why don't you want what I want? How to win support for your ideas without hard sell, manipulation, and power plays.* Bard Press, Atlanta, GA, 2002.

McCullagh, P. and Nelder, J.A. *Generalized linear models.* Chapman & Hall, London, 1989.

McCullough, B.D. Assessing the reliability of statistical software: Part I. *American Statistician* 1998; 52: 358–366.

McCullough, B.D. Assessing the reliability of statistical software: Part II. *American Statistician* 1999; 53: 149–159.

McCullough, B.D. and Wilson, B. On the accuracy of statistical procedures in Excel 97. *Computational Statistics & Data Analysis* 1999; 31: 27–37.

McLachlan, G.J. On bootstrapping the likelihood ratio test for the number of components in a normal mixture. *Applied Statistics* 1987; 36: 318–324.

McLean, R.A. and Sanders, W.L. Approximating degrees of freedom for standard errors in mixed linear models. In: *Proceedings of the Statistical Computing Section.* American Statistical Association, New Orleans, 1988, pp. 50–59.

McLeod, J.w.C. *Computer modeling and simulation: Principles of good practice.* Society for Computer Simulation, La Jolla, CA, 1982.

Merino, J.A., de Biasi, J., Plusquellec, Y., and Houin, G. Minimal experimental requirements for structural identifiability in linear compartmental models: The software 'IDEXMIN'. *Arzneimittel Forschung/Drug Research* 1996; 46: 324–328.

Mesterton-Gibbons, M. *A concrete approach to mathematical modelling.* Addison Wesley, Reading, MA, 1989.

Meyer, R.R. and Roth, P.M. Modified damped least squares: an algorithm for nonlinear estimation. *Journal of the Institute of Mathematical Applications* 1972; 9: 218–233.

Meyer, U.A. Genotype or phenotype: The definition of a pharmacogenetic polymorphism. *Pharmacogenetics* 2001; 1: 66–67.

Meyer-Barner, M., Meineke, I., Schreeb, K.H., and Gleiter, C.H. Pharmacokinetics of doxepin and demethyldoxepin: An evaluation with the population approach. *European Journal of Clinical Pharmacology* 2002; 58: 253–257.

Mirochnick, M., Capparelli, E., Dankner, D., Sperling, R.S., Van Dyke, R., and Spector, S.A. Zidovudine pharmacokinetics in premature infants exposed to human immunodeficiency virus. *Antimicrobial Agents and Chemotherapy* 1998; 42: 808–812.

Mooney, C.Z. and Duval, R.D. *Bootstrapping: A nonparametric approach to statistical inference.* Sage, Newbury Park, CA, 1993.

Moore, K.H., Yuen, G.J., Hussey, E.K., Pakes, G.E., Eron, J.J., Jr., and Bartlett, J.A. Population pharmacokinetics of lamivudine in adult human immunodeficiency virus-infected patients enrolled in two phase III clinical trials. *Antimicrobial Agents and Chemotherapy* 1999; 43: 3025–3029.

Moore, M.J., Bunting, P., Yuan, S., and Theissen, J.J. Development and validation of a limited sampling strategy for 5-fluorouracil given by bolus intravenous administration. *Therapeutic Drug Monitoring* 1993; 15: 394–399.

Mordenti, J. Man versus beast: Pharmacokinetic scaling in mammals. *Journal of Pharmaceutical Sciences* 1986; 75: 1028–1040.

Mordenti, J., Chen, S.A., Moore, J.A., Ferraiola, B., and Green, J.D. Interspecies scaling of clearance and volume of distribution data for five therapeutic proteins. *Pharmaceutical Research* 1991; 8: 1351–1359.

Morrell, C.H., Pearson, J.D., and Brant, L.J. Linear transformations of linear mixed effect models. *Journal of the American Statistical Association* 1997; 51: 338–343.

Mosteller, R.D. Simplified calculation of body surface area. *New England Journal of Medicine* 1987; 317: 1098.

Mould, D.R., Holford, N.H.G., Schellens, J.H.M., Beijen, J.H., Hutson, P.R., Rosing, H., ten Bokkel Huinink, W.W., Rowinsky, E., Schiller, J.H., Russo, M., and Ross, G. Population pharmacokinetic and adverse event analysis of topotecan in patients with solid tumors. *Clinical Pharmacology and Therapeutics* 2002; 71: 334–348.

Moye, L.A. *Multiple analyses in clinical trials: fundamentals for investigators.* Springer-Verlag, New York, 2003.

Myers, R.H. *Classical and modern regression with applications.* Duxbury, Boston, 1986.

Naber, K.G., Westenfelder, S.R., and Madsen, P.O. Pharmacokinetics of the aminoglycoside antibiotic tobramycin in humans. *Antimicrobial Agents and Chemotherapy* 1973; 3: 469–473.

Nath, C.E., McLachlan, A.J., Shaw, P.J., Gunning, R., and Earl, J.W. Population pharmacokinetics of amphotericin B in children with malignant diseases. *British Journal of Clinical Pharmacology* 2001;52: 671–680.

National Cancer Institute Cancer Therapy Evaluation Program. *Common Toxicity Criteria Manual, Version 2.0.* National Cancer Institute, Rockville, MD, 1999.

National Institutes of Health. *Clinical Guidelines on the Identification, Evaluation, and Treatment of Overweight and Obesity in Adults.* U.S. Department of Health and Human Services, National Institutes of Health, National Heart, Lung, and Blood Institute, Bethesda, MD, 1998.

Nelder, J.A. and Mead, R. A simplex method for function optimization. *The Computer Journal* 1965; 7: 308–313.

Nesterov, I. Sensitivity analysis of pharmacokinetic and pharmacodynamic systems: I. A structural approach to sensitivity analysis of physiologically based pharmacokinetic models. *Journal of Pharmacokinetics and Biopharmaceutics* 1999; 27: 577–596.

Neter, J., Kutner, M.H., Nachtsheim, C.J., and Wasserman, W. *Applied linear statistical models.* Irwin, Chicago, 1996.

Nguyen, L., Tranchand, B., Puozzo, C., and Variol, P. Population pharmacokinetics model and limited sampling strategy for intravenous vinorelbine derived from Phase I clinical trials. *British Journal of Clinical Pharmacology* 2002; 53: 459–468.

Niedzwiecki, D. and Simonoff, J.S. Estimation and inference in pharmacokinetic models: The effectiveness of model reformulation and resampling methods for functions of parameters. *Journal of Pharmacokinetics and Biopharmaceutics* 1990; 18: 361–377.

Nocedal, J. and Wright, S.J. *Numerical optimization.* Springer-Verlag, New York, 1999.

Noreen, E.W. *Computer-intensive methods for testing hypotheses: An introduction.* Wiley, New York, 1989.

Olson, S.C., Bockbrader, H., Boyd, R.A., Cook, J., Koup, J.R., Lalonde, R.L., Siedlik, P.H., and Powell, J.R. Impact of population pharmacokinetic-pharmacodynamic analyses on the drug development process. *Clinical Pharmacokinetics* 2000; 38: 449–459.

Parks, R.E. Estimation with heteroscedastic error terms. *Econometrica* 1966; 34: 888.

Pearson, K. Notes on the history of correlation. *Biometrika* 1920; 13: 25–45.

Pharsight Corporation. *WinNonlin Professional User's Guide, Version 2.* Pharsight Corporation, Palo Alto, CA, 1997.

Pharsight Corporation. *WinNonlin Reference Guide, Version 3.2.* Pharsight Corporation, Mountain View, CA, 2002.

Phillips, L., Grasela, T.H., Ágnew, J.R., Ludwig, E.A., and Thompson, G.A. A population pharmacokinetic-pharmacodynamic analysis and model validation of azimilide. *Clinical Pharmacology and Therapeutics* 2001; 70: 370–383.

Pigeot, I. The jackknife and bootstrap in biomedical research—Common principles and possible pitfalls. *Drug Information Journal* 2001; 35: 1431–1443.

Pinheiro, J.C. and Bates, D.M. Model building in nonlinear mixed effect models. In: *ASA Proceedings of the Biopharmaceutical Section.* American Statistical Association, Alexandria, VA, 1994, pp. 1–8.

Pinheiro, J.C. and Bates, D.M. Approximations to the log-likelihood function in nonlinear mixed-effects models. *Journal of Computational and Graphical Statistics* 1995; 1: 12–35.

Pinheiro, J.C. and Bates, D.M. *Mixed-effect models in S and S-Plus.* Springer-Verlag, New York, 2000.

Pitsiu, M., Hussein, Z., Majid, O., Aarons, L., de Longueville, M., and Stockis, A. Retrospective population pharmacokinetic analysis of cetirizine in children aged 6 months to 12 years. *British Journal of Clinical Pharmacology* 2004; 57: 402–411.

Pitt, M.A. and Myung, I.J. When a good fit can be bad. *Trends in Cognitive Science* 2002; 6: 421–425.

Pool, J.L., Cushman, W.C., Saini, R.K., Nwachuku, C.E., and Battikha, J.P. Use of the factorial design and quadratic response models to evaluate the fosinopril and hydrochlorothiazide combination in hypertension. *American Journal of Hypertension* 1997; 10: 117–123.

Port, R.E., Daniel, B., Ding, R.W., and Hermann, R. Relative importance of dose, body surface area, sex, and age in 5-fluorouracil clearance. *Oncology* 1991; 48: 277–281.

Preston, S.L., Drusano, G.L., Berman, A.L., Fowler, C.L., Chow, A.T., Dornseif, B., Reichl, V., Nataranjan, J., and Corrado, M. Pharmacodynamics of levofloxacin: A new paradigm for early clinical trials. *Journal of the American Medical Association* 1998; 279: 125–129.

PricewaterhouseCoopers. *Pharma 2005: Silicon rally: The race to e-R&D.* PriceWaterHouseCoopers, New York, 1999.

Proost, J. Do computational results depend on PC processor? *Clinical Pharmacology and Therapeutics* 1999; 65: 460.

Purves, R.D. Multiple solutions, illegal parameter values, local minima sum of squares, and anomalous parameter estimates in least-squares fitting of the 2-compartment pharmacokinetic model with absorption. *Journal of Pharmacokinetics and Biopharmaceutics* 1996; 24: 79–101.

Racine-Poon, A. and Wakefield, J. Statistical methods for population pharmacokinetic modeling. *Statistical Methods in Medical Research* 1998; 7: 63–84.

Rajagopalan, P. and Gastonguay, M.R. Population pharmacokinetics of ciprofloxacin in pediatric patients. *Journal of Clinical Pharmacology* 2003; 43: 698–710.

Ramakrishnan, R., DuBois, D.C., Almon, R.R., Pyszczynski, N.A., and Jusko, W.J. Fifth-generation model for corticosteroid pharmacodynamics: Application to steady-state receptor down-regulation and enzyme induction patterns during seven-day continuous infusion of methylprednisolone in rats. *Journal of Pharmacokinetics and Biopharmaceutics* 2002; 29: 1–24.

Rao, S.S. *Engineering optimization: Theory and practice.* New Age International Limited, New Delhi, 1996.

Ratain, M.J., Robert, J., and van der Vijgh, W.J.F. Limited sampling models for doxorubicin pharmacokinetics. *Journal of Clinical Oncology* 1991; 9: 871–876.

Reich, J. Parameter redundancy in curve fitting of kinetic data. In: *Kinetic data analysis: Design and analysis of enzyme and pharmacokinetic experiments.* (Endrenyi, L., Ed.). Plenum, New York, 1981, pp. 39–50.

Reklaitis, G.V., Ravindran, A., and Ragsdell, K.M. *Engineering optimization: Methods and applications.* Wiley, New York, 1983.

Rescigno, A., Beck, J.S., and Thakur, A.K. The use and abuse of models and commentary. *Journal of Pharmacokinetics and Biopharmaceutics* 1987; 15: 327–344.

Retout, S., Mentre, F., and Bruno, R. Fisher information matrix for nonlinear mixed-effects models: Evaluation and application for optimal design of enoxaparin population pharmacokinetics. *Statistics in Medicine* 2002; 30: 2623–2629.

Ribbing, J. and Jonsson, E.N. Power, selection bias and predictive performance of the population pharmacokinetic covariate model. Presented at Population Analysis Group in Europe Annual Meeting, Verona, Italy, 2003.

Ribbing, J. and Jonsson, E.N. Power, selection bias, and predictive performance of the population pharmacokinetic covariate model. *Journal of Pharmacokinetics and Pharmacodynamics* 2004; 31: 109–134.

Rice, J.A. *Mathematical statistics and data analysis.* Wadsworth & Brooks/Cole, Pacific Grove, CA, 1988.

Risch, N., Burchard, E., Ziv, E., and Tang, H. Categorization of humans in biomedical research: Genes, race, and disease. *Genome Biology* 2002; 3: comment2007.1–comment2007.12.

Ritschel, W.A. and Kearns, G.L. Pediatric pharmacokinetics. In: *handbook of basic pharmacokinetics.* (Ritschel, W.A., 5th Ed(s).). Drug Intelligence Publications, Inc., Hamilton, IL, 1998

Ritschel, W.A., Vachharajani, N.N., Johnson, R.D., and Hussain, A.S. The allometric approach for interspecies scaling of pharmacokinetic parameters. *Comparative Biochemistry & Physiology* 1992; 103C: 249–253.

Rockhold, F.W. and Goldberg, M.R. An approach to the assessment of therapeutic drug interactions with fixed combination drug products. *Journal of Biopharmaceutical Statistics* 1996; 6: 231–240.

Rodman, J.H. and Silverstein, M.H. Comparison of two-stage and first-order methods for estimation of population parameters in an intensive pharmacokinetic study. *Clinical Pharmacology and Therapeutics* 1990; 47: 151.

Roe, D.J. Comparison of population pharmacokinetic modeling methods using simulated data: Results from the population modeling workgroup. *Statistics in Medicine* 1997; 16: 1241–1262.

Rosario, M.C., Thomsen, A.H., Jodrell, D.I., Sharp, C.A., and Elliot, H.L. Population pharmacokinetics of gentamicin in patients with cancer. *British Journal of Clinical Pharmacology* 1998; 46: 229–236.

Rosenberg, N.A., Pritchard, J.K., Weber, J.L., Cann, W.M., Kidd, K.K., Zhivotovsky, L.A., and Feldman, M.W. Genetic structure of human populations. *Science* 2002; 298: 2381–2385.

Roses, A.D. Phamacogenetics and the practice of medicine. *Nature* 2000; 405: 857–865.

Ross, G.J.S. *Nonlinear estimation.* Springer-Verlag, Berlin, 1990.

Royston, P. and Thompson, S.G. Comparing nonnested regression models. *Biometrics* 1995; 51: 114–127.

Rubin, D.R. *Multiple imputation for nonresponse in surveys.* Wiley, New York, 1987.

Ruppert, D., Cressie, N., and Carroll, R.J. A transformation/weighting model for estimating Michaelis–Menten parameters. *Biometrics* 1989; 45: 637–656.

Sakia, R.M. Box–Cox transformation technique: A review. *The Statistician* 1992; 41: 169–178.

Sale, M.E. Model fitness measures for machine learning based model selection. Presented at American Association of Pharmaceutical Scientists, Denver, CO, 2001.

Savic, R., Jonker, D.M., Kerbusch, T., and Karlsson, M.O. Evaluation of a transit compartment model versus lag-time model for describing drug absorption delay. Presented at the Population Analysis Group Europe, Uppsala, Sweden, 2004.

Sawyer, W.T., Canaday, B.R., Poe, T.E., Webb, C.E., Gal, P., Joyner, P.U., and Berry, J.I. Variables affecting creatinine clearance prediction. *American Journal of Hospital Pharmacy* 1983; 40: 2175–2180.

Schabenberger, O. Mixed model influence diagnosists. Presented at SAS Users Group Proceedings, Paper 189–29, 2003.

Schaefer, H.G., Stass, H., Wedgwood, J., Hampel, B., Fischer, C., Kuhlmann, J., and Schaad, U.B. Pharmacokinetics of ciprofloxacin in pediatric cystic fibrosis patients. *Antimicrobial Agents and Chemotherapy* 1996; 40: 29–34.

Schafer, J. *Analysis of incomplete multivariate data.* Chapman & Hall, London, 1997.

Schenker, N. Qualms about the bootstrap confidence intervals. *Journal of the American Statistical Association* 1985; 80: 360–361.

Schilling, M.F., Watkins, A.E., and Watkins, W. Is human height bimodal? *American Statistician* 2002; 56: 223–229.

Schiltmeyer, B., Klingebiel, T., Schwab, M., Murdter, T.E., Ritter, C.A., Jenke, A., Ehninger, G., Gruhn, B., Wurthwein, G., Boos, J., and Hempel, G. Population pharmacokinetics of oral busulfan in children. *Cancer Chemotherapy and Pharmacology* 2003; 52: 209–216.

Schmith, V.D., Fiedler-Kelly, J., Phillips, L., and Grasela, T.H., Jr. Prospective use of population pharmacokinetics/pharmacodynamics in the development of cisatracurium. *Pharmaceutical Research* 1997; 14: 91–97.

Schrack, G. and Borowski, N. An experimental comparison of three random searches. In: *Numerical methods for nonlinear optimization.* (Lootsma, F.A. Ed.). Academic, New York, 1972, pp. 137–147.

Schumitsky, A. Nonparametric EM algorithms for estimating prior distributions. *Applied Mathematics and Computation* 1991; 45: 141–157.

Schwartz, R.S. Racial profiling in medical research. *New England Journal of Medicine* 2001; 344: 1392–1393.

Schwarz, G. Estimating the dimension of a model. *Annals of Statistics* 1978; 6: 461–464.

Scott, D.W. On optimal and data-based histograms. *Biometrika* 1979; 66: 605–610.

Scott, D.W. *Multivariate density estimation*. Wiley, New York, 1992.

Seber, G.A.F. and Wild, C.J. *Nonlinear regression*. Wiley, New York, 1989.

Seebauer, E.G. and Barry, R.L. *Fundamentals of ethics for scientists and engineers*. Oxford University Press, New York, 2001.

Shao, J., Chow, S.C., and Wang, B. The bootstrap procedure in individual bioequivalence. *Statistics in Medicine* 2000; 19: 2741–2754.

Shargel, L. and Yu, A. *Applied biopharmaceutics and pharmacokinetics*. McGraw-Hill, New York, 1999.

Sheiner, L. and Peck, C. Hypothesis: A single clinical trial plus causal evidence of effectiveness is sufficient for drug approval. *Clinical Pharmacology and Therapeutics* 2003; 73: 481–490.

Sheiner, L.B. and Beal, S.L. Evaluation of methods for estimating population pharmacokinetics parameters. I. Michaelis–Menten model: Routine clinical pharmacokinetic data. *Journal of Pharmacokinetics and Biopharmaceutics* 1980; 8: 553–571.

Sheiner, L.B. and Beal, S.L. Evaluation of methods for estimating population pharmacokinetic parameters. II. Biexponential model and experimental pharmacokinetic data. *Journal of Pharmacokinetics and Biopharmaceutics* 1981a; 9: 635–651.

Sheiner, L.B. and Beal, S.L. Some suggestions for measuring predictive performance. *Journal of Pharmacokinetics and Biopharmaceutics* 1981b; 9: 503–512.

Sheiner, L.B. and Beal, S.L. Evaluation of methods for estimating population pharmacokinetic parameters. III. Monoexponential model: Routine clinical pharmacokinetic data. *Journal of Pharmacokinetics and Biopharmaceutics* 1983; 11: 303–319.

Sheiner, L.B. and Beal, S.L. Pharmacokinetic parameter estimates from several least squares procedures: Superiority of extended least squares. *Journal of Pharmacokinetics and Biopharmaceutics* 1985; 13: 185–201.

Sheiner, L.B., Rosenberg, B., and Marathe, V.V. Estimation of population characteristics of pharmacokinetic parameters from routine clinical data. *Journal of Pharmacokinetics and Biopharmaceutics* 1977; 5: 445–479.

Sheiner, L.B. and Steimer, J.L. Pharmacokinetic/pharmacodynamic modeling in drug development. *Annual Review of Pharmacology and Toxicology* 2000; 40: 67–95.

Shen, M., Schilder, R.J., Obasaju, C., and Gallo, J.M. Population pharmacokinetic and limited sampling models for carboplatin administered in high dose combination regimens with peripheral blood stem cell support. *Cancer Chemotherapy and Pharmacology* 2002; 50: 243–250.

Schoemaker, R.C., and Cohen, A.F. Estimating impossible curves using NONMEM. *British Journal of Clinical Pharmacology* 1996; 42: 283–290.

Shrader-Frechette, K. *Ethics of scientific research*. Rowman & Littlefield, Lanham, MD, 1994.

Simon, S.D., and Lesage, J.P. The impact of collinearity involving the intercept term on the numerical accuracy of regression. *Computer Science in Economics and Management* 1988; 1: 137–152.

Simonoff, J.S., and Tsai, C.L. The use of guided reformulations when collinearities are present in nonlinear regression. *Applied Statistics* 1989; 38: 115–126.

Simonsen, L.E., Wahlby, U., Sandstrom, M., Freijs, A., and Karlsson, M.O. Haematological toxicity following different dosing schedules of 5-fluorouracil and epirubicin in rats. *Anticancer Research* 2000; 20: 1519–1526.

Singh, B.N. Effects of food on clinical pharmacokinetics. *Clinical Pharmacokinetics* 1999; 37: 213–255.

Slob, W., Janssen, P.H.M., and van den Hof, J.M. Structural identifiability of PBPK models: Practical consequences for modeling strategies and study designs. *Criticial Reviews in Toxicology* 1997; 27: 261–272.

Smith, B.P., Vandenhende, F.R., DeSante, K.A., Farid, N.A., Welch, P.A., Callaghan, J.T., and Forgue, S.T. Confidence interval criteria for assessment of dose proportionality. *Pharmaceutical Research* 2000; 17: 1278–1283.

Smith, D., Humphrey, M.J., and Charuel, C. Design of toxicokinetic studies. *Xenobiotica* 1990; 20: 1187–1199.

Smith, M.K. Software for nonlinear mixed effects modelling: A review of several packages. *2* 2003; 69: 75.

Sonnichsen, D.S., Hurwitz, C.A., Pratt, C.B., Shuster, J.J., and Relling, M.V. Saturable pharmacokinetics and paclitaxel pharmacodynamics in children with solid tumors. *Journal of Clinical Oncology* 1994; 12: 532–538.

Sparreboom, A., van Tellingen, O., Nooijen, W.J., and Beijen, J.H. Tissue distribution, metabolism, and excretion of paclitaxel in mice. *Anti-Cancer Drugs* 1996a; 7: 78–86.

Sparreboom, A., van Tellingen, O., Nooijen, W.J., and Beijnen, J.H. Nonlinear pharmacokinetics of paclitaxel in mice results from the pharmaceutical vehicle Cremophor EL. *Cancer Research* 1996b; 56: 2112–2115.

Sparreboom, A., van Zuylen, L., Brouwer, E., Loos, W.J., de Bruijn, P., Gelderblom, H., Pillay, M., Nooter, K., Stoter, G., and Verweij, J. Cremephor EL-mediated alteration of paclitaxel distribution of human blood: Clinical pharmacokinetic implications. *Cancer Research* 1999; 59: 1454–1457.

Spendley, W., Hext, G.R., and Himsworth, F.R. Sequential application of simplex designs in optimization and evolutionary operation. *Technometrics* 1962; 4: 441–461.

St.Laurent, R., and Cook, R.D. Leverage and superleverage in nonlinear regression. *Journal of the American Statistical Association* 1992; 87: 985–990.

St.Laurent, R., and Cook, R.D. Leverage, local influence and curvature in nonlinear regression. *Biometrika* 1993; 80: 99–106.

Stefanski, L.A., and Cook, J.R. Simulation-extrapolation: The measurement error jackknife. *Journal of the American Statistical Association* 1995; 90: 1247–1256.

Steimer, J.-L., Mallet, A., Golmard, J.-L., and Boisvieux, J.-F. Alternative approachs to estimation of population pharmacokinetic parameters: Comparison with the nonlinear mixed-effect model. *Drug Metabolism Reviews* 1984; 15: 265–302.

Stewart, W.H. Application of response surface methodology and factorial designs for drug combination development. *Journal of Biopharmaceutical Statistics* 1996; 6: 219–231.

Stigler, S.M. *The history of statistics: The measurement of uncertainty before 1900.* The Belknap University Press of Harvard University, Cambridge, MA, 1986.

Stine, R. An introduction to bootstrap methods: examples and ideas. In: *Modern methods of data Analysis.* (Fox, L. and Long, J.S. Eds.). Sage, Newbury Park, CA, 1990, pp. 325–373.

Stine, R.A. Bootstrap prediction intervals for regression. *Journal of the American Statistical Association* 1985; 80: 1026–1031.

Stram, D.O., and Lee, J.W. Variance components testing in the longitudinal mixed effects model. *Biometrics* 1994; 50: 1171–1177.

Sturges, H.A. The choice of a class interval. *Journal of the American Statistical Association* 1926; 21: 65–66.

Sun, H., Ette, E.I., and Ludden, T.M. On the recording of sample times and parameter estimation from repeated measures pharmacokinetic data. *Journal of Pharmacokinetics and Biopharmaceutics* 1996; 24: 637–650.

Svensson, C.K. Ethical considerations in the conduct of clinical pharmacokinetics studies. *Clinical Pharmacokinetics* 1989; 17: 217–222.

Swabb, E.A., Singhvi, S.M., Leitz, M.A., Frantz, M., and Sugerman, A. Metabolism and pharmacokinetics of aztreonam in healthy subjects. *Antimicrobial Agents and Chemotherapy* 1983; 24: 394–400.

Swallow, W.H., and Monahan, J.F. Monte Carlo comparison of ANOVA, MIVQUE, REML, and ML estimators of variance components. *Technometrics* 1984; 26: 47–57.

Takahashi, N., Takahashi, Y., Blumberg, B.S., and Putman, F.W. Amino acid substitutions in genetic variants of human serum albumin and in sequences inferred from molecular cloning. *Proceedings of the National Academy of Science USA* 1987; 84: 4413–4417.

Tett, S., Holford, N.H.G., and McLachlan, A.J. Population pharmacokinetics and pharmacodynamics: An underutilized resource. *Drug Information Journal* 1998; 32: 693–710.

Thakur, A.K. Model: Mechanistic versus empirical. In: *New trends in pharmacokinetics.* (Rescigno, A. and Thakur, A.K., Eds.). Plenum, New York, 1991, pp. 41–51.

Theil, H. *Principles of econometrics.* North-Holland, Amsterdam, 1971.

Thron, C.D. Linearity and superposition in pharmacokinetics. *Pharmacology Reviews* 1974; 26: 3–31.

Tod, M., Lokiec, F., Bidault, R., De Bony, F., Petitjean, O., and Aujard, Y. Pharmacokinetics of oral acyclovir in neonates and in infants: A population analysis. *Antimicrobial Agents and Chemotherapy* 2001; 45: 150–157.

Tremmel, L. The visual separability of plotting symbols in scatterplots. *Journal of Computational and Graphical Statistics* 1995; 4: 101–112.

Tufte, E.R. *The visual display of quantitative information.* Graphics, Chesire, CT, 2001.

Tukey, J.W. *Exploratory data analysis.* Addison-Wesley, Reading, MA, 1977.

Turing, A.M. Computer machinery and intelligence. *Mind* 1950; 59: 433–460.

United States Department of Health and Human Services, Food and Drug Administration, Center for Drug Evaluation and Research, and Center for Biologics Evaluation and Research. *Draft Guidance: General Considerations for Pediatric Pharmacokinetic Studies for Drugs and Biological Products,* 1998.

United States Department of Health and Human Services, Food and Drug Administration, Center for Drug Evaluation and Research, and Center for Biologics Evaluation and Research. *Guidance for Industry: Population Pharmacokinetics,* 1999.

United States Department of Health and Human Services, Food and Drug Administration, Center for Drug Evaluation and Research, and Center for Biologics Evaluation and Research. *Guidance for Industry: Statistical Approaches to Establishing Bioequivalence,* 2001.

United States Department of Health and Human Services, Food and Drug Administration, Center for Drug Evaluation and Research, and Center for Biologics Evaluation and Research. *Guidance for Industry: Food–Effect Bioavailability and Fed Bioequivalence Studies: Study Design, Data Analysis, and Labeling,* 2002.

United States Department of Health and Human Services, Food and Drug Administration, Center for Drug Evaluation and Research, and Center for Biologics Evaluation and Research. *Guidance for Industry: Collection of Race and Ethnicity Data in Clinical Trials,* 2003a.

United States Department of Health and Human Services, Food and Drug Administration, Center for Drug Evaluation and Research, and Center for Biologics Evaluation and Research. *Guidance For Industry: Exposure–Response Relationships: Study Design, Data Analysis, and Regulatory Applications,* 2003b.

Van Buskirk, P. Saving corporations millions: The benefits of modeling. *PCAI* 2000;July/August: 38.

van den Bongard, H.J.G.D., Mathot, R.A.A., Beijne, J.H., and Schellens, J.H.M. Pharmacokinetically guided administration of chemotherapeutic agents. *Clinical Pharmacokinetics* 2000; 39: 345–367.

van Houwelingen, J.C. Use and abuse of variance models in regression. *Biometrics* 1988; 44: 1073–1081.

van Warmerdan, L.J.C., Bokkel Huinink, W.W., and Beijnen, J.H. Limited sampling strategies for anticancer agents. *Journal of Cancer Research and Clinical Oncology* 1994; 120: 427–433.

Van Wart, S., Phillips, L., Ludwig, E.A., Russo, R., Gajjar, D.A., Bello, A., Ambrose, P.G., Costanzo, C., Grasela, T.H., Echols, R., and Grasela, T.H. Population pharmacokinetics and pharmacodynamics of garenoxacin in patients with community-acquired respiratory tract infections. *Antimicrobial Agents and Chemotherapy* 2004; 48: 4766–4777.

van Zuylen, L., Karlsson, M.O., Verweij, J., Brouwer, E., de Bruijn, P., Nooter, K., Stoter, G., and Sparreboom, A. Pharmacokinetic modeling of paclitaxel encapsulation in Cremephor EL micelles. *Cancer Chemotherapy and Pharmacology* 2001; 47: 309–318.

Venables, W.N., and Ripley, B.D. *Modern applied statistics with S-PLUS*. New York, Springer-Verlag, 1997.

Verbeke, G. and Lesaffre, E. A linear mixed effects model with heterogeneity in the random effects populations. *Journal of the American Statistical Association* 1996; 91: 217–221.

Verbeke, G. and Lesaffre, E. The effect of misspecifying the random effects distribution in linear mixed models for longitudinal data. *Computational Statistics & Data Analysis* 1997; 23: 541–556.

Verbeke, G. and Molenberghs, G. *Linear mixed models in practice: A SAS-oriented approach*. Springer-Verlag, New York, 1997.

Verbeke, G. and Molenberghs, G. *Linear mixed models for longitudinal data*. Springer-Verlag, New York, 2000.

Verme, C.N., Ludden, T.M., Clementi, W.A., and Harris, S.C. Pharmacokinetics of quinidine in male patients: A population analysis. *Clinical Pharmacokinetics* 1992; 22: 468–480.

Verotta, D. Building population pharmacokinetic-pharmacodynamic models using trees. In: *The population approach: Measuring and managing variability in response, concentration, and dose*. (Balant, L.P. and Aarons, L., Eds.). Commission of the European Communities, European Cooperation in the field of Scientific and Technical Research, Brussels, 1997

Vonesh, E.F., Chinchilli, V.M., and Pu, K. Goodness-of-fit in generalized nonlinear mixed-effects models. *Biometrics* 1996; 52: 575–587.

Wade, J.R., Beal, S.L., and Sambol, N.C. Interaction between structural, statistical, and covariate models in population pharmacokinetic analysis. *Journal of Pharmacokinetics and Biopharmaceutics* 1994; 22: 165–177.

Wade, J.R., Kelman, A.W., Howie, C.A., and Whiting, B. Effect of misspecification of the absorption process on subsequent parameter estimation in population analysis. *Journal of Pharmacokinetics and Biopharmaceutics* 1993; 21: 209–222.

Wagner, J.G. Do you need a pharmacokinetic model and, if so, which one? *Journal of Pharmacokinetics and Biopharmaceutics* 1975; 3: 457–478.

Wagner, J.G. *Pharmacokinetics for the pharmaceutical scientist*. Technomic, Lancaster PA, 1993.

Wahlby, U., Bouw, M.R., Jonsson, E.N., and Karlsson, M.O. Assessment of Type I error rates for the statistical submodel in NONMEM. *Journal of Pharmacokinetics and Pharmacodynamics* 2002; 29: 251–269.

Wahlby, U., Jonsson, E.N., and Karlsson, M.O. Assessment of actual significance levels for covariate effects in NONMEM. *Journal of Pharmacokinetics and Pharmacodynamics* 2001; 28: 231–252.

Wahlby, U., Jonsson, E.N., and Karlsson, M.O. Comparison of stepwise covariate model building strategies in population pharmacokinetic-pharmacodynamic analysis. *AAPS PharmSci* 2002; 4: Article 27.

Wainer, H. How to display data badly. *American Statistician* 1984; 38: 137–147.

Wallace, W.A. *Ethics in modeling*. Elsevier, New York, 1994.

Wand, M.P. Data-based choice of histogram bin width. *American Statistician* 1997; 51: 59–64.

Wang, Y., Moss, J., and Thisted, R. Predictors of body surface area. *Journal of Clinical Anesthesiology* 1992; 4: 4–10.

Wastney, M.E., Siva Subramanian, K.N., Broering, N., and Boston, R. Using models to explore whole-body metabolism and accessing models through a model library. *Metabolism* 1997; 46: 330–332.

Wastney, M.E., Wang, X.Q., and Boston, R.C. Publishing, interpreting, and accessing models. *Journal of the Franklin Institute* 1998; 335B: 281–301.

West, J.B. *Best and Taylor's physiological basis of medical practice*. Williams & Wilkins, Baltimore, 1985.

Westlake, W.J. Bioavailability and bioequivalence of pharmaceutical formulations. In: *Biopharmaceutical statistics for drug development*. (Peace, K.A. Ed.). Marcel Dekker, New York, 1988, pp. 329–352.

White, D.B., Walawander, C.A., Tung, Y., and Grasela, T.H. An evaluation of point and interval estimates in population pharmacokinetics using NONMEM analysis. *Journal of Pharmacokinetics and Biopharmaceutics* 1991; 19: 87–112.

Wierkin, P.H., Schwartz, E.L., Strauman, J.J., Dutcher, J.P., Lipton, R.B., and Paietta, E. Phase I clinical and pharmacokinetic study of taxol. *Cancer Research* 1987; 47: 2486–2493.

Wiernik, P.H., Schwartz, E.L., Einzig, A., Strauman, J.J., Lipton, R.B., and Dutcher, J.P. Phase I trial of taxol given as a 24-h infusion every 21 days: Responses observed in metastatic melanoma. *Journal of Clinical Oncology* 1987; 5: 1232–1239.

Williams, D.R. Race and health: Basic questions, emerging directions. *Annals of Epidemiology* 1997; 7: 322–333.

Wilson, J.F., Weale, M.E., Smith, A.C., Gratiz, F., Fletcher, B., Thomas, M.G., Bradman, N., and Goldstein, D.B. Population genetic structure of variable drug response. *Nature Genetics* 2001; 29: 265–269.

Winker, M.A. Measuring race and ethnicity: Why and how. *Journal of the American Medical Association* 2004; 292: 1612–1614.

Winslade, N.E., Adelman, M.H., Evans, E.J., and Schentag, J.J. Single-dose accumulation pharmacokinetics of tobramycin and netilmicin in normal volunteers. *Antimicrobial Agents and Chemotherapy* 1987; 31: 605–609.

Wolfe, J. H. *A Monte Carlo study of the sampling distribution of the likelihood ratio for mixtures of multinormal distributions*, 1971.

Wolfinger, R. Covariance structure selection in general mixed models. *Communications in Statistics Series—Simulation A* 1993; 22: 1079–1106.

Wolfinger, R.D. Heterogeneous variance–covariance structures for repeated measures. *Journal of Agricultural, Biological, and Environmental Statistics* 1996; 1: 205–230.

Wu, G. Sensitivity analysis of pharmacokinetic parameters in 1-compartment models. *Pharmacological Research* 2000; 41: 445–453.

Wu, H. and Wu, L. A multiple imputation method for missing covariates in nonlinear mixed-effects models with application to HIV dynamics. *Statistics in Medicine* 2001; 20: 1755–1769.

Wu, H. and Wu, L. Identification of significant host factors for HIV dynamics modelled by nonlinear mixed-effects models. *Statistics in Medicine* 2002a; 21: 753–771.

Wu, L. and Wu, H. Missing time-dependent covariates in human immunodeficiency virus dynamic models. *Applied Statistics* 2002b; 51: 297–318.

Xu, R. Measuring explained variation in linear mixed effects models. *Statistics in Medicine* 2003; 22: 3527–3541.

Xuan, D., Lu, J.F., Nicolau, D.P., and Nightingale, C.H. Population pharmacokinetics of tobramycin in hospitalized patients receiving once-daily dosing regimen. *International Journal of Antimicrobial Agents* 2000; 15: 185–191.

Yafune, A. and Ishiguro, M. Bootstrap approach for constructing confidence intervals for population pharmacokinetic parameters. I: A use of bootstrap standard error. *Statistics in Medicine* 1999; 18: 581–599.

Yamaoka, K., Nakagawa, T., and Uno, T. Application of Akaike's information criterion (AIC) in the evaluation of linear pharmacokinetic equations. *Journal of Pharmacokinetics and Biopharmaceutics* 1978; 6: 165–175.

Yano, Y., Beal, S.L., and Sheiner, L.B. Evaluating pharmacometric/pharmacodynamic models using the posterior predictive check. *Journal of Pharmacokinetics and Pharmacodynamics* 2001; 28: 171–192.

Yeo, I.-K. and Johnson, R. A new family of power transformations. *Biometrika* 2000; 87: 954–959.

Yin, Y. and Chen, C. Optimizing first-time-in-human trial design for studying dose proportionality. *Drug Information Journal* 2001; 35: 1065–1078.

Yukawa, E., Hokazono, T., Yukawa, M., Ichimaru, R., Maki, T., Matsunaga, K., Ohdo, S., Anai, M., Higuchi, S., and Goto, Y. Population pharmacokinetics of haloperidol using routine clinical pharmacokinetic data in Japanese patients. *Clinical Pharmacokinetics* 2002; 41: 153–159.

Zar, J.H. *Biostatistical analysis, 2nd edn.* Prentice-Hall, New York, 1984.

Zelterman, D. *Models for discrete data.* Clarendon, Oxford, 1999.

Zhang, L.-Q., Collins, J.C., and King, P.H. Indistinguishability and identifiability analysis of linear compartmental models. *Mathematical Biosciences* 1991; 103: 77–95.

Zhi, J. Unique pharmacokinetic characteristics of the 1-compartment first-order absorption model with equal absorption and elimination rate constants. *Journal of Pharmaceutical Sciences* 1990; 79: 652–654.

Zuideveld, K.P., Rusic-Pavletic, J., Maas, H.J., Peletier, L.A., van der Graaf, P.H., and Danhof, M. Pharmacokinetic-pharmacodynamic modeling of buspirone and its metabolite 1-(2-pyrimidinyl)-piperazine in rats. *Journal of Pharmacology and Experimental Therapeutics* 2002a; 303: 1130–1137.

Zuideveld, K.P., van Gestel, A., Peletier, L.A., van der Graaf, P.H., and Danhof, M. Pharmacokinetic-pharmacodynamic modelling of the hypothermic and corticosterone effects of the 5–HT1A receptor agonist flesinoxan. *European Journal of Pharmacology* 2002b; 445: 43–54.

INDEX

Printed in the United States of America.